T

5

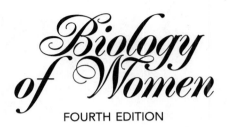

Biology of Women

FOURTH EDITION

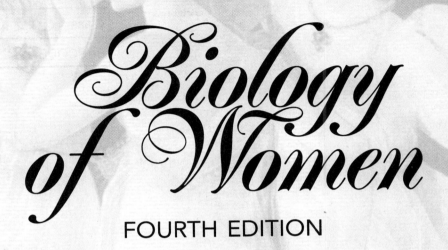

Biology of Women

FOURTH EDITION

Ethel Sloane

DELMAR

THOMSON LEARNING™   Australia   Canada   Mexico   Singapore   Spain   United Kingdom   United States

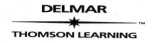

DELMAR

THOMSON LEARNING™

Biology of Women, 4E
Ethel Sloane

Health Care Publishing Director:
William Brottmiller

Executive Editor
Cathy L. Esperti

Acquisitions Editor:
Matthew M. Kane

Editorial Assistant:
Terry Lynne Brown

Executive Marketing Manager:
Dawn Gerrain

Channel Manager:
Tara Carter

Executive Production Manager:
Karen Leet

Project Editor:
Mary Ellen Cox

Production Coordinator:
Nina Lontrato

Art/Design Coordinator:
Mary Colleen Liburdi

For permission to use material from this text or product, contact us by
Tel   (800) 730-2214
Fax   (800) 730-2215
www.thomsonrights.com

Library of Congress Cataloging-in-Publication Data
Sloane, Ethel.
    Biology of women / Ethel Sloane. — 4th ed.
        p. cm.
    Includes bibliographical references and index.
    ISBN 0-7668-1142-5
    1. Women—Health and hygiene.   2. Women—Physiology.
3. Gynecology—Popular works.   I. Title.
    RG121 .S637 2002
    613'.04244—dc21   00-065690

NOTICE TO THE READER

Publisher does not warrant or guarantee any of the products described herein or perform any independent analysis in connection with any of the product information contained herein. Publisher does not assume, and expressly disclaims, any obligation to obtain and include information other than that provided to it by the manufacturer.

The reader is expressly warned to consider and adopt all safety precautions that might be indicated by the activities herein and to avoid all potential hazards. By following the instructions contained herein, the reader willingly assumes all risks in connection with such instructions.

The Publisher makes no representation or warranties of any kind, including but not limited to, the warranties of fitness for particular purpose or merchantability, nor are any such representations implied with respect to the material set forth herein, and the publisher takes no responsibility with respect to such material. The publisher shall not be liable for any special, consequential, or exemplary damages resulting, in whole or part, from the readers' use of, or reliance upon, this material.

FOREWORD

During the final preparation of the fourth edition of *Biology of Women,* Ethel Sloane died of an illness she had lived with and fought for many years. In the last months of her life, she was working diligently at her computer to update this book. When that no longer was easy for her, a group of extraordinary colleagues from the University of Wisconsin-Milwaukee stepped in to help her, making contributions to several chapters to ensure that the information covered was accurate and up to date. This edition of *Biology of Women* could not have been completed without the expert assistance and great generosity of the following people at the University of Wisconsin-Milwaukee: Rene Gratz, professor, Department of Health Sciences; Donna Van Wynsberghe, professor, Department of Biological Sciences; Ruth E. Williams, assistant vice chancellor; Leslie Schulz, professor, Clinical Laboratory Sciences program; and Reinhold Hutz, professor, Department of Biological Sciences. Later, after Ethel Sloane's death, Rene Gratz, Donna Van Wynsberghe, and Ruth E. Williams put in hours of work to make sure the manuscript was complete and prepared exactly as Ethel would have wished it to be. Cathy Esperti, executive editor at Delmar Thomson Learning, was committed to making sure this edition would be published without a hitch, and marshaled all the resources at her disposal to bring it to print.

After her death, a generation of Ethel Sloane's students wrote or spoke to us, members of her family, to describe the powerful impact this book and the course it was written for had on their development as health care professionals or as health care consumers. All of them described the feeling of empowerment it gave them, a consequence of learning how to better understand their bodies in sickness and in health, and how to better communicate with health care providers. Many of them shared stories of how that knowledge changed their lives or helped them bring about change in the lives of their mothers, sisters, or daughters.

Ethel's friends, family, colleagues, and editor wanted to ensure that the fourth edition of this book would be available to yet another group of students, instructors, and readers. It is a testimony to Ethel that *Biology of Women* continues to enrich people's lives.

The family of Ethel Sloane

CONTENTS

PREFACE

The goal for the fourth edition of *Biology of Women* is the same as for previous editions: to provide a comprehensive look at the human female throughout her entire life span. The book explains biological sex differentiation, fetal development, and reproductive anatomy. It is concerned with all the events of a woman's reproductive life from menarche to menopause. It deals with sexuality, birth control, infertility, and pregnancy. It discusses sexually transmitted diseases, gynecological problems, breast cancer, and controversies in treatment. It examines sociological and cultural factors that influence a woman's nutrition, physical activity, and use of cosmetics.

This book is also about health care. Health care today is complex. Consumers are confronted with traditional, alternative, and controversial methods, all purporting to help them become and stay healthy. How are decisions to be made? What *are* the facts when newspapers almost daily report new health information different from information published the week before, when magazine articles refute one another on what is right and wrong for our health? We all must know enough to choose the methods of being and staying healthy that are appropriate for us.

Since the publication of the first edition, there have been many changes in medical research and in the treatment of sickness and disease. Not only has medicine advanced since the first edition of this book, the consumer's relationship to health care resources has also changed. It is increasingly common today for people to take a more active role than ever before in their own health care by empowering their knowledge through books and television programs, magazine articles, newsletters, and perhaps most significantly, by information obtained via the Internet. Because the health resources available via the media and the Internet are so vast, and so varied in quality, it is more important than ever that people are able to recognize good health care information and to avoid the dubious and inaccurate information and advice that appears in published material and on many Internet sites. This book, which through its various editions has helped women become better consumers of health care information, now in its fourth edition provides what the author feels are the most accurate and well-maintained medical, health, and support-group Internet sites available to consumers and students. With these, readers can stay completely up to date on the research being done on women's health and sickness and stay fully apprised of treatments, medications, and supportive resources for an array of physical and emotional needs. To further this knowledge and provide a current view of all aspects of the biology of women, the fourth edition has been fully revised and updated. New research is presented on subjects that continue to seriously affect women's lives, such as the detection and treatment of breast cancer and other reproductive cancers; sexually transmitted diseases and infertility; and crucial updates on women and heart disease, osteoporosis, and treatments for problems of menopause. Material on contraception and abortion has all been fully updated as well.

As important, this fourth edition has been greatly updated with new illustrations and photography. Anatomical illustrations have been redrawn for clarity and ease of understanding, and most photographs have been changed or added to reflect new technologies and advances in health care and diagnosis. New to this edition are also the addition of key terms and a glossary—crucial terms are highlighted in context within every chapter and also defined in the glossary. This should be an important element for improving students' understanding of the material and an aid to instructors.

What has *not* changed since the first edition of this book is that many questions, concerns, and controversies remain in the field of women's health. Women still need to be vigilant health care consumers to understand which treatments, procedures, contraceptives, or medicines are beneficial to them; to understand which research the medical profession is now concentrating on and why; and to help them make sense of lifestyle choices that affect their health and bodies, today and tomorrow. Over the nearly 20 years this book has been in print, I believe women have learned to interact more intelligently with health care professionals. Bolstered with information, women increasingly understand the functioning of their own bodies and take ever-greater responsibility for maintaining and

enhancing their health. They take a more active role in partnership with their doctors and health care providers. More and more, women make health and lifestyle decisions that reflect their own knowledge and personal preferences, and they have become better at communicating their ideas to the members of the medical profession who treat them.

It has always been my intention that this book be of value both to people with little or no background in biology and to students in health professions who have taken many science courses. I have tried to achieve both broadness of scope and inherent flexibility in order to provide a book adaptable to various needs: for class use in such courses as biology of women and human reproduction; as a resource in courses in maternity nursing and gynecological nursing for health professionals in training or continuing education programs; or as a basis for discussion on women's studies courses. But in addition, my goal has been to write a book that can be meaningful to any woman at different times of her life—one that any woman can share with her mother, her friend, her husband. It is exactly this sharing of knowledge that is so very important to all of us—women with peer women, women and the generation of women who gave birth to them, women and men, and, most certainly, women and their daughters. It is in this spirit, finally, that I wrote *Biology of Women* and its subsequent editions.

Ethel Sloane

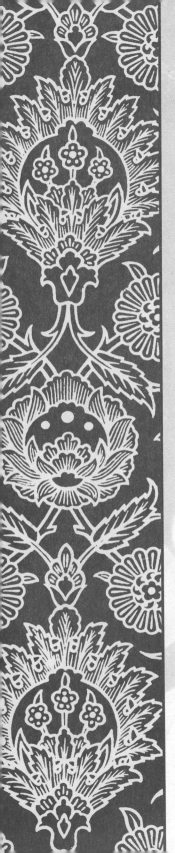

1

Women and Their Health: From Early Feminism through the Millennium

KEY TERMS

American Medical
  Association (AMA)
Health maintenance
  organizations (HMOs)
National Institutes of
  Health (NIH)

OB/GYN
Preferred provider
  organizations (PPOs)
Women's Health Initiative

The height of the women's movement was in the late 1960s and early 1970s. There was at least recognition, if not remedy, for the fact that women did not have equal rights—they were not receiving equal pay for equal work, and they could not get the types of jobs they wanted. More fundamentally, it also was perceived that women's personal and social experiences, history, accomplishments, and ideas largely had been ignored or suppressed and were missing from most aspects of American political and social institutions. Although antifeminism existed—the

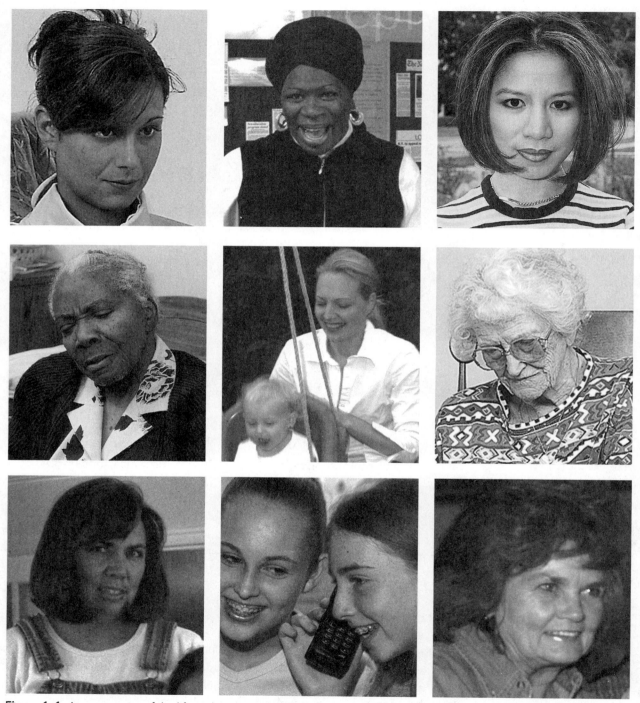

Figure 1–1 At every stage of the life cycle, women have special health needs and interests. They must have the factual information to aid them in maintaining and promoting their own health as well as easy access to high-quality health care.

stereotypical mocking image of a feminist was the bra-burning, strident, man-hating, angry radical—the movement was strong and reforms began to take place. Huge strides toward equality and justice for women were made through federal and state legislation.

In this enlightened environment of the late 1960s and early 1970s, groups of women's health activists, under the impetus of the larger women's movement, called attention to the failure of traditional medicine to deliver quality health services to women and began to organize into the women's health movement. The movement grew rapidly and involved increasing numbers of women. Banding together to provide themselves and other women with health information and advocacy services, they formed local groups of grassroots health collectives. Women would meet together to share their health experiences, to increase their knowledge concerning female anatomy and physiology, to learn enough about medicine to try to improve doctor-patient relationships, and to understand and evaluate what constitutes quality health care so that it could be expected and demanded. By the middle of the 1970s, there were more than 1,200 such health collectives in the United States, some publishing newsletters and pamphlets. A handful of women's health activists combined to form the National Women's Health Network, a Washington-based public interest group. The Network continues to provide the most significant national voice for women's health needs, acting as a watchdog on health policies affecting women and distributing health information through a speaker's bureau, appearances on radio and TV programs, and the publication of a newsletter and resource guides on various aspects of women's health.

A number of the women's health advocates hired their own physicians and started their own women-controlled feminist health centers. Some offered a wide range of gynecological, contraceptive, childbearing, and feminist therapy services. In some of the collectives, the goals expanded beyond consciousness raising, the development of better-informed patients, and improved patient-practitioner relationships, to more radical self-help activity. Self-help emphasized self-examination with the conviction that increased knowledge is the way to increased power and control.

A movie produced in 1974 by Cambridge Documentary Films, Inc. is a wonderful example of the self-help and self-health philosophy of the women's health collectives. Called *Taking Our Bodies Back,* the film made an eloquent and powerful statement about women's dissatisfaction with the health care they were receiving and expressed women's developing assertiveness in trying to regain control of their bodies. In a series of vignettes, the movie illustrated many of the women's health issues of the time—unnecessary surgery; the lack of options in breast cancer treatment; the way women generally, and teenagers in particular, were not given the information or the opportunity to make informed choices about birth control; and the demeaning way in which minority women often experience medical treatment. But perhaps the most graphic depiction of the way things were in the early days of the women's health movement occurs at the beginning of the film, when a young woman demonstrates how to perform vaginal self-examination. In the opening scene, she is standing on a platform in front of a large audience and showing and describing a plastic speculum, an instrument that is inserted into the vagina to spread apart the vaginal walls. She jokes about its "duck-bill" bivalves and says she had to buy one for her little boy as well as herself because he wanted it as a "quack-quack" toy. The audience laughs, and she goes on, talking rapidly. Moving very quickly now, she climbs up on a table, puts herself into the familiar gynecological examination position, inserts the speculum, and the movie camera and lights focus in to frame . . . of all things! The audience is being invited to look at her cervix! The women in the film solemnly file past her, their excitement and interest apparent on their faces. They are fascinated and, surprisingly, there is no embarrassed laughter. All the women are seeing a part of a woman's body they have never seen before, a portion of their reproductive tracts that until that moment has been visible only to their doctors—and they evidently are captivated by the sight.

To doctors and many others, such a demonstration on film of how to look at your own cervix was a prime example of the lunatic fringe of the women's health movement. Peering into body orifices always had been the prerogative of the physician. Why would a woman want to look at her own or another woman's cervix? For a woman to buy a plastic speculum and twist herself into a pretzel to do a vaginal examination—what a strange idea! Why would she do it?

The reason for a woman's desire or need for self-examination, however, was not just in seeing the cervix; she can look at a drawing in an anatomy book. The importance of *looking* was in the demystification of her own body. Vaginal examination was the initial symbol of self-help, the way women began to take their bodies back from the medical profession. Many women, even after studying human reproduction in school, still are fairly ignorant and maybe uncomfortable about their own reproductive anatomy. Most men are not. The genital organs of a man are exposed, easily visible; they can be seen and touched. If any changes occur, the man can note and describe them himself. But in a woman, the reproductive organs cannot be seen. They are internal and not easily subject to examination. What women are, reproductively, remains hidden to them, enigmatic and strange.

If all women took a mirror and a diagram of their anatomy and then viewed and examined their own external genitalia, they would progress tremendously in self-awareness and in the reassurance that everything is "normal." Inserting a plastic speculum and looking at the cervix, for many women, is a way of feeling more comfortable about their reproductive organs, a way of dispelling much of the mystique that surrounds them. But the choice of whether or not to look at the cervix is up to the woman. For many, knowing *about* the reproductive organs is enough, and we really do not choose to examine them. Besides, there may be strong cultural taboos stemming from childhood that discourage touching or tampering with one's self "down there." And so, once or twice a year, a woman is encouraged to see her doctor for her pelvic examination, when the position, size,

shape, and general health of her reproductive organs are checked.

The specialist in obstetrics and gynecology **(OB/GYN)** is the acknowledged expert, the authority within the medical profession on the aspect of a woman's life so highly valued in our society—that pertaining to the sexual organs. Women consult their OB/GYN for their routine gynecological examination. A woman may also rely on her OB/GYN for an evaluation of her general health. She may ask her physician for advice about any medical problem, sexual matter, becoming pregnant, or avoiding pregnancy. She exposes her most intimate self and her most intimate problems to her OB/GYN—the doctor a healthy woman visits most frequently. The experience can be informative and reassuring, or it can be an ordeal. It depends on the physician.

Most OB/GYNs today will explain exactly what they are doing or even offer a mirror to the woman to let her see what they see. Such physicians, sensitive to a woman's possible embarrassment or anxiety about having a "pelvic," will not perform it in complete silence, or, in the alternative, make chatty, off-hand remarks such as "Hmmmm . . . you have a tipped uterus," or ". . . your cervix is a little eroded,"★ without offering further explanation. The woman is made to feel more comfortable, that she is a real person, and more than just a set of reproductive organs to be poked and prodded. After the examination, when the woman is dressed and sees the doctor in the office, she senses that *her* concerns, as well as the doctor's, are important. She gets the opportunity to ask all of her questions and then gets a full explanation of her condition and any proposed therapy.

Not all women have a similar positive experience with their OB/GYN. Some doctors are threatened by

---

★One young woman indicated that after hearing "eroded," she visualized her cervix, which she thought was located somewhere up around her navel, looking like the side of a mountain after a rainstorm. Another young woman was told. "My, your vagina is long and narrow," and wanted to respond, "Well, doctor, maybe your hand is short and fat." She now regrets not having said it.

even mild assertiveness or are irked by questions they perceive as challenging to their authority or self-esteem. Such physicians may be brusque, hurried, and unable to communicate with their patients. A woman is made to feel that the attention given to her is perfunctory, that she is taking up too much of the doctor's valuable time, and she forgets most of the questions she had prepared. When she does get a response, the doctor may make judgmental recommendations concerning her lifestyle, her decisions about becoming pregnant, or what kind of contraceptive she should use. Some men and women doctors (gender bias is not confined to men) evidently make their decisions about a woman's physiological and psychological needs based not only on her actual health status but also on what the doctor presumes that she is or thinks that she should become. Lack of dignity and respect in medical treatment often is felt even more keenly by minority women, lesbian women, teenage and older women, and poor women.

ℬASIC ISSUES IN WOMEN'S HEALTH

The women's health movement brought a number of significant women's health issues to national attention. Even women who shrank from the label of "feminist" could not help but recognize that women were not getting the quality of health care they wanted and needed and that something was wrong with traditional medicine. The success of the barrier-breaking *Our Bodies, Ourselves,* by the Boston Women's Health Book Collective, soon was followed by the publication of a shelfful of books, hundreds of articles in magazines, and television specials on women's health. Women were frustrated by the paternalistic, traditional doctor-patient relationship and objected to the medicalization of normal events such as menstruation, pregnancy and childbirth, and menopause.

Most of women's dissatisfaction and anger was directed at the OB/GYN, the arbiter of women's health care. Women had trusted their doctors completely, and they believed that their physicians had been giving them the kind of health care they wanted and needed. Instead, what they saw was a women-exploiting tradition of health care in which their basic health rights virtually had been ignored and their treatment was inherently hazardous. Women had been given hormones for birth control, for menopause, or to prevent miscarriage, and were not informed about the potential risks of such treatment. Surgery on women's bodies was sometimes unnecessary and excessive, and women were not given the opportunity to consider alternatives. Pregnancy and childbirth, natural and normal functions, had been turned into medical problems to be technologically "managed," frequently for the convenience of the hospital and medical staff and to the possible detriment of the child—certainly to the psychological detriment of the mother. And women's mental health was defined in terms of the social and cultural expectations of the stereotyped feminine role. Their illnesses were frequently perceived as psychosomatic, their reproductive disorders as manifestations of psychiatric disorders, and their demands for treatment as neurotic. The medical panacea for women's emotional problems was pills, and there was evidence of the overprescribing of tranquilizing and mood-elevating drugs.

The increased attention to women's health issues and the shortcomings of traditional medical practice obviously resulted in some change. Federal guidelines protect human subjects from being used without their knowledge or consent in clinical investigations of drugs or medical devices. In response to the demands of pregnant women, there are alternatives to the usual hospital-based delivery of infants. And as part of the legacy of those "crazy radicals" who looked at their own and other women's vaginas, women also now know more about their bodies. Armed with greater knowledge, many are more assertive, reserving the right to reject advice or to seek a second opinion. There are now more enlightened doctors and other health care professionals who treat women with greater respect and sensitivity and explain more to the patient about procedures and therapies. For many women, however, underlying health concerns are unchanged. The problems in the areas of reproductive rights, hormonal therapy, unnecessary surgery, prescription drug abuse, pregnancy and childbirth interventions, and mental health treatment remain to be solved. There still is no assurance of the complete safety of many of the pills or products prescribed for women or taken over the counter. The safety of some medical devices is unknown. It is still unlikely that some commonly performed major surgical procedures in the United States today such as cesarean section and hysterectomy (surgical removal of the uterus) need be so common. Hormone replacement therapy in the menopause currently is being advocated routinely by many doctors for menopausal women. And while virtually every hospital now has birthing rooms and is "family centered," pregnancy and childbirth are even more high tech than they were previously. Additional issues have emerged—the health of women in the labor force, especially when they are single parents coping with the stresses of work and child care; environmental effects on women's health; the necessity for basic research on the causes of breast cancer and other reproductive cancers; the epidemic of sexually transmitted diseases in women and the special needs of women with AIDS; the impact of eating disorders in women; the disparities between the treatment of men and women with cardiovascular disease; and the enormous gap between the quality and access of health care services for the privileged and that existing for poor women, rural women, older women, women of color, lesbians, and disabled women.

In the United States, scientific inquiry into the health needs of women was, for many years, shortchanged, but this is rapidly changing. The **National Institutes of Health (NIH),** the primary federal granting agency for research, reported in 1999 that 16% of its research budget was allocated for "gender-specific research for women," 6% was allocated for "gender-specific research for men," and 78% of the budget was allocated for diseases that affect *both* men and women.

Every year, women suffer half of the fatal heart attacks in the United States. The only difference is that

the onset of heart disease is earlier in men, who are more likely to show it by a heart attack between the ages of 40 and 50. According to the American Heart Association 1997 Bio-Statistical Report, a heart attack in women is more likely to occur between the ages of 65 and 84. Although the problem of heart disease is thus as serious in women as in men, it apparently has not been taken as seriously by clinical researchers. Virtually all of the data on heart disease have been accumulated for men, and there is little understanding of the disease in women. For example, many doctors advise men over 50 to take low-dose aspirin to reduce the risk of heart attack. Should women take aspirin as well? It is difficult to know for certain because the evidence for aspirin in primary prevention of cardiovascular disease was provided by 22,071 *male* doctors in the Physician's Health Study (1989). A reduction in blood cholesterol levels by 1% also lowers the risk of heart attack by 2%. Is this true for women? Presumably, but the data reported in 1990 came from more than 10 years of observation of mortality rates from coronary heart disease in 12,866 *men* participating in the Multiple Risk Factor Intervention Trial (known as Mr. FIT!).

The lack of research on cardiovascular disease in women has resulted in major omissions in medical knowledge. It is not known why the first heart attack is more often fatal to women than to men, why women who have coronary bypass surgery have twice the risk of dying from the procedure, or why balloon angioplasty (a procedure to flatten the fatty deposits that block the coronary arteries) is less successful in women, especially if they are premenopausal. Is there something in women's biology that produces the differences, or could there be other factors—nonbiological but gender based—that are involved? Two reports involving tens of thousands of patients showed clear evidence of sexist bias in the treatment of women with heart disease. The studies showed that doctors treated women less aggressively than they treat men, even though the women in the studies generally had more advanced heart disease than the men (Ayanian & Epstein, 1991; Steingart et al., 1991). More recently, a study of 720 physicians reinforced previous data from epidemiological studies by showing that both gender and race, independently, influenced the way the physicians treated the possibility of cardiac disease in their patients. Doctors were 60% as likely to order cardiac catheterization for chest pain in women and blacks as for men and whites, respectively. Black women were 40% less likely to be referred for catheterization (Schulman et al., 1999).

In a 1991 report titled "Gender Disparities in Clinical Decision Making," the Council on Ethical and Judicial Affairs of the **American Medical Association (AMA)** documented the differences in diagnosis and treatment among men and women, specifically in regard to kidney dialysis and treatment, lung cancer, and cardiac catheterization for coronary bypass surgery. The Council concluded that while biological differences such as the longevity of women may account for some of the disproportionate use of medical services by women, biology cannot explain the gender differences, to women's disadvantage, in the diagnosis and treatment of certain conditions.

After increased public attention to the inequities in research on women's health and illness, and additional political prodding from the Congressional Caucus for Women's Issues and the House Subcommittee on Health, the NIH took some concrete action. A new agency, the Office of Research on Women's Health, was created in 1990, and one of its responsibilities was to make certain that the already 5-year-old NIH recommendations to include women in clinical studies actually would be implemented. Following the establishment of the Office of Research on Women's Health, headed by Vivian Pinn, NIH strengthened and revitalized its guidelines for the inclusion of women in clinical studies. To ensure the implementation by NIH, Congress enacted this into law through a section in the NIH Revitalization Act of 1993 titled "Women and Minorities As Subjects in Clinical Research," and in 1994 NIH revised its policy and published guidelines. The NIH Revitalization Act of 1993 mandates that women and underrepresented minorities and their subpopulations must be included in all NIH clinical research studies and in numbers adequate to allow for valid analyses. Cost is not acceptable for exclusion. Although this legal mandate now exists, issues that make it difficult for women to participate in studies need to be considered. To ensure recruitment and retention of women in research studies, sensitivity to women's needs must be paramount, and potential barriers such as lack of child care, transportation, financial constraints, and cultural differences must be addressed (Office of Research on Women's Health, 1995). Another major change in 1992 was the mounting of the largest community-based clinical intervention and prevention trial ever conducted. Known as the **Women's Health Initiative,** it is a $625 million study involving between 100,000 and 200,000 women to gather data on the prevention and treatment of the major causes of death in middle-aged and older women, including cardiovascular disease, cancer, and osteoporosis. Interventions such as smoking cessation, low-fat diets, vitamin and calcium supplements, exercise, and hormone therapy will be studied to assess their effect on women's health. Moreover, the Society for the Advancement of Women's Health Research had been established in 1990 to bring attention to serious shortcomings and unmet needs in women's health research in the United States. The five goals of the Society include the following:

1. Identifying areas of research that will have an impact on the health of women
2. Promoting and encouraging both public and private financial support for women's health research
3. Effecting changes in policies and behavior based on research outcomes
4. Creating an environment for change by informing policy makers, the public, and educators of research outcomes
5. Advancing women as leaders in the health professions

These goals were developed with the intent of increasing research in women's health. Since 1992, the Society has published the *Journal of Women's Health,* and the definition of its research and policy agenda for the improvement of women's health research and the actions necessary to ensure that it remains a permanent priority for policy makers have been detailed. There is a focus on the study of diseases that affect only women and the secondary influence of reproduction on other physiological systems. Researchers also are beginning to look at the differences between men and women in terms of "gender-based biology" (Haseltine & Jacobson, 1997). Thanks to insistent congresswomen, women's health activists, pressure from advocacy groups like the National Women's Health Network and the Public Citizen's Health Research Group, women's health issues have again risen to the public consciousness.

Our society's focus on breast cancer illustrates how important women's health issues have become and how it is possible for women to garner public attention and financial support for a specific disease. Women's experiences with the life-threatening illness of breast cancer, which formerly had been hidden and certainly were not talked about publicly, were nationally spotlighted in the early 1980s when two president's wives, Betty Ford and Nancy Reagan, as well as a number of actresses and other celebrities, revealed that they had survived breast cancer. Also in the 1980s, the Susan G. Komen Breast Cancer Foundation, based in Dallas, Texas, was founded by Nancy Brinker in commemoration of her sister Susan, who had died of the disease at 36. The Foundation became a leader in breast cancer research funding, education, and legislative advocacy. Since its inception, it has raised millions of dollars and currently is the nation's largest private funder of research dedicated solely to breast cancer. Throughout the 1990s, lessons learned from the activists who drew attention to AIDS research were applied by women activists. Government funding for breast cancer research and education increased and so did financial support for research on other cancers in women. Although women patients and activists have been successful in instigating public awareness and increased funding for health issues such as breast cancer, Belkin (1996) wisely pointed out the necessity for women to recognize what it may take to remain a "cause" in the world of many causes and dwindling research dollars. Women's health issues and women's diseases compete for attention and money with the health issues and diseases of men, children, minorities, the elderly, the poor, and all other groups in the general public. The Office of Research on Women's Health, the Society for the Advancement of Women's Health Research, and the inclusion of women in clinical studies are strides forward but have not minimized the greater need today for women to be informed consumers of the health care system.

Women As Health Care Consumers

There is an almost universal dissatisfaction with the cost, quality, and kind of health care that people receive, and, as the predominant consumers of health care, women are more frequently at the receiving end. By all indices of measurement of illness, women evidently get sick more often than men. They have more days of restricted activity associated with acute conditions, more days of bed rest, more physician visits, and more discharges from short-stay hospitals than men. They take more prescription drugs in all categories and receive two-thirds of all the prescriptions for psychoactive (mood-elevating or tranquilizing) drugs. It is not, however, to be inferred that women are less healthy than men. Women live longer—a female baby born in 1998 has a life expectancy at birth of 79.6 years, exceeding that of a male baby by nearly 7 years—and women experience lower death rates than men for all causes except diabetes mellitus. However, women do report symptoms of both physical and mental illness more frequently than men. Of course, it may be that they report more illness than men because it is culturally more acceptable for them to do so. Women are thought of as the weaker sex, and illness is perceived as weakness, whereas strength, vigor, and good health are typically macho qualities, and men are held to a more rigid standard. There also are speculations that doctors are more likely to attribute health complaints of women to emotional rather than physical causes, even when scientific evidence clearly indicates a physiological reason for their disorders. Women's greater use of health services thus has been attributed to their greater concern, their "overanxiousness" about their health. As the AMA Council Report pointed out, decision making by doctors is based not only on scientific indications but also on "social attitudes, including stereotypes, prejudices, and other evaluations based on gender roles." A number of studies have attempted to document such physician prejudice, but as pointed out by Verbrugge and Steiner (1981), it is very difficult to scientifically prove sex bias in health care, even when it seems apparent. It is evident, however, that for whatever reasons, males and females utilize health services differently.

Health care policy is set by a small group of doctors, hospital administrators, medical school deans, and pharmaceutical and insurance industry executives. These workers in the medical-industrial complex are extremely well organized through their professional organizations, are able to mount extensive lobbying efforts, and are very well paid—their incomes having increased inordinately over the salaries of other health care workers in the past decades.

Women As Health Care Providers

The National Science Foundation, which supports nonmedical basic research in science, engineering, and mathematics, in a groundbreaking move appointed the first woman, a microbiologist, as director in 1998. Although the two top positions in health in the government, the surgeon general and the head of the National Institutes of Health, have been female, women are practically nonexistent in the power positions of the rest of the health care system. Women tend to form the large group of nurses, dietitians, occupational and physical therapists, social workers, and medical technologists and the even larger group of clerical and service workers. The participation of women in the health care labor force has been highly segregated and chiefly limited to supportive or auxiliary positions.

If the status of women as both consumers and providers of health care is to improve, a major change will be necessary—the admittance of women to the prestigious health professions and the participation of women from all economic levels in decision-making jobs in the health care system.

There is evidence that substantial change has occurred in the former "my son-the-doctor, my daughter-the-nurse-therapist-dietitian, etc." tradition. In 1970, women made up only 8% of the students entering medical schools. According to the Association of American Medical Colleges, however, by 1997–98, 41% of the freshmen were women, and in about 20 schools, women constituted 50% of the class. Even more promising is the trend among OB-GYN doctors. In 2001, the American College of Obstetricians and Gynecologists reported that women now fill 70.3% of all OB-GYN residencies. As the number of women in medical schools continues to increase, the processes of medical education that socialize physicians toward sexist attitudes should be modified. Moreover, these women should have considerable influence on medical practice, with a resulting improvement of medical services for women and all of society.

Currently, however, women medical students still face difficulties, although they may be finding that their increased numbers have made their medical training easier for them than it was for their counterparts a decade ago. There is less overt discrimination in recruitment, admissions, financial aid, health services, and lodging. Such bias is unquestionably illegal and specifically prohibited by Title IX of the 1972 education amendments to the Civil Rights Act. Women students encounter problems, but perhaps now in a more subtle way. They may be teased, baited, called on in class too much or not at all, or they may be asked how many hours they will work, or how many years they will take off for childbearing and rearing. They gained equal opportunity to become physicians, but once they graduate, they may find that certain subspecialty residencies are virtually closed to them.

The traditional expectation that women will want to link family responsibilities with their professional duties has resulted in the specialty orientation of women in areas of pediatrics, allergy, psychiatry, public health, and anesthesiology, which are viewed as being more compatible with the traditional female image.

Women graduates themselves, aware of the potential conflicts produced by marriage, motherhood, and medicine, may self-select into those residencies. Although women are training in virtually every specialty, they continue to be aggregated in the less prestigious, lower-paying areas. And when they have finished a residency, according to a number of surveys of physician compensation, the average incomes of women physicians lag considerably behind those of men physicians even within the same specialty (Angier, 1999). Partial explanation for the discrepancy could be that there are fewer women doctors to participate in the surveys, which skews the statistical results, and that the number of patients seen and the time spent with each patient generally differ between men and women doctors. Seeing more patients means more money, of course. Further reasons for the discrepancy could include the fact that female doctors want more flexibility and fewer hours of work if they have children, given that society views child rearing as primarily a maternal responsibility.

A topic debated among women physicians throughout the past decade with no resolution as yet is whether a separate specialty in women's health should be initiated. Although such a specialty could meet the health needs of women patients, it could also further isolate women's health issues from mainstream medicine. Lila Wallis (1992) stated that a comprehensive curriculum on women's health is needed and must be legitimized as an area of knowledge and skills. Others think it is better to integrate women's health issues into existing research and practice, that there should be more emphasis on women's health throughout the medical curriculum, and that it should be a priority for all physicians, not just a few specialists.

Although much progress has been made by women in gaining access to medical school, residency programs, and successful practices, they have as yet made few gains in the leadership positions in the medical world. In fact, one of the most insidious forms of discrimination against women medical students is the lack of role models during their medical education because of the few, if any, senior faculty women as instructors or administrators. Any expectation that the increasing numbers of women doctors will eventually infiltrate medical faculty ranks thus far is belied by the data. Although the number of female physicians has quadrupled in the past two decades, a corresponding increase in the number of women physicians on medical school faculties has not occurred. Moreover, those female physicians who want to do research and teach in medical academia are clustered in the nontenured, lower academic ranks. Although somewhat more women hold the positions of assistant or associate deans, they are most often in student or minority affairs.

It is hardly news that gender-based unfair treatment, gender-related obstacles to career advancement, discomfort from sexist remarks or "humor," or unwanted sexual advances are facts of life for women doctors and medical students. A woman working in any male-dominated profession is likely to have encountered such sexism, if not outright harassment.

Now that half of medical students are women, and probably more vocal and assertive women than their predecessors of a generation ago, blatantly sexist offenses by male faculty or peers may diminish. But it probably will take more than just additional women in medicine to surmount the difficulties of their climbing the academic ladder or getting financial equity with males. Dr. Anne E. Bernstein, writing in the *Journal of the American Medical Women's Association,* argued that the increased numbers of women students actually could work against women in medicine and that women physicians must fight against the possible "feminizing" of medicine as a woman's profession, . . . where, as in teaching and nursing, women are used, abused, and underpaid" (1989). It is clear from examples in European countries where numerically there are more women doctors than men doctors, that numbers alone do not ensure a share of the power and wealth at the top. Medical activity has long been a male activity, based on the male model and tailored to the image of the energetic workaholic man, free of any family responsibilities because he has a wife to take care of that aspect of his life. Many women physicians believe that the only way for women to succeed in the power structure is for the structure to change. For women as well as men to rise to positions of influence, the system will have to incorporate such innovations as extending the tenure clock for women, or considering alternative models of career development that recognize the differences between the lives of women and men. It seems logical, however, that as more activist women join the ranks of physicians, administrators, and research scientists, they will not continue to remain invisible. Changes in the system that increase women's status are inevitable.

Moreover, formerly submissive groups such as nurses, nurse-midwives, and nurse-practitioners, with a growing assertiveness of their professional status and rights, are insisting on their significant impact on the composition of policy-making bodies. A key factor in nurses' strength during the 1990s was the shortage of nurses, which resulted in their first major salary increase in history. Although their income is still not in line with professionals with similar degrees, such as engineers, chemists, or accountants, being in a seller's market benefited the profession in both wages and clout. As the head of a nursing program, quoted in Emily Friedman's (1990) report on the past, present, and future of nursing, states, ". . . nurses finally have the power to speak. They resent being forced aside, and as a result they are making trouble; and they will likely be doing so for a great long time." The system of control and governance will improve with the more vocal presence of women—doctors, nurses, administrators—in the health hierarchy who are "making trouble." Health care then is going to be more responsive to those women who receive it and those who work in it.

ᴛHE HEALTH CARE INDUSTRY

All segments of society have a great deal to gain by changing the health care system. The emphasis through the years has shifted from the "caring" to the "system," and the medical care industry has become the biggest business in the United States. In 1950, the cost of health care was $12 billion, but it was more than a trillion dollars by the end of the century, having risen faster than any other item in the cost of living. Despite the exorbitant bills, however, the system has failed for many citizens. About 43 billion people at the Census Bureau's last count are denied access to health care because they lack insurance. But even if people do have health insurance, their coverage may be limited because companies profit not by providing insurance but by trying to avoid paying for its use. The costs of the enormously complicated health care industry—the doctors, the health workers, the hospitals, the clinics, the nursing homes, the prescription drug industry— continue to increase. Although patients are referred to as health care consumers, they are not the ones to decide, as they may with other services and products, what and how much medical care to buy. Generally they take what they can get.

Managed Care or Managed Costs

After decades of incredible escalation of spending on health care, by the end of the century the majority of Americans with private health insurance (66%) were enrolled in "managed care" plans. Such plans were supposed to cut costs while increasing quality and access to health care. In managed care plans, the enrollees receive their health care from a group of approved doctors and hospitals called "providers" within a provider network. The two predominant types of plans are **health maintenance organizations (HMOs)** and **preferred provider organizations (PPOs).** An HMO generally employs its own doctors and operates its own clinics and hospitals. For a fixed monthly premium, an HMO requires that all health care is received from its providers. Most HMOs require that enrollees see a primary care physician (less expensive "gate-keeper"), who delivers routine care and must give approval for a patient to see a (more expensive) specialist. A PPO contracts with selected doctors, clinics, and hospitals, which then constitute the PPO's preferred network. A patient has the option of going to a doctor outside the network but pays more for it. A third kind of managed care plan is the rapidly growing point of service (POS) program. POS is like an HMO in requiring an inside primary-care physician, but like the PPO, patients may go outside the network for a price. For those who can afford it, traditional health insurance—"indemnity" or "fee-for-service" coverage—is available but is considerably more expensive than managed care plans. Through a traditional fee-for-service plan, the insurance company pays all or part of the bill for any health care provider a person chooses but generally requires annual deductible payments before payment.

Many people are satisfied with their managed care plans. These tend to include healthy individuals with little need for specialists and for whom the covered services are sufficient. Others are less happy with HMOs and PPOs when access to physicians of choice or referral to specialty care by the gatekeeper/physician is difficult or denied. A number of national polls have indicated that 40%–50% of Americans believe that insurance companies have a greater effect on their health care than doctors do. As for doctors, the majority are distinctly dissatisfied with managed care techniques and some have referred to managed care as "mangled care." Given that more than 90% of U.S. physicians have at least one contract with a managed care company, many doctors, like the public, believe that managed care can rob them of medical decision-making authority as well as their customary reimbursement rates. At this writing, Congress is debating six bills on managed care regulation, but with 80% of recent physician graduates taking salaried positions with HMOs (Greenhouse, 1999) instead of setting up a private practice, the health care industry continues to move toward managed care.

Medical Incompetency or Misconduct

Poor-quality medical care, that which falls far below acceptable standards and is delivered by careless or inept physicians, can cause serious damage and actually be life threatening. All people—men and women, children and adults—can suffer from bad medical practice. There are indications that billions of dollars are wasted on unneeded hospitalizations and that thousands of lives may be needlessly lost as a result of unnecessary surgery, useless and ineffective treatment, and adverse drug reactions from excessive and irrational prescribing.

According to the American Medical Association, between 7% and 9% of the nation's doctors are chemically dependent, that is, in some state of alcoholism or other drug addiction. This figure, based on the known rates of drug addiction and alcoholism in professional groups and on cases reported by patients, pharmacists, narcotics agents, or doctors themselves, means that, potentially, more than 30,000–40,000 physicians may be impaired because of some degree of dependency. This number does not reflect or take into account the doctors who are incompetent and unfit to practice medicine because they are suffering from mental illness, physical disability, or senility. In recognition of the problem of incompetency, the AMA sponsored a model bill aimed at "providing for the restriction, suspension, or revocation of the license of any physician to practice medicine because of his inability to practice medicine with reasonable skill and safety to patients, due to physical or mental illness, including deterioration through the aging process or loss of motor skill, or abuse of drugs, including alcohol." Most of the states have passed such "disabled doctor" legislation, but in 1996 only 0.3% of the nearly 700,000 nonfederal physicians were subject to serious disciplinary action annually by state licensing boards.

The thoroughly unfit doctors are presumably guilty of great damage to their unsuspecting patients, but there may be inestimable harm done by the much greater number of doctors who, for whatever reasons, do not practice the very best medicine they can. Doctors who are arrogant or careless, who ignore recent medical advances, whose prescribing practices reflect medical advertising more than scientific evaluation, who give the wrong drug or the right drug in the wrong dosage, who operate too much or not soon enough, or who bungle the surgery when it is performed—these are examples of substandard medical practices frequently unrecognized because consumers are ignorant of what actually constitutes quality and competence in health care. Two

Women and Their Health: From Early Feminism through the Millennium   •   **13**

studies that examined more than 31,000 hospital records in New York State found that almost 4% of all patients were injured at the hands of a doctor, and that more than a quarter of those were the result of substandard care, either by negligence or by error. About half of the problems occurred in patients undergoing surgery: 14% of the injuries were fatal and slightly less than 3% resulted in permanent disability (Brennan et al., 1991; Leape et al., 1991).

Even if people who are healthy get sick, or if people who are sick get worse or die because of the medical treatment they have received, there is still not much formal recourse available to the survivors or relatives. The number of medical malpractice suits has increased as people attempt to attain a favorable verdict and compensation for damages; however, cases of malpractice by physicians and hospitals are difficult to evaluate and prove. Unfortunately, physicians now view each patient who walks in the door as a potential litigant, and they practice more defensive medicine. By ordering even more diagnostic tests and more hospitalizations, doctors pass these costs along to the patients, who then pay even more for their health care.

Monitoring of Quality by the Medical Profession

Doctors affirm that they have always had a major interest in policing their own profession. In hospitals, for example, there have always been peer review committees that surveyed the treatment delivered and the surgeries performed, and it has been maintained that the medical societies have adequate mechanisms to control incompetence. Physicians conventionally claim that the percentage of incompetent professionals and the magnitude of abuses are highly exaggerated by the mass media and government agencies, and these physicians probably make such claims in good faith. Doctors, however, inherently lack objectivity. They are evaluating their own colleagues and, in the medical societies, their own dues-paying members. They have no particularly effective disciplinary sanctions to impose if they find abuses, and they generally do not actively search

them out. Responding to public complaint, legislators in many states have demanded that doctors take a more active role in protecting the public against medical incompetency. New statutes have been passed, or old ones have been revised to put more clout in physician-policing laws. There are additional grounds for disciplining doctors, a greater flexibility in penalties so that various degrees of punishment may be used and, in general, stricter sanctions.

But according to Wolfe, from Public Citizen Health Research Group, the health advocacy group that in 1998 published a list of 16,638 doctors nationwide who had been formally disciplined by state or federal agencies, the system for protecting the public from doctors guilty of incompetence, substance abuse, or patient abuse is uncoordinated, ineffective, and highly inadequate. State medical boards, often underfunded and understaffed, may have a backlog of 400–600 cases and are unable to give attention to new ones. Even if a physician's license is revoked, the physician can appeal the board's actions in the courts, a process that can take years, and in the meantime the doctor continues to practice.

Some state boards use an informal hearing process and plea bargaining—action on the license will be stayed if the doctor voluntarily seeks therapy, for example. Disabled doctors' programs with goals of prevention, intervention, and rehabilitation of impaired physicians have been initiated by a number of state medical societies. The effectiveness of such activities is controversial.

"Physician helping physician" is one solution to the problem of medical incompetency, but identification of the impaired physician remains the difficulty. There are several reasons why the medical staff may procrastinate or refuse to take action against an incompetent physician. An impaired doctor's popularity and the nurses' and aides' unwillingness to cause personal or professional harm may result in silence. The medical staff members could be reluctant to set a precedent; someone may blow a whistle on them next. Moreover, fellow professionals are generally not directly affected by incompetency; it is the patients who fall prey to the actions of the impaired physician. Finally, physicians may not want to get involved because it is they who might be vulnerable to economic reprisals from the impaired physician and his/her friends by a change in the way they make referrals.

Get a Second Opinion

Surgeons have always been the prima donnas of the medical world, having long enjoyed greater prestige and financial success than other physicians. The number of surgeons has nearly tripled since 1970 and, necessarily, the more surgeons there are, the more surgeries are done. In recent years, however, the supply of surgeons has tended to exceed the demand for their services, and the average general surgeon now feels the pressure of an increasingly competitive market. Especially in crowded urban areas, there are no longer enough operations for the expanded number of surgeons to perform. Many conditions involving the stomach, colon, kidneys, gallbladder, heart, and blood vessels that were formerly treated by surgery currently can be, and should be, treated with drugs or lesser procedures than major surgery. Now that some of the surgeons' bread-and-butter business has been taken over by other specialists, the result has been a 25% decrease in operations done by the average general surgeon (Rosenthal, 1989).

Too many surgeons for too few operations has a number of potential ramifications for patients. One is that surgeons may not be getting enough practice in certain procedures to maintain their skills at peak proficiency. Some surgeons have both protected their income and maintained their skills by limiting their practice to one type of surgery, such as hernias or gallbladders. This can benefit patients because studies suggest that for complicated surgical procedures, adverse consequences, including mortality, can be decreased by as much as 40% by having the surgery done by someone who performs the operation often. But some surgeons may respond to the competition by expanding the number of major surgeries they perform or scheduling more minor procedures, either of which could result in a greater number of unnecessary surgeries. The amount of surgery performed that is medically unwarranted is difficult to assess, however, because

even the most conscientious and competent doctors might disagree on the need for a particular operation at a particular time. Also, whether an expansion of surgical rates that has occurred in the past decade means that a certain proportion is unnecessary is unclear. There is no completely acceptable method available that has been developed to assess what proportion of surgery is essential, or effectively to decrease the number of operations even if they are deemed unnecessary. A good example is the controversy that surrounds hysterectomy, or removal of the uterus.

The United States is the hysterectomy capital of the world. The number of such surgeries performed annually, mostly on women between the ages of 35 and 45, is about three times more than in any other country. It seems unlikely that the uteri of American women have three times the pathology of European women's uteri. A 10% decrease in rate occurred at the height of the women's health movement, between the middle 1970s and 1980, but since then the national rate has dropped only slightly. Moreover, huge and inexplicable disparities for hysterectomy rates exist among various parts of the country. A woman living in the South or in California may be twice as likely to get a hysterectomy as a woman living in New York. According to the Agency for Health Care Policy and Research in 1999, by the time they reach 60 years of age, one woman in three in the United States will have had a hysterectomy.

The operation is one of the most controversial of surgical procedures, with disagreement existing among doctors both on when and how it should be done. Hysterectomy is clearly necessary for cancer of the uterus, ovaries, and fallopian tubes, but only about 10% are performed for cancer. Most of the other reasons for hysterectomy are considered "elective," and it is these that have created the greatest debate about necessity. Hysterectomy may be performed to remove benign tumors (fibroids) of the uterus or for endometriosis, a sometimes painful condition in which the uterine lining is found in and around other tissues in the abdominal cavity. Large fibroids that cause heavy bleeding, abdominal distension, and pressure on the urinary bladder or rectum may not be life threatening as is cancer, but for many women this kind of discomfort interferes with the quality of life and could justify hysterectomy. Whether asymptomatic fibroids should be the reason for removing the uterus is controversial. They often can be either left alone or treated conservatively by more limited procedures than hysterectomy. In many instances, so can endometriosis, uterine prolapse, pelvic pain, and some of the other reasons why so many hysterectomies are performed.

During the early 1970s, Eugene McCarthy and Geraldine Widmer (1974) at Cornell University Medical College made an extensive study of the need for elective, nonemergency surgery in a group of union members in New York. They set up a screening program in which a person who had been recommended for an operation would go to a board-certified physician as a consultant in order to get a second opinion on the need for the operation. It was discovered that when a second gynecologist examined the patients recommended for hysterectomies, nearly one out of three, 32%, were not confirmed as being necessary. A subsequent investigation of the New York Hospital-Cornell Medical Center patients studied through 1980 produced similar results—41.3% of the women who voluntarily sought a second opinion and 30.7% of those who were required to seek a second opinion were not confirmed for the necessity of the hysterectomy by the board-certified consultant (Finkel, McCarthy, & Ruchlin, 1982).

Some feminist groups have claimed that women are frightened into having hysterectomies and are exploited to make money for the doctors, even though there are alternative methods of treatment. Some doctors, however, maintain that there has been an increasing demand on the part of women for hysterectomies. These doctors claim that more women request the operation as a means of sterilization or because they are unwilling to put up with the "nonsense" of menstruation each month, and that if one doctor will not remove their uteri, these women will find one who will. If this is actually a trend, it is another indication of how ill-informed women are about their own bodies and major medical procedures. Using hysterectomy to achieve sterilization is excessive for the purpose and somewhat equivalent to using decapitation to cure a migraine.

It seems clear that second-opinion programs for all surgeries might decrease the number of operations. After all, some people get several estimates on their cars before undergoing a major repair job; their own bodies deserve no less. Many health insurance companies, including managed care, will pay for consultants to verify a diagnosis recommending surgery. Both the patient and the doctor can then be more certain about the decision to operate, and the final choice is up to the patient.

Consumerism in Health Care

The second-opinion-in-surgery plan, a process by which a patient can make an informed choice concerning a proposed treatment, is one step toward a different kind of doctor-patient relationship, different from the traditional one in which the doctor makes all the decisions and the patient rarely questions them. To many people, the old way is no longer tenable. They view doctors not as deities with superhuman powers, but as highly skilled, highly educated human beings who provide services that are purchased by consumer-patients. They believe that all individuals have the right to decide what shall be done with or to their bodies and their personalities and that the essence of a just and adult physician-patient relationship in a democratic society is the sharing of information and opinion to reach an intelligent judgment together. Patients do not want the entire burden of decision making placed on them, but they do want to be invited to participate in the process. They assume that a mature and competent physician has no desire for total control but feels a responsibility to proceed in the best interest of the patient.

Some members of the medical profession have a great deal of difficulty accepting the idea of sharing decision making with nonprofessionals. Hippocrates himself advised doctors to conceal most things from their patients and to reveal nothing of the patient's present and future condition. This attitude on the part of physicians has frequently resulted in having mature, taxpaying citizens relegated to the status of passive, childlike individuals with less-than-normal intelligence. Women in particular have felt themselves in a double bind because they have been treated not only within such an authoritarian paternalistic relationship but also within the social framework of the stereotyped feminine role—dependent, unquestioning, accepting.

Irrevocable changes have already intruded upon the customary and age-old personal relationship between doctor and patient. Modern medicine is fragmented, highly specialized, institutionalized, and enormously expensive—a condition considered counterproductive and actually "sickening" for patients by many social critics. But the original goals of the women's health movement—self-care, medical self-awareness, patient decision making, improvement and change in the health care delivery system—now have become part of a general social trend for all consumers of health care. Through forums and conferences, lectures, community "know-your-body" courses and "health fairs," through university and community college courses on biology of women and women's health, through magazine and newspaper articles and television programs and the Internet, women and men are being given the information they need to interact with the health professionals and not be acted upon. As improved public education further demystifies medical practices, and individuals realize that health is also their own responsibility and not the sole responsibility of the medical profession, patients can become their own consumer advocates and demand and understand the following:

- What the doctor is doing, and why the doctor is doing it

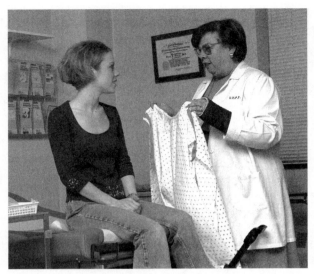

Figure 1–2 Lack of knowledge can make a woman feel vulnerable and afraid. Knowing how the body functions in health and disease can give women the self-confidence to participate in the decisions concerning their own health care.

- A complete examination of their medical condition and the right to privacy and confidentiality
- Participation as a partner in decisions concerning their treatment, all the alternatives to treatment, and their right to refuse treatment

People will no longer tolerate being patronized or treated with condescension; they will insist on being treated with dignity, respect, and consideration. In this way, a further positive modification of the traditional doctor-dominant, patient-subordinate role will occur to the mutual benefit of both (Figure 1–2).

ℛEFERENCES

Angier, N. (1999, January 12). Among doctors, pay for women still lags. *The New York Times,* p. D7.

Ayanian, J. Z., & Epstein, A. M. (1991). Differences in the use of procedures between women and men hospitalized for coronary heart disease. *New England Journal of Medicine, 325*(4), 221–225.

Belkin, L. (1996, December 22). Charity begins at the marketing meeting, the gala event, the product tie-in. *The New York Times,* section 6.

Bernstein, A. E. (1989). Gender equity. *Journal of the American Women's Medical Association, 44*(3), 84–85.

Brennan, T. A., Leape, L. I., Laird, N. M., et al. (1991). Incidence of adverse events and negligence in hospitalized patients. Results of the Harvard Medical Practice Study I. *New England Journal of Medicine, 324*(6), 370–376.

Council on Ethical and Judicial Affairs. (1991). American Medical Association. Gender disparities in clinical decision making. *Journal of the American Women's Medical Association, 266*(4), 559–562.

Finkel, M. L., McCarthy, E. G., & Ruchlin, H. S. (1982). The current status of surgical second opinion programs. *Surgical Clinics of North America, 62*(4), 705–719.

Friedman, E. (1990). Nursing: Breaking the bonds. *Journal of the American Women's Medical Association, 264*(24), 3117–3122.

Greenhouse, S. (1999, February 4). Angered by HMO's treatment, more doctors are joining unions. *The New York Times*, p. A1.

Grobbee, D. E., Rimm, E. B., Giovannucci, E., et al. (1990). Coffee, caffeine, and cardiovascular disease in men. *New England Journal of Medicine, 323,* 1026–1032.

Haseltine, F., & Jacobson, B. G. (1997). (Eds.). *Women's health research: A medical and policy primer.* Washington, DC: Health Press International.

Leape, L. L., Brenna, T. A., Laird, N. M., et al. (1991). The nature of adverse events in hospitalized patients. Results of the Harvard Medical Practice Study II. *New England Journal of Medicine, 324*(6), 377–384.

McCarthy, E. G., & Widmer, G. (1974). Effects of screening by consultants on recommended elective surgical procedures. *New England Journal of Medicine, 288*(6), 288–292.

Office of Research on Women's Health. (1995). *Recruitment and retention of women in clinical studies* (NIH Publication No. 95-3756). Bethesda, MD: NIH Office of Communications.

Rosenthal, E. (1989, November 7). Innovations intensify glut of surgeons. *The New York Times.*

Schulman, K. A., Berlin, J. A., Harless, W., et al. (1999). The effect of race and sex on physicians' recommendations for cardiac catheterization. *New England Journal of Medicine, 340*(8), 618–626.

Steering Committee of the Physician's Health Study Group. (1989). Final report on the aspirin component of the ongoing physician's health study. *New England Journal of Medicine, 321,* 129–135.

Steingart, R. M., Packer, M., Hamm, P., et al. (1991). Sex differences in the management of coronary artery disease. *New England Journal of Medicine, 325*(4), 226–230.

The Multiple Risk Factor Intervention Trial Research Group. (1990). Mortality rates after 10.5 years for participants in the Multiple Risk Factor Intervention Trial: Findings related to a priori hypotheses of the trial. *Journal of the American Medical Association, 263*(13), 1795–1801.

Verbrugge, L. M., & Steiner, R. P. (1981). Physician treatment of men and women patients. Sex bias or appropriate care? *Medical Care, 19,* 609–632.

Wallis, L. (1992). Women's health: A specialty? Pros and cons. *Journal of Women's Health, 2*(1), 107–108.

Wolfe, S. (1998). *16,638 questionable doctors.* Washington, DC: Public Citizen Health Research Group.

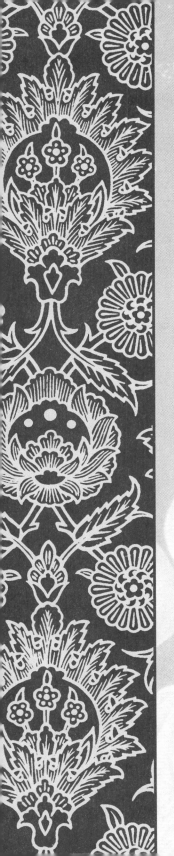

2

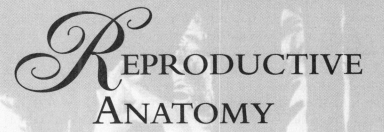

REPRODUCTIVE ANATOMY

KEY TERMS

Cervix	Oviducts
Clitoris	Prostate
Fallopian tubes	Semen
Hymen	Seminal vesicles
Labia majora	Testes
Labia minora	Vagina
Mons pubis	Vulva

Historically, the female body and, more specifically, the female reproductive tract, because it is internal and therefore hidden, has always been subject to much romanticism, fantasizing, and descriptive error. Until the publication of the writings and illustrations of the most outstanding anatomist of the Renaissance, Andreas Vesalius, there was virtually no anatomically correct knowledge of female structure. The reason for the lack of information until the sixteenth century has been attributed to the lack of material for dissection. Even when courses in human anatomy were recognized as part of the curriculum in medical schools all over Europe, corpses for dissection were difficult to obtain because only the bodies of executed criminals who came from an area at least 30 miles away could be used. One or two dissections a year were performed, and female cadavers were rarely available. Vesalius's unprecedented graphic visualization of anatomy, *De Humani Corporis Fabrica,* was not only an accurate representation of the structure of males but was based on the dissections of at least nine female cadavers as well and, therefore, formed the foundation for modern anatomical knowl-

edge of both men and women. In the 400 years since Vesalius, if there were any women physicians and anatomists who contributed to the advancement of knowledge concerning the female reproductive tract, it would not be obvious from the nomenclature. The discoverers of the female anatomical parts; the recognizers of clinical syndromes, signs, tests, and phenomena; the developers of instruments, techniques, operations, and therapies were evidently all men or, at any rate, only men have received acknowledgment (Table 2–1).

Even after anatomical knowledge of the human female was available, there was relatively scant knowl-

TABLE 2–1	Some Contributions to Nomenclature in Gynecology and Obstetrics	
Individual	**Eponym**	**Description**
Caspar Bartholin 1655–1738	Bartholin's glands	Greater vestibular glands
James Read Chadwick 1884–1905	Chadwick's sign	Color changes in the pregnant vulvovaginal mucosa
Albert Döderlein 1860–1941	Döderlein's bacilli	Lactobacilli of vagina
Gabriele Fallopius 1523?–1562	Fallopian tubes	Oviducts
Regnier de Graaf 1641–1673	Graafian follicle	Preovulatory follicle
Alfred Hegar 1830–1914	Hegar's sign	Softening of the lower uterine segment during pregnancy
John Braxton Hicks 1823–1897	Braxton Hicks contractions	Contraction of the pregnant uterus
Hugh Lenox Hodge 1796–1873	Hodge pessary	Vaginal support of uterine displacement
Max Huhner 1873–1947	Huhner test	Postcoital semen examination
William Fetherstone Montgomery 1797–1859	Montgomery's tubercles	Breast areolar changes during pregnancy

(continues)

TABLE 2–1 *(continued)*

Individual	Eponym	Description
Johannes Müller 1801–1858	Müllerian ducts	Embryonic paired ducts; give rise to uterus and vagina
Martin Naboth 1675–1721	Nabothian cysts	Cervical mucous cysts
Franz Carl Nägele 1777–1851	Nägele's rule	Formula for estimation of date of delivery
Anton Nuck 1650–1692	Canal of Nuck	Inguinal canal
George Papanicolaou 1883–1962	Pap smear	Cervical cancer detection
Isidor Rubin 1883–1958	Rubin test	Tubal insufflation
Alexander Skene 1838–1900	Skene's ducts	Paraurethral ducts
Friedrich Trendelenburg 1844–1924	Trendelenburg position	Elevated pelvic position
Henry Turner 1892–1970	Turner's syndrome	Ovarian dysgenesis
Thomas Wharton 1614–1673	Wharton's jelly	Umbilical cord mucous matrix
Caspar Wolff 1733–1794	Wolffian duct	Embryonic mesonephric duct

edge about her physiology until more recently, and the dissemination of such information to men and women has been minimal. Some of the myths that have arisen concerning the physical and mental abilities of women have had remarkable persistence among educators and physicians who presumably should know better. Fallacies and generalizations about female anatomy, physiology, and sexuality have arisen based more on cultural assumptions than on accurate observations. Even when it is pointed out that insufficient evidence exists for a belief, or that scientific data invalidate a previously held opinion, there is a tendency to cling to outmoded misinformation. The ignorance of men and women concerning the female body has helped to perpetuate the continuation of fallacy and superstition; this chapter provides the anatomical basis to distinguish the myths from the realities.

THE PELVIC GIRDLE

One widely held notion, for example, is that there is greater risk in participation in contact sports for

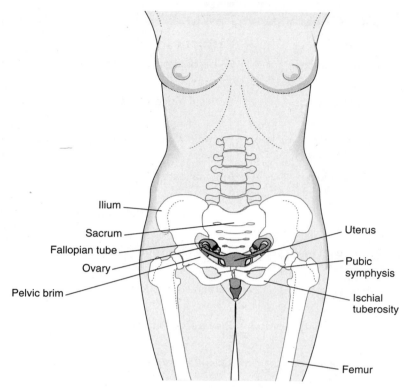

Ilium

Sacrum

Fallopian tube

Ovary

Pelvic brim

Uterus

Pubic symphysis

Ischial tuberosity

Femur

Figure 2–1 Position of the reproductive organs within the pelvic girdle.

females because they are more vulnerable to injury than males and because their internal reproductive organs are more vulnerable to damage. Actually, there are differences in the susceptibility of females and males to the impact of direct contact in sports, but the resultant injuries are to ligaments and muscles, for reasons to be described later, and not to the internal organs. A protective cage for the sexual organs of women is formed by the strong bony pelvic girdle, and the pelvic viscera are seldom damaged, even in the crushing injuries of accidents (see Figure 2–1). The exposed genitalia of the male are far more likely to be injured in contact sports.

The pelvic girdle is the general name given to the two broad, heavy hip bones that provide an attachment for the leg and support the lower spine in order to transmit the weight of the body from the vertebral column to the limbs. Each hip bone, also called the *os coxae,* is composed of three fused bones: the *ilium,* the *ischium,* and the *pubis.* A cup-shaped socket, the *acetabulum* (Latin for little saucer that holds vinegar), receives the head of the thigh bone or femur to form the hip joint (Figures 2–2, 2–3).

Ilium

The large ilium flares upward and outward from the acetabulum. When hands are placed on hips, one is feeling the broad and thick crest of the ilium. Follow it forward along the forefinger. The tip of the forefinger is on the *anterior superior iliac spine.* The tip of the thumb is approximately in the region of the *posterior superior iliac spine,* easily palpable through the skin of a

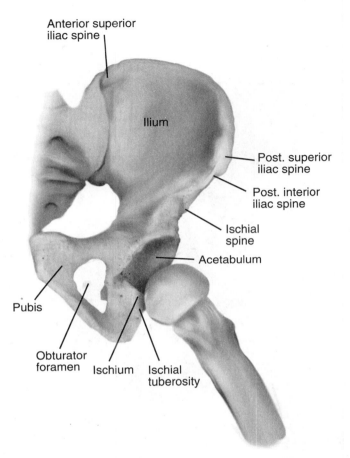

Figure 2–2 Lateral aspect of left os coxae.

thin person and always marked by a dimple. The inner surface of the iliac bones is concave and forms the origin of a powerful muscle of thigh and trunk movement, the *iliacus*. On the right side, the concavity in the iliac bone, the iliac *fossa*, accommodates the *cecum*, which is the pouchlike, blind end of the large intestine formed at its junction with the small intestine. From the cecum extends the vermiform (wormlike) appendix, and because of its anatomical position, the pain of acute appendicitis is felt in the right iliac fossa. The fallopian (uterine) tubes or oviducts are also in anatomical proximity to the concavities of both iliac bones, and pain originating from the tubes when they are

inflamed or infected is often referred to (i.e., felt in) the fossae.

The rear or posterior part of the inner surface of each ilium has an *auricular* (ear-shaped) *surface* that forms an articulation or junction with the *sacrum*, the fused vertebrae at the lower end of the spinal column. When one bone articulates with another, a joint is formed, whether or not it is movable. The joint here is the *sacroiliac joint*, one of the most important joints of the body because the body's full weight is transmitted through it to the legs when a person is standing upright. The great load placed on the sacrum by the entire vertebral column would tend to cause it to rock

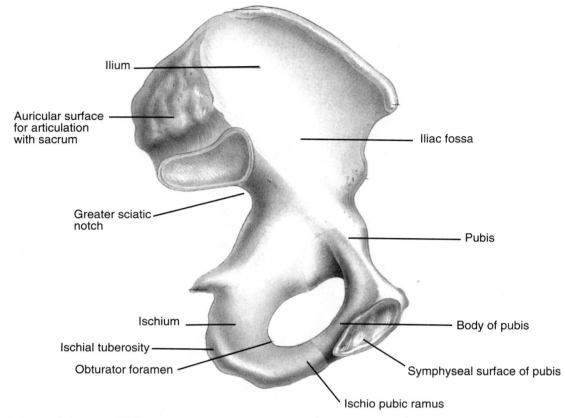

Ilium

Auricular surface
for articulation
with sacrum

Iliac fossa

Greater sciatic
notch

Pubis

Ischium

Body of pubis

Ischial tuberosity

Obturator foramen

Symphyseal surface of pubis

Ischio pubic ramus

Figure 2–3   Medial aspect of left os coxae.

back and forth between the hip bones if it were not for enormously strong ligaments that surround the sacroiliac joint to form an interlocking mechanism to brace and reinforce it.

Ischium

Below the sacroiliac joint, the rear border of each ilium indents to form a huge *greater sciatic* notch through which pass blood vessels and nerves. The lower part of the greater sciatic notch is formed by the *ischium,* which ends in a large knob, the *ischial tuberosity.* When one is sitting up straight, one sits on the ischial tuberosities, and they, instead of the legs, receive the weight of the body through the sacroiliac

joints. The hamstrings, that group of large muscles on the back of the thigh, are attached to the ischial tuberosities.

Pubis

From the tuberosity of the ischium extends a flattened *ischial ramus,* or bar, which meets the flattened ramus of the *pubis.* The ramus of the pubis flares out to form the body of the pubis, which meets the other pubic bone from the opposite side. The union of the two pubic bones is called the *pubic symphysis,* a joint that is united by cartilage and held together by strong ligaments. During pregnancy, both the symphysis and the sacroiliac joints are softened and stretch as a result of the tremendous amounts of hormones that are produced. The joints become mobile and make delivery easier.

Bony Pelvis

The term bony pelvis refers to the bowl-like structure (pelvis means "basin" in Latin) that is formed by the hip bones at the sides and the front and the sacrum and coccyx at the back. It is divided anatomically into the following:

1. False or greater pelvis, made up of the upper flared parts of the two iliac bones with their concavities, and by the two wings of the base of the sacrum

2. True or lesser pelvis, formed by the rest of the ilium, pubis, and ischium on both sides, and the sacrum and the coccyx

The boundaries of the opening to the true pelvis, or *pelvic inlet,* are called the *pelvic brim.* The diameters of the pelvic brim have particular obstetric significance. The dimensions of the *pelvic outlet,* bounded by the ischial tuberosities, the lower rim of the pubic symphysis, and the tip of the coccyx, are also of great importance obstetrically (Figure 2–4).

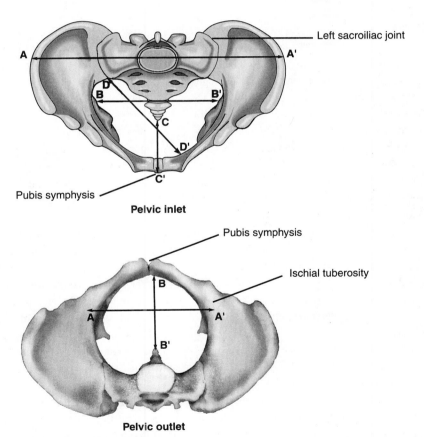

Figure 2–4 Diameters of the pelvic inlet and the pelvic outlet. Inset: A–A' = false pelvis; B–B' = true pelvis, transverse diameter; C–C' = anterior-posterior diameter, from the tip of the coccyx to the pubic symphysis; D–D' = oblique diameter from sacroiliac joint to the iliopubic eminence. Outlet: A–A' = transverse diameter, between inner edges of ischial tuberosities; B–B' = anterior-posterior diameter, from pubic symphysis to tip of coccyx.

At birth, the three parts of the hip bone—the ilium, ischium, and pubis—are composed mainly of cartilage and are separate bones. The ischium and the pubis become bony and fuse at approximately 7 or 8 years of age, but total ossification of all the cartilaginous portions is not completed until sometime between 17 and 25. Although pregnancy is possible after puberty, the pelvic ring may not be as capable of withstanding the stresses and strains of childbearing until all the weaker cartilaginous links among the three bones have fused and become bony.

SEX DIFFERENCES IN THE PELVIS

The body measurements (stature, sitting height, head circumference, and so on) of an adult female average approximately 92% of the body measurements of the adult male. This same proportionality may be applied to skeletal measurements. Generally, the male pelvis as a whole is larger than the female pelvis, except for the dimensions of the *true pelvis,* which has to accommodate the dimensions of the full-term fetal head, since 95% of babies are born head first. Pelvic measurements, however, show considerable variation (as do all other measurements in humans), and there is actually as much variation in the size and shape of the pelvis among women as there is between women and men. No two pelves are alike; it is the individual pelvis and the particular fetal head involved that become important obstetrically.

Sexual differences in the adult pelvis have been studied extensively, and there are different classifications that have been used to describe the normal range of variation in the morphology of the male and female pelvis. The most commonly quoted are those described by W. E. Caldwell and H. C. Moloy, based on x-ray determinations of the dimensions of the pelvic inlet, or superior opening of the true pelvis. These authorities said that female pelves are divided into four main groups:

1. The *anthropoid* pelvis is common in men and occurs in 20%–30% of white women and nearly 50% of black women. The pelvic inlet is oval and the sacrum is long, producing a deep pelvis.
2. The *android* pelvis is also common in men, but one-third of white women and 10%–15% of black women also have this type, in which the inlet is heart shaped and the side walls are narrow. This classification, also called the "funnel" pelvis, produces difficulty in delivery of the baby.
3. The *gynecoid,* or true female, pelvis is less common in males. About 50% of all women have this type. The inlet is round, the outlet is roomy, and the subpubic angle or pubic arch is almost a 90° angle. The gynecoid is the best pelvic type for an easy, normal delivery and is the one selected for contrast with the android pelvis in anatomy books to depict typical male and female pelvic differences.
4. The *platypelloid,* or flat, pelvis is the least common type of pelvic structure among most men and women. In this rare type, the pelvic cavity is shallow but widens at the pelvic outlet, permitting a delivery that is not difficult, as long as the fetal head can pass through the pelvic inlet (Figure 2–5).

Many women have a combination of these four basic types, and the anterior part of the pelvis may be one classification, whereas the posterior segment is another. These classifications are based on average values obtained from skeletal material and, as indicated, are obviously not as important as the individual woman's measurements compared to the measurements of the head of the child she is bearing. Measuring the dimensions of the true pelvis is called pelvimetry, and it is usually performed as part of the physical examination of a pregnant woman to determine whether she will have any difficulty in delivery.

Pelvimetry can be done by x-ray, by external measurements made with a *pelvimeter,* and by internal examination through the vagina. Because of the dan-

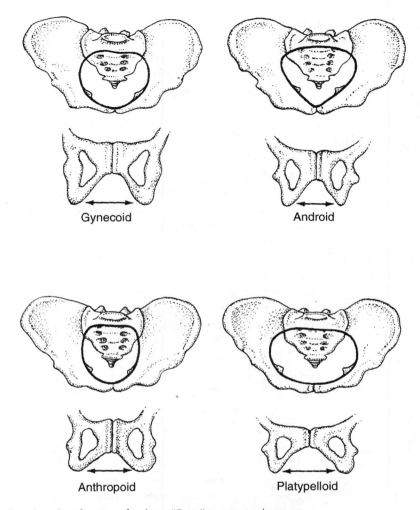

Gynecoid

Android

Anthropoid

Platypelloid

Figure 2–5 Caldwell-Moloy classification of pelves. "Pure" types are shown.

ger of radiation to the ovaries of the mother and the fetus, radiography is used rarely, delayed until the time of delivery, and then done only if there is some apparent difficulty in labor. Most x-ray pelvimetry has currently been replaced by ultrasonography.

If a woman has very narrow pelvic dimensions or if some distortion of the normal pelvis has occurred as a result of poor nutrition, injury, or disease, the decrease in size may be enough to interfere with normal labor. Such a pelvis is said to be contracted and could cause *dystocia,* or long, difficult labor. It may be necessary for the fetus to be removed by an incision into the uterus, or *cesarean section.*

Pelvic Tilt

When we stand in an upright position, the whole pelvis is tipped forward so that the plane of the pelvic brim forms an angle of approximately 50°–60° with the horizontal. The plane of the pelvic outlet, an imaginary line drawn from the tip of the coccyx to the inferior part of the pubic symphysis, forms an angle of about 15° with the horizontal. This means that the pelvic surface of the pubic symphysis faces upward as much as it does backward, and the concavity of the sacrum is directed both downward and forward. If one were to stand upright, facing flat against a wall, the anterior superior iliac spines and the upper border of the pubic symphysis would both almost touch the wall; that is, they would be in the same vertical plane. This tilt of the pelvis is called the angle of pelvic inclination, and although subject to great individual variation, it is frequently exaggerated in women due to the difference in dimensions of the true pelvis. As a result of the greater tilt of the pelvis in females, the spinal curvature in the lumbar region of the spine is increased in an anterior (forward) direction to compensate and maintain the center of gravity. Otherwise, a woman might fall forward and be unable to maintain an erect posture. Because this forward lumbar curve is greater in some women, their buttocks are usually more prominent than those of men, depending, of course, on the shape of the pelvis and amount of the pelvic tilt (Figure 2–6).

Another general statement, again subject to great individual variation, is that women are more frequently seen with knock-knees than are men. This is true because the head of the femur fits into the cup-shaped acetabulum to form a femoral angle of approximately 125° at the neck of the femur so that the shaft of the thighbone can swing clear of the pelvis when the leg moves. That angle determines the position of the knees. The more oblique the angle, the more the shafts of the femur will slope inward, and the closer the knees will meet. In women, the pelvis is generally wider and the femurs shorter, and hence the greater tendency to have knock-knees (Figure 2–7). Some orthopedic physicians have maintained that because of

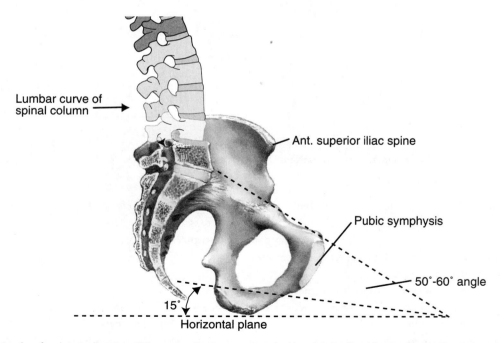

Figure 2–6 Angle of pelvic inclination. When standing erect, the whole pelvis is tilted forward, and the pelvic canal is directed backward relative to the abdominal cavity and the torso. The greater the pelvic tilt of the pelvis, the greater the curve in the lower back.

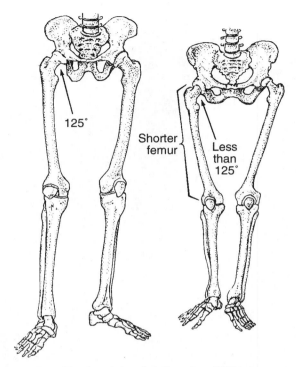

Figure 2–7 The female angle is less than 125° in some women, giving them a greater tendency to have knock-knees.

the above mentioned body mechanics, women's knees are much more vulnerable to injury and that they should, therefore, avoid participation in contact sports. This may be true for some women who have a gynecoid pelvis and a smaller, lighter bone structure. It may be equally valid for some men.

Backache and Its Relation to the Pelvis

If a woman has a greater angle of pelvic inclination, she will also have a greater increase in the curvature of the lumbar spine. Then anything that places further strain on the lumbar area, such as the protruding abdomen of pregnancy or obesity, is almost certain to result in lower back pain. There are estimates that 50%–60% of the population has had back trouble at one time or another, but more females than males suffer with chronic backache.

Sometimes the very process of delivering a baby, particularly if the labor is long and difficult, puts unusual strain on the muscles and ligaments surrounding the sacroiliac joints, which have "unlocked" and stretched under hormonal action to have much more mobility at full term than in a nonpregnant woman. Although these sacroiliac joint changes regress in the period after the birth of the baby, it can take a long time for them to get back to normal, and the woman will have chronic low back pain in the interim.

With the exception of the period of *puerperium* (after delivery of a baby), most backaches in women are muscular aches resulting from poor posture and are not gynecological in origin. If lower back pain is a result of pelvic pathology, it is felt in the area over the sacrum; postural backache is higher—between the top of the sacrum and the bottom of the rib cage.

When one is standing erect with good posture, the weight of the body is passed down the lumbar vertebrae through the sacrum, divided through each sacroiliac joint to the acetabula of the hip bones, and then to the legs. The most important supporting spinal muscles, those that keep the line of gravity in appropriate balance, arise from the front and back of the pelvis. When good posture is disturbed, those muscles are placed under stress, and they become sore and ache. Numerous factors can act to destroy good posture. One, mentioned previously, is the strain on the muscles of the spinal column caused by pregnancy, labor, and the puerperium. Maybe the muscles are weak because of lack of exercise. Or there may be congenital (present at birth) defects in the spine, pelvis, or feet. Sometimes sleeping on the wrong kind of mattress, walking or standing in shoes with high heels or rigid soles, or spending long periods of time in a fixed position—sitting all day in a particular type of chair or driving hundreds of miles without a break—can result in backache. These types of factors, once recognized, should not be difficult to eliminate.

If poor posture and weak muscles are the result of minor defects in the spine, hips, knees, or feet, there are exercises that strengthen the tone and increase the flexibility of abdominal, back, and thigh muscles so that the

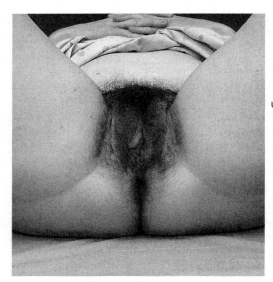
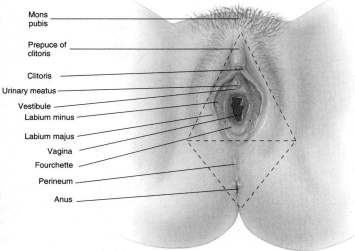

Mons pubis

Prepuce of clitoris

Clitoris

Urinary meatus

Vestibule

Labium minus

Labium majus

Vagina

Fourchette

Perineum

Anus

Figure 2–8 Female genitalia.

spine can be supported in a corrected position. Although many cases of low back pain will respond to a home exercise plan, it is important to check with a knowledgeable professional first (orthopedist, neurologist, rheumatologist, physiatrist, physical therapist) and never to continue an exercise that causes pain.

When the ligaments and tendons that support the spinal column are traumatically stretched, the sudden strain can produce muscle spasm and backache. This happens when heavy objects are lifted incorrectly by bending forward with the knees straight. Bed rest and moist heat will relax the muscles and relieve the pain. Another cause of back pain is osteoarthritis or degenerative joint disease, which usually occurs after the fourth decade of life. Should the intervertebral disc between two adjacent vertebrae begin to degenerate, great stress is placed on the surrounding ligaments. If the disc herniates or protrudes it may impinge on the nerves that exit in between the vertebrae. A "slipped disc" may also be associated with numbness or weakness in one or both legs because of the pressure on the spinal nerves. These types of symptoms may require hospitalization, physical therapy, or even surgery for treatment.

The point is, most backaches arise in the back; that is, they are musculoskeletal in origin. They are much more rarely the result of ulcers, kidney disease, or pelvic pathology. Some of the gynecological difficulties that do result in back pain will be covered later.

EXTERNAL GENITALIA

The Vulva

The **vulva,** sometimes called the pudendum, is the term for the visible external genitalia. The name vulva means "covering" in Latin and refers to the area bounded by the *mons pubis* anteriorly, the *perineum* posteriorly, and the *labia minora* and *majora* laterally. The vulva is erotic and highly sensitive to touch; it also serves to protect the urethral and vaginal openings (Figure 2–8).

Mons Pubis

Another name for the **mons pubis** is the *mons veneris,* literally, "the mountain of Venus"—suitably named, the ancients thought, because Venus was the goddess of love (venereal disease has the same linguistic root). It is the cushion of fatty tissue and skin that lies over the pubic symphysis and, after puberty, is covered with pubic hair. Pubic hair varies in texture, as does the hair on the head, depending on the race of the individual. In many women, the upper border of pubic hair is straight across, forming a triangle, and this is the so-called female escutcheon. In males, the pubic hair supposedly grows upward toward the umbilicus as a result of androgenic activity, thus defining maleness and femaleness in the configuration of pubic hair growth. In actuality, some 25% of women and most men do have an apparent upward continuation of pubic hair to the umbilicus; it is not pubic hair proper, but ordinary body hair. Some people are just genetically hairier than other people. When a woman has this abdominal growth of hair, it is very rarely a sign of some virilizing hormonal influence.

Labia Majora

Extending down from the mons pubis are two longitudinal folds of skin, narrowing to enclose the vulvar cleft, and meeting posteriorly in the *perineum,* that area of skin between the junction of the labia major and the anus.

These **labia majora** (major lips) protect the inner parts of the vulva. The outer surface of the labia is covered with pubic hair. The inner surface is not, but has many sebaceous and sweat glands. The tissue inside the labia majora is loose connective tissue with pads of subcutaneous fat. The fat, like the fat on the hips and in the breasts, is particularly sensitive to estrogen. This is why the labia and the rest of the vulva become enlarged (hypertrophy) from puberty on and shrink (atrophy) after the menopause. Underneath the subcutaneous fat and deep within the substance of the labial tissue are masses of erectile tissue, tissue filled with large blood spaces that engorge with blood during sexual excitement. These masses, which encircle the vaginal opening, are called the *bulbs of the vestibule;* they are equivalent to the *corpus spongiosum* of the male penis.

Under the skin of the labia majora, there are fibers of smooth muscle that are similar to the dartos muscle of the male scrotum. This subcutaneous muscle is temperature sensitive and causes the labia to wrinkle up when exposed to cold and to appear larger and softer in warm weather.

Labia Minora

The **labia minora** are the delicate inner folds of skin that enclose the urethral opening and the vagina. They are also called *nymphae,* from the Greek word for "maiden," referring to the goddesses of the fountain.★ The labia minora grow down from the anterior inner part of the labia majora on each side. Each fold joins above and below the *clitoris.* The joining of the folds above the clitoris forms the *prepuce;* the junction below the clitoris forms the *frenulum.* Each labium minus then extends downward to surround the vagina and join again at the posterior end of the vagina, where it blends into the skin of the labia majora. At this junction, there is a slightly raised ridge of skin, the *fourchette.* After the birth of a baby, the fourchette flattens out. There are no pubic hairs on the labia minora, but there are many sebaceous glands that feel like tiny grains of sand when pressed between the thumb and forefinger.

The large numbers of sebaceous glands on the vulvar skin produce sebum, a mixture of oils, waxes, triglycerides, cholesterol, and cellular debris. Sebum lubricates the skin, and in combination with the secretions from the sweat glands and the vagina forms a waterproofing protective layer that enables the vulvar skin to repel urine, menstrual blood, and bacterial infections. Because of the many sebaceous glands, however, the labia minora, particularly in the area of the clitoris, are frequently the site of sebaceous cysts: painful nodules about the size of a pea in the skin. A vulvar sebaceous cyst usually spontaneously drains and

---

★Everyone knows that a nymphomaniac is a woman with an excessive sex drive. Why is it that hardly anyone knows the same condition in males is satyriasis? Think about it.

disappears within a few days; however, it may become secondarily infected and require treatment or removal.

There are wide variations in the size and shape of the labia minora, and one is generally larger than the other. Sometimes they are completely hidden by the labia majora, or they may be enlarged so that they project forward. Enclosed within the skin of the labia minora are venous sinuses or blood spaces that become engorged with blood during sexual excitement, causing a color change and an increase in the thickness of the labia, sometimes as much as two to three times their diameter.

Vestibule

The vestibule is the area enclosed by the labia minora. Opening into the vestibule are the urethra from the urinary bladder, the vagina, and the two ducts of *Bartholin's glands,* also called the greater vestibular glands. Bartholin's glands produce a few drops of mucus during sexual excitement in the female in order to moisten the vestibule in preparation for intercourse. This amount of secretion is not significant in the lubrication of the vagina. The duct of a Bartholin's gland may become obstructed for no apparent reason, and the gland continues to secrete behind the duct. The result is a large Bartholin's cyst, which usually produces no symptoms, but which occasionally may form an abscess and have to be removed. A gonorrhea infection may sometimes cause a Bartholin's cyst.

Clitoris

The word **clitoris** is from the Greek word for *key,* indicating that the ancient anatomists considered it the key to a woman's sexuality, a perception that had been largely ignored until recently. It is always referred to as the homologue of the penis, that is, similar in embryological origin and structure but not necessarily in function. Some texts describe the clitoris as a *vestigial* homologue of the penis—a vestige being a small, degenerate, or incompletely developed structure. This is a truly erroneous statement except for one thing—

the clitoris is smaller than the penis and is usually more easily felt than seen. It has, however, for its size, a generous blood and nerve supply relatively greater than that of the penis. There are more free nerve endings of sensory reception located on the clitoris than on any other part of the body, and it is, unsurprisingly, the most erotically sensitive part of the genitalia for most females.

The clitoris consists of two *crura,* or roots; a *shaft,* or body; and a *glans.* The two crura arise from the lower borders of the ischiopubic rami and join at the pubic symphysis to form the shaft of the clitoris. Within the shaft are the two *corpora cavernosa,* the "cavernous bodies," consisting of erectile tissue that, when engorged with blood, causes the clitoris to become erect and double in size. At the end of the shaft is the rounded glans, extremely sensitive to the touch.

There are two muscles on each side important in clitoral erection. The *ischiocavernosus* muscles arise from the ischium and insert into the corpora cavernosa, and the *bulbocavernosus* muscles arise from the area around the vestibular bulbs of the labia majora and also insert into the corpora cavernosa of the clitoris. During sexual excitement, these muscles contract and compress the dorsal vein of the clitoris, the only vein that drains the blood from the spaces in the corpora cavernosa. The arterial blood continues to pour in and, having no way to drain out, fills the venous spaces until they become turgid and engorged with blood. This mechanism causes the stiffening and erection of the clitoris (Figure 2–9). That there is more erectile tissue associated with the clitoris than generally described in standard anatomical texts was reported by Australian urologist Helen O'Connell and her colleagues (1998). In investigating the relationship between the urethra and surrounding erectile tissue, the researchers performed dissections on the genital anatomy of 10 adult female cadavers who ranged in age from 22–88 years. When they compared the arrangement and amount of erectile tissue in the urethra and genitalia of the cadavers with current anatomical descriptions, they found that the age of the woman made a difference. That is, there was more erectile tissue associated with the

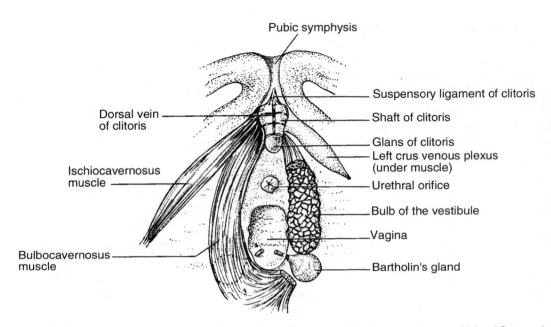

Pubic symphysis

Suspensory ligament of clitoris

Dorsal vein of clitoris

Shaft of clitoris

Glans of clitoris

Left crus venous plexus (under muscle)

Ischiocavernosus muscle

Urethral orifice

Bulb of the vestibule

Vagina

Bulbocavernosus muscle

Bartholin's gland

Figure 2–9 Mechanism of clitoral erection. Tactile stimulation of the clitoris results in an increased blood flow to the erectile tissue (corpora cavernosa) in the shaft of the clitoris. The contraction of the two clitoral muscles (bulbocavernosus and ischiocavernosus) compresses the only vein that drains the corpora cavernosa. The blood, trapped in the erectile spaces of the cavernous bodies, causes their engorgement and thus the enlargement and erection of the clitoris.

clitoris in younger women than is described in modern anatomical texts and diagrams. The workers concluded, although the sample size was small, that dissections upon which modern and older anatomical descriptions of female human urethral and genital anatomy relied were inaccurate because they were likely to have been performed on elderly women in which the erectile tissue had shrunk. The investigators recommended that because the erectile tissue of the vestibular bulbs actually is more related to the clitoris and urethra than to the labia majora, the bulbs of the vestibule should be renamed the bulbs of the clitoris. But in addition to calling attention to the inaccuracy of anatomical textbooks, an important implication of this research led by a female urologist (an uncommon specialty for women until recently) is that when women have operations for bladder problems, hysterectomy, or other surgery in the vicinity of the urethra, there could be potential damage to the erectile

tissues involved in sexual function unless the findings are considered.

The bulbocavernosus muscles compress the vestibular bulbs during sexual excitement, and they become congested and erect as well, contributing to what Masters and Johnson call the "orgasmic platform" (Chapter 6). Like the penis, the clitoris is suspended from the lower border of the pubic arch by a ligament called the *suspensory ligament*. The prepuce, or foreskin, is a little hood over the glans formed by the anterior junction of the labia minora. As in the male, a sebaceous gland secretion is produced under the prepuce and can cause irritation and itching if not washed away.

Urethra

Approximately 2.5 cm below the clitoris, there is a small elevation like a dimple. In its center is the opening of the urethra, called the *external urethral orifice*. The urethra is the passageway for urine from the urinary bladder to the outside. When a catheterization is performed to empty the bladder or to obtain an uncontaminated urine specimen, a flexible tube or catheter is inserted into the external orifice and passed upward into the bladder.

On either side of the midline, just posterior to the external urethral orifice, are the openings from the paraurethral or Skene's glands, the female homologue to the prostate glands in the male. They secrete a small amount of mucus and, along with the secretion of other small mucus-secreting glands in the wall of the urethra, function to keep the opening moist and lubricated for the passage of urine.

When Skene announced his discovery of the glands that bear his name in the 19th century, they had already been described by de Graaf 200 years earlier as the producers of "female semen," the lubricating fluid discharged during sexual stimulation. That in some women these glands may produce a secretion emitted from the urethra during coitus was momentously "rediscovered" in 1982 by Ladas, Whipple, and Perry. The three reported in their instant best-selling book, *The G Spot & Other Recent Discoveries about Human Sexuality,* that the secretion, dubbed the female ejaculate, occurred in response to stimulation of the alleged Grafenberg spot, an approximately 2-inch area on the anterior wall of the vagina near the urinary bladder. Ernst Grafenberg, a German gynecologist, had been, until then, better known for the Grafenberg ring, the first widely used intrauterine device. His 1950 description of a "zone of erogenous feeling located along the anterior vaginal wall" was largely ignored, but the publication of Ladas, Whipple, and Perry's book revived controversial inquiry about the phenomenon during the early 1980s and still surfaces occasionally on talk shows and in newspaper and magazine articles about the "G spot."

There is no convincing evidence that the so-called G spot exists, and whether it has profound and wide-ranging implications for female sexual response remains to be demonstrated. In some women there may be a sensitive area on the anterior vaginal wall that produces pleasurable sensations when it is pressed. Other women who look for the G spot with their fingers may find a place that produces a sensation of having to urinate; it is, after all, close to the bladder. But there are women who are concerned about expelling what seems to be a small gush of urine during intercourse, especially at orgasm. They are not urinating but are probably experiencing a greater discharge from the paraurethral (Skene's) glands and the vulvovaginal (Bartholin's) glands—for them, a normal sexual response.

The female urethra, in contrast to that of a male, is short: only about 4 cm in length when a woman is standing erect. This anatomical difference predisposes a woman to bladder infection much more frequently than a man, whose urethra is 18–20 cm in length. Not only is the external opening exposed to vaginal discharges containing bacteria, but organisms like *Escherichia coli* from the rectum can easily ascend up the short urethra and multiply tremendously within hours, leading to a condition called *cystitis,* or urinary tract infection (UTI). For this reason, women should always wipe from front to back after moving their bowels to avoid transferring the bacteria from the anus to the urethra. For similar reasons, internal tampons inserted into the vagina are preferable to external pads as long as they are changed frequently. Although a tampon can be associated with other health problems, a pad can provide a direct link from the anus and vagina to the urethra, as well as an environment in which microorganisms can thrive.

"Honeymoon cystitis," a term that has lost considerable relevance to current lifestyles, is the name given to the bladder infections that occur within a short time after the initiation of regular intercourse in a woman, particularly after a period of little sexual activity. The proximity of the urethra and the base of the bladder to the anterior vaginal wall can cause those structures to become swollen and irritated as a result of repeated coitus, causing an urge to urinate more frequently. Vigorous thrusting movements of the penis can also be responsible for forcing microorganisms up into the urethral orifice and into the bladder to cause cystitis, which must be treated with an antibiotic. One way of preventing or at least decreasing susceptibility to this cause of bladder infection is to maintain a high fluid intake and to urinate before and after sexual intercourse.

Symptoms of cystitis are burning pain on urination, and an urge to urinate frequently, even immediately after voiding. The urine is cloudy and dark and contains pus cells, red blood cells, and many bacteria. There may be fever, backache, and lower abdominal pain. If the bladder infection is not treated, it can spread to the kidneys and cause a condition called *pyelonephritis,* which is a potentially very serious complication. Additional causes, prevention, and treatment of cystitis and UTI are discussed in Chapter 9.

Hymen

Below the external urethral orifice in the vestibule is the opening to the vagina. Around the vaginal opening there is a small, insignificant membrane with no known function called the **hymen,** after Hymen, the god of marriage in Greek mythology. There are probably few other parts of the female reproductive tract as subject to folklore and misconception as this little membrane. Most people do not even know where it is—they think it is somewhere up in the vagina near the cervix. It is commonly believed that it tears at the first coitus, that copious and visible bleeding occurs, and that the virgin has been "deflowered," defloration being a curious and romantic term for rupture of the hymen. If no bleeding occurs, this is taken as evidence of nonvirginity. Many also believe that the hymen makes it impossible for a virgin to wear tampons during the menstrual period, or that if the attempt is made, this sign of virginity will disappear.

All of this is nonsense. An intact hymen is not proof of virginity; a ruptured hymen is not indicative that sexual intercourse has occurred, and no one, including a doctor, can tell whether or not there has been initial coitus by just looking at the vaginal opening. It is usually possible to determine with accuracy whether or not a woman has had a child but generally impossible to say whether or not she is a virgin. This is because the hymen may be as follows:

- Thin as a spiderweb, or thick and fleshy
- Quite vascular, with a good blood supply, or relatively avascular
- Extremely variable in how much of the vaginal opening is covered
- Sometimes so pliable and flexible that it never ruptures but only stretches, even after childbirth

The hymen very rarely completely occludes the opening to the vagina. This is called an *imperforate* hymen and is usually discovered during adolescence. A girl with an imperforate hymen will menstruate into the vagina month after month, and the discharge will accumulate in the vagina, a condition called hematocolpos. If it is not recognized, menstrual blood may fill the uterus and the fallopian tubes as well. Cutting of the hymen cures the problem, and there is no further difficulty.

Another variation is the septate hymen. If the septum is not too thick and is stretchy enough, intercourse is not hampered. There is usually no problem with insertion of tampons, although there may be some difficulty encountered in removal.

After childbirth, the hymen usually no longer has a continuous rim but remains as isolated remnants with gaps in between. These are referred to as *carunculae hymenales.* The hymen is present throughout life, has no function, and is merely an embryological vestige. Its only significance, if one believes the mythology, is psychological, sociological, or cultural.

Vagina

The **vagina** is a tube that passes upward to the uterus at an approximate 45° angle from the vulva.

The size of the vagina is so variable and so capable of distension that it is difficult to measure its dimensions. This great distensibility enables the vagina to withstand vigorous stresses during intercourse or childbirth. Despite all the stories, a normal vagina can accommodate any size penis with ease. There is no relationship between the size of a woman's vagina and her general body size or shape; the same is true of the size of the penis of a man.

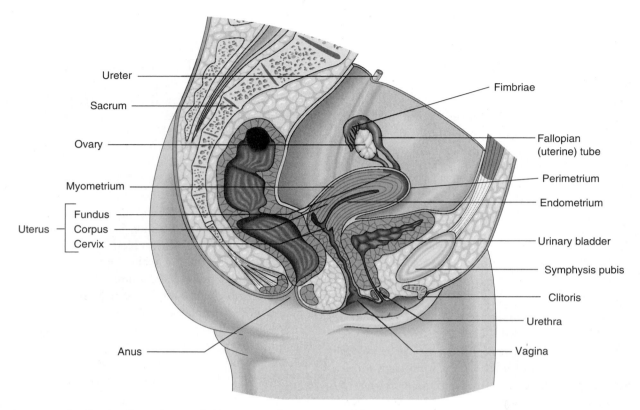

Figure 2–10   Section through reproductive organs showing vaginal fornices.

Actually, the tube of the vagina is only a potential space because its anterior and posterior walls are thrown up into transverse folds that are in close apposition. In a woman who has never had a child, there are many folds and the vaginal walls are firm. After parturition (giving birth), the walls are more or less smoothed out, but they retain their firmness, especially near the opening of the vagina. This is not always true for women who have had many children.

Projecting into the upper part of the vagina is the lower part of the uterus, the conical *cervix.* The circular gutter formed all around the cervix is anatomically divided into the *anterior, posterior,* and *lateral fornices* (Figure 2–10). The walls of the fornices are thin because they consist only of the vaginal wall with the pelvic cavity on the other side. During an internal pelvic examination,

the position and relations of the various pelvic viscera can be palpated and outlined through the fornices. Normally, the posterior fornix is empty, and the body of the uterus can be felt through the anterior fornix; the fallopian tubes and the ovaries, through the lateral fornices.

The posterior fornix extends deeper into the pelvis and is, therefore, larger and longer than the anterior fornix. This anatomical arrangement favors the passage of sperm into the cervix during intercourse because when a woman lies on her back, the opening in the cervix is not only directly exposed to the male ejaculation, but the pool of ejaculated semen collects in the posterior fornix and bathes the cervix, which is resting in it (Figure 2–11). The posterior fornix also takes the brunt of penile thrusting during coitus and thus prevents injury or jarring of the cervix.

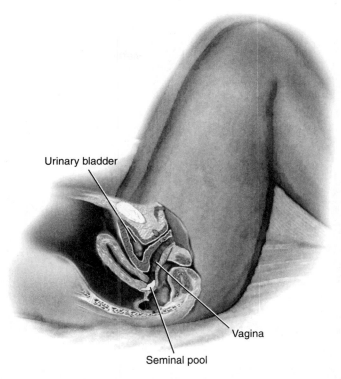

Urinary bladder

Vagina

Seminal pool

Figure 2–11   When a woman is on her back during intercourse, the semen collects in the posterior fornix, providing sperm with easy access to the cervical opening.

Only a thin partition of vaginal wall separates the posterior fornix from the lining *(peritoneum)* of the pelvic cavity, which dips down to form the *pouch of Douglas,* or the rectouterine pouch. The posterior fornix, therefore, forms the route for several kinds of diagnostic and surgical procedures. In *culdocentesis,* a needle is inserted into the pouch of Douglas to determine the nature of any fluid that might be present—blood, pus, excess tissue fluid. *Colpotomy* is surgical incision through the posterior fornix into the peritoneum of the pelvic cavity. Through this opening, the pelvic viscera can be visually explored by means of a *culdoscope,* which is a tube equipped with optical devices and light—a sort of internal microscope.

The Vaginal Lining.   The lining of the vagina is called the vaginal epithelium and consists of layers (as many as 40) of cells resting on connective tissue, containing blood vessels and nerves. This epithelium is like skin but has no hair follicles, sweat glands, or sebaceous glands to weaken it or provide a passageway for entrance of microorganisms. It is, therefore, a very tough, resistant protective lining (Table 2–2). The deeper basal layers of the cells are closer to the blood vessels in the connective tissue underneath and proliferate faster, pushing up to replace the superficial layers that are sloughed off. Estrogen, the female sex hormone, stimulates the growth of the cells. Before puberty and after menopause when there is little estrogen present, the vaginal epithelium is thin and made

TABLE 2–2 Changes in the Vaginal Epithelium with Age

	Newborn Child	One Month Old	Puberty	Sexually Mature Childbearing Years	Post-menopause
Amount of estrogen present (causes changes in)	Much estrogen from placenta	None	Begins to appear	High levels	Relatively very low levels
Appearance of epithelium	Similar to mature	Very thin	Develops thickness	Thick, 20–40 layers	Thinner, may be atrophied
Amount of glycogen in cells (causes)	Moderate	None	Goes from none to much	Much	Little or none
Acidity of vaginal secretions (when acted upon by)	Acid, pH 4–5	Alkaline, pH 7	Becomes acid	Acid pH 4–5	Neutral, may be alkaline
Type of bacteria present	Sterile but Döderlein's bacilli present after 12 hours, from mother	Very sparse, some cocci	Goes from sparse varied to Döderlein's bacilli	Döderlein's bacilli and other microorganisms	Various bacteria

up almost entirely of basal cells. When the ovaries are actively producing estrogen during the reproductive years, a smear of cellular material taken from the thick vaginal epithelium will show large numbers of sloughed-off cells, and it is possible to recognize phases of the menstrual cycle by the shape and staining qualities of these cells. An index of estrogenic activity can, therefore, be determined by the relative numbers of basal, intermediate, or superficial cells present in a stained smear of the vaginal lining. The appearance of cells of the vaginal lining is also utilized in tests for cancer detection (Pap test, Schiller test), to be described later.

Vaginal Discharge.   The contents of the vagina after puberty and before menopause are normally quite acid, with a pH of approximately 3.5–5.5 (pH is a measure of the acidity or alkalinity of a solution on a scale of 1–14. The lower numbers indicate acidity, the higher numbers, alkalinity, and 7 is neutral). The mechanism for the production and maintenance of this acidity is that the estrogen produced by functioning ovaries during sexual maturity causes rapid proliferation of the basal cells of the vaginal epithelium. These actively growing cells accumulate glycogen granules, the stored form of glucose, in their cytoplasm. Certain bacteria called Döderlein's bacilli (after Albert Döderlein, a German obstetrician) that are normal residents of the vagina are *lactobacilli;* that is, they have the ability to break down the glycogen to form lactic acid. The presence of the lactic acid is responsible for the lowered pH of the vaginal contents.

The normal vaginal discharge is a clear acid material consisting of fluid arising from the capillaries in the vaginal walls with lesser amounts contributed from the cervical glands, the uterine cavity, and the fallopian tubes. In the fluid are mucus; superficial sloughed-off cells; Döderlein's bacilli; other microorganisms (streptococci, staphylococci, yeasts); and various fat, protein, and carbohydrate compounds. The acid discharge combined with the toughness of the thick epithelium protects the vagina from infection by harmful bacteria and makes the vagina much more vulnerable to infec-

tion before puberty and after menopause. Döderlein's bacilli are absolutely essential to normal vaginal physiology. If they are disturbed or destroyed by chemical contraceptives, antibiotics, or excess douching, vaginal infections will occur more easily.

Douching.   Douching is a procedure of vaginal irrigation in which fluid in a bag is permitted to run through a tube, entering the vagina under slight pressure and ballooning it out slightly. As the fluid runs out or is expelled through muscular action, the vaginal contents are washed out. Douching to prevent pregnancy after intercourse is totally ineffective because it has been determined that sperm can be recovered from the uterus within seconds after being deposited in the vagina—and no woman can get the douche bag apparatus set up and going that fast.

Some women like to douche after their menstrual period because it makes them feel clean. As long as the bag is not suspended too high so that the fluid enters the vagina at too great a pressure, there is no harm in occasional douching for general hygiene. Habitual and vigorous douching may force fluid, and a possible infection, upward into the uterus and into the fallopian tubes. Douching is seldom essential for normal health because the vagina is self-cleansing through the process of normal discharge. But if sexual intercourse is frequent, and gels, foams, or creams are used for contraception, there may be vaginal leakage, which can feel unpleasantly wet. The spermicidal gel used with a diaphragm nightly may have to be douched out weekly, for example. To douche more than every 4 or 5 days is excessive, however, and it will destroy the normal physiology of the vagina.

For a douching medium, plain warm water or water with 1 tablespoon of vinegar (or bicarbonate of soda) to a quart is certainly as effective as the commercial solutions and certainly less expensive. Perfumed, colored, and flavored solutions are not only a waste of money but could cause an allergic reaction. The manufacturers of such products prey on a woman's concern, reinforced by massive advertising campaigns, that natural genital odor is offensive, and that to feel "fresh and confident" one must use perfumed and deodorizing douches, suppositories, or feminine hygiene sprays.

There is a specific odor produced by the healthy female genitalia that comes from the secretions of the sebaceous and apocrine sweat glands of the vulva, the secretions of Bartholin's and Skene's (urethral) glands, and from the vaginal discharge. It is not an unpleasant odor and is in no way unclean, unless it has been permitted to remain on the skin too long or there is an infection in the vagina causing an abnormal discharge. Feminine hygiene deodorant products, meant to be sprayed on the external vaginal area, are particularly unnecessary and should not be used. If vaginal infection is the source of a perceived malodorous condition, the spray cannot possibly get to the source of the odor and may only cover it up and delay treatment. In some women, allergic sensitivity to the sprays may result in a very painful reaction to their use. Some of the early versions of such products were taken off the market and others were required to include labels with printed warnings about their use. Currently, products are likely to be advertised as hypoallergenic, nonirritating, and completely safe, which may or may not be true for an individual woman. The best "feminine wash" or "intimate cleanser" is neutral, nonperfumed soap and water.

Europeans, particularly in France and Italy, have always been more advanced than Americans in sensible genital hygiene for both men and women. There is, in most home and hotel bathrooms, a bidet. The bidet, which most Americans think is a funny-looking toilet (or perhaps a footbath), is a porcelain basin that one straddles so that a stream of warm water flows over genital and perineal areas after urination or bowel movement. This provides an excellent and convenient method of cleansing the small folds and crevices of the genitalia.

Vaginal Odor. Chemical compounds secreted by an organism into the environment to evoke various developmental, behavioral, or reproductive responses in another member of the same species are called *pheromones.* Sex attractant pheromones have been studied extensively in insects, and synthetic pheromones or their analogues are increasingly being used in biological (rather than pesticide) control of insect pests. Nonhuman mammals have glands that produce a variety of secretions, some odor free and some distinctly malodorous, and the importance of such pheromones in establishing territoriality or in affecting reproductive behavior is well known. Ask anyone with a male dog near an unspayed female in heat. But while the evidence for the existence of sex attractant pheromones in nonprimates is clear-cut, the case for such a phenomenon operating in primates such as rhesus monkeys and humans is controversial and has been studied by scientists for decades. It has been determined that both human women and female monkeys have the same kind of organic acids (short-chain carbon aliphatic acids, such as lactic, butyric, pentanoic, and hexanoic) present in their vaginal secretions and that levels of these acids change during the menstrual cycle. Although the fluctuation of these vaginal acids is reportedly dependent upon fluctuating ovarian hormone levels in the monkeys, any attempts to correlate changing acid levels with hormonal changes in women have, thus far, been unsuccessful. The possibility that vaginal acids may act as sex attractant pheromones in humans was pursued by some workers (Doty, Ford, & Preti, 1975; Keith et al., 1975). Their investigations, although based on small sample sizes, suggested that changes in vaginal odor could be related to the day of the menstrual cycle, with qualities of mildness and pleasantness being perceived around the time of ovulation and objectional odors observed just prior and after menstruation. The evidence for vaginal odors actually having an influence on human sexual behavior was slim, and that line of research appears to have been abandoned. Further intriguing bits of information on "human pheromones" were provided by studies on "bad breath." Although most normal bad breath is related to diet, bad breath is often noted during menstruation and pregnancy. But Tonzetich and colleagues in 1978 studied the volatile sulfur compounds in the mouth ("bad breath") throughout the menstrual cycle in five subjects and determined that bad breath not only increased during menstruation but also increased fourfold near ovulation. These researchers speculated that increases in the compounds involved in mouth odor could be related to estrogen levels. The paradox of why nature would provide for "good" smells in the vagina and "bad" smells in the mouth at ovulation, the time most conducive to conception, further illustrates how little is known of the role, or even the very existence, of human response to body odors. There have been suggestions that if chemical (pheromonal) communication exists in humans, it may not even involve conscious odor perception but instead may operate via neural pathways that are separate from main olfactory nerves. Many other species have an accessory olfactory system in the nose called the vomeronasal organ with its own neural connections to the brain, which processes the pheromone and directs a response. In the Asian elephant, for example, an identified pheromone chemical in the urine of female elephants who are about to ovulate is detected through the vomernasal organ of the male elephant and tells him that the female is ready to mate. This chemical compound is identical to the sex attractant in more than a hundred species of insects. Some pheromone researchers have postulated the existence of a residual vomeronasal organ in humans that could elicit reproductive physiological or behavioral responses similar to that in other species, but others find such reports highly speculative and controversial (Ben-Ari, 1998).

Laypersons have probably always been aware of the individuality of what has been termed the *olfactory signature* of a person. Even with our relatively underdeveloped olfactory systems, we recognize that different people smell different. Although the existence of human pheromones acting as chemical communicators is unproven, the erotic potential of odor is well known to the manufacturers and advertisers of perfumes and incense. So is the word *pheromone*. An expensive women's fragrance produced in the United States has been named "Pheromone" and sells very well. One enterprising British firm went further in putting sex appeal in a gold-plated bottle by marketing an even more costly scent for men and women that contains a synthetic pheromone. Just what the "synthetic" pheromone is derived from is not disclosed. Perhaps users, who might get amorous advances from insects or dogs, should be cautious.

Musk oil-based scents are very popular with both men and women, and to many people musk smells very much like healthy body odor. Although armpit aroma generally is thought to produce negative behavioral responses, the commercial possibilities have not been ignored. The same product that claims to "mask" or eliminate body odor actually mimics natural body odor, such as musk-scented products. Investigation continues regarding human pheromones, whether they exist, their chemical nature, how they act, and the role of human odors and nonodors in human behavior. Perhaps the "body chemistry" often referred to in sexual attraction is real and genetically determined. See "Menstrual Synchrony" in Chapter 3 for research indicating that women produce compounds that have the ability to affect the menstrual cycles of other women.

Vaginal Lubrication. There is always a certain amount of lubrication of the vagina from vaginal discharge, but sexual stimulation produces considerable wetness, which is usually noticeable. Since the vaginal epithelium has neither sweat glands nor sebaceous glands, where does this moisture come from? Before the observations of Masters and Johnson, it was always incorrectly assumed that Bartholin's glands and cervical mucus from the cervical glands produced the vaginal lubrication. Now it is believed that the blood vessels of the wall of the vagina actually play the essential role. The wall of the vagina is supplied with arterial blood by four branches of the internal iliac artery: the vaginal, uterine, internal pudendal, and middle rectal arteries. They branch into capillary networks, and the blood then drains from the vagina through veins that are large, thin walled, and form an interweaving plexus at the sides of the vagina. This venous plexus ultimately drains through the vaginal veins into the internal iliac vein. Under the conditions of sexual stimulation, the veins around the vagina become engorged with blood. The resulting congestion of blood in the venous plexus results in pressure that forces a mucoid kind of liquid, or *transudate,* to pass from the veins through the epithelium of the vagina. This liquid at first forms individual droplets and then, as the droplets coalesce, forms a coating for the entire vagina. Because this appeared to sex researchers William Masters and Virginia Johnson as similar to drops of perspiration beading on a forehead, they called this the "sweating phenomenon" of the vagina. This occurs very early in the sexual response of the female and provides sufficient lubrication for intercourse. The vaginal response tends to be prevented when certain kinds of vaginal infections are present, and some women who are on the pill may also find that their ability to lubricate is diminished. Without lubrication, of course, penetration during coitus may be very uncomfortable.

Nerves of the Vagina. The upper two-thirds of the vagina is supplied almost entirely by nerve fibers from the autonomic nervous system, which means that they control the constriction and dilation of blood vessels in the walls of the vagina. There are very few sensory receptors for touch or pain located in the vagina. Sensations of awareness or pressure within the vagina are mainly received by nerve receptors in the rectum or urinary bladder and not in the vagina itself. The upper part of the vagina is hence relatively insensitive. The lower third of the vagina does contain some touch and pain receptors from the pudendal nerve, but such innervation is scanty. In contrast, the vulva has a rich supply of fibers from the pudendal nerve and is very sensitive. If the internal wall of the vagina is inflamed or infected (vaginitis), although the site of the irritation is inside, the itching or pain is referred to the outside on the vulva because of the way that the nerves are distributed. If the area around the vaginal opening itches and burns and an abnormal discharge is present, it very likely means that undesirable organisms are inhabiting the vagina.

*U*TERUS

From the medical records that have remained intact, it is evident that the uterus, a hollow, muscular organ in which a fetus develops, more than all the female reproductive organs, was the most subject to fanciful and erroneous description by ancient physicians. Evidently unwilling or unable to credit women for owning an organ in which the fetus developed, early accounts described the uterus as an independent animal capable of independent activity. A Greek physician in the fourteenth century A.D. wrote:

> *In the middle of the flanks of women lies the womb, a female viscus, closely resembling an animal, for it is moved of itself hither and thither in the flanks . . . and in a word, is altogether erratic. It delights also in fragrant smells and advances toward them, and it has an aversion to fetid smells and flees from them; and on the whole the womb is like an animal within an animal.★*

Centuries earlier, Hippocrates had written that the uterus went wild unless it was often fed with male semen. Even by the 14th century, the descriptions of the uterus were equally inaccurate but perhaps more ingenious. The prevailing opinion of female anatomy was still that it was a poor second to the obviously superior architecture of the male, and a French surgeon compared the uterus to a male organ turned inside out! "It has in its upper part two arms with the testicles . . . like the scrotum," he wrote, and went on to compare the body of the uterus, with a canal in it, to the shaft of the penis with the urethra running through it.

It is not surprising that extravagant errors were made in explaining the "mysteries of the womb"—the uterus is a very unique organ. Every month it prepares to receive a fertilized ovum; if it does not, it sheds its lining and starts all over again. If it does receive a fertilized ovum, it shelters it, nourishes, and protects it dur-

---

★From *A Pictorial History of Gynecology and Obstetrics,* by H. Speert, 1973, Philadelphia: F. A. Davis Co.

ing its development for 9 months, and then expels it at the end of pregnancy. The actual mechanism for doing all this is still unknown. The uterus has the ability to grow from a weight of about 2 oz when nonpregnant, to 2 lb, its weight immediately after delivery, and then shrink back to its original size by 6 weeks after delivery.

Hollow and muscular, the uterus has an upper expanded portion called the body or *fundus* and a lower constricted part called the neck or *cervix*. The cervix projects down into the vagina and has an opening, the *external os*. As with all other parts of the reproductive tract, there is considerable variation in the size of the normal, nonpregnant uterus, but on average it is 3 in. long, 2 in. wide at the fundus, 1 in. thick at its thickest part, and the wall of the uterus is ½ in. thick. The exact size of the uterus can be measured only with an instrument called a uterine sound, which is inserted through the external os. Clinical impressions of size derived from pelvic examination are very deceptive, making physicians' remarks such as "you have an infantile uterus" not only unnecessarily disturbing but usually erroneous.

The walls of the uterus are solid and made of involuntary smooth muscle. They enclose a cavity that is lined with epithelium called the *endometrium,* which undergoes cyclic changes during menstruation and forms the site for implantation of the fertilized egg if pregnancy occurs.

Positions of the Uterus

The normal uterus is a very mobile organ, and its position between the rectum and the bladder varies, depending on posture, how full the bladder or the rectum is, and how many children have been borne. As seen in Figure 2–12, the body of the uterus is typically inclined forward: When the urinary bladder is distended, the backward movement of the uterus is called *retroversion;* when the rectum is distended, the forward movement of the body of the uterus is called *anteversion.* Further and marked anteversion with relation to the cervix is called acute flexion; marked retroversion

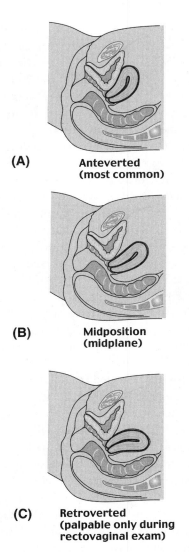

(A)   **Anteverted (most common)**

(B)   **Midposition (midplane)**

(C)   **Retroverted (palpable only during rectovaginal exam)**

Figure 2–12 The normal uterus can vary in position. (A) Uterus is anteverted. (B) Uterus in midposition. (C) Uterus retroverted.

is called *retroflexion.* The uterus is normally anteverted and anteflexed. It may also be retroverted and retroflexed and still be normal; a "tipped" uterus is of no clinical significance and results in no symptoms. Backache, constipation, menstrual cramps—none of these can be related to retroversion or retroflexion.

During the 19th century, gynecologists collected a great deal of money for inserting vaginal pessaries, which are devices used to correct retrodeviations of the uterus. During the early part of the 20th century, there was much unnecessary surgery performed to "correct" the position of the uterus to relieve the symptoms ascribed to its nontypical but perfectly normal position. Of course, it is important for the size, shape, and position of the uterus to be known if any procedure like an abortion or a D and C is to be performed (D and C: *dilatation*, or enlargement of the cervical opening with dilators, to permit *curettage*, or scraping of the uterine lining with an instrument called a curette).★ Otherwise, an instrument inserted into a markedly anteflexed or retroflexed uterus may perforate the wall.

The lower part of the uterus, the cervix, projects into the vagina and is circumferentially attached to it, thus dividing the uterus into an upper, or supravaginal part, and a lower, or vaginal portion. The vaginal part of the cervix is called the *portio vaginalis.* In an adult woman who has not delivered any children (nullipara), the cervix comprises approximately one-half the length of the uterus; in a woman who has given birth to at least one child (primipara; more than one child, multipara), it may be only one-third the length of the uterus. In its typical position in most women, the cervix is directed downward and backward, with its long axis making an angle of between 80° and 120° in relation to the forward-inclined body of the uterus. This position is supported and maintained by fibrous muscular bands called ligaments, described later.

External Os

The opening of the cervix into the vagina is the *external os.* The opening into the uterine cavity is the *internal os.* The canal between the external and the internal

★Dilation and dilatation are synonymous; the dilation of the cervical opening is customarily referred to as dilatation.

os is the *endocervical canal,* lined with the endocervical epithelium. It contains many mucus-secreting glands and is approximately 1 in. long.

There is a very visible difference between the nulliparous os and the multiparous one. Before childbirth, the external os is a little round dimple, approximately 3 ml in diameter. It is sometimes called the *os tincae,* or "mouth of a small fish." This tiny canal dilates during labor and delivery to accommodate the passage of the head and body of a full-term infant; after parturition, it never again returns to its previous shape but becomes a transverse slit with irregular margins. Enlarging the cervical opening with dilators to perform an abortion or a D and C has the same effect. Note that although it is not possible to determine whether or not a woman is a virgin, an examiner can tell whether she has had a baby or an abortion. No matter how small the trauma, very minute lacerations and abrasions occur that change the appearance of the os (Figure 2–13).

Cervix

The **cervix** is predominantly composed of fibrous connective tissue with many smooth muscle fibers. It is firm to the touch except after approximately 6 weeks of pregnancy, when it softens, owing to the increased blood supply to the uterus and cervix. The feel of the nonpregnant cervix has been compared to the feel of the tip of the nose, or to the glans of the erect penis.

The epithelium on the surface of the vaginal aspect of the cervix is pale pink, whereas the epithelium of the endocervical canal leading into the uterus from the external os is redder in color. Because of this color difference, inflammations (cervicitis), extensions of the endocervical epithelium onto the vaginal aspect of the cervix (erosions), benign polyps, or cysts are highly visible on the surface of the portio vaginalis, even though these conditions originate on the mucous membrane of the endocervical canal. The glands on the endocervical canal are highly branched and burrow deeply into the recesses and folds of the cervical mucosa. Once organisms get into this desirable envi-

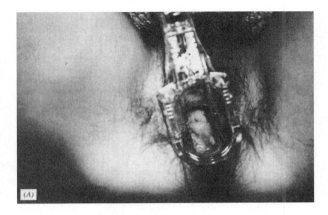

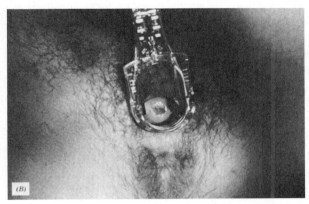

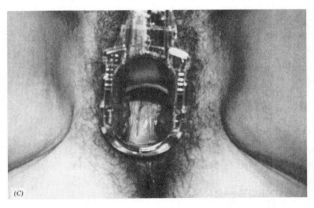

Figure 2–13 Appearance of the cervix and the external os. (A) Nulliparous os. (B) Parous os. (C) Appearance of the vaginal vault after the cervix has been removed in conjunction with a hysterectomy performed through the vagina. The vertical line represents the location of the suturing of the vaginal mucosa.

ronment, they remain hidden and can stubbornly resist most attempts to get rid of them. This is why infections of the cervix tend to become chronic.

Cervical Mucus. The endocervical glands secrete cervical mucus, which is composed mostly of water; electrolytes like sodium and potassium ions dissolved in the water; blood proteins, including immunoglobulins; and mucins, a complex group of glycoproteins. Glycoproteins are compounds made up of carbohydrates and proteins, and in cervical mucus they have been found to contain an extremely high percentage of carbohydrates. During the menstrual cycle, the physical properties of the cervical mucus change as a result of the differing levels of circulating hormones. Before and near the time of ovulation, the mucus is dilute, secreted in greatest quantity, and when it is spread out on a slide it will undergo "ferning" or "arborization"; that is, it forms a distinct pattern as it dries and looks like ferns or tree branches. After ovulation, the mucus becomes much thicker, reaches a gel state, and no longer demonstrates ferning. These changes form the basis for tests of both hormonal activity and determination of the time of ovulation.

The thinner, more fluid cervical secretion enhances sperm migration up to the uterine cavity; the gel-like mucin in the latter half of the menstrual cycle acts as a barrier to sperm motility. It is possible that the cervical mucus may function as a bacteriocide to protect the upper reproductive tract from invasion by harmful bacteria. It has also been suggested that it may form a mechanical protection at the junction of the external os and the endocervical canal against the development of cancer.

$\mathcal{O}$VIDUCTS OR FALLOPIAN TUBES

The **oviducts** or **fallopian tubes** and the ovaries are frequently referred to as the *adnexa* because they are adjacent or next to the uterus. The fallopian tubes are named after the 16th-century anatomist Gabrielle Fallopius, who thought they resembled tubas or curved trumpets and believed they released noxious fumes from the uterus. More ancient anatomists thought the oviduct looked like a straight trumpet, and they called it the *salpinx* (Greek for tube). That prefix appears in the words describing conditions of the oviducts, such as *salpingitis,* or inflammation of the oviducts, or *salpingectomy,* removal of a tube, among other salpingo-type procedures.

The fallopian tube is anatomically divided into four sections:

1. The *interstitial* or uterine portion: very short, very narrow in diameter, and lying completely within the muscle of the uterus
2. The *isthmus:* the straight part with a thick muscular wall and a narrow lumen (passageway); the section that is the usual site of a tubal ligation, a surgical procedure that prevents the sperm from meeting the ovum by cutting or ligating the oviduct
3. The *ampulla:* occupying about one-half the entire length of the tube, thin walled, with a highly folded lining
4. The *infundibulum:* nearest the ovary, a trumpet-shaped expansion with finger-like projects called fimbriae that wave back and forth through muscular action to attract the ovum into the opening, or *ostium;* one fimbria is longer, closer to the ovary, and is called the ovarian fimbria (Figure 2–14)

The walls of the tubes contain many blood vessels and much longitudinally and circularly arranged smooth muscle. The lining of the tubes is thrown up into folds that almost fill the lumen, but the number of the folds varies with each segment and is most extensive in the infundibulum. The epithelium of the lining consists of those cells that secrete a nutrient fluid to provide an environment necessary for movement, fertilization, and sustenance of the ovum, and other cells that bear cilia, little hairlike processes that beat toward the uterus to create a current to help the egg progress into the uterine cavity. The transport of the egg into the uterus is mainly accomplished by contraction of the circular and longitudinal muscle that creates peristaltic waves, which move the ovum along. This muscular activity is influenced by hormones and is greatest at the time of ovulation.

When an ovum is released from the ovary, it is not in direct contact with the end of the fallopian tube, and the exact mechanisms that keep the egg from falling into the pelvic cavity and getting lost are still not completely known. Culdoscopic observations at the time of ovulation have revealed that the fimbriae are brought closer to the ovary to curve around it by contraction of muscle fibers in the connective tissue, which covers and suspends the fallopian tubes from the abdominal wall. It has also been suggested that muscular contractions in the walls of the fimbriae, coupled with suction action from the ciliary movement of their lining cells, actually actively engulf the ovum, swallowing it up as though the end of the tube were a vacuum cleaner hose.

It is possible that scar tissue resulting from previous pelvic surgery or fallopian tube infection can interfere with the mechanism of picking up the ovum at the time of ovulation, and thereby cause infertility. On the other hand, there are cases on record in which women had a tube removed (salpingectomy) on one side, an ovary removed (ovariectomy) on the other side, and still had several children. Somehow these ova crossed over the uterus to enter the ostium of the opposite side.

Once in the infundibulum of the tube, the egg is rapidly transported through the ampulla until it reaches the ampullary-isthmus junction, where its transport is delayed for about 30 hours. This restraint of movement is referred to as the "tube-locking" mechanism, or the "isthmic block," and if sperm are present, fertilization occurs here. If conception occurs, the new embryo divides and develops, nurtured and sustained by the secretions of the tubal lining, and passes fairly rapidly through the isthmus and interstitial portion into the uterine cavity. No fewer than 45 nor more than 80 hours elapse between the time of ovula-

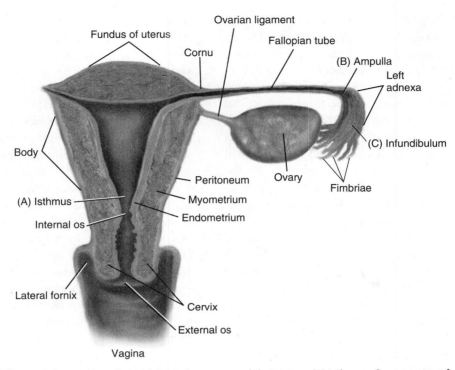

Figure 2–14 The fallopian tube and its relationship to the ovary and the uterus. (A) Isthmus. One-quarter of ectopic pregnancies occur in this area. The thick muscular wall permits little distension, and early rupture is likely. (B) Ampulla. More than half of ectopic pregnancies implant in this portion of the tube, which is more distensible. The pregnancy is further advanced before rupture. (C) Infundibulum. Fewer than 10% of tubal pregnancies occur here or in the fimbriated end.

tion and the ovum's entry into the uterus. Two to three more days pass before the timing is optimal for the joining of the embryo and the uterine lining, the process called implantation.

If the egg is not fertilized, it disintegrates, and its remains are cleaned up by those ubiquitous scavenger cells of the body, the macrophages.

Ectopic Pregnancy

After the conceptus (the collective name for the egg and all its derivatives from the time of fertilization until birth of the baby) arrives into the uterine cavity, it normally implants in the upper part of the cavity. If, for some reason, it fails to get to that destination, it may implant in some other place, like the fallo-

pian tube, the ovary, the cervix, or (rarely) even the abdominal cavity. Such ectopic, or out-of-place, pregnancies are a major public health problem, and their incidence has been increasing dramatically. One in 100 pregnancies is reported to be an ectopic pregnancy, and 98% occur in the fallopian tubes (a tubal pregnancy). The tubes are not distensible enough to permit adequate development of the embryo and subsequent increase in size, particularly the closer the tubal implantation is to the uterus. The embryo, therefore, must always be removed surgically before the tube bursts, which can cause severe hemorrhage and infection in the abdominal cavity. Difficulty and delay in diagnosis and treatment have made ectopic pregnancy the major cause of death during the first 3 months of pregnancy.

Symptoms of an Ectopic Pregnancy.   Unfortunately, the early diagnosis of tubal pregnancy is difficult because the early symptoms of an ectopic pregnancy are no different from the symptoms of a normal uterine pregnancy—a missed period, slight uterine enlargement, and softening of the cervix. If the tubal implantation is situated so that fetal tissue is in contact with maternal blood vessels, the hormone tested in pregnancy tests will appear in maternal blood and will yield a positive result. It is possible, however, for the fetal tissue to become separated from the tubal wall, and then a pregnancy test will prove negative, which of course does not exclude the possibility of ectopic pregnancy. A tender and distended tubal mass, palpable on pelvic examination, is a classic symptom, but it is not always detectable. The signs and symptoms of a tubal implantation vary greatly; differentiating it from threatened miscarriage, urinary tract infection, appendicitis, salpingitis, or an ovarian cyst is sometimes very difficult.

Lower abdominal or pelvic pain, with or without vaginal bleeding, is one of the most common symptoms. When there is bleeding or spotting accompanied by the sudden onset of pain after one period has been missed—corresponding to 6–8 weeks of gestation—it certainly warrants investigation. Pain and bleeding may be an indication that the tube has ruptured and that there is hemorrhage into the uterus and body cavity. The pain may be increased when a Valsalva maneuver (increasing abdominal and thoracic pressure by a forced expiration against a closed glottis) is performed. If the internal bleeding irritates the peritoneal lining of the body cavity, the pain may be referred to the shoulder.

Special means for diagnosis, such as laparoscopy, ultrasonic imaging, and immunoassay pregnancy tests, have made earlier determination possible, but it could take all three tests to diagnose a questionable ectopic pregnancy. Ultrasound usually cannot determine whether implantation has occurred in the fallopian tube; it can, however, rule out a tubal pregnancy if a clearly defined gestational sac or even more specifically, a fetal beating heart is seen in the uterus. If a highly sensitive pregnancy test, such as the human chorionic gonadotropin beta-subunit immunoassay, is positive for pregnancy, and there is no uterine pregnancy visible with ultrasonography, laparoscopic examination to permit visualization of the internal organs can make it possible to diagnose ectopic pregnancy before rupture occurs. One other marker is the serum progesterone level, which is considerably lower in an ectopic extrauterine pregnancy than in a normal intrauterine pregnancy. A progesterone level less than 5 nanograms/ml is suggestive of an ectopic pregnancy.

An ectopic pregnancy must always be terminated because there is no way for the embryo to develop to full term without rupturing the tube. In very rare instances, a fertilized ovum escapes through the ostium of the fimbriated end of the tube, implanting itself and developing in the abdominal cavity. Some of these pregnancies have actually been successful, and a nearly full-term baby can be delivered by an abdominal incision. Even more rarely, a fertilized ovum implants itself directly on the surface within the abdominal cavity, without ever having entered the tube.

If the isthmus of the tube is the site of the implantation, however, an early rupture is more likely to take place because here the thick muscle of the tubal wall permits little distension. In the infundibular part of the fallopian tube or in the ampulla portion, it is possible for the pregnancy to continue longer, but it always ultimately terminates in rupture, usually into the pelvic cavity.

Causes of Ectopic Pregnancy.   The cause of many ectopic pregnancies is unknown, although endocrine dysfunction has been suggested. In some instances, there are conditions in or around the fallopian tube that prevent the fertilized ovum from getting to the uterine cavity. Thus, a tubal implantation results.

One such condition can occur when a gonorrhea or chlamydia infection that has spread to the fallopian tubes causes a further narrowing, through scar-tissue formation, of the already-narrow lumen. The tiny opening may permit the sperm to get up to the egg, but the fertilized developing egg, larger than a sperm, may not be able to descend to the uterus, and implants in the tube. Actually, it is more likely that infection of the upper reproductive tract results in infertility because the destructive changes in the lining of the oviducts usually do not permit the passage of sperm at all.

Another cause of ectopic pregnancy may be related to the presence of an intrauterine device (IUD) that has been placed in the uterus for purposes of contraception. It has been observed that tubal pregnancy occurs more often in women with IUDs, and it may result from an alteration in tubal motility, causing a delay in the descent of the conceptus, which then goes ahead and implants in the tube. At any rate, since the function of an IUD is not to prevent the sperm from getting to the egg, but somehow to prevent uterine implantation, any woman with a previous history of sexually transmitted disease (and a possibly narrowed tube) should never have an IUD inserted. It places her in double jeopardy for the possibility of an ectopic pregnancy.

Tubal pregnancy has also been associated with a history of tubal surgery, including sterilization by tubal ligation ("tying the tubes"). The incidence is rare, however, and may be related to the method of tubal occlusion used. Other factors that have been suggested as increasing the risk of ectopic pregnancy include tubal ligation reversal, previous pelvic surgery, ovulation-inducing drugs, and smoking.

It is entirely possible and probable that many tubal pregnancies, like many uterine pregnancies, spontaneously regress or abort at a very early stage, and the woman may never suspect she was pregnant at all.

Treatment of Ectopic Pregnancy. Before 1975, nearly 80% of ectopics ruptured before diagnosis. As a result of the newer diagnostic techniques, currently fewer than 30% rupture before they are recognized, despite the increased incidence of tubal pregnancy. Diagnosed, unruptured ectopic pregnancy allows the surgical procedure of salpingostomy (making an incision in the tube and removing its contents) rather than the former salpingectomy (removal of the entire tube), frequently accompanied by oophorectomy (removal of the ovary on the affected side). Such conservative treatment permits preservation of the fallopian tube for future fertility. An alternative to a major surgical incision through the abdominal wall (laparotomy) is the removal of a small ectopic pregnancy using a laparascope, an internal telescope for viewing the pelvic organs. With laparoscopy, a small incision is made just under the umbilicus. The tubal incision and removal of the contents may be accomplished by electrocautery, scissors, and/or laser surgery. Laparoscopic surgery strikingly decreases hospitalization and recuperation time but should be performed only by gynecologists who have done it many times.

Nonsurgical medical management of tubal pregnancy usually consists of intramuscular injection of methotrexate, a folic acid analogue that prevents synthesis of DNA. The low doses of methotrexate, which can be given only if rupture has not occurred, cause few side effects and have a greater potential for maintaining future fertility. After a single dose, the woman is usually monitored on an outpatient basis. The success rate is said to be 90%–95%.

Despite attempts to preserve the tube, women who have had an ectopic pregnancy have a 12% incidence of recurrence, and 40% are unable to conceive again. Of the 60% who do become pregnant, approximately 15%–20% will miscarry (DeCherney, 1990).

Peritonitis: More Likely in Women

The body cavity is not a cavity at all but is a potential space that exists between the abdominopelvic viscera, which are covered by a membrane called the *visceral peritoneum,* and the body wall, lined by a continuation of that same membrane, which is reflected backward and called the *parietal peritoneum.* When bacteria like gonococci, staphylococci, and streptococci gain access to that space and attack the peritoneum, the resulting inflammation and infection is called *peritonitis,* and it can be life threatening. While one may think that all body openings lead into the body cavity, they actually do not. The mouth opening leads into the long tube of the digestive tract and ultimately exits at the other end in the anus; the urethral opening at the tip of the penis in males permits exit of spermatozoa from the testis and urine from the urinary bladder. In females, the urethral opening is for the passage of urine only and leads to the bladder. The only way, in both males and females, that harmful organisms can get into the body cavity is through an opening in the body wall by surgery, by accidental perforation, by rupture of an organ (like a ruptured appendix), or through the bloodstream (blood poisoning). In females, however, there *is* another route, which results in a unique anatomical disadvantage. Because the end of the fallopian tube at the ostium opens directly into the pelvic or body cavity, the outside of the body, by way of the vaginal opening, is in contact with the inside of the body cavity via the fallopian tube.

Women, therefore, are much more subject to pelvic peritonitis than men. Fortunately, the acidity of the vaginal secretions and the cervical mucus act as a bacteriocide for most harmful organisms, with the exception of the gonococci of gonorrhea. But whenever the cervix is dilated for procedures such as an abortion, a D and C, a uterine biopsy (a small bit of tissue is taken for examination), or the insertion of an IUD, the possibility of peritonitis exists unless sterile techniques are very carefully observed.

*O*VARIES

The ovaries are two glands in the pelvic cavity that produce ova and sex hormones. The ovaries are the size and shape of almonds in the shell; that is, they are approximately 3 cm long by 1½ cm wide by 1 cm thick, although the size varies. They are suspended in the pelvic cavity three ways: attached to the peritoneal covering over the back of the uterus (the broad ligament) by connective tissue called the mesovarium; attached to the uterus by the ovarian ligament; and attached to the lateral body wall by the suspensory ligament of the ovary. The actual position of the ovaries is variable, especially after the birth of a child because

at that time they are displaced from their original position and may never return to it.

The ovaries are the only organs in the pelvic cavity that are not covered with peritoneum, and they are a dull gray color in comparison to the pink, shiny, smooth uterus. The surface of the ovaries is covered with the *germinal epithelium,* a flattened layer of cells that was misnamed because it was thought that it gave rise to ova throughout life. Under the germinal epithelium is a zone or region called the *cortex,* the area in which the ova develop. Inside the cortex is the region called the *medulla,* with many large blood vessels, lymphatic vessels, and nerves. The connective tissue of the ovary is called the *stroma,* a framework of fibrous cells.

When a female baby is born, her ovaries contain a fixed number of primary ovarian follicles, and the ova she is destined to produce throughout her reproductive life will develop from them. These primary follicles arose from special cells called *primordial germ cells,* which were segregated from the rest of the body cells by as early as 10 days after fertilization. After migrating to the side of the primitive ovary, the germ cells, now called *oogonia,* become surrounded with a layer of cells called follicle cells, and the combination is known as the primary follicle. The primary follicles in the fetal ovary divide at a prodigious rate, and by 20 weeks of fetal life, there are more than 7 million. After that, there is no further division either before birth or after it; from that time on and for the next 50 years or so, the majority of ova undergo a process of regression and degeneration called *atresia.*

Various investigators differ in their estimates of the number of follicles remaining at birth. Some say that 150,000 exist, others maintain that about 1 million are present to form the stock from which all future eggs to be ovulated will be selected. At birth, the primary follicles contain an ovum arrested in the stage of development known as primary oocyte. By puberty, the number of follicles is further decreased to 50,000 (or fewer), and only one of these is ovulated each month—a total of approximately 400 from puberty to menopause.

A woman is, therefore born with all the eggs she will ever have. If she is still ovulating at the age of 50, that ovum has been in her ovary for some 50 years and 4 months. All the rest have become atretic. If this seems like an inordinate waste of cells with talent, consider that when a male ejaculates approximately 3 ml of seminal fluid, each ml contains 40–250 million sperm—yet only one sperm is necessary to fertilize an egg! This apparent overkill is not at all unusual in nature, whose interest is perpetuation of the species.

After puberty, those primary oocytes that will be ovulated go through a monthly scheme of development called the ovarian cycle. The hormones produced by the ovary during its cycle govern the activity of the endometrium of the uterus and result in cyclic menstruation. What is going on in the ovaries and the uterus is determined by hormones released by the anterior pituitary gland, and the anterior pituitary, in turn, is controlled by secretions called releasing hormones from a part of the brain, the hypothalamus. This constitutes the hypothalamic-pituitary-gonadal-uterine axis described in detail in the next chapter.

Anatomically, the ovarian cycle is diagrammed in Figure 2–15. At the beginning of each cycle, a group of follicles begins to undergo development, but only one will completely differentiate and mature. The rest become atretic. The follicle cells around the ovum multiply, form many layers, and become known as the granulosa cells. The stroma cells become organized into two layers, the *thecae interna* and *externa,* which produce hormones. The ovum itself enlarges and becomes surrounded by a membrane, the *zona pellucida,* a noncellular clear zone that lies between it and the granulosa cells. The zona pellucida functions during fertilization, permitting the entrance of only one sperm and blocking all others.

The next stage of follicular development is called the *secondary* or *antral* follicle. The granulosa cells, initially, and later the theca layers, secrete a viscous follicular fluid that accumulates in between the granulosa cells, forming cavities that eventually coalesce to form one large fluid-filled space called the antrum. The primary oocyte stays embedded at one side surrounded by a mound of granulosa cells called the *cumulus oophorus* (Latin for heap of egg cells). When the ovum is ovulated, the two or three adhering layers of granulosa cells shed with it form the *corona radiata,* or crown of cells. Perhaps 20–50 primary follicles reach the antral stage, but only one goes on to ripen fully to ovulation. That dominant one is called the mature *Graafian follicle.* In the follicles that do not fully mature, the granulosa layers become disorganized, the cells deteriorate, the follicular cavity shrinks, and the ovum itself degenerates.

The mature Graafian follicle moves toward the outer part of the ovary and forms a bulge on its surface. It manages to move mostly because of its increased size (2.5 cm or about 1 in. in diameter) and because the theca layers somehow facilitate a pathway. The area on the surface where the bulging follicle has caused a thinning out that looks like a blister is called the *stigma.* At the time of ovulation, the follicle bursts, and the egg, surrounded by its protective and nourishing corona radiata, floats out into the peritoneal cavity on a rush of follicular fluid. There is slight bleeding into the center of the follicle, and some of the blood may escape into the pouch of Douglas to produce the ovulatory pain called *mittelschmerz* (German for middle pain), which some women experience.

The ovulated egg (now a secondary oocyte) is swallowed up by the fimbriated end of the fallopian tube and begins to travel down it. It will die if it is not fertilized within 24 hours. Meanwhile, back in the ovary, the wall of the ruptured follicle collapses and the granulosa cells greatly increase in size, accumulating a yellow lipid-rich pigment called lutein in their cytoplasm. The cells are now called luteal cells, and the former follicle is called the *corpus luteum,* which produces hormones. The corpus luteum reaches its peak of activity approximately 5–7 days after ovulation, and if the ovum is not fertilized, begins to regress on the 10th day. Its life is over by the 15th day. The entire corpus begins to be invaded by connective tissue and, ultimately, is transformed into the *corpus albicans,* the white scar. After puberty, the formation of white scars from previous corpora lutea each

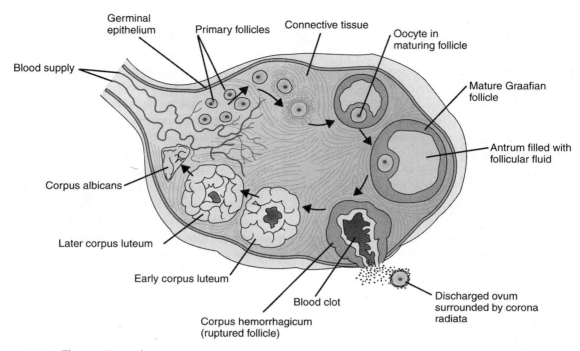

Germinal epithelium

Primary follicles

Connective tissue

Oocyte in maturing follicle

Blood supply

Mature Graafian follicle

Antrum filled with follicular fluid

Corpus albicans

Later corpus luteum

Early corpus luteum

Blood clot

Discharged ovum surrounded by corona radiata

Corpus hemorrhagicum (ruptured follicle)

Figure 2–15   The ovarian cycle.

month give the ovary its characteristic pitted, convoluted surface. Before these monthly cycles begin, the ovary in a prepubertal female is smooth; afterward, it looks something like a peach pit. The complete absorption of corpora albicantes takes a year or more, so the ovary always has a few in various stages of disappearance if a microscopic section is examined.

How the one follicle destined for ovulation is chosen while all the others die is not completely known. It takes an estimated 25 days for a small antra follicle to grow into a mature Graafian preovulatory follicle—considerably longer than the period from the beginning of menstruation to ovulation. There must be, therefore, continuous development of a number of primary follicles progressing along to the antral stage independent of hormonal support. Most of them will become atretic, but it is suspected that the follicle most likely to be saved from atresia by the increasing pituitary hormone levels at the onset of a new ovarian cycle is the one best developed at that time. This

advanced follicle, rescued by hormones at a later stage than the others because of its increased development, goes on to become the successful ovulatory follicle. The other antral follicles, less mature and lacking the ability to respond to hormones, become atretic.

There must also be some kind of quantitative relationship functioning between antral follicles doomed to atresia and those ordained to ovulate because even one tiny bit of ovarian tissue left after surgery still manages to produce an ovum each month. There is some evidence from animals that in that situation, fewer follicles become atretic than in a woman with two fully functioning ovaries.

When all the follicles are gone from the ovary by atresia or ovulation, ovarian activity ceases, and that period in a woman's life is called menopause. For the great majority of women, the nonactivity of the ovaries in menopause has been highly overrated; it need not be particularly significant to their well-being, sex lives, or general health.

𝒮UPPORT OF THE PELVIC VISCERA

That we stand erect and walk on two legs instead of four has been of primary importance in the development and progress of human society. There are many marvelously ingenious evolutionary modifications that have taken place to produce and maintain this posture. These anatomical modifications have significantly influenced our sex lives and the way in which women bear and deliver children. They also have contributed greatly to the development of some human ills, like backaches, sinus trouble, headaches, hernias, impacted wisdom teeth, fallen and weak arches, varicose veins, and hemorrhoids, to mention only a few. Most authorities agree that these malfunctions are signs of how inadequately the human body has adapted to a vertical biped stance instead of a quadruped posture.

The difficulty with standing erect is that gravity is always trying to pull everything down, and the older one gets, the harder it becomes to maintain all structures in their appropriate balanced arrangement of bone, muscle, and soft tissue. The way in which injury or congenital defects can compromise this balance to produce backache has already been discussed. Similarly, there are potential weaknesses that exist in the support of the internal organs. In a four-footed animal, the abdominal and pelvic viscera hang suspended from a horizontal backbone and are supported by the abdominal wall without much trouble, but in humans the abdominal and pelvic organs are constantly subjected to the downward pull of gravity. Even when a person is standing motionless, the viscera exert pressure on the muscles and connective tissue of the pelvic floor. Any movement increases abdominal pressure, as the viscera are squeezed against each other and against the pelvis. When the abdominal pressure is deliberately increased by contraction of the abdominal muscles during such ordinary activities as respiration, urination, and defecation, the stress placed on the pelvic supports that keep the viscera from falling out of the pelvis is enormous.

There are three kinds of supports for the abdominopelvic organs. One is provided by the bony bolstering of the spinal curvatures and the flaring of the ilia of the pelvis. These form shelves to brace portions of the digestive tract. Second, there are folds of the peritoneal lining of the body cavity and packings of connective tissue that attach to the viscera and hold them in place. The major support for the viscera, however, is from underneath—the muscles and connective tissues that make up the *pelvic diaphragm,* which stretches like a hammock across the bones of the pelvic outlet.

The inherent weakness in the pelvic diaphragm is that openings in it must exist for the exits of the urethra and the rectum, and in women, for the vagina. In females, childbearing and childbirth can strain the integrity of the pelvic support systems, and sometimes, after many pregnancies, the organs actually may slide out, or *prolapse* from the pelvis.

Structure of the Pelvic Floor

The pelvic floor consists of all the soft tissues that close the pelvic outlet, from the skin on the outside to the peritoneum on the inside, and all the muscles in between. When skin and superficial connective tissue are removed, the next layer is that of the superficial or *perineal muscles.* They include the ischiocavernosus muscles, important in erection of the clitoris; the bulbocavernosus muscles, which form the external vaginal sphincter and also function in clitoral erection; the superficial and the deep transverse perineal muscles; and the muscles of the external anal sphincter (Figure 2–16).

Underneath the perineal muscles are the *levator ani muscles,* major component (and the largest) of the pelvic diaphragm. In animals, these are the tail-wagging muscles. In humans, because we have no tails to wag, it would be expected that these muscles be diminished and vestigial. Instead, the levator ani muscles are bigger, stronger, and more powerful because their function in us is support, and that makes them the most important muscles in the pelvic floor. They are further strengthened by very strong connective tissue sheaths, the

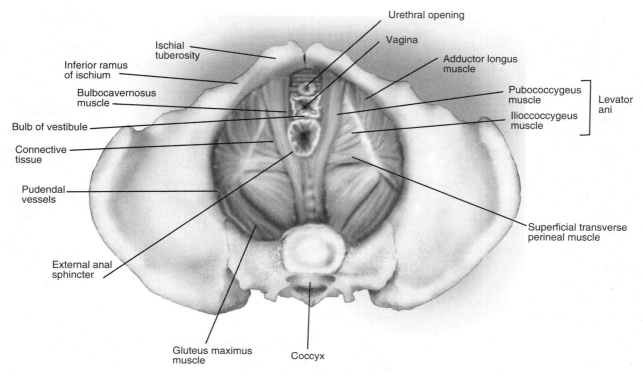

Figure 2–16 Muscles of the pelvic floor, from below.

inferior and *superior levator fascia*. Each half of the levator ani meets its partner from the other side in the midline to surround the urethra, the vagina, and the rectum with fibers that form sphincter muscles, which can powerfully constrict those hollow organs. Of the three component parts of the levator ani, the *pubococcygeus* is the one performing the main sphincteric action.

Sphincter Actions of the Pubococcygeus on Urinary Control

The pubococcygeus muscle fibers around the base (or trigone) of the urinary bladder form a sphincter mechanism that compresses the urethra as it exits and pulls it upward behind the pubic symphysis so that a sharp angle called the urethrovesical angle is formed between it and the neck of the bladder. Even if the bladder is very full and the pressure within it is much greater than

normal, urine can be retained. When the pubococcygeus muscle is voluntarily relaxed, the urethrovesical angle can straighten out and descend. Then the bladder muscle, called the *detrusor,* involuntarily contracts to let the urine enter the urethra and proceed until the bladder is empty. If the pubococcygeus is voluntarily contracted during urination, the sharp angle between the urethra and the bladder is restored to its previous elevated position, and urination stops. It is, therefore, possible to repeatedly stop and start urinary flow by contracting and relaxing the pubococcygeus muscle.

However, if the fibers of the pubococcygeus muscle are traumatized, stretched, or torn during childbirth, they no longer meet in the midline around the base of the bladder to maintain the integrity of the urethrovesical angle. Then, any increase in intra-abdominal pressure, like sneezing, coughing, or laughing, pushes the viscera against the bladder and results in a dribble or even a gush of urine that cannot be controlled by the now lax pubococcygeus muscle. This annoying and embarrassing situation is experienced by some multiparous women to a slight extent at the time of menstruation and is called *stress incontinence*. In a more severe form, it is present throughout the month. Some women never experience incontinence until menopause. There are estimates that nearly 40% of women over 60 are affected.

Although urinary incontinence may also be a result of a neurological disorder or a mechanical obstruction to the bladder or urethra, the most common cause of difficulty is injury to the soft tissues during delivery. The role of the obstetrician present at a delivery is to minimize the possibility of injury to the mother or to the baby, and the doctor's gentle and presumably expert assistance is certainly required in difficult labors. While it is not reasonable to blame all stress incontinence on incompetent or negligent behavior by the obstetrician, there are some procedures performed by physicians that tend to encourage trauma and tissue injury rather than to decrease it. For example, when labor is induced with hormones for no other reason than the convenience of the physician, the result may be a precipitous delivery that can injure both the baby and the mother. Another example is neglecting to catheterize the bladder during labor if the woman is unable to void on her own. The resultant pressure may then injure the bladder neck area. However, many cases of mild and uncomplicated stress incontinence are unavoidable, even with the best and most conscientious obstetrical help, particularly when large infants are delivered through a small bony pelvis. It is likely that the number of births (parity) of a woman is more significant in causing stress incontinence than any perineal damage associated with an individual delivery.

Urinary incontinence produces not only social and psychological distress but also may result in a substantial economic burden for affected women and the nation's health care costs. Obviously, any treatment other than drugs or surgery that can help control incontinence should be considered, especially in older women for whom the risks of surgery and the side effects of drug therapy may be greater.

Kegel Exercises.   Most surgical treatment for stress incontinence is aimed at restoring the integrity of the pubococcygeus muscle and the urethrovesical angle. Voluntary contractions of the pubococcygeus, commonly called Kegel exercises, can alleviate and even cure many cases of mild to moderate stress incontinence and are certainly worth trying before resorting to surgery. The exercises, as described by Kegel, the physician who advocated them, are meant to strengthen the pelvic diaphragm. Fifty to 100 times a day, said Kegel, the pubococcygeus should be contracted for at least 3 seconds and the anus and vagina drawn up into the pelvis. No one can observe that these exercises are being performed and they can be done in any position—standing, sitting, lying down. An easy regimen to follow would be to perform the contractions for 15 repetitions, 6 times a day (i.e., first thing in the morning, midmorning, lunchtime, midafternoon, dinnertime, and bedtime). Also, whenever voiding, the flow of urine should be stopped and started several times. For many women Kegel exercises will strengthen the pubococcygeus muscle enough to pull up the neck of the bladder and increase the urethrovesical angle, thereby preventing leakage of urine. Reductions of incontinent episodes by 50%–60% as a result of such pelvic floor exercises have been reported (Burns et al., 1990; Bo, Talseth, & Holme, 1999).

Bladder Training.   Another nonmedical possibility to restore urinary control involves "bladder training" or "bladder discipline," a program that involves educating a woman about bladder function and then having her follow a mandatory voiding schedule. A study utilizing bladder training recruited 123 women 55 years or older who had at least one episode of urinary incontinence a week. Sixty of the women formed the experimental group and were enrolled in a 6-week bladder training program. They were educated about how the brain controls urinary tract function and how the bladder and the urethra work. They were also told to follow a regular voiding schedule that was progressively lengthened and to resist the urge to void at other times by distraction or relaxation techniques. The rest of the women formed the control group. Although the researchers have no real explanation for the physiological or psychological mechanisms of action of the training program, they reported that it was effective. After the program, 12% of the treated women had no incontinent episodes and 75% had at least a 50% reduction in involuntary urine loss (Fanti et al., 1991). Clearly, the use of nonmedical low- or no-cost treatments of urinary incontinence can work for some women.

Action of the Pubococcygeus on the Vaginal Wall

Kegel exercises have also been advocated for the improvement of sexual relations between couples because they increase the ability of the vaginal sphincter to contract. The vaginal sphincter is responsible for the clasping action of the vagina around the penis during sexual intercourse, and the sphincter is formed by the fibers of the pubococcygeus muscles blending into those of the superficial perineal muscles around the walls of the vagina.

The involuntary spasm of the pubococcygeus muscle that may occur during sexual intercourse or perhaps during a pelvic examination in a doctor's office is called *vaginismus*. Here, the constrictive action of the pubococcygeus actually shuts off the vaginal opening so that introduction of the penis during coitus or of a speculum during examination produces pain and makes penetration impossible. Vaginismus can be a result of anticipated pain, or it may be caused by fear, guilt, or nervousness. It sometimes develops in a rape victim, particularly if sexual assault has produced severe lacerations to the genital area. Intercourse may then be severely painful to a woman long after the physical damage has healed.

Sometimes a mild and temporary vaginismus, enough to delay penetration or make it uncomfortable, however, may occur as a result of a previously painful intercourse during an episode of vaginitis. A temporary vaginismus can also be associated with a lack of sufficient lubrication.

It is possible to alleviate mild discomfort during intercourse with a surgical, water-based lubricant like K-Y Jelly, but if vaginismus is the primary response to sexual stimulation, some type of therapeutic counseling may be helpful.

No one has ever seen it happen, but almost everyone has heard the story about the couple that became "locked" together during sexual intercourse as a result of vaginismus and had to be separated in the emergency room of the local hospital. There is no medical basis or case on record to verify this persistent myth, called *penis captivus*. It can occur in animals, most frequently in dogs, and this is probably the source of the fantasy.

Action of the Pubococcygeus on the Rectal Wall

The pubococcygeus muscles also have an effect on the walls of the rectum. When strongly contracted, the pubococcygeus pulls the rectum and anus forward toward the pubic symphysis and supplements the action of the anal sphincter.

Other Muscles of the Levatores Ani

In addition to the pubococcygeus muscles, the lateral components of the levator ani are the *iliococcygeus* muscles, which extend (as their name indicates) from the ilium to the coccyx. Posteriorly, the triangular *coccygeus* muscles complete the pelvic diaphragm. The iliococcygeus muscles and the coccygeus muscles are supportive only; they have no sphincteric action.

Internal Support of the Pelvic Viscera

The uterus, the tubes, the ovaries, the urinary bladder, and the rectum are connected to each other and to the walls of the true pelvis by a number of "ligaments," some of which are not ligamentous structures at all but are merely folds of the peritoneal lining of the pelvic basin. Others do function as ligaments, combinations of smooth muscles and fibrous connective tissue, that tie the pelvic organs together, or function as ropes to suspend them from the body wall. Some additional support for the viscera is actually accomplished by their positions: being all crowded together provides pressure to hold them in place.

The peritoneum is the membrane that lines the body wall and is reflected back to cover all the viscera. The lining part is the *parietal* peritoneum, and the part that covers the organs is the *visceral* peritoneum. In between is the peritoneal cavity, also referred to as the pelvic cavity. It is actually only a potential space, since the parietal and visceral layers are in close contact.

The arrangement of the peritoneum in the abdominopelvic cavity is complicated. Trying to trace it from one organ to another or to the body wall is frustratingly difficult because in their embryonic development the organs pushed into the peritoneum from behind, acquiring for themselves a visceral peritoneal covering but leaving behind a complex scheme of folds and reflections of the parietal peritoneum. The reflected and folded peritoneal lining forms the route for blood vessels and nerves that supply the organs.

If one imagines the pelvic basin as a huge bowl lined with a membrane, the pelvic peritoneum, it is possible to visualize how the urinary bladder pushes up into it anteriorly, the rectum pushes up into it posteriorly, and the uterus pushes up into it in the middle. The viscera of the pelvis are only partially covered by the peritoneum. They lie mostly underneath it, surrounded by abundant connective tissue, the endopelvic fascia. It is apparent how the two pouches of peritoneum are formed in front and in back of the uterus. The one between the uterus and the bladder is the vesicouterine pouch. The one between the uterus and the rectum is the rectouterine, the pouch of Douglas, or the cul-de-sac, easily reached through the posterior fornix of the vagina.

Each fallopian tube extends laterally from the uterus like an arm, and the peritoneum is draped like a blanket over the uterus and the tubes. Each tube is covered with the blanket except at the ostium, which opens directly into the body cavity. The draped tent of reflected peritoneum is called the *broad ligament*. The ovaries are not covered by the broad ligament but are suspended from its back (posterior) surface by an extension called the *mesovarium*.

Inside the broad ligament is the connective tissue containing the blood vessels and nerves that supply the pelvic organs. Two cordlike condensations of this connective tissue, the *ovarian ligaments* and the *round ligaments,* are found in the apex of the broad ligament; The ovarian ligaments contain smooth muscle fibers and extend between the ovaries and the lateral angle of the uterus. At the time of ovulation, the fibers contract to change the position of the ovaries and bring them closer to the ends of the fallopian tubes. The round ligaments, almost completely composed of smooth muscle, are flat, narrow bands that extend from the lateral angle of the uterus on either side, cross over many blood vessels and nerves, and travel down through the inguinal canal (a passageway through the anterior abdominal wall) to insert into the tissues of the labia majora. The round ligaments hold the uterus forward in its typical anteverted position over the urinary bladder. As they traverse the inguinal canal, these ligaments become surrounded with connective tissue coverings and are accompanied by blood vessels, nerves, and lymphatic vessels. The lymphatics drain from the upper part of the uterus where the tubes enter and connect with the superficial inguinal lymph nodes, providing easy access for the spread of a possible malignancy from the uterus to the nodes.

Inside the base of the broad ligament, near the cervix, are masses or condensations of connective tissue associated with peritoneum, which extend out to the pelvic wall from the cervix and the wall of the vagina like spokes of a wheel. These are the main supports of the uterus, bladder, and vagina. They are the *cardinal* ligaments, extending from the cervix laterally to the pelvic wall, and the *uterosacral* ligaments, extending from the cervix posteriorly to the sacrum.

All the supports that have been described, the muscular components of the pelvic diaphragm and the broad, round, cardinal, and uterosacral ligaments, do their job of retaining the pelvic viscera inside the pelvis as long as they are strong and firm. If they are repeatedly traumatized in childbirth or if they are lacerated or atrophied, or in any way impaired in their action, they progressively weaken, and the uterus, bladder, or rectum will be displaced downward and begin to protrude or drop out of position. This dropping down or falling of an organ is called *prolapse.* When the urinary bladder prolapses into the anterior wall of the vagina and causes a bulge, it is called a *cystocele.* When the anterior wall of the rectum bulges into the posterior wall of the vagina, it is called a *rectocele.* Even though the uterus has more supporting structures than the other organs, it is the most likely to prolapse.

All the pelvic organs with their associated connective tissue and muscle are sensitive to estrogen. During pregnancy, when hormone levels are at a maximum, all the tissue greatly increases in size (hypertrophies). After menopause, when estrogen levels are low, muscle and connective tissue are likely to shrink (atrophy). The supports are weakened, and there is an increasing predisposition to prolapse, particularly with a previous history of childbirth damage to the supports. Like a stretched-out rubber band, there may be no tension left. The degree of prolapse may be mild, with the cervix only moderately descended into the vaginal canal (first degree), or the cervix may protrude through the vaginal opening (second degree). In extreme or complete prolapse, the cervix and the entire body of the uterus is pushed outside the vaginal opening.

Treatment depends on the extent of the prolapse but it most usually involves surgical correction and shortening and tightening of the cardinal ligaments and repair of the pelvic diaphragm. If the uterus has actually prolapsed out of the vagina, the cervix extends outside the vaginal opening, and the vaginal canal is inside out. A hysterectomy may then be a necessary part of the surgical procedure. In this situation, in which a woman is virtually walking around with her uterus between her legs, there is justification for the removal of a histologically normal uterus.

For the great majority of women, childbearing and delivery are completely normal physiological processes that result in no permanent injury to the reproductive organs or the surrounding soft tissues. Even after several pregnancies, the uterine supports remain firm and intact, having recovered their full functional capacity even though ligaments were stretched and soft tissues lacerated during delivery. Not all women heal as well as others, however, and some may develop subsequent difficulties. There are women who may have what is called a congenital soft tissue deficiency; that is, they were born with a pelvic support mechanism that is just not as strong as it could be. Despite every effort to eliminate trauma during delivery, these women are predisposed to experience some of the problems that have been described, after they have delivered several children. Occasionally, nulliparous women (i.e., those who have never delivered a baby) also experience stress incontinence or uterine prolapse.

THE MALE REPRODUCTIVE TRACT

The reproductive tract of the adult female is adapted for its purpose: to produce ova capable of fertilization by a spermatozoon and then to nourish and protect the rapidly growing conceptus until its birth. The reproductive tract of the adult male is adapted for its purpose: to produce large numbers of spermatozoa capable of fertilizing an ovum and to insert those sperm into the female's body so that one of them may encounter the ovum. What follows is a brief description of the male reproductive structure and function along with some comparisons of the homologues of female and male anatomy. Homologous organs or parts have the same evolutionary or embryological origin. They are similar in structure but not necessarily in function (Figure 2–17).

Testes

Spermatozoa are produced in the **testes,** oval smooth organs about 4–5 cm long and 2.5 cm in diameter. The testes are suspended in the *scrotum,* a loose pouch

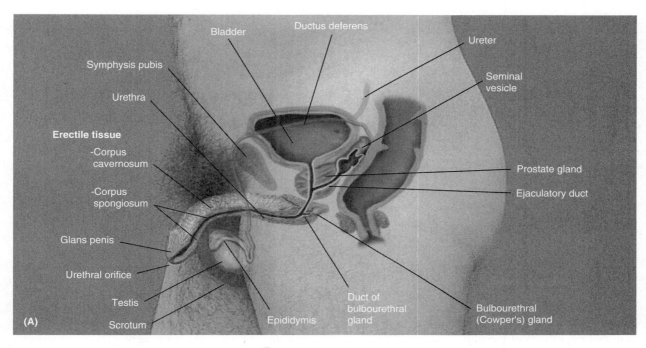

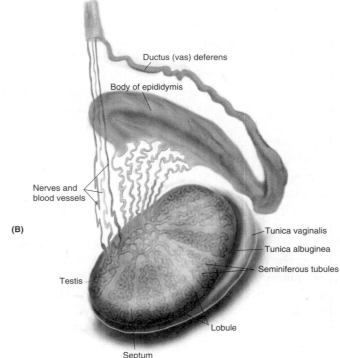

Figure 2–17   (A) Side view of male reproductive tract. (B) Testicle.

of skin divided by a septum into a right and left half, each containing a testis. The right and left scrotal sacs are homologous to the right and left labia majora. As in the labia, a sheet of dartos muscle lying just under the skin causes skin wrinkling in response to cold weather. Contraction of the smooth muscle also can change the closeness of contact of the testes with the body in order to conserve body heat.

Although the testes are carried in the scrotum, they originated during fetal life as the primordial germ cells in the abdominal cavity, just as in the female. In the last months of fetal life, however, the testes descend along with their ducts, nerves, blood vessels, and lymphatics through the inguinal canal, out of the abdominal cavity, and into the relatively cooler scrotal sacs. This is necessary because growth and development of viable sperm can take place only at several degrees less than body temperature. To help maintain the lower temperature, the scrotum lacks insulating fat under the skin and has many sweat glands.

In a small percentage of male babies, one or both testes may not descend and remain in the body cavity, a condition known as cryptorchidism (from the Greek for "hidden testis"). Cryptorchidism sometimes corrects itself during childhood, or hormone administration may be used to encourage testes descent. If uncorrected by the time of puberty, irreversible infertility could result.

Spermatogenesis (the production of sperm) occurs within the long, highly convoluted *seminiferous tubules* of the testes. The differentiation process, from the progenitor germ cell (spermatogonium) to a mature spermatozoon, takes about 74 days (plus or minus 4 days), begins at puberty, and continues throughout the life of the male. Every day a healthy male makes hundreds of millions of sperm. If they are not ejaculated, they die and are disposed of through phagocytosis, the normal scavenger activity of certain white blood cells and the *Sertoli cells,* which are scattered between the cells destined to become sperm. In addition to cleaning up unwanted germ cells, Sertoli cells mechanically support and nurture maturing sperm and produce hormones. Between the seminiferous tubules are clumps

of *interstitial cells,* which produce androgens, the male sex hormones. The most potent androgen is testosterone.

Male Accessory Genital Ducts

The accessory duct system transports the sperm from the testes to the outside of the body and includes the epididymis, ductus deferens, and urethra. In each testis the seminiferous tubules lead into straight tubules (tubuli recti), which lead into a network of canals, the rete testis, which lead into about 15–20 efferent ducts that emerge from the upper part of the testis. The *epididymis* is a 20-foot-long coiled tube that receives the sperm from the efferent ducts. It runs alongside the testis and is a storage site for sperm, which may be retained in the epididymis for up to 6 weeks while they acquire motility and fertilizing capacity. The *ductus (vas) deferens* is the continuation of the epididymis on each side. It is a straight tube that leaves the scrotum to ascend upward through the inguinal canal into the body cavity. The end of each ductus deferens expands into an enlargement, which joins with a duct from a seminal vesicle to form a short *ejaculatory duct*. The two ejaculatory ducts from either side penetrate the prostate gland to join the *urethra* as it exits from the urinary bladder. The urethra extends from the bladder to the end of the penis.

Male Accessory Glands

Semen consists of sperm suspended in a semigelatinous fluid that contains substances to nourish and protect the sperm and facilitate their movement. Only about 5% of the volume of semen is spermatozoa; the rest of the ejaculate is a mixed secretion of several accessory glands. The **seminal vesicles,** located at the base of the bladder, produce a viscous, alkaline fluid rich in fructose to provide a direct source of energy for sperm. More than half of the bulk of semen comes from the seminal vesicles. The **prostate** is a single gland that surrounds the urethra as it leaves the bladder. The prostate secretes a milky, alkaline fluid to neutralize the acidity of the vagina during intercourse and enhance sperm motility, which is best at a pH of 6.0–6.5. The prostate is the homologue of the paraurethral or Skene's glands in the female. Although small in childhood, it begins to grow at puberty and reaches adult size at age 20 and remains stationary until about the age of 50. At that age in some men the prostate may slowly begin to grow larger or hypertrophy and may eventually cause urinary obstruction.

The two small *bulbourethral (Cowper's) glands* secrete an alkaline mucus-containing fluid that is lubricating and protective. Their equivalent in the female is the right and left Bartholin's glands.

Penis

The penis and the scrotum form the external genitalia in the male. The penis is the organ for copulation and also serves as the outlet for urine. It has an attached root, a body or shaft, and a glans, the same as in its female homologue, the clitoris. The skin of the penis is thin with no hairs except near the root of the organ. The prepuce (foreskin) is a circular fold of skin that extends over the glans unless it is removed by circumcision shortly after birth, a procedure that formerly was routine and has become much more controversial.

The body of the penis contains three cylindrical masses of erectile tissue—two corpora cavernosa on the top side of the penis and one corpus spongiosum that lies below them and surrounds the urethra. The bulbs of the vestibule are the female homologue to the corpus spongiosum. As the vestibular bulbs contribute to vulvar clasping or "erection," so does the corpus spongiosum contribute to penile erection. The bulbo-cavernosus muscles in the female and the bulbospongiosus muscles in the male are counterparts and serve a similar function during intercourse. The corpora cavernosa in the male and the ischocavernosus muscles are mainly responsible and behave identically in erection of the penis as do these same erectile tissue masses and muscles in erection of the clitoris.

Ejaculation

Ejaculation is the culmination of the male sex act. Under involuntary nervous control, muscle contractions in the testes and the reproductive ducts move the sperm into the urethra. Simultaneous contractions in the seminal vesicles, prostate, and bulbourethral glands expel seminal fluid along with the sperm. The volume of ejaculate averages 3 ml (about a teaspoon) but can normally range from 1–10 ml. The number of sperm in a single ejaculate is subject to individual variation and may be anywhere from 100 million sperm to half a billion sperm, but the normal average is 300–400 million. The first fraction of ejaculate contains most of the sperm, which have better motility and survival ability than those in the later portions. In addition to the sperm, semen contains many of the substances ordinarily found in blood plasma with the addition of chemicals such as prostaglandins, enzymes, enzyme inhibitors, and hormones that play a role in sperm vitality, motility, migration, and fertilizing capacity. Immediately after ejaculation, the fluid semen coagulates and then spontaneously liquefies within 15–20 minutes. The sperm do not reach their full motility until liquefaction occurs, so the rate of coagulation and liquefaction can be significant in the clinical evaluation of male fertility.

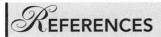

REFERENCES

Ben-Ari, E. T. (1998). Pheromones: What's in a name? *Bioscience, 48*(7), 505–511.

Bo, K., Talseth, T., & Holme, I. (1999). Single blind, randomised controlled trial of pelvic floor exercises, electrical stimulation, vaginal cones, and no treatment in management of genuine stress incontinence in women. *BMJ, 318*(7182), 487–493.

Burns, P. A., Pranikoff, K., Nochajski, T., et al. (1990). Treatment of stress incontinence with pelvic floor exercises and biofeedback. *Journal of the American Geriatric Society, 38,* 341–344.

Caldwell, W. E., & Moloy, H. C. (1933). Anatomical variations in the female pelvic and their effect on labor with a suggested classification. *American Journal of Obstetrics and Gynecology, 26,* 479–482.

DeCherney, A. H. (1990). Ectopic pregnancy. In N. G. Kase, A. B. Weingold, & D. M. Gershenson (Eds.), *Principles and practice of clinical gynecology* (2nd ed., pp. 465–469). New York: Churchill Livingstone.

Doty, R., Ford, M., & Preti, G. (1975). Changes in the intensity and pleasantness of human vaginal odors during the menstrual cycle. *Science, 190,* 1316–1317.

Fanti, J. A., Wyman, J. F., McClish, D. K., et al. (1991). Efficacy of bladder training in older women with urinary incontinence. *Journal of the American Medical Association, 265*(5), 609–613.

Keith, L., Stromberg, P., Krotszynski, B. K., et al. (1975). The odors of the human vagina. *Archiv für Gynakologie 220*(1), 1–10.

Ladas, A., Whipple, B., & Perry, J. (1982). *The G Spot & Other Recent Discoveries about Human Sexuality.* New York: Holt, Rinehardt, & Winston.

O'Connell, H. E., Hutson, J. M., Anderson, C. R., & Plenter, R. J. (1998). Anatomical relationship between urethra and clitoris. *Journal of Urology, 159*(6), 1892–1897.

Tonzetich, J., Preti, G., & Huggins, G. R. (1978). Changes in concentration of volatile sulphur compounds of mouth air during the menstrual cycle. *Journal of International Medical Research, 6,* 245–254.

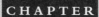

THE MENSTRUAL CYCLE AND ITS HORMONAL INTERRELATIONSHIPS

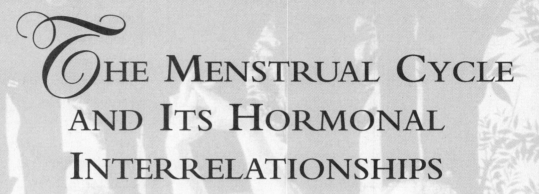

KEY TERMS

Activin

Adrenal glands

Androgens

Cholesterol

Conjugated equine
  estrogens

Corpus luteum

Corticosteroids

Endocrine glands

Endometrial cycle

Endometrium

Enzyme-linked
  immunosorbent assay
  (ELISA)

Estradiol

Estriol

Estrogen-receptor-alpha
  (ER-alpha)

Estrogen-receptor-beta
  (ER-beta)

Estrogens

Estrone

Follicles

Follicle-stimulating
  hormone (FSH)

Follicular phase

"Gonadostat" hypothesis

Gonadotropin-releasing
  hormone (GnRH)

Granulosa cells

Growth hormone (GH)

Hormones

Hypothalamus

Inhibin

Luteal phase

Luteinizing hormone (LH)

Menarche

Menstrual phase

Menstrual
  synchronization

Menstruation

Oocyte maturation
  inhibitor

Ovulation

Oxytocin

Pituitary gland

Progestational phase

Progesterone

Progestins

Proliferative phase

Prostaglandins (PGs)

Puberty

Receptors

Reproductive
  neuroendocrinology

Secretory phase

Sepsis

Steroid

Steroid hormones

Testosterone

Theca externa

emale primates menstruate. Every month the endometrial lining of the uterus is prepared by hormones to receive and nurture a fertilized egg. If fertilization and implantation does not occur, the superficial two-thirds of the lining is shed, and periodic bleeding takes place, emerging through the cervix and out the vagina.

Women, like female monkeys and apes, are primates, but some of them find themselves reluctant to admit the existence and the normality of **menstruation.** Instead, they get "sick," get "the curse," get their "period," the "monthlies," a "visit from a friend," "hoist the red flag," "fall off the roof"—the euphemisms are many.

It is not surprising that many women have difficulty talking about "that time of the month" and feel much more comfortable using such euphemisms. Throughout the course of history, society has been less than kind to the menstruating woman. Depending on the area and the culture, she has been regarded with fear and awe, with derision and distaste. Even primi-

tive peoples recognized that blood was essential to life; to bleed and not to die, indeed, to lose blood cyclically and still remain healthy, must be supernatural. Magical powers were ascribed to menstruation and menstrual blood, and superstitions and taboos surrounding the completely natural physiological function of menstruation endured for centuries.

Some of these myths have persisted in modern society. Few people today, except for the truly uneducated, still believe that a menstruating woman can blight crops, curdle milk, sour wine, wilt flowers, or be responsible for natural disasters like floods or tornadoes. Many, however, find it completely plausible that a menstruating female should be excused from sports at school, should not take showers after gym, should not get a permanent or have hair tinted because it won't "take," is more vulnerable to illness, and, still believing in the uncleanness of menstrual blood, should not have sexual intercourse. All of these attest to the "sickness" of menstruation, and sickness implies suffering. If a young woman learns that to menstruate is to be sick, that it is a burden she must suffer for 40 years or more, that it is at best an unfortunate and uncomfortable nuisance, and that it is physically and psychologically incapacitating, she has then inherited the modern version of the ancient myths, taboos, and superstitions.

Of course, not all women view menstruation in the same way because they do not all experience menstruation in the same way. But even if women were to regard their own menstrual periods ideally, that is, as a normal, neutral, unremarkable biological given, the rest of the world does not. We get much more information from women's magazines and newspaper articles on menstrual disorders and problems. The prevailing attitudes toward the event could be, but are generally not, positive. Despite increased candor about sexuality on film and TV, any discussion of menstruation openly is still, for the most part, uncommon except by stand-up comedians who do deprecating tampon or premenstrual syndrome (PMS) jokes. Several books by feminist authors have attempted to chronicle and change our learned attitudes toward menstruation and bring it out of the closet, so to speak. (Particularly good is the revised edition of *The Curse,* by Delaney, Lupton, and Toth.) But the reluctance to speak openly about women's physiological processes is founded in entrenched attitudes toward women's "otherness" in a male-dominated world, and these attitudes are not easily unlearned. When 80 college women, who might be expected to have a better understanding of their bodies than the average, were queried about their knowledge of the menstrual cycle, researchers found that their basic knowledge of menstruation and menopause was mostly incorrect, generally incomplete, and distinctly negatively biased (Koff, Rierdan, & Stubbs, 1990). The authors of the paper speculated that if negative attitudes and misconceptions were present in educated college women, those women with even fewer opportunities for accurate information would demonstrate even less knowledge and more negative bias toward menstruation. Perhaps if

women, who all share the experience of menstruation, more fully understood the nature, meaning, and function of it, they could more freely talk about it, perhaps develop more positive attitudes toward their reproductive cycles, and be less likely to find them difficult or disturbing.

The female reproductive cycle, less accurately called the menstrual cycle, refers to the rhythmic changes that occur in the ovaries and uterus under hormonal influences. Although the existence of hormones has been known since the turn of the 20th century, the recognition that there is a complex relationship between the organs of reproduction and the endocrine system did not occur until the early 1920s. Thereafter, in an amazing burst of research progress, within the next 10 years all of the sex steroid hormones were identified, their functions were recognized, and they were purified to be available for research and therapy. The next big discovery, in the mid-1950s, was the certainty that a part of the brain, the hypothalamus, plays a dominant role in the regulation of reproductive function and that the brain could perhaps be viewed as another endocrine organ. **Reproductive neuroendocrinology,** the study of the integration of the nervous system and the endocrine organs of reproduction, continues to be a rapidly expanding area of biological and medical research. Much of the research focus is at the submicroscopic or molecular level and utilizes approaches that require highly sophisticated instrumentation. Despite rapid progress, however, there is yet much that is theorized or unknown. For this reason, the gynecologist-obstetrician (OB/GYN) is probably even more of a medical empiricist than other specialists; that is, a gynecologist administers hormones as a treatment (as contraceptives, at menopause) because they work and not because there is a clearly defined understanding of their action in the body.

The major efforts in reproductive endocrinology today are focused on greater understanding of how hormones are formed, how they get into and work within the cell, how they can cause synthesis of other substances, and how they are metabolized.

ℰNDOCRINE SYSTEM

The endocrine system was the last organ system to be recognized, probably because there is no anatomical continuity between its parts. The classic **endocrine glands** are the pituitary gland, the thyroid gland, the parathyroid glands, the adrenal glands, the islets of Langerhans of the pancreas, and the ovaries and the testes (Figure 3–1). The concept of "hormones" and the glands that secrete them has been broadened to include the hypothalamic hormones regulating the pituitary gland; the placental hormones; the gastrointestinal tract (gut) hormones; regulatory neurotransmitters from some brain neurons; the pineal gland, which secretes melatonin; and the thymus gland, which influences the immune response. The glands of greatest importance to the reproductive cycle and to the physical differences that exist between males and females are the anterior pituitary gland and the ovaries and testes, but all of the endocrine organs have interrelating physiological effects that are necessary to the proper growth, development, and function of the reproductive system.

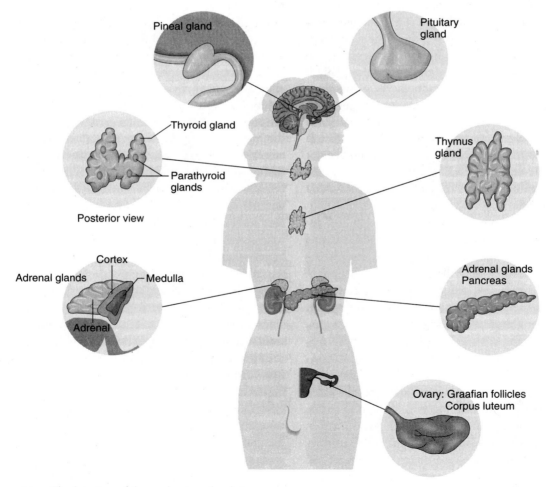

Figure 3–1   The location of the endocrine glands in a woman.

Endocrine glands have no ducts; they secrete directly into the tissue fluid that surrounds their cells. The secretion passes into the bloodstream to be transported elsewhere in the body, sometimes a considerable distance from the original gland. Because they secrete into the blood capillaries that surround them, all endocrine glands generally have a very good blood supply. Viewed microscopically, they consist of cords or clumps of cells surrounded by many capillaries and supported by connective tissue.

Hormones

Endocrine secretions are called **hormones** from the Greek word, *horman,* meaning "to urge on." Hormones secreted by the glands of the endocrine system are all different, and the cells on which they exert their effects are different; however, they are, generally speaking, all of the urging-on type, although exactly how they accomplish this action is still speculative. Some hormones have an effect on the growth and metabolism of all cells of the body; others have an action on just certain tissues, which are then called *target* tissues or cells. More than 60 human hormones have been identified. New ones are being found in a variety of body sites.

Chemical Composition of Hormones. There are two major types of hormones chemically:

1. Proteins, or derivatives of proteins, such as polypeptides, peptides, glycoproteins (carbohydrate-protein complexes), and amines (structurally similar to amino acids)
2. Steroids, which are fat-soluble compounds, and part of a large family of substances with the same chemical skeleton; the ovaries, testes, placenta, and the outer part of the adrenal glands produce steroids

Control of Hormone Secretion. Some endocrine glands are directly connected with the nervous system. Nerve fibers ending on gland cells cause the gland to release its hormones in response to nerve impulses, or the nerve cells themselves produce neurosecretions, which are stored in the gland. Neuroendocrine control may also be indirect, as in the hypothalamic hormonal regulation of the anterior pituitary gland.

The rate and quantity of hormone secretion from an endocrine gland may be controlled by blood levels of another hormone or by levels of organic or inorganic substances other than hormones, like glucose or calcium. If the message of the second hormone or substance is to *inhibit* the further secretion of the endocrine gland, it is said to be a *negative feedback* mechanism; when the message transferred back to the original gland is to *increase* the rate or quantity of secretion, it is called *positive feedback*.

Mechanisms of Hormone Action. Hormones basically control the activities of the cells they affect, and there has been very extensive investigation of the mechanisms by which they provide this control function. Once the mode of action of a hormone at the cellular level is known, it may be possible to interfere with or manipulate it in some way—to cure an endocrine defect, to produce a more effective contraceptive, or to increase fertility.

Because hormones circulate in the bloodstream in such very low concentrations compared with some other biologically active substances, such as glucose, there has to be some way for the target cells to recognize, receive, and retain the hormone molecules as they pass by in the capillaries. Accordingly, there are specific receptor sites for specific hormones located on the cell membranes or in the cytoplasm of the target cells. The job of the receptor is to transmit the message of the hormone's arrival to the area of the cell that is involved in the response, either to initiate chemical activities within the cytoplasm or to activate the genes in the nucleus to synthesize intracellular proteins that, in turn, result in specific cellular functions. The cell receptors, almost always composed of glycoprotein, are highly sensitive to the hormones they recognize and bind. It takes only a few molecules of the bound hormone to initiate the full cellular response. Some hormones are even able to regulate the number and activity of their own and other hormone receptors. For example, the pituitary gonadotropins, follicle-stimulating hormone (FSH) and luteinizing hormone (LH) (hormones that act on the gonads), cause the granulosa cells of the primary follicles to develop receptors for FSH and estrogen and stimulate the theca cells to develop LH receptors.

The molecules of protein, peptide, or amine hormones are water soluble and cannot diffuse easily through the cell membrane, and, therefore, their receptors are located on the surface of the cell membrane, outside the cell itself. Once a protein hormone (the "first messenger") unites with its receptor, it interacts with one or more membrane-bound regulatory G-proteins (so called because they can bind the high-energy nucleotide GTP, or guanosine triphosphate), which through additional chemical reactions allow the activation of an enzyme within the cell membrane, adenylate cyclase. Adenylate cyclase passes the message to the inside of the cell by causing the formation of a hormone mediator named cyclic AMP, which becomes the "second messenger." Cyclic AMP (3'5' adenosine monophosphate) is formed from the conversion of ATP (adenosine triphosphate). ATP is the high-energy compound stored within all cells to provide a source of energy for cellular activities. Cyclic AMP (sometimes cyclic GMP, guanosine mononucleotide), working together with intracellular calcium, moves into the cytoplasm to combine with and activate a cyclic AMP-dependent enzyme, protein kinase. Protein kinase catalyzes specific phosphorylation reactions (that is, transfers phosphate groups) to key protein enzymes in the cytoplasm. This leads to the cellular response to the hormonal message, depending on the cell's inherent nature. If the cell is in the ovary, testis, or adrenal cortex, cyclic AMP ultimately results in production of steroid hormones (Figure 3–2).

When **steroid hormones** circulating in the blood reach their target cells, their smaller, fat-soluble

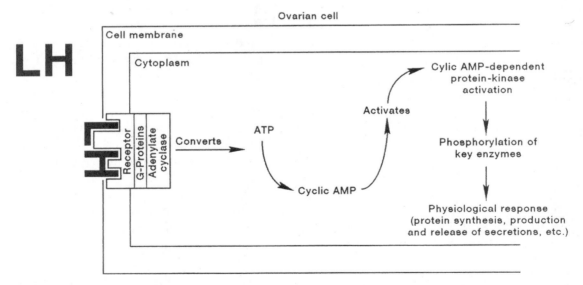

Figure 3–2 The cyclic AMP mechanism by which protein hormones exert their action. A stimulating protein hormone, such as LH, unites with a specific receptor at the cell membrane of an ovarian cell. The combination of hormone and receptor activates adenylate cyclase, which causes the conversion of ATP to cyclic AMP within the cytoplasm. Cyclic AMP, called the second messenger (because the original stimulating hormone is the first messenger), initiates cellular activities that lead to estrogen release.

molecules diffuse across the cellular membranes where they bind to a receptor specific for that particular steroid, either in the cytoplasm or the nucleus. For example, receptors specific for estrogen, a steroid hormone, exist in the cells of the breast, the uterus, the vagina, the pituitary gland, the brain, the bone, the liver, the skin, the blood vessels—virtually all tissues of the body. When estrogen arrives at these sites, it crosses the cell membrane and moves to the nucleus, where it becomes loosely bound to its receptor. After a process of activation, the estrogen-receptor complex binds tightly to a specific section of DNA, the genetic material of the cell that encodes the information to control all cell activities. The coded message from the DNA is copied, or transcribed, onto messenger RNA, which leaves the nucleus to move out into the cytoplasm, where it initiates the synthesis of proteins with specific cellular functions (Figure 3–3).

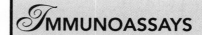

IMMUNOASSAYS

Cells in the body not only have **receptors** for protein and steroid hormones but also possess specific binding sites for a wide variety of natural and introduced substances that may be present in the body fluids. For example, lymphocytes, a type of white blood cell, are known to have surface receptors for viruses, bacterial toxins, histamine, nerve impulse transmitters, and various cell-to-cell communication products affecting growth, cell division, or self-recognition, as well as hormone receptor sites. It is now possible to employ the binding capacity of such cell surface receptors to measure incredibly small concentrations of the substances they bind. The radioimmunoassay, introduced in 1960 by Yalow and Berson (for which Rosalyn S. Yalow received the Nobel Prize in 1977), is based on the technique in which radioactive or "labeled" molecules of a

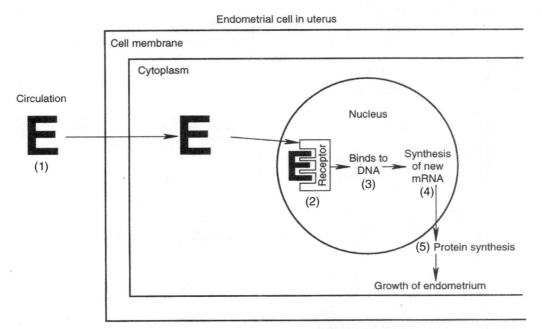

Figure 3–3 Mechanism of action for steroid hormones. In this example, the steroid estrogen (1) diffuses across the cell membrane and through the cytoplasm to the nucleus where it binds with a receptor (2). The estrogen-receptor complex binds to nuclear DNA (3), activating specific genes to form messenger RNA (4). The MRNA passes into the cytoplasm to result in protein synthesis (5).

substance and nonlabeled molecules of the same substance compete for a limited number of sites on a receptor protein specific for the substance. The development of this method has made obsolete the hormone analyses that had formerly been made by biological (animal) techniques, in which the hormone was injected into a test animal and the amount of response was noted. Bioassays are relatively reliable but are time consuming and expensive to perform because they require a day or more wait and the destruction and dissection of the animals. Today, it is possible to measure routinely (but not necessarily inexpensively) levels of hormones in billionths of a gram (nanogram), trillionths of a gram (picogram), or even, in the case of estrogen receptor assays, quadrillionths (femtomols) bound per gram.

A radioimmunoassay (RIA) uses the binding sites on immune bodies or antibodies as the binding protein reagent. When the binding protein is not part of the immune system but is a structural component of a cell, the technique is actually a radioreceptor assay (RRA). RIA has virtually become generic, however, for any assay technique that uses radioactive agents that bind to a protein, regardless of whether antibodies or cell receptors are used.

To measure the concentration of a pituitary hormone like LH in the blood, for example, a known quantity of (1) LH antibodies (produced by injecting the antigen LH into animals to cause antibody formation) is mixed with (2) the blood sample containing an unknown amount of LH and (3) a known amount of purified LH that has been labeled with a radioisotope like carbon 14 or iodine 125. The mixture of the three substances is then incubated until the reactions are presumed to have reached equilibrium. Because both the labeled and unlabeled LH in the mixture *compete* for the fixed number of active binding sites on the antibodies, the amount of labeled LH antibody complex formed, as determined by counting the emissions in a scintillation counter, is a function of the LH concentration in the blood sample. That is, the more radioactive LH that was bound, the less natural LH there must have been in the sample. Conversely, if just a small amount of radioactive LH has been bound, there must have been more natural hormone present (Figure 3–4). The concentration of LH in the sample can be read directly from a previously constructed standard curve.

Control of normal or abnormal levels of hypothalamic hormones, pituitary gonadotropins, and ovarian steroids can be studied by RIA techniques, and the method has led to a more complete understanding of the endocrine events associated with the menstrual cycle. Radioimmunoassays are so extremely sensitive that they also are commonly used for the detection of trace amounts of drugs. Other kinds of immunoassays employ fluorescent dyes or enzymes coupled to antibodies as labels and are fast, sensitive, and very specific. Fluorescent-antibody tests can identify microorganisms in clinical specimens and detect the presence of either antigens or specific antibodies in blood serum. The enzyme-linked immunoassay (EIA) is similar to the RIA but uses a labeled enzyme instead of a radioactive-labeled molecule. The **enzyme-linked immunosorbent assay (ELISA)** is used to diagnose many bacterial, viral, and parasitic infections. Because of its relative simplicity, the ELISA test is widely used to screen for the presence of antibodies to HIV virus proteins. The method of choice now for many hormone measurements is the immunometric assay. In these

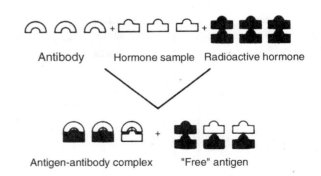

Figure 3–4 The radioimmunoassay technique. A fixed amount of antibody is mixed with an unknown amount of hormone and a known amount of radioactive hormone. The unlabeled nonradioactive hormone competes with the radioactive hormone for attachment to the antibody binding sites. (Sloane, E., Reprinted with permission from *The Science Teacher,* a publication of the National Science Teachers Association.)

assays, unlabeled hormone is added to antibody, and a secondary antibody is then added to the resultant antigen-antibody complex. It is this second antibody that carries a labeled compound to provide the signal for detection. The immunofluorometric assay (IFMA), immunoradiometric assay (IRMA), and the immuno-chemiluminometric assay (ICMA) are examples.

$\mathcal{O}$THER CHEMICAL MESSENGERS— PROSTAGLANDINS

Prostaglandins (PGs) are a closely related group of fatty acid derivatives with a variety of effects and belong to a group of compounds called *eicosanoids*. They include prostaglandin (PG) D_2, E_2, F_{2a}, thromboxane, prostacyclin, and the leukotrienes. Almost all cell membranes of the body can synthesize prostaglandins by oxygenation

of arachidonic acid, a 20-carbon polyunsaturated fatty acid commonly found in food, but the particular type and activity of the prostaglandin formed depends upon the nature and function of the cell producing it. Although they have regulatory effects and are sometimes classified as hormones, prostaglandins are not technically hormones because they are produced by all tissues rather than by special glands. Neither are they transported like hormones in the bloodstream to target cells; most prostaglandins are immediately deactivated by enzymes once they get into the circulation so that they affect cells only a short distance away from their site of production.

These compounds, originally discovered in human semen, were named "prostaglandins" in 1935 by Nobel laureate Von Euler because small amounts were found in the prostate gland. Originally recognized for their potent effects on uterine muscle contraction, subsequent prostaglandin research has now determined their great biological importance as well as their chemical structure and the mechanisms of biosynthesis. Figure 3–5 is a

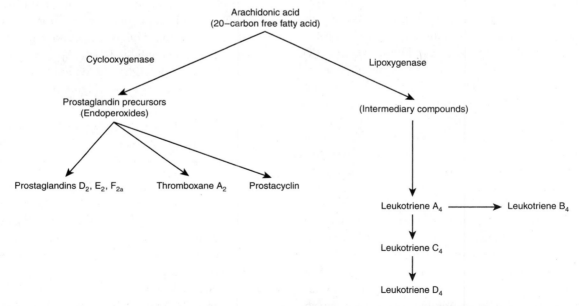

Figure 3–5 Metabolic pathways leading to the synthesis of prostaglandins and leukotrienes. Prostaglandin inhibitors block the enzyme cyclooxgenase and prevent the conversion of arachidonic acid to endoperoxides. The leukotrienes are involved in inflammation and possibly in bronchial asthma. The anti-inflammatory effects of corticosteroids are believed to be due to their inhibition of leukotriene synthesis.

schematic diagram of their formation. There are two main pathways: one, catalyzed by the enzyme cyclooxygenase and leading to prostaglandin, prostacyclin, and thromboxanes, and the other using the enzyme lipoxygenase to eventually form the leukotrienes. Aspirin and similar anti-inflammatory drugs inhibit the cyclooxygenase enzyme, and a number of other compounds are now known to block synthesis or antagonize the actions of PGs.

The ubiquitous PGs have amazingly diverse physiological effects, ranging from regulatory control in a number of body organs to more general activities associated with pathology, response to trauma, and body defense mechanisms. They may be involved in the maintenance of blood pressure and the rate of blood flow. F-prostaglandins and thromboxane stimulate blood platelet aggregation necessary for initiation of the clotting mechanism and cause constriction of tiny blood vessels. Prostacyclin and the E-prostaglandins, produced by the cells lining blood vessels, inhibit platelet aggregation and cause vasodilation. Leukotrienes are produced by cells of the immune system and participate in allergic reactions. PGs of the E-group inhibit gastric secretion and may be protective against ulcer development. High levels of PGs have been shown to be associated with pain and inflammation and possibly with fever. In low concentrations, PGs inhibit transmission of impulses in the nervous system. The earliest work on the nature of PGs, however, was concerned with their effects on the reproductive system. Primarily deriving from their ability to stimulate smooth muscle contraction, prostaglandins are closely associated with reproduction. They may be involved in ejaculation in men and in facilitation of sperm transport in the uterus and fallopian tubes after ejaculation has occurred. They are now known to be responsible for dysmenorrhea, or menstrual cramps, and play a role in "ripening" of the cervix at the end of pregnancy, as well as in labor and delivery. PGs may be responsible for determining the life span of the corpus luteum and affect hypothalamic and pituitary hormones that trigger ovulation. They are used clinically to induce labor and to cause abortion in the second 3 months of pregnancy. At the cellular level, PGs can cause both stimulation and inhibition of adenylate cyclase, leading to greater or lesser formation of cyclic AMP and suggesting the mechanism for the molecular action of PGs.

The Pituitary Gland

The **pituitary gland,** oval and about the size of a pea, is attached to the hypothalamus of the brain by a stalk called the infundibulum. The pituitary rests in a depression of the sphenoid bone of the skull and is protected by the bone and by the same tough connective tissue that covers the brain. The anterior part of the pituitary gland (i.e., the section closer to the face) is called the *anterior lobe,* or *adenohypophysis;* the posterior part is the *posterior lobe* or *neurohypophysis.* An intermediate lobe is present in many mammalian species, human fetuses, and pregnant women but is absent in adult humans. Each of these parts has a different embryological origin. The adenohypophysis arises from an upgrowth of the roof of the mouth, while the neurohypophysis develops from a downgrowth of the brain. This is why, under the microscope, the neurohypophysis looks like nervous tissue and the adenohypophysis has the typical cell cords and clumps of an endocrine organ (Figure 3–6).

Hormones of the Pituitary Gland.   It is known currently that there are seven hormones synthesized by the cells of the anterior pituitary gland:

1. **Growth hormone (GH),** or somatotropin controls the growth of all the cells of the body capable of growth, resulting in an increase in the numbers of cells and in enlargement of existing cells.
2. Thyrotropin, or thyroid-stimulating hormone (TSH), controls thyroid gland activity.
3. Adrenocorticotropic hormone, or adrenocorticotropin (ACTH), is responsible for the activity of the cortex portion of the adrenal glands.
4. Melanocyte-stimulating hormone (MSH), may stimulate pigment formation and dispersal in the

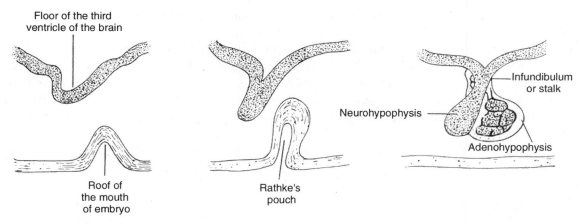

Figure 3–6 Development of the pituitary gland. The neurohypophysis, or part of the gland that arises from the brain tissue, never loses its connection and remains attached by the stalk or infundibulum. The portion of the gland that forms from the roof of the primitive mouth of the embryo becomes the adenohypophysis.

pigment-producing cells of the epidermis. Its exact hormonal role in humans is uncertain.

Both ACTH and MSH are derived from a large precursor protein called proopiomelanocortin, or POMC. POMC is produced by many different tissues, but its highest concentration is in the pituitary gland, where it is processed into different end products depending upon the region of the gland. The POMC in the anterior lobe is the source of ACTH and beta lipotropin (B-LPH). Beta lipotropin is the prohormone source of MSH and can be cleaved into the biologically active fragments known as the enkephalins and the alpha, beta, and gamma endorphins that have natural pain-killing abilities. The discovery of endorphins, called endogenous opiates because they are innate in the body and mimic the effect of heroin and morphine, created as much excitement among neuroendocrinologists as did the discovery of PGs. Investigations have linked endorphins not only with natural pain relief but also with obesity, epilepsy, drug addiction, schizophrenia, the explanation of the effects of hypnosis and acupuncture, and jogger's high or runner's second wind.

5. Prolactin is responsible for the initiation and sustaining of milk production from the breasts when they have been previously readied for lactation by the action of other hormones.

6. **Follicle-stimulating hormone (FSH)** stimulates the growth and development of the primary follicles and results in hormone production in ovaries and sperm production in testes.

7. **Luteinizing hormone (LH)** is responsible for ovulation, corpus luteum formation, and hormone production in the ovaries and is the stimulus for hormone production from the interstitial cells of the testes.

The last two hormones, FSH and LH, are called gonadotropins because they regulate the activities of the organs of reproduction. FSH and LH are glycoproteins with a carbohydrate content varying from 13%–31%.

There are two hormones that are synthesized by nerve cells in the hypothalamus and stored in the posterior pituitary gland:

1. Antidiuretic hormone (ADH), also called vasopressin, affects the excretion of water by the kidneys and increases blood pressure.

2. **Oxytocin** is a very powerful stimulant of uterine contraction, especially of a pregnant uterus. Oxytocin is believed to participate in uterine contractions during the process of delivery, although the actual mechanism of the initiation of labor is not known. Oxytocin also affects the flow of milk from the breasts in a nursing mother in response to the sucking stimulus from the baby. To a lesser extent than vasopressin, oxytocin affects blood pressure.

Relationship between the Pituitary Gland and the Hypothalamus

In the basal region of the brain, located underneath the cerebral hemispheres, is the **hypothalamus,** a part of the brain that consists of neuron cell bodies, fibers, and supporting tissue that make up the floor and part of the side walls of the third ventricle. The hypothalamus is a key portion of a group of brain structures collectively called the *limbic system,* which is believed to be the part of the brain concerned with emotional behavior—fear, anger, feelings of depression and elation, sexual desires, and feelings of reward and pleasure or punishment and pain. The different areas of the limbic system perform different functions, but overall it is thought to be responsible for our emotional and behavioral patterns. The hypothalamus is connected by nerve fiber tracts to all parts of the limbic system, which is in turn connected to practically every other section of the brain. The hypothalamus, therefore, can be regarded as the pathway through which neural inputs not only from the limbic system but also from the higher brain centers in the cerebrum can influence and control many major functions of the body.

Located in the hypothalamus are groups of nerve cells that control the involuntary activities of the body that are necessary for life, such as regulation of appetite and satiation, body water, body temperature, blood pressure, and heart rate. Moreover, the hypothalamus controls all pituitary gland secretion. Years ago, the pituitary gland was always called the master gland of the body because its hormones were responsible for the activities of many other endocrine glands. The view now is that part of the brain itself—that is, the hypothalamus—is the master gland, providing the integration of the nervous and the endocrine systems. Neurons in the hypothalamus produce *neurosecretions,* which are themselves the hormones, or which cause the pituitary to release its tropic hormones (that is, those that stimulate the growth and function of other endocrine glands). So the pituitary is really the servant of the hypothalamus.

But the question of who is the real boss is complicated by the evidence that regions of the brain outside of the hypothalamus contain peptide hormones. ACTH, MSH, β-LPH, and β-endorphin are all derived from a large precursor protein molecule present not only in the pituitary and hypothalamus but, to a lesser extent, in the rest of the brain, including the limbic areas, the midbrain, the cortex, and the cerebellum. Evidently, the cells of the pituitary gland and the brain are able to process and split up the same precursor molecule differently in order to produce the different component hormones, each with different activities. Moreover, hormones formerly believed to be secreted only by endocrine cells, such as insulin from the pancreas or cholecystokinin and gastrin from the secretory cells of the intestine, also have been discovered in the brain. What pituitary and gut hormones are doing in the brain, and why the brain, in addition to all its other functions, appears to be another endocrine organ, are still not completely known. Some researchers think brain hormones may act as local neuron-to-neuron communicators or as modulators of signals from other transmitters, thus affecting behavioral responses.

Hypothalamus to Posterior Pituitary. The influence of the hypothalamus on posterior pituitary lobe secretions is very direct and evident. Nerve fibers from two groups of neuron cell bodies in the anterior wall of the hypothalamus, the *supraoptic* and the *paraventricular nuclei,* extend down the infundibular stalk and terminate in little bulbous endings in the substance of the neurohypophysis. ADH and oxytocin are secreted by these supraoptic and paraventricular neurons, and these substances pass down their long axon fibers to be stored in the cells of the neurohypophysis. These hormones, therefore, are secretions of the hypothalamic neurons, not of the posterior lobe, and are released into the bloodstream on nerve signals from the hypothalamus.

Hypothalamus to Anterior Pituitary. In contrast to the direct nervous connection of the hypothalamus with the posterior pituitary gland, the message for control or hormone release by the anterior pituitary arrives from the brain in a rather indirect way. It involves a series of blood vessels called the *hypothalamic-hypophyseal portal system,* which consists of two capillary beds, one in the hypothalamus and one in the adenohypophysis, and the veins that connect them. The neurons that secrete the neurosecretory *releasing* and *inhibiting* factors are roughly in the same regions as the supraoptic and paraventricular nuclei, that is, in the medial and lateral parts of the basal hypothalamus. But the fibers of these neurons are not long, and they do not extend down the infundibular stalk. Instead, the axons are short, and they terminate on nearby loops of a capillary bed within the hypothalamus. The releasing and inhibiting factors, actually hormones, are deposited in these capillaries, whose venules drain down the infundibulum and empty into another capillary bed in the anterior lobe of the pituitary gland. The neurosecretions produced by the hypothalamic neurons never get into the general blood circulation but go first to the anterior pituitary and cause or inhibit the release and synthesis of the hormones of the gland. Figure 3–7 shows the relationship of neurosecretory cells in the hypothalamus to the anterior and posterior pituitary glands.

The hypothalamus currently is known to produce nine releasing or inhibiting hormones regulating pituitary gland secretions. They include corticotropin-releasing hormone (CRH); prolactin-releasing hormone (PRH) and prolactin-inhibiting hormone (PIH) (actually dopamine, a neurotransmitter related to adrenaline); and growth hormone-releasing hormone (GHRH) and growth hormone-inhibiting hormone (GHIH or

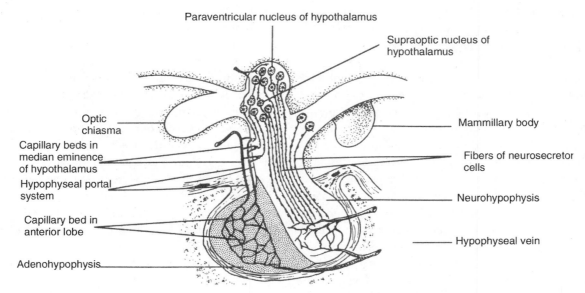

Figure 3–7 The anatomical relationship between the hypothalamic neurons, the hypothalamic-hypophyseal portal system, and the pituitary gland.

somatostatin). Thyrotropin-releasing hormone (TRH) stimulates the release of thyroid-stimulating hormone. **Gonadotropin-releasing hormone (GnRH)** causes the release of both FSH and LH. Two hypothalamic hormones, melanocyte-stimulating hormone-releasing hormone (MRH) and melanocyte-stimulating hormone-inhibiting hormone (MIH), regulate the release of MSH.

What Causes the Release of the Releasing Hormone?

The monthly rhythmic functioning of the female reproductive cycle is totally dependent on the changing concentrations of the steroid hormones estrogen and progesterone, which are secreted in response to the changing concentrations of the pituitary gonadotropins FSH and LH, which are in turn secreted in response to hypothalamic GnRH. GnRH is secreted in a rhythmic, pulsatile fashion, one pulse every 60–90 minutes throughout most of the cycle, decreasing in frequency closer to menstruation. This highly complex and intricate relationship is based on both positive and negative feedback mechanisms. For a long time it has been known that variations in the release of FSH and LH are the result of feedback from gonadal steroids, but just where the feedback effects occur—whether at the hypothalamic level or the pituitary level or both—has been extensively investigated.

The classic concept is that the site for feedback control by estrogen and progesterone is in the hypothalamus and it is based upon evidence from experiments with rodents. In rats and mice, the feedback centers, called tonic and cyclic centers, are located in the hypothalamus and consist of a group of steroid-sensitive neurons. The tonic center is responsible for a continuous day-to-day basal release of GnRH in males and females and is responsive to the negative feedback effects of sex steroids; the cyclic center, present in the female brain, is responsible for an additional periodic release of GnRH, resulting from the positive stimulatory effect of estrogen, which causes a midcycle outpouring of the gonadotropins FSH and LH from the anterior pituitary. This concept is still accurate for rodents but becomes confusing and controversial as to how it may operate in higher primates.

Direct evidence for a hypothalamic site of feedback control in humans could be obtained by the same kinds of experiments done in rodents, that is, those that involve destroying the hypothalamic areas where GnRH is produced, cutting the connection between the hypothalamus and the pituitary, implanting steroids directly into the hypothalamus to assess the effects, or sampling the GnRH levels in the portal blood vessels. Obviously these studies cannot be performed in women, so most of the research has taken place in female monkeys. According to the current concept of the neuroendocrine control of the menstrual cycle, the role of the hypothalamus is permissive, that is, its pulsatile secretion is a necessary prerequisite for normal pituitary and ovarian function. In response to each GnRH pulse, a pulse of FSH and LH is discharged by the pituitary to get into the general circulation and reach the ovaries. If the pulses are slowed down or slightly increased, follicles do not develop properly and hormone production is disturbed. GnRH release is mediated through the brain neurotransmitter, dopamine, which inhibits GnRH, and the neurotransmitter norepinephrine, which is thought to have stimulatory effects.

Under normal physiological conditions, then, the GnRH pulses cause gonadotropin (FSH and LH) pulses. Under the influence of gonadotropic hormone stimulation, the ovarian follicles develop and produce estrogen, which increases in the circulation, reaches the pituitary gland, and affects the amounts of FSH and LH secreted without significantly affecting the pulse frequency (negative feedback). When the estrogen level gets high enough, the negative feedback effect on the pituitary is reversed. Now estrogen causes a midcycle positive feedback effect on the pituitary, which results in a surge of LH and FSH and causes ovulation. Under LH influence, the ruptured follicle becomes the corpus luteum and secretes progesterone. Although progesterone reduces the frequency of the hypothalamic GnRH pulses, the amount of LH released from the pituitary is proportionally increased to sustain the corpus luteum and the production of progesterone. In the absence of pregnancy, the corpus luteum degenerates, progesterone levels decline, and menstruation occurs. The GnRH pulses return to their frequency at the beginning of the follicular phase and a new cycle begins.

This model of the control system for the ovarian cycles of higher primates is the hypothesis currently accepted. It assumes that the main target of negative and positive feedback effects of estrogen and progesterone is the anterior pituitary but also recognizes a number of additional inputs (from higher brain centers, the autonomic nervous system, ovarian factors) to the GnRH pulse-generating system. These modulate the pulsatile pattern and influence the signal.

Psychic Effects on Menstruation.

Apparently, GnRH can be affected by other internal and external factors. How emotional distress, reaction to a new and strange situation, or concern over a possible unwanted pregnancy can translate itself into a hormonal effect is not clear, but most women are aware that such things exist because the visible effect is delay or cessation of menstrual periods. The clue may be the relationship of the hypothalamus to the entire limbic system of the brain. The amygdala, that part of the limbic system that receives signals from all parts of the cerebral cortex and transmits those signals not only back to the cerebral cortex but also especially to the hypothalamus, is thought to be the monitor of all emotional stimuli that control the overall patterns of behavior. In the situation of stopped or missed periods that are not a result of pregnancy, it can be theorized that emotional stress may be mediated through the amygdala to suppress GnRH in the hypothalamus. If GnRH is inhibited, LH from the anterior pituitary is not released, ovulation from the ovary does not occur, and menstruation may not take place.

Another explanation for how stress causes missed or absent periods involves the effect of endogenous opiates on GnRH pulses. As described previously, normal menstrual function is dependent on GnRH pulsatile secretion, which is mediated via two brain neurotransmitters—inhibitory dopamine and stimulatory norepinephrine. In turn, this double neurotransmitter system can be modified by the influence of gonadal steroids and endorphins, particularly beta-endorphin. Since there is evidence that the endogenous opiates inhibit FSH and LH release by suppressing the hypothalamic release of GnRH (Speroff, Glass, & Kase, 1994) and that the levels of endogenous opiates increase with stress, this may be a pathway by which stress interrupts the menstrual cycle. Also, in a review of opiates in exercise physiology, Cumming & Wheeler (1987) concluded that many studies indicate an increase in endorphins with strenuous exercise. It is possible that "runner's high" could play a role in the amenorrhea frequently found in women runners.

STEROID HORMONES

Chemical Composition

All steroid hormones in the body are produced by the ovaries, the testes, the cortex of the adrenal glands, and the placenta during pregnancy. Steroid hormones are usually divided into four groups: the **estrogens,** the **androgens, progesterone,** and the **corticosteroids.** The first three are called the sex steroids because they are responsible for the physical and physiological differences that exist between males and females. Estrogens and progesterone are the female sex hormones, and androgens are the male sex hormones.

Steroid is a general term applied to a group of substances that all have a common structural nucleus. Steroids are found in both plants and animals and include a large number of body constituents, vitamins, and drugs, as well as sex hormones. The chemical nucleus they all have in common is called the *cyclopentanoperhydrophenanthrene ring,* which is really not as intimidating as it looks and sounds. Three rings have 6 carbon atoms each and make up the phenanthrene part; one has 5 carbon atoms and is the cyclopentane. Conventionally, the rings are designated A through D, and the carbon atoms are numbered C_1 through C_{17}, as shown.

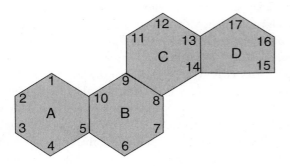

When there is an 18th carbon atom in the form of a methyl group attached at C_{13}, the resulting nucleus is called *estrane* and is the source of all the natural estrogens.

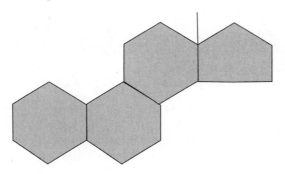

Estrane

All androgens derive from the *androstane* nucleus, which has a 19th carbon atom attached at C_{10}.

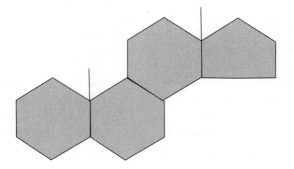

Androstane

Steroids that have 21 carbon atoms are known as the *pregnane* nucleus and give rise to progesterone, its derivatives, and the corticosteroids.

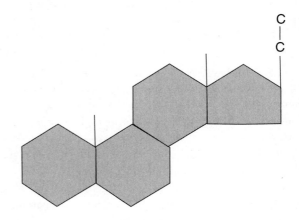

Pregnane

Synthesis of the Steroid Hormones

The basic building block for the synthesis of steroids is **cholesterol,** a 27-carbon compound with the steroid nucleus. Cholesterol has negative associations for most people in relation to its link to hardening of the arteries and cardiovascular disease, and everyone is aware of the implications of a high plasma cholesterol level. Although high dietary intake of cholesterol-containing foods can lead to elevated blood cholesterol levels, cholesterol is formed endogenously in all the cells of the body because it is part of their membrane structures, and it is likely that cell synthesis of cholesterol is inversely related to dietary consumption. All the endocrine tissues that produce sex hormones assemble them bit by bit through a biosynthetic pathway, starting with cholesterol.

The ovaries produce all three types of sex steroids: the estrogens, progesterone, and the androgens. The follicular structures (the **theca externa** and the **granulosa cells**) tend preferentially to produce estrogens, the **corpus luteum** cells produce progesterone, and the ovarian stroma or connective tissue, the androgens. Androgens are produced in females by both the ovaries and, to a greater extent, by the **adrenal glands.** In the ovaries, some androgens are precursors in the pathway to the synthesis of estrogens. In the male, the interstitial cells between the seminiferous tubules of the testes produce androgen, but some estrogen is synthesized by the testes and the adrenals.

The pathways for the synthesis of all four types of steroids are shown in Table 3–1. Cholesterol gives rise to pregnenolone, a compound with little known biological activity, which gives rise to progesterone, androgens, and estrogens. The route for the synthesis of estrogens diverges from that of progesterone at pregnenolone. All the steps require energy in the form of ATP and involve enzymes located in the mitochondria of the cells. The reactions that result in the forma-

tion of corticosteroids do not take place in gonadal tissue, but only in the adrenal glands.

Estrogens

Estrogen is a general term. It is used for all those substances that produce the biological effects characteristic of estrogenic hormones. Although there are many naturally occurring estrogens in the body, the three, in order of greatest potency, are **estradiol, estrone,** and **estriol.** There are other types of estrogens that are administered clinically, such as the **conjugated equine estrogens,** derived from the urine of pregnant mares, and synthetic estrogens like diethylstilbestrol (DES), tamoxifen, and raloxifene, which do not

TABLE 3–1   The Synthesis of Estrogens, Progestins, Androgens, and Corticosteroids from Cholesterol

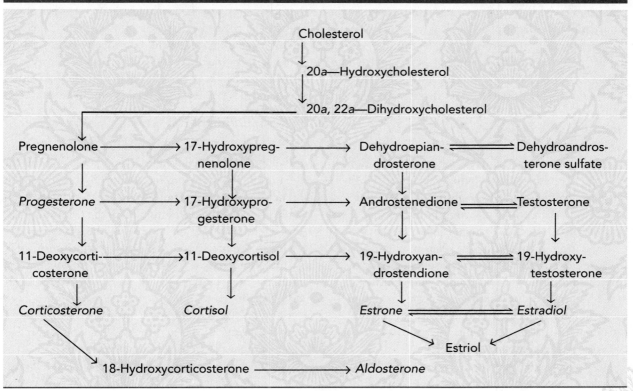

have a steroid structure but still have an estrogenic effect. Because it has been known only since the late 1990s that there are two estrogen receptors, one called **estrogen-receptor-alpha (ER-alpha)** and the other **estrogen-receptor-beta (ER-beta),** and that the distribution of the two types varies in the many different cells of the body sensitive to estrogen, the mechanism of action of administered estrogen and related synthetics is clearly more complex than previously thought.

Physiological Effects of Estrogens. Estrogens cause the growth of a thick, folded vaginal epithelium, differentiated into layers, and resistant to trauma and infections. The cells accumulate glycogen, which is acted on by lactobacilli to produce the acidic vaginal secretions. As a result of estrogen stimulation, cervical glands produce a clear, watery secretion with little mucus and low viscosity, which facilitates sperm passage into the uterus. In addition, the uterine endometrium is stimulated to grow, resulting in both an increase in the numbers of cells (hyperplasia) and an increase in the size of existing cells (hypertrophy). The muscle of the uterus shows an increased tendency to contract. Furthermore, estrogens cause the lining of the fallopian tubes to increase in thickness and there is an enhanced ability of the cilia to beat toward the uterus. In the breasts, estrogen causes growth of the duct tissue and increases fat deposition, thereby enlarging breast size.

Estrogen causes an increase in bone formation. In girls, the growth spurt at puberty is enhanced by it, but estrogen also causes the closing of the epiphyseal cartilages at the ends of the long bones so that cessation of growth occurs. Estrogen influences total body configuration, not only in the skeleton, but also in the increased deposition of fat in all subcutaneous tissue, particularly in the buttocks, thighs, and breasts.

The strength of capillary walls is increased by estrogen, and when estrogen levels are low before and during menstruation, there may be a greater tendency to bruise and have nosebleeds.

Estrogen causes a reduction in blood cholesterol levels and a decrease in the cholesterol-rich fraction of the plasma lipoproteins known as low-density lipoproteins (LDLs).

Liver cells are stimulated by estrogen to produce greater amounts of some blood proteins, particularly those involved in blood clotting, red blood cell formation, and certain of the globulins that bind to some hormones to transport them through the bloodstream.

The steroid-sensitive areas of the hypothalamus are affected by estrogen so that the production of GnRH is enhanced or inhibited. The temperature-regulating and vasomotor centers of the hypothalamus controlling the nerves that cause the dilation and constriction of blood vessels are also affected, and the basal body temperature is lowered during the first, or estrogen, half of the menstrual cycle.

Progestins

Progestins is a general term referring to chemical agents, both natural and synthetic, that produce changes in the uterine endometrium after it has previously been primed by estrogen. In vertebrates, the naturally occurring progestin is progesterone, and in women it produces the characteristic secretory and glandular changes in the endometrium after ovulation has occurred. Progesterone is used synonymously with progestin; another term is progestogen.

Physiological Effects of Progesterone. Progesterone prepares the endometrial lining of the uterus for the implantation of a fertilized ovum. To this end, it also inhibits uterine contractions so that an implanted ovum is retained. It also reduces motility in the fallopian tubes. Progesterone causes an increase in the glandular elements of the breasts, but the actual production of milk by the mammary glands is a function of the influence of prolactin after the breasts have been prepared for lactation by estrogen and progesterone. Progesterone causes cervical mucus to become viscous, which tends to prevent the passage of sperm through the cervical os. It also causes a slight rise in basal body temperature.

Progesterone causes an increase in the excretion of water and sodium from the kidneys. This makes it unlikely that progesterone alone is responsible for the water retention and swelling that occur in many women in the second, or progesterone, half of the menstrual cycle.

Androgens

Androgen is a term generally used synonymously with male sex hormone, but functionally it means any compound that has certain masculinizing effects. The androgen produced by the interstitial cells of the male testes is testosterone, but the adrenal glands produce at least five other androgens.

In the same way that estrogens are responsible in women for those physical and physiological features that distinguish femaleness, androgens are responsible for those features in men that are characteristically male.

Physiological Effects of Androgens.
The **testosterone** secreted by the fetal testes during prenatal development causes male differentiation of the embryonic reproductive tract.

After puberty, testosterone produced by the testes causes an increase in the growth and development of the male genitalia. It is responsible for the distribution of hair in the male pattern—increased on the body and decreased on the top of the head. Testosterone causes enlargement of the larynx and an increase in the length and thickness of the vocal cords, thereby causing a deeper voice. The thickness and texture of the skin is increased, and the skin tone is darkened. Another skin effect is an increase in sebaceous gland secretion, and testosterone is believed to be involved in acne in both males and females. The male sex hormone causes an increase in muscle mass and an increase in the size and strength of the skeleton in general, resulting in the larger body configuration of the male. It causes an increase in the rate of metabolism, heightening activity of all body cells, and results in greater numbers of red blood cells, thus resulting in a greater oxygen capacity in males. Both the ovaries and the adrenals in females produce testosterone, and various precursors to testosterone are produced by those glands and can be metabolized to testosterone by other organs. When plasma levels of testosterone approach the male range—a situation that can result from diseases of the ovary or adrenals—there are masculinizing effects on females. These can include excessive development and distribution of hair, voice and skin changes, and changes in fat distribution.

𝒫UBERTY

Puberty is the transition period between childhood and adulthood when physical and psychological changes that are associated with the ability to reproduce take place. **Menarche** is the term for the onset of the menstrual periods, but ovulation generally does not take place for a year or more afterward. Menarche, then, is not the indication of full sexual maturity.

The physical changes associated with puberty will be described later. The endocrine events that control the onset of puberty have been extensively investigated, and there are several hypotheses that attempt to explain it. Of course, attention focuses on the hypothalamus, but the onset of puberty is influenced by genetic factors, social and economic factors relating to nutrition and general health, and possibly (although research is scant) on external environmental factors mediated through the limbic system and the hypothalamus.

The hypothalamus controls more than gonadal function; it also regulates many body activities and a variety of behavioral functions. It may be that all of these activities are integrated with each other to provide a combination of events in addition to the onset of the hypothalamic–hypophyseal–ovarian function that controls the onset of sexual maturity.

One theory of control of puberty in girls has been called the **"gonadostat" hypothesis,** a play on words from a thermostat device for controlling temperature. It postulates that the immature hypothalamic-pituitary unit functions during childhood as a "gonadostat," is set at a particular level, and is extremely sensitive to the feedback action of the small amounts of circulating estrogen produced by the ovaries and to inhibin, a glycoprotein produced by ovarian granulosa cells. Accordingly, FSH and LH are not produced in appreciable amounts by the anterior pituitary prior to puberty. Then, for undetermined reasons, the gonadostat matures. Its sensitivity to circulating hormones decreases and the anterior pituitary becomes progressively responsive to pulsatile GnRH. The FSH and LH levels rise, ovarian steroids subsequently increase, and the transition into puberty is triggered. The factors involved in this maturing and desensitization of the gonadostat are unknown. There may be some kind of internal timekeeping mechanism in another part of the brain, possibly the limbic system, that recognizes age and growth and reverses the inhibition of pulsatile GnRH. A role for adrenal gland dehydroepiandrosterone (DHEA) has been suggested because DHEA secretion typically rises in children preceding puberty.

HORMONES AND THE MONTHLY CYCLES

The menstrual cycle involves the rhythmic fluctuations of the hormones of the hypothalamus, anterior pituitary, and ovaries, and the morphological changes that occur in the ovaries and the **endometrium** of the uterus. The endometrium is the mirror of the ovaries; whatever is going on in the uterus during the cycle is precisely correlated with whatever is occurring in the ovaries. The purpose of the ovarian cycle is to produce an ovum; the purpose of the endometrial cycle is to prepare a haven to nourish and maintain that ovum should it become fertilized. The ovarian cycle can be divided into three phases: the **follicular phase, ovulation,** and the **luteal phase.** The **endometrial cycle** can be divided into the menstrual and proliferative phases (which correspond to the follicular phase in the ovaries) and into the **secretory phase** or **progestational phase,** which is synchronized with the luteal phase of the ovaries (Figure 3–8).

All that most studies have indicated about the length of the menstrual cycle is its extreme variability. For purposes of description, a 28-day cycle is generally used, with ovulation occurring on the 14th day before menstruation.

Ovarian Cycle

Follicular Phase. The primary follicles in the ovary contain the stored oocytes, arrested in the prophase stage of meiosis with all 46 chromosomes still enclosed by a nuclear membrane. As indicated in Chapter 2, throughout the reproductive life of a woman, and without any help from FSH and LH, every day a small number of primary follicles begin to recommence growth. Most of them will undergo atresia, but what happens to a group of developing follicles at any point in time depends on whether adequate levels of FSH and LH in the circulation coincide with the development of receptors for FSH and LH on the granulosa and theca cells of the **follicles.** At the beginning of the ovarian cycle, the cells of the anterior pituitary respond to the signal of GnRH from the hypothalamus by secreting FSH and LH. The best developed follicles, that is, those with enough granulosa cells, develop receptors for estrogen and FSH on the cells of the granulosa layers and LH receptors on the theca cells. The initial role of FSH is to induce an increase in the development of its own receptors on the granulosa cells so that they can produce estrogen. The initial role of LH is to stimulate theca cell production of androgens, which are then converted to estrogen by the granulosa layers. Thus, estrogen production during the follicular phase is explained by the so-called two-cell (theca and granulosa) and two-gonadotropin (FSH and LH) mechanism.

The increasing levels of estrogen tend to suppress FSH because of the negative feedback effect. The decline in FSH tends to inhibit the further development of the follicles, but by then a dominant follicle has been selected. This follicle was chosen for ovulation as early as day 5 because its rate of granulosa proliferation exceeded that of all the others, and it has the

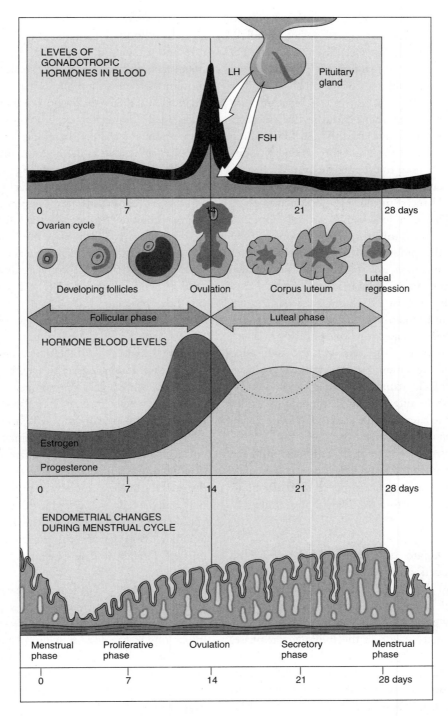

Figure 3–8 The hormonal levels and events of the endometrial and ovarian cycles in the absence of fertilization.

capacity for continued growth despite the decreased levels of FSH because its greater number of granulosa cells necessarily gives it greater FSH and estrogen receptor content. The dominant follicle produces more estrogen than the combined efforts of all the other developing follicles. Its estrogen, in combination with FSH, induces the development of more LH receptors on the outermost granulosa layers. These LH-binding sites are critical for ovulation and for subsequent conversion of the follicle to the corpus luteum.

Increased levels of estrogen are not the only inhibitors of FSH secretion during the follicular phase of the cycle. The granulosa and theca cells secrete a peptide hormone called **inhibin,** which suppresses FSH secretion from the pituitary gland. **Activin,** another peptide hormone, enhances FSH secretion, but follicular fluid contains more inhibin than activin. One hypothesis for the function of inhibin is that early in the cycle, the inhibin produced by all the newly developed follicles limits FSH release from the pituitary and sets the stage for one follicle—the one with the slight edge on development—to emerge as the dominant follicle. The dominant follicle maintains its superiority and continues to flourish despite the initial inhibition of FSH by inhibin and the later negative feedback effect on FSH by the increasing amounts of estrogen.

Final maturation of the dominant follicle until the time of ovulation is suppressed by **oocyte maturation inhibitor,** a peptide hormone in follicular fluid. Its effect ends hours before the LH surge described as follows.

Ovulation. Despite the waning FSH levels, the accelerated production of estrogen from the dominant follicle continues. Although low levels of estrogen cause a decrease in LH, high levels of estrogen result in a positive stimulatory effect and cause an increase in LH. As estrogen levels increase during the midfollicular phase, they ultimately attain the critical blood level of approximately 200 picograms/ml that is maintained for up to 50 hours. This surge of estrogen affects the pituitary and hypothalamus and is followed by a peak burst of LH,

which causes ovulation. The LH surge causes a number of changes in the follicle that has been selected for rupture and growing about 1 mm/day. First, the nuclear membrane around the oocyte breaks down, the chromosomes progress through the rest of the first meiotic division, and the egg moves on to the secondary oocyte stage. At this point, for some unknown reason, meiosis stops again and will continue only if the ovum is fertilized. LH also results in the luteinization of the granulosa cells, and they begin to produce progesterone, which enhances the positive feedback effect of estrogen on the LH surge. Progesterone also is responsible for encouraging the activity of enzymes in the follicular fluid capable of digesting the follicle wall. Next, the high levels of LH cause the synthesis of prostaglandins of the E and F type, which reach a peak concentration in the follicular fluid at ovulation and are essential for follicle rupture. Just how prostaglandins induce the expulsion of the oocyte is unknown, but their role in ovulation is so well known that women who want to become pregnant probably should avoid the use of drugs (aspirin, ibuprofen) that inhibit prostaglandin synthesis.

Thus, at midcycle, the estrogen surge produces the LH surge, which, in turn, stimulates a series of events leading to ovulation about 34–36 hours later. The follicle wall becomes stretched and thinned out, proteolytic enzymes in the follicular fluid are activated, prostaglandins exert their influence, and the ovum (actually the oocyte), accompanied by its protective and nourishing cumulus cells, is expelled to be sucked up by the ciliated, fingerlike fimbriae of the fallopian tube. The granulosa cells left in the ruptured follicle enlarge, undergo luteinization, and become the corpus luteum.

Luteal Phase. The corpus luteum produces progesterone and estrogen and reaches a peak of activity 8 days after ovulation. If there is a fertilized ovum, it is implanting in the endometrium of the uterus at about that time. If fertilization does not occur and there are no hormones from the developing embryo to increase its life span, the corpus luteum regresses. After 14–16 days, its life is over.

In the human, it is not yet known what causes the demise of the corpus luteum, or even precisely what sustains it before it declines. During the luteal phase, the FSH and LH in the blood are at their lowest levels at the same time estrogen and progesterone levels are at their highest, which would appear to be the consequence of negative feedback effects of the steroids on gonadotropin secretion. Although FSH and LH levels are low, however, they do not completely disappear, and there is always the continuous presence of small amounts of LH throughout the cycle. There is some evidence that the estrogen produced by the corpus luteum hastens its decline and that local concentrations of prostaglandin may be involved. Some researchers believe that the corpus luteum is autonomous and has an inherent life span of 2 weeks unless pregnancy takes place.

With the decline of the corpus luteum, the levels of estrogen and progesterone decrease rapidly, their negative feedback effect is diminished, and the FSH and LH can again increase to initiate a new cycle.

Endometrial Cycle

The endometrium consists of two layers: a superficial one that contains glands and occupies two-thirds of the endometrium, and a thin basal layer. The superficial layer is the one that responds to steroids, changes to a great extent during the cycle, and is almost completely lost during menstruation. The basal layer does not change in character during the cycle.

From day 1 to day 4, the endometrium is in the **menstrual phase.** After day 4 until a day or two after ovulation, the endometrium is in the **proliferative phase.** Even while menstruation is occurring, estrogen from the developing follicles in the ovaries causes cell division that repairs the denuded areas in the uterine lining. Regeneration of the sloughed-off superficial layer occurs rapidly. Within a few days of menstruation, the entire uterine cavity is covered with new epithelial cells. The gland cells of the superficial layer proliferate rapidly but do not accumulate much secretion at this time.

The second half of the endometrial cycle is called the *secretory phase* because the glands of the endometrium become dilated as they fill up with secretions of substances like glycogen and fats. The endometrium becomes twice as thick as it was in the previous phase, cushiony and nutritive, thereby forming a hospitable site for implantation of a fertilized ovum. It is also called the *progestational phase* because the changes that occur in the superficial layer of the endometrium are the result of the action of progesterone.

Toward the end of the secretory phase, if pregnancy has not occurred, the endometrium begins to regress. It is no longer supported by the high levels of progesterone and estrogen that are now undergoing rapid decline. The breakdown of the superficial layer of the endometrium is caused by lack of estrogen and progesterone stimulation, but the actual bleeding has to do with the special type of arteries present in the endometrium. The endometrium of the human female and the uteri of other female primates contain particular coiled spiral arteries, and only female mammals with this unique kind of spiral blood vessel are able to menstruate. As the endometrium regresses, these arteries become even more tortuously coiled in the rapidly thinning layer. The blood circulation through them slows down. Some of the arteries intermittently constrict, cutting off the blood flow to the areas they supply, and the tissue dies from lack of blood. Prostaglandins, especially PGF_{2a}, may play a role in inducing arterial constriction. When the arteries dilate again, the blood escapes from the top where the tissue has already disintegrated. The little pools of blood rupture through the endometrial surface into the uterine cavity. The same sequence occurs in other arteries during the next few days. As more of the superficial layer disintegrates, small pieces of endometrium become detached, and glandular secretions and blood slowly ooze into the uterine cavity.

For 4 or 5 days, approximately 50 ml of blood, glandular secretions, and some tissue fragments flow from the uterine cavity through the cervical os and out the vagina. That amounts to 3½ tablespoons of blood.

Menstrual blood does not clot because some of the clotting factors ordinarily found in blood have been lysed by lysosomal enzymes in the uterus. The clots that may appear to form with a heavier flow are a combination of red blood cells, mucus, glycogen, and glycoproteins and form in the vagina rather than in the uterus, possibly because the amount of flow is too great for the amount of lysing enzymes.

MENSTRUAL HYGIENE

Menstrual blood is sterile and in no way unclean. Many women are overly concerned with hygiene and odor during the period of flow. Even the word *sanitary* in sanitary napkin implies a certain uncleanliness and reinforces the association of menstruation with impurity and **sepsis**—an association recognized by manufacturers who no longer use the term and now call their products mini- or maxi- "pads" or "shields." Actually, pads may be quite unsanitary, particularly if changed infrequently, because they form a breeding ground for bacteria as well as a potential pathway for organisms to migrate from the rectum to the vagina or urethra. Since menstrual blood develops an odor only after being exposed to air, an alternative means of protection against potential vaginitis, urethritis, and odor would appear to be internal absorption of the menstrual flow by tampons. The possible correlation between tampon usage and toxic shock syndrome, however, has created a quandary for women who are reluctant to give up the convenience of tampons but have qualms about the potential risk. A complete discussion of toxic shock and tampon usage follows in Chapter 4.

Any woman who chooses to use tampons can do so. There are no normal vaginas that cannot accommodate them. Difficulty in insertion usually turns out to be more emotional than physical. If necessary, lubrication with sterile jelly can assist in insertion. If the hymenal aperture is very small in adolescence, it is possible to accomplish painless stretching by using a tampon with a cardboard applicator and a little lubricating jelly. After a few months, there should be no problem in inserting tampons, and visible evidence of virginity will still exist if that need is important.

MENSTRUAL SYNCHRONY

An interesting phenomenon, which mothers and daughters in the same house may have noticed but never really thought about, was reported first in 1971 by a Harvard graduate student. Martha McClintock observed that females living in close proximity tended to menstruate at approximately the same time. When the time of onset of the menstrual flow was studied in 135 young women 17–22 years of age who were living together in a dormitory, the menstrual cycles were synchronized as to day of onset in a significant number of women who were close friends but not roommates. But when they were close friends and roommates, the simultaneous onset was even more highly significant. Stranger yet, when the young women were asked to keep track of their menstrual cycles and dating frequency, it was observed that those who dated most often had shorter cycles. Two Scottish researchers subsequently confirmed that **menstrual synchronization** occurred among women who were not roommates but close friends and who spent a lot of time together. In contrast to McClintock's data, however, they found no significant correlation between cycle length and the amount or type of interaction with men (Graham & McGrew, 1980.) Quadagno, Subeita, Deck, and Francoeur (1981) reported that menstrual synchrony occurred among three and four women living together as well as between pairs but also saw no effect of socialization with males. Veith et al. (1983), however, found that women who spent at least two or more nights with men during a 40-day period had more frequent occurrence of ovulation than women who had no nights or only one night of sleeping with a man. Because the women's cycle length was unaffected by their sleeping arrangements, the investigators concluded that the mechanism was unknown, but speculated that it may have something to do with odor.

Over the past several decades, a number of studies confirmed the existence of menstrual synchrony, while others refuted it. Sociologists, anthropologists, psychologists, and biologists investigated the possibility of the phenomenon with varying results. Trevathan, Burleson, and Gregory (1993) found no evidence for menstrual synchrony in cohabiting lesbian couples, a result confirmed by Weller and Weller (1998). The Wellers, who are Israeli psychologists who studied Bedouin women, reported in 1997 that they did find a definite but very moderate shift toward menstrual synchrony (20% to 25%) in Bedouin women between 13 and 50 years of age who shared living space. The Wellers, however, as well as other researchers, have published critiques of menstrual synchrony research based on methodological issues (Wilson, 1992; Weller & Weller, 1997; Miller, 1998).

There are believers and nonbelievers concerning the existence of menstrual synchrony, and definitive answers await future research. But since McClintock's original publication, there have been suggestions that human odors play a role in why it occurs.

Russell, Switz, and Thompson (1980) tried to find out whether underarm perspiration could be a stimulus for synchronous cycles. For a period of 4 months, they had five female volunteers daily rub on their upper lips cotton pads containing the perspiration odor from a donor female with regular cycles, while six controls rubbed plain cotton pads on their upper lips. At the end of the experiment, there was no change in the onset dates of menstrual flow between the control subjects and the "sweat donor," but the average difference in date of onset of menstruation between the experimental group (the women who rubbed sweat on their lips) and the donor was reduced from 9.3 days to 3.4 days, suggesting that synchronization had occurred. This study was criticized for lacking a double-blind research procedure (a double-blind experiment is one in which neither the experimenter nor the subjects know which part of the experiment is the control, and prevents bias in recording the data) and was

replicated by Preti, Cutler, Garcia, Huggins, and Lawley (1986) using more subjects and a double-blind protocol. Their results were similar to the earlier study in that the women who received applications of the axillary extracts had a significant alteration in the time of the onset of menstruation that matched the cycles of the donor females. Although the methodology of the Preti et al. study was also criticized (Wilson, 1987), it conforms with the earlier work and does appear to provide a clue as to how the menstrual synchrony phenomenon can occur. The idea that people, like animals from insects to elephants (see Chapter 2), can influence each other by odorless chemical signals, or pheromones, also has produced believers and nonbelievers.

Winnifred Cutler and her colleagues (1979, 1986) are believers. These investigators found that shorter (closer to "normal") menstrual cycles as well as higher levels of plasma estradiol appeared to be associated with regular weekly sexual intercourse, at least in small samples of college women. To check the possibility that a chemical signal from males could be involved, the experiments described previously were repeated using underarm extracts from donor males instead of females. It was found that compared to the controls who received blank applications, the women who received applications of sweat derived from male donors for 12–14 weeks had reduced cycle length variability and a decrease in the number of aberrant length cycles, that is, more regular cycles. Although correlations between sexual behavior and cycle length are provocative, obviously it would be a giant leap at this point to infer that there is scientific evidence that having weekly heterosexual sex would benefit irregular menstrual cycles. More recently, Cutler, Freidmann, and McCoy (1998) tested whether synthesized human male pheromone, advertised as "designed to improve the romance in their lives," increased the sexual behavior of men when compared with a placebo. Although the investigators admitted that the initial data need replication, they reported that a significantly larger proportion of pheromone users than placebo users increased sociosexual behaviors such as kissing, petting, or sexual intercourse with women but that there was no increase above baseline in solitary behaviors such as male masturbation. They concluded that human male pheromones thus had an effect on the sexual attractiveness of men to women.

The study that has provided to many the most compelling evidence of the existence of human pheromones was published by Kathleen Stern and Martha McClintock in 1998. The experiment involved 20 recipient women and 9 donor women. The donors wore cotton pads under their armpits for at least 8 hours, and pieces of the pads, which the recipients said were odorless, were wiped under the noses of the recipient women every day for four consecutive menstrual cycles. When the donors were in the follicular phase of their menstrual cycles, the armpit secretions accelerated the LH surge in the recipients, who ovulated earlier and their menstrual cycles were shortened. When the underarm secretions from the same donors were taken later at ovulation and were applied to the recipients, the recipients ovulated later and their menstrual cycle was lengthened. Secretions taken even later, during the luteal phase of the menstrual cycle, had no effect. Although the shortening or lengthening of the cycle did not occur in all the recipients—it occurred in about two-thirds of them—the results were certainly statistically significant. It appears from this study that human pheromones exist and that the timing of ovulation can be manipulated by them. Why this should happen at all or what the purpose of pheromones is in daily life remains a puzzle.

REFERENCES

Cumming, D. C., & Wheeler, G. D. (1987). Opioids in exercise physiology. *Seminars in Reproductive Endocrinology, 5,* 171–176.

Cutler, W. B., Freidmann, E., & McCoy, N. L. (1998). Pheromonal influences on sociosexual behavior in men. *Archives of Sexual Behavior, 27*(1), 1–13.

Cutler, W. B., Garcia, C. R., Huggins, G. R., & Preti, G. (1986). Sexual behavior and steroid levels among gynecologically mature premenopausal women. *Fertility and Sterility, 45*(4), 496–502.

Cutler, W. B., Garcia, C. R., & Krieger, A. M. (1979). Sexual behavior frequency and menstrual cycle length in mature premenopausal women. *Psychoneuroendocrinology 4,* 297–309.

Cutler, W. B., Preti, G., Krieger, A., Huggins, G. R., Garcia, C. R., & Lawley, H. J. (1986). Human axillary secretions influence women's menstrual cycles: The role of donor extract from men. *Hormones and Behavior, 20*(4), 463–473.

Delaney, J., Lupton, M. J., & Toth, E. (1988). *The Curse: A cultural history of menstruation.* Urbana, IL: University of Illinois Press.

Graham, C. A., & McGrew, W. C. (1980). Menstrual synchrony in female undergraduates living on a coeducational campus. *Psychoneuroendocrinology, 5,* 245–252.

Koff, E., Rierdan, J., & Stubbs, M. I. (1990). Conceptions and misconceptions of the menstrual cycle. *Women and Health, 16*(3–4), 119–136.

McClintock, M. K. (1971). Menstrual synchrony and suppression. *Nature, 229,* 244–245.

Miller, E. (1998). Menstrual synchrony: A methodological comment. *Mankind Quarterly, 38*(4), 363–481.

Preti, G., Cutler, W. B., Garcia, C. R., Huggins, G. R., & Lawley, H. J. (1986). Human axillary secretions influence women's menstrual cycles: The role of donor extract of females. *Hormones and Behavior, 20*(4), 474–482.

Quadagno, D. M., Subeita, H. E., Deck, J., & Francoeur, D. (1981). Influence of male social contacts, exercise, and all female living conditions on the menstrual cycle. *Psychoneuroendocrinology, 6,* 239–244.

Russell, M. J., Switz, G. M., & Thompson, K. (1980). Olfactory influences on the human menstrual cycle. *Pharmacology, Biochemistry, and Behavior, 13,* 737–738.

Speroff, L., Glass, R. H., & Kase, N. G. (1994). *Clinical gynecologic endocrinology and infertility* (5th ed.). Baltimore: Williams & Wilkins.

Stern, K., & McClintock, M. K. (1998). Regulation of ovulation human pheromones. *Nature, 392*(6672), 177–179.

Trevathan, W. R., Burleson, M. H., Gregory, W. L. (1993). No evidence for menstrual synchrony in lesbian couples. *Psychoneuroendocrinology, 18*(5–6), 425–435.

Weller, A., & Weller, L. (1997). Menstrual synchrony under optimal conditions: Bedouin families. *Journal of Comparative Psychology, 111*(2), 143–151.

Weller, A., & Weller, L. (1998). Prolonged and very intensive contact may not be conducive to menstrual synchrony. *Psychoneuroendocrinology, 23*(1), 19–32.

Weller, L., & Weller, A. (1997). Menstrual variability and the measurement of menstrual synchrony. *Psychoneuroendocrinology, 22*(2), 115–128.

Wilson, H. C. (1987). Female axillary secretions influence women's menstrual cycles: A critique. *Hormones and Behavior, 21*(4), 536–546.

Wilson, H. C. (1992). A critical review of menstrual synchrony research. *Psychoneuroendocrinology, 17*(6), 565–591.

Wilson, H. C. (1992). A critical review of menstrual synchrony research. Comment. *Psychoneuroendocrinology, 18*(7), 533–539.

Veith, J. L., Buck, M., Getzlaf, S., et al. (1983). Exposure to men influences the occurrence of ovulation in women. *Physiology and Behavior, 31*(3), 313–315.

CHAPTER

4

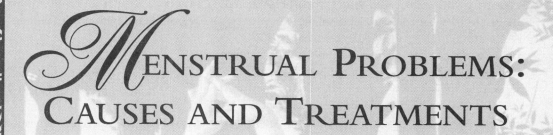

MENSTRUAL PROBLEMS: CAUSES AND TREATMENTS

KEY TERMS

Abnormal uterine bleeding

Amenorrhea

Dysfunctional uterine
   bleeding (DUB)

Dysmenorrhea

Endometriosis

Nonsteroidal
   anti-inflammatory drugs
   (NSAIDs)

Premenstrual syndrome
   (PMS)

Toxic shock syndrome (TSS)

What is "normal?" What is "regular?" The one unvarying aspect of the menstrual cycle is how extremely variable it is. The studies that have produced data concerning length and duration of the menstrual cycle are as variable as the cycles themselves. They have been made on women of different nationalities, occupations, nutritional status, and age. The extent to which these and other social variables produce variations has not been determined. The method of selecting samples of women who are included in the studies differ, and so do the methods of data analysis. Some investigations may have excluded women who do not "menstruate normally," whatever that

91

means. In some studies, all the cycles may have been lumped together for analysis; in others, the individual cycle for each woman may have been analyzed separately. It may be that the women who agree to participate in a study do so because they menstruate more regularly than women who refuse to participate, and this results in data of questionable validity.

It is important to recognize that the statistics that follow are based on such investigations. The figures generally pertain to what is considered average and not necessarily typical. With that admonition, they can provide a basis for distinguishing between what is regular and what is irregular, and, within a broad range, what is considered normal and abnormal.

MENSTRUAL STATISTICS

The mean length of the menstrual cycle is 25–30 days. Only about 10%–15% are exactly 28 days, and anywhere from 20–40 days is still considered within normal range. When cycles are shorter than 3 weeks, the woman is said to have *polymenorrhea*. If the cycles are longer than 40 days, the condition is *oligomenorrhea*. These short or long cycles may indicate a disturbance that is not serious and is of little functional significance. Two-thirds of all cycles vary in length by 6 days, and one-third have greater variability. There is more regularity to the menstrual cycles that occur between the ages of 20 and 40. The preovulatory phase in a longer cycle is the one that is more variable. The postovulatory phase is generally constant and lasts 13–15 days. That means that a woman with a 21-day cycle ovulates on day 7 and not halfway through the cycle.

The duration of menstrual flow is 4–6 days, although a flow for as few as 2 days or as many as 8 days is considered normal. *Hypomenorrhea* refers to a normal interval for the cycle, but the duration of the flow is short and the amount is scant. In *hypermenorrhea,* again the interval is normal, but the bleeding is excessively heavy for a normal length of time. When the menstrual bleeding time is prolonged, it is called *menorrhagia*. If bleeding occurs between periods and is unrelated to the cycle, it is termed *metrorrhagia*.

The amount of blood that is lost at each period is variable as well. It makes up only about half of the total menstrual flow, and while the average is 50 ml, it may be as little as 20 ml or as much as 80 ml and still be considered within normal range.

MENSTRUAL DISORDERS

Many women experience deviations from the average in their menstrual cycles during their reproductive years. Since feelings about one's maturity, being a normal woman, and being able to bear children, for example, are likely to focus on the visible evidence that everything is all right, most women are understandably anxious about delayed periods, missed periods, periods that are too scant, too profuse, or too frequent. But since there is so much variation in frequency of cycles, amount of flow, and duration of flow, how is a woman to know when it is necessary to seek medical attention? Generally, a change in bleeding pattern from what is normal and usual for her that persists for several months is an indication that there may be a problem.

All women who are not of the regular-every-28-days-like-a-clock type should keep a menstrual chart (Figure 4–1). Even if a woman is very regular, a change in the frequency, duration, or amount of the menstrual flow can easily be determined from such a chart.

Abnormal Uterine Bleeding

A variation over time in the normal pattern of menstrual cycles in terms of too much, too often, or too prolonged a flow could be an abnormality and require investigation. Or, it may be bleeding that occurs intermenstrually between what are otherwise regular periods. There are a variety of possible reasons for abnormal bleeding. The cause may be an endocrine disturbance because the hormones of the hypothala-

MENSTRUAL CHART

Month	1	2	3	4	5	6	7	8	9	10	11	12	13	14	15	16	17	18	19	20	21	22	23	24	25	26	27	28	29	30	31	No. of days from start of period to beginning of next
JANUARY																																
FEBRUARY																																
MARCH																																
APRIL																																
MAY																																
JUNE																																
JULY																																
AUGUST																																
SEPTEMBER																																
OCTOBER																																
NOVEMBER																																
DECEMBER																																

TYPE OF FLOW

Normal [X]

Exceptionally light [O]

Exceptionally heavy [■]

Figure 4–1 A menstrual record chart.

mus, the pituitary gland, the ovaries, the adrenal cortex, and the thyroid can all have an effect on the menstrual cycle. A physical disturbance of the tissues of the vagina, cervix, or uterus—what a physician calls an "organic lesion"—may also result in a change in bleeding pattern. Such a lesion could be benign (fibroids) or a malignant growth in the reproductive tract and will be discussed later.

Generally, **abnormal uterine bleeding** is considered in two categories: as occurring in conjunction with regular, ovulatory cycles or as bleeding that occurs in the absence of ovulation (anovulatory cycles). If abnormal bleeding is interspersed at times along with what are otherwise regular ovulatory menstrual cycles, confirmed by basal body temperature determinations or diagnostic tests, there are a number of possibilities. Light spotting that occurs just before or at the time of ovulation could be the result of the change in estrogen level just before the luteinizing hormone (LH) surge. Such midcycle bleeding is often accompanied by ovulatory pain *(mittelschmerz)*. Abnormal bleeding may also be the result of acute infection, a blood or liver disease, hormone or drug ingestion, or the presence of an intrauterine device. It may be caused by a complication of pregnancy—a spontaneous abortion (miscarriage) or an ectopic (out-of-place) pregnancy. Another bleeding abnormality that could occur in the presence of normal ovulation is caused by an inadequacy of the corpus luteum, also known as a luteal phase defect and sometimes associated with infertility. The cause of this condition, in which the corpus luteum secretes a very low level of progesterone, is essentially unknown and suspected to be multifactorial.

Dysfunctional Uterine Bleeding

After ruling out, through diagnostic tests and physical examination, all the other possible reasons for unpredictable, excessive, frequent, and/or prolonged bleeding, the problem is often called **dysfunctional uterine bleeding (DUB)** and believed to be due to hormonal abnormalities. Although DUB can occur during ovulatory cycles, it is usually associated with anovulatory cycles. In a cycle in which ovulation has not occurred, the endometrium is not stimulated by progesterone because a corpus luteum has not formed. The endometrium continues to grow in the proliferative phase. It becomes very thick but, lacking progesterone stimulation, never becomes secretory or receives the structural support that progesterone provides. When the ovarian theca and granulosa cells eventually disintegrate, the estrogen level decreases, causing menstruation. The bleeding from an estrogen-only stimulated endometrium is prolonged and heavy, and parts of it are shed irregularly. The bleeding continues until a new crop of follicles in the ovary produces enough estrogen to stimulate new endometrial cell growth. Cell regeneration then stops the bleeding.

Anovulatory cycles are most frequent during the two transitional periods of a woman's life, just after menarche and just before menopause, and DUB also commonly occurs during these periods. Irregularity in an adolescent girl is almost considered normal—about half of teenagers do not ovulate during their initial menstrual cycles—so mild dysfunctional bleeding may occur and resolve itself after several months to a year. It is treated only if the menstrual periods are distressingly heavy, frequent, unpredictable, and the adolescent becomes anemic as a result. Heavy and frequent menstruation also is not unusual in premenopausal women, but it is particularly important to be certain that no pathology exists. The incidence of uterine cancer increases with age, and any woman who has abnormal bleeding in the perimenopausal period or after she has completely stopped having menstrual periods should see a physician immediately for a complete diagnostic evaluation, especially if she is taking estrogen. Obese women are also prone to DUB because excess fat tissue can result in excess extraovarian estrogen production via the biochemical conversion of androstenedione to estrone.

Treatment of Abnormal Uterine Bleeding

Abnormal uterine bleeding is probably one of the most frequently encountered conditions in gynecological practice. The decision of how or whether to treat it is related to establishing the reason for it, the age of the woman, and the severity of the bleeding. Diagnostic tools during childbearing years should include using the basal body temperature and vaginal smear to establish whether ovulation has occurred; getting a complete blood count, a Pap smear, and a pregnancy test; determining blood and urine levels of hormones or their metabolites; testing for possible blood coagulation disorders, sexually transmitted diseases, and thyroid dysfunction; and/or using outpatient hospital procedures such as transvaginal ultrasonography to determine the thickness of the uterine endometrium, and endometrial biopsy if the endometrium is thicker than 5 mm. When a nonpregnant woman appears to have a pelvic mass on pelvic examination, an abdominal ultrasound, a CT scan, or if necessary, a laparoscopic examination is required for evaluation.

There are two basic ways to control, stop, or at least regulate abnormal uterine bleeding—by administering steroids or **nonsteroidal anti-inflammatory drugs (NSAIDs)** or by surgery. In adult women, especially around the time of the menopause, there is a greater chance of endometrial cancer or other uterine pathology, so an endometrial biopsy or a *dilatation and curettage* (D and C) usually is the first step to rule out that possibility. In the absence of anything dire, when the endometrium is removed surgically by a D and C, abnormal bleeding does not recur for some reason, or at least does not recur for several months. There should be little reason to perform a D and C in young girls, however. Not only are adolescents seldom subject to endometrial malignancies, but D and C rarely alleviates the anovulatory dysfunctional bleeding (Altchek, 1991).

Nonsurgical treatment is effected with the administration of oral or injected steroids. Oral contraceptive pills containing estrogen and progestins, given four times a day, often will stop excessive bleeding within 12–24 hours. Subsequently, it is possible to mimic normal cycles. and reduce abnormal bleeding by the administration of one combination birth control pill daily for 3–4 months. In a woman experiencing DUB just prior to menopause, an oral progestin taken in the second half of the menstrual cycle is likely to regulate the endometrial buildup. A commonly used oral progestin is medroxyprogesterone acetate (Provera) 10 mg/day, which may be prescribed for 10–14 days each month. When the progestin is discontinued, withdrawal bleeding (sometimes known as medical curettage) occurs. Natural progesterone may be given by injection or by vaginal suppositories. If progesterone or progestin does not correct DUB after two or three cycles, further diagnostic evaluation should take place.

Other nonhormonal and hormonal agents used to control DUB include NSAIDs, danazol used for endometriosis, and the administration of synthetic GnRH to suppress ovarian function. The nonsteroidal anti-inflammatory drugs are prostaglandin inhibitors. Their antiprostaglandin effect improves platelet aggregation responsible for blood clotting and increases constriction of the blood vessels in the uterus. Menstrual cramps (dysmenorrhea) often accompany excessive bleeding, and NSAIDs are effective for this problem as well, as is discussed later in the chapter.

Obviously, hysterectomy or removal of the uterus is the most definitive treatment for dysfunctional uterine bleeding. During their reproductive years, women should never agree to a hysterectomy for DUB except as a last resort after all other means of therapy have been tried.

As an alternative to hysterectomy in treatment of DUB that is unresponsive to hormonal therapy, physicians may use *endometrial ablation,* the total removal of the upper or functional layer and coagulation of the basal layer from which it grows, by laser; cautery; or thermal balloon, a less invasive, newer technique. The procedure was developed as a nonsurgical alternative for women who have excessive bleeding. Endometrial ablation allegedly prevents regeneration of the endometrium and the recurrence of DUB, although the endometrium does regenerate in some women who have undergone the procedure. The treatment, which requires general anesthesia or a spinal block, necessarily results in amenorrhea or very scant flow. Also, because most of the time there is not enough endometrium left to allow implantation, it tends to eliminate the possibility of pregnancy. Some women, therefore, have requested endometrial ablation as a form of birth control or to do away with their periods. As yet there are no long-term controlled studies to evaluate the safety, efficacy, or permanence of endometrial ablation.

Amenorrhea

Amenorrhea is the lack of menstruation during a woman's reproductive years. It is normal only during pregnancy. Amenorrhea itself is a symptom, not a disease. Once it has been established that there is no life-threatening underlying cause for the lack of menstruation, it is not medically serious. Psychologically, however, it can certainly be a major cause of anxiety in a girl who has not started to menstruate when all of her friends have. And when periods stop occurring after several years of reasonable regularity, there are so many possible etiological factors that, while it may not be ultimately important to treat it medically, it is obviously necessary to try to establish some reason for it.

Causes of Amenorrhea.   When menarche does not appear until the age of 16, it is called delayed menstruation and is most likely the result of a familial tendency to late maturation. Actual *primary amenorrhea* is the failure to menstruate by age 18. In more than 40% of cases, it is related to chromosomal abnormalities, malformation of the reproductive tract, or both. Less frequently, primary amenorrhea is caused by disorders of the thyroid, adrenal cortex, or (even more rarely) diseases of the pituitary gland. It can also result from extreme malnutrition.

Cryptomenorrhea (Greek: *kryptos,* hidden) is a term for "silent" menstruation. Uterine bleeding occurs, but it is blocked from exiting from the cervix or vagina. The most common reason for the condition is an imperforate hymen, but an infection that causes subsequent scar tissue formation in the vagina or cervix may result in cryptomenorrhea. It is rarely the result of total absence of the vagina, a genetic malformation. Cryptomenorrhea is usually diagnosed several years after puberty, and it is treated surgically.

Secondary amenorrhea is a term applied to the cessation of menstrual periods any time between menarche and menopause when the cause is not pregnancy. In the same unknown way that emotional factors can cause abnormal bleeding, an abrupt failure to menstruate may also have a psychological basis.

Secondary amenorrhea has often been traced to psychogenic factors such as stress, fear, anxiety, or trauma. A great fear of pregnancy or a tremendous desire for pregnancy can cause it; so can a change in environment or a death in the family. It also can result from an oversecretion of prolactin from the anterior pituitary (hyperprolactinemia). Although the exact mechanism is unknown, high levels of prolactin apparently inhibit the pulsatile secretion of GnRH and may also interfere with ovarian steroid modulation of pituitary function. Hyperprolactinemia is treated with bromocriptine, a drug that inhibits pituitary prolactin secretion.

Nutrition also has an effect on menstruation. Limited amenorrhea can result from a quick weight loss after a crash diet or it may be related to obesity. Some of the reasons for secondary amenorrhea are listed in Table 4–1. A more complete list could fill several pages.

Many of the cases of psychogenic secondary amenorrhea are temporary and self-limiting. No one ever died from not menstruating; it is not in itself dangerous or life threatening. The only significance over a long period of time in a young woman is that the lowered estrogen level might set the stage for osteoporosis by causing a loss of bone density. But because there is no evidence that administering hormones or inducing ovulation has any effect on the return of normal cycles if there is a psychological basis for amenorrhea, there is no reason to use hormone therapy to induce ovulation unless the woman wants to become pregnant. Generally speaking, excessive bleeding is always of greater concern than absence of bleeding.

An explanation of the hypothalamic amenorrhea associated with weight loss was proposed by Frisch and Revelle in 1970. The investigators postulated that there is a critical body weight (around 105–106 lb) that is

Table 4–1 Some Causes of Secondary Amenorrhea

Physiologic (Normal)	Anatomic	Central Nervous System (Hypothalamic)
Pregnancy	Chromosome disorders	Psychogenic
Lactation	Hysterectomy	Environmental
Menopause	Cryptomenorrhea	Nutritional
	Destruction of endometrium	Sudden weight loss
	Trauma (overly enthusiastic curettage)	Anorexia nervosa
	Disease (e.g., TB)	Obesity
	Irradiation	Iatrogenic (medically induced)
	Ovarian	Oral contraceptives ("post-pill amenorrhea")
	Disease (cysts, tumors, etc.)	
	Ovarian failure, premature menopause	Psychotropic drugs
	Destruction, through surgery, infection, irradiation	Thyroid dysfunction
		Adrenocortical dysfunction
	Pituitary	Chronic systemic disease
	Tumors, disease	Hyperprolactinemia
	Pituitary insufficiency	

associated with menarche and the maintenance of menstrual cycles. Frisch (1985) modified the hypothesis and suggested critical fatness—as indicated by a fatness index or the body composition of fat as a percentage of body weight—as the significant factor and Frisch, as well as other investigators, continues work on the critical fatness hypothesis (1993, 1994, 1996, 1997). According to the theory, 17% body fat is the minimum for the initiation of cycles at menarche, and 22% body fat is necessary to sustain menstrual cycles. After the start of regular menstrual cycles, a weight loss of 10%–15% of normal weight for height would represent a loss of body fat below the 22% level and may result in amenorrhea. Although there has been criticism of the critical weight/fatness theory, and investigators have subsequently found numerous examples where low body weight or percentage of fat appeared to be no deterrent to menarche, menstrual cycles, conception, pregnancy, or even repeated pregnancies, the relationship between weight loss and amenorrhea is valid for many women. Frisch (1985, 1987) has suggested at least four mechanisms whereby fatness influences menstruation: (1) Androgens produced by the ovaries are chemically converted to estrogen by fat tissue. Thus, body fat becomes an additional source of estrogen. (2) Body fat influences the way estrogen is metabolized; lean women make more of a less potent form of estrogen. (3) Obese women and fat young girls exhibit a decreased estrogen-binding capacity with sex-hormone-binding-globulin, a blood plasma transport protein that serves as a carrier of estrogen and testosterone into selected cells. (4) Fat tissue can store steroid hormones.

Normal menstruation is a complex process, however, and body weight, while important, is not likely to be the sole factor that influences it. While there is a strong association between thinness and disrupted menstruation, the currently favored theory is that a combination of physical, psychological, genetic, nutritional, and other, as yet unknown, factors act together to determine the time of onset of menarche, continued menstrual function, and fertility.

That there is a relationship between weight and hypothalamic GnRH function is supported by evidence that indicates that when a weight loss is self-imposed and severe, especially when coupled with physical or psychological stress, hypothalamic GnRH pulse frequency and gonadotropin release are disrupted. At first the endocrine changes may be subtle, as in luteal phase defect. Eventually oligomenorrhea or amenorrhea may result (Reame et al., 1985; Reid & Van Vugt, 1987; Warren et al., 1999).

Women who literally exercise off most of their excess body fat also have been discovered to have irregular or absent menstrual periods, and the term *athletic amenorrhea* has been used. Surveys of women long distance runners participating in National Amateur Athletic Union cross-country championships showed that a significant number were found to have fewer than two cycles a year. Wakat, Sweeney, and Rogot (1982) found that half of the cross-country runners studied had oligomenorrhea, and there have been similar findings of menstrual dysfunction in marathoners, gymnasts, and professional ballet dancers, who train as hard as football players and also worry more about their weight and appearance. Weight loss in itself, although common with intensive training, is apparently not the determining factor because not all athletes or ballerinas have dysfunctional periods, and those that do are often no different in height and weight than those who menstruate normally. They may differ, however, in their specific body composition, having greatly decreased subcutaneous fat and greatly increased lean muscle mass. Female athletes have generally been found to have body fat ranging between 5% and 6% of their body weight compared with an average fat range in women of 24%–34%. At any rate, when the grueling exercise stops, so does menstrual irregularity. Several studies (Warren, 1985; Abraham, Beumont, Fraser, & Llewellyn-Jones, 1982) of ballet dancers found that cessation of exercise (usually due to injury) brought a return of normal cycles but that when the young women went back to training, the menstrual dysfunction returned without any change in body weight. Unsurprisingly, however, there is no simple explanation for the relationship between strenuous exercise and disrupted or absent menstrual periods. Stress, a change in metabolism (an "energy drain" that modulates hypothalamic function), a self-imposed dietary restriction, pre-exercise menstrual irregularity, could all play independent roles. The underlying mechanism probably is hypothalmic GnRH inhibition, but although the suppression of LH-pulse frequency and amplitude reportedly occurs in some oligomenorrheic or amenorrheic women athletes, it does not occur in all (Veldhuis et al., 1985; Cumming, Vickovic, Wall, & Fluker, 1985). And while endogenous opiate secretion, known to suppress gonadotropins by inhibiting GnRH, is increased in exercise and may be responsible for a "high," or feelings of exhilaration and elation, the role of endorphins and menstrual dysfunction remains to be proved.

Although exercise is the most common cause of secondary amenorrhea in women athletes, especially those engaged in endurance sports, those athletes who participate in sports in which their appearance and weight are considered important are particularly vulnerable to what is termed the *female athlete triad* by sports medicine physicians (Furia, 1999). The components of the triad are abnormal eating patterns (not necessarily the same as eating disorders, a psychiatric diagnosis described in Chapter 17) that may lead to amenorrhea, and the amenorrhea may lead to osteoporosis or decreased bone mass and increased risk of bone fracture. Long recognized as a problem for some postmenopausal women, osteoporosis currently is seen as a possible concern for amenorrheic women athletes who may have low bone mineral density and be at increased risk for fractures during their competitive years. The American Academy of Sports Medicine has recommended that women athletes with exercise-induced amenorrhea also be screened for the other elements of the triad—disordered eating habits and osteoporosis (Drinkwater et al., 1997).

It is not known whether the decreased bone mineral density in some amenorrheic women athletes is completely reversible or whether they later will be at greater risk for postmenopausal osteoporosis. There is no evidence, however, that menstrual irregularity associated with hard exercise has any lasting effects on later reproductive ability. It should also be pointed out that menstrual dysfunction is associated only with the intensive physical training that accompanies competitive sports, marathon running, or professional ballet—and not walking, jogging, aerobics, or any other kind of recreational sport. Even if moderately vigorous exercise were to result in body leanness to the point of menstrual irregularity, the overall benefit of exercise outweighs any disadvantage unless immediate fertility is desired. Exercise maximizes health. It decreases the risk of developing heart disease and may decrease susceptibility to other diseases, according to Rose Frisch. Frisch, Wyshak, Albright, Albright, and Schiff (1989), who have done a number of studies comparing former college athletes with nonathletic women, found that strenuous exercise early in life is linked to a lower incidence of diabetes, breast cancer, and other reproductive and nonreproductive cancers later in life. Because a decrease in body fat is apt to result in amenorrhea, the occurrence of irregular cycles with obesity becomes even harder to explain. One theory suggests that because fat tissue can synthesize estrogen, the excess production may interfere with the hypothalamic-pituitary-gonadal regulation of menstruation. Another possible explanation is that the amenorrhea is stress induced, the stress resulting from the obesity or being present as its initial cause.

DYSMENORRHEA

The medical term for pelvic pain or cramps that occur during menstruation is **dysmenorrhea.** It is called primary dysmenorrhea when a woman has had painful menstrual periods since menarche, and there is no organic pathology. It is termed secondary dysmenorrhea when it first occurs months or years after menarche, when it could be the result of some organic pelvic pathology.

Symptoms of Dysmenorrhea

Many girls and women experience moderate to severe discomfort just before the menstrual period starts or on the first day of menstruation. The pain generally lasts for 24 hours but in some cases continues for several days. Cramping is felt in the lower pelvic area together with a drawing sensation in the thighs and a mild backache. The intensity of the pain varies and can be incapacitating in some women, although individual response to discomfort could be a factor in how seriously the pain is perceived.

The actual prevalence of dysmenorrhea is unknown. Statistical studies that have been attempted to determine the frequency of menstrual cramps among large groups of women have produced inconsistent results. A 1957 survey of adolescent girls indicated that 50% were affected, but it was 21.9% in a 1981 epidemiological study of American teenagers. It is a rare woman who has no idea of what menstrual cramps are, but the number of women who have pain severe enough to limit normal activities or to stay home from school or work is thought to be about 5%.

Severe, incapacitating menstrual cramps accompanied by headache, nausea, and vomiting may be "normal" in the sense that there is no underlying pathology but should not be tolerated by any woman as merely being her lot in life. This kind of symptomatology demands a complete history and physical examination to determine whether existing uterine or ovarian problems are responsible. If not, and the pain is from primary dysmenorrhea, the suffering may be needless in view of the recent availability of more effective therapy.

Etiology of Dysmenorrhea

The causes of primary dysmenorrhea are not definitively known, although there are a number of theories that try to explain it. Psychological, anatomical, and hormonal reasons have been proposed, but none of these has provided an adequate explanation for all cases. There was a time when it was thought that psychogenic causes were at the root of dysmenorrhea were predominant. Many practicing physicians, taught to believe that the pain is in the head and not in the lower pelvis, did not take it seriously and, thus, were not particularly concerned with its alleviation or treatment.

It may be possible that in some women severe dysmenorrhea is a sign of an underlying emotional disturbance, but then presumably menstrual cramps would not be its only manifestation. It is equally possible that many women respond to monthly episodes of sharp and painful cramps by developing real anxieties and fears about their menstrual periods, which could then increase the severity and persistence of the pain. To the person experiencing it, pain is pain, whether or not there is any organic basis for its origin.

The anatomical theory holds that an occluded cervical opening is a major cause of menstrual pain because for many women, having their first baby decreases or eliminates dysmenorrhea. But because as many women are cured by cesarean births as by vaginal delivery, it is not likely that it is the cervical dilatation alone that accounts for the alleviation of menstrual cramps. It may be that the greatly increased blood supply to the uterus during pregnancy and the subsequent vasculature that remains are factors.

Other theories that have been advanced about the causes of dysmenorrhea are too much estrogen, not enough estrogen, imbalance in the estrogen/progesterone ratio, too much progesterone, a food allergy, or a reaction to some chemical factor in menstrual blood. The idea that some sort of menstrual factor was involved in uterine contractions had been theorized for many years. The factor was later identified as being prostaglandin, (PG), and a recognition of the role of PGE_2 and PGF_{2a} has resulted in the currently accepted theory of why it often hurts to menstruate.

The nonpregnant uterus is a far from quiet organ, since the smooth muscle of the myometrium undergoes continuous contractions. During menstruation, the frequency of the contractions decreases but the intensity increases, and they are described as "labor-like." In severely dysmenorrheic women, there is exaggerated uterine contractility and a significantly higher prostaglandin content in the menstrual blood with a twofold to tenfold increase when compared with women who do not have menstrual pain. The proposed physiological mechanism to explain the pain is as follows: During menstruation, PGs are produced locally by the uterine endometrium. Their function is to mediate normal contractions to ease endometrial shedding. In women with dysmenorrhea, for unknown reasons, PGs are produced in excessive amounts. Increased uterine contractility and increased pain result. Pain may also be a consequence of a reduction of arterial blood flow to the uterus (uterine ischemia) mediated by PGs.

One shortcoming of the prostaglandin-uterine contractility-ischemia-pain theory is that it may not apply in all cases. Some severely dysmenorrheic women have neither increased contractility nor increased PG levels. Moreover, studies of uterine PG content have included only adult women with severe dysmenorrhea, omitting adolescent girls in whom the greatest prevalence of dysmenorrhea presumably exists.

One other factor in dysmenorrhea, although the mechanism is obscure, is that it almost always occurs from a secretory endometrium, that is, when ovulation has occurred. That is not to say that absence of menstrual cramps means an anovulatory cycle, but just that when the progesterone effect is absent, the cycles always terminate in painless flow.

Treatment of Dysmenorrhea.   For about 80% of women with primary dysmenorrhea, the miracle drugs for their menstrual cramps are the nonsteroidal anti-inflammatory drugs (NSAIDs) or PG inhibitors. Their known effect is to block the enzyme cyclooxygenase, thus interfering with the transformation of arachidonic acid into the intermediate endoperoxides. The most commonly prescribed and studied NSAIDs are in two classes of drugs: the fenamates mefenamic acid (Ponstel) and flufenamic acid (Arlef), and the arylproprionic acid derivatives ibuprofen (Motrin), naproxen (Naprosyn), and naproxen sodium (Anaprox). Aspirin has a weaker prostaglandin-inhibiting effect than the other compounds but can be effective for mild dysmenorrhea, although heavier menstrual bleeding has been observed in some women. All of the NSAIDs have possible side effects, which may include blurred vision, headaches, or dizziness. Gastrointestinal distress

is common, so the medication should be taken with food and not on an empty stomach. The choice of which type to use is subjective. Mefenamic acid has been shown to substantially reduce menstrual blood loss. Naproxen sodium is more rapidly absorbed and reaches a higher peak plasma level than naproxen in the acid form.

In 1984, the FDA approved ibuprofen for over-the-counter sales. Under the trade names Advil (produced by American Home Products, the makers of Anacin), Nuprin (manufactured by Bristol-Myers, the company that makes Excedrin and Bufferin), and Medipren (McNeil Consumer Products), for example, the nonprescription drug is available in 200-mg tablets, half the dosage of the widely prescribed ibuprofen, Motrin (Upjohn). In 1998 and 1999, the FDA also approved two new prescription "super" NSAIDs, Celebrex (celecoxib) and Vioxx (rofecoxib), for women with severe menstrual pain as well as for adults with other types of acute pain such as arthritis. The other NSAID painkillers work by suppressing the COX enzyme, or cyclooxygenase, the enzyme that initiates prostaglandin formation. The two new drugs more specifically block the form of the enzyme known as COX-2, associated with inflammation, and bypass COX-1, which has an effect on normal functioning of the digestive tract. Thus, the COX-2 inhibitors result in less gastric discomfort, a serious side effect of the older drugs, especially in arthritis patients. Celebrex and Vioxx, however, are much more expensive than ibuprofen, naproxen, or aspirin.

Prostaglandins are produced by nearly all body cells and are likely to influence their function in many as-yet-unknown ways. Prostaglandin inhibitors do not discriminate between blocking prostaglandins in the uterus and preventing prostaglandin synthesis throughout the body, so the long-term effect of these drugs is still unevaluated. They do have the potential for prolonging bleeding time, causing gastrointestinal irritation and ulceration, and producing kidney disease. Fortunately, treatment of dysmenorrhea requires only once-a-month therapy of short duration. Aspirin and acetaminophen (Tylenol) may have a lesser potential for relief and a greater potential (in the case of aspirin) for gastrointestinal side effects, but if they work, they also have a more proven safety record than the more potent NSAIDs.

If PG inhibitors are unsuccessful in providing relief, and since anovulatory cycles rarely result in painful menstruation, an effective way to eliminate dysmenorrhea may be to eliminate ovulation. Suppressing ovulation with oral contraceptives should result in almost uniform success in producing painless menstruation. If a woman wants to become pregnant or is concerned about the other effects of hormonal therapy, she must weigh the potential risk against the benefit to her. Sometimes, if normal periods are allowed to resume after several months of hormone treatment, they are more comfortable, and dysmenorrhea may never recur.

Several surgical techniques have been used to alleviate menstrual pain. One is cervical dilatation, but it produces relief only 25% of the time and the problem frequently returns for that percentage. A very drastic surgical procedure is presacral neurectomy, in which all the autonomic nerves to the uterus, both sensory and motor, are severed. Obviously, such denervation of the uterus relieves dysmenorrhea, but just as obviously, no woman or her doctor should consider this form of alleviation of pain when other methods are available.

Home Remedies.   Some women may be unable to tolerate the antiprostaglandins or be unwilling to take them or oral contraceptives. For centuries, women have been advocating remedies for menstrual pain to each other. Because there are many factors that can be involved in the cause of dysmenorrhea, it should not be surprising that there are many ways in which it can be treated without using drugs or hormones. But what works for one woman may not work for another; each may have her own particular problems.

Heat, in the form of a hot water bottle, a heating pad, or a soak in a hot tub, has been effective. Heat promotes an increase in blood flow and decreases muscle spasm. A hot drink, such as spiced or herbal tea or soup, is soothing and relaxing and may help to break the pain-tension/more pain–further tension circle.

Exercise relieves menstrual cramps in many women. It has been noted that physically fit women generally suffer less menstrual distress. Few women would want to do push-ups or knee bends when having cramps, but a brisk walk is frequently more helpful than going to bed with the pain.

Dysmenorrhea produces tension and anxiety. Two mechanisms that are used to relieve the stress and tense muscles accompanying cramps are yoga and transcendental meditation (TM). Yoga is a method of mind and body control that uses physical and breathing exercises as well as meditation. *Hatha Yoga* is the most popular form and is concerned with *pranayamas,* or breath-control exercises, and *asanas,* the postures or physical exercises. Several of the postures work specifically on the abdominal and lower back muscles and are recommended for women experiencing dysmenorrhea, both as a preventive measure and at the time of the pain.

Meditation is a method of altering one's mental activities and autonomic functions. In meditation, energy and concentration are directed inward rather than outward to achieve relaxation. Transcendental meditation is a technique that produces total body relaxation, a number of metabolic changes, and a state of restful alertness of the mind. TM advocates claim less anxiety and a more relaxed attitude.

Biofeedback involves learning to control physiological responses not normally under conscious control such as heart rate, breathing, and blood pressure. The technique is used widely to reduce stress and pain.

During orgasm, the uterus undergoes spontaneous contractions beginning at the fundus and terminating at the cervix, and immediately after orgasmic response, the external os of the cervix dilates slightly, remaining somewhat opened for 5–10 minutes. This may be a physiological basis for the reports of some women that orgasm attained by intercourse or masturbation is very helpful in alleviating menstrual cramps.

TOXIC SHOCK SYNDROME

Toxic shock syndrome (TSS) is not a new disease, not necessarily a tampon disease, and not associated exclusively with menstruation. TSS has been recognized as a rare childhood disease since 1927, when it was described and called staphylococcal scarlet fever associated with *Staphylococcus aureus* instead of streptococcus organisms. The reason for its dramatic emergence in 1979 as a potentially fatal disease affecting menstruating women is unknown, but its recognition was the result of astute observations by a medical detective, epidemiologist Jeffrey P. Davis of the Wisconsin Division of Health. In 1978, Todd, Fishaut, Kapral, and Welch published an article in *Lancet* that described TSS in seven children aged 8–17 years. All had sudden onset of high fever, sore throat, diarrhea, a sunburnlike skin rash, and associated kidney failure, liver abnormalities, and a rapid drop in blood pressure leading to shock. One child died and all of the survivors had skin peeling of the hands and feet during convalescence. Little attention was paid to Todd's article until Davis (1980) noted a curious similarity—that between July 1979 and January 1980 seven patients with the same clinical symptoms were hospitalized in Madison, Wisconsin. All were women and six of the seven were menstruating at the time of the onset of the illness. Suspecting an association with menstruation, Davis initiated a surveillance system among physicians for identification and reporting of TSS in Wisconsin. A similar system was established in the neighboring state of Minnesota, and other states also began active surveillance for TSS.

In interviews with the seven Wisconsin women, Davis discovered that most of them had used tampons during the menstrual period corresponding to the onset of illness, and he suspected an association. As other reports came in, more data suggesting a relationship between tampon use and toxic shock accumulated, and in June 1980, a report from the federal Centers for Disease Control (CDC), verifying the apparent link, was released and received national media attention. Almost daily publicity followed, and there was frequent mention of the possible association of TSS and the new type of highly absorbent tampon, such as Rely, manufactured by Procter & Gamble. After the issuance of a second CDC report showing a statistically significant association between tampons and TSS, with the highest risk occurring in users of Rely tampons, Procter & Gamble was persuaded to voluntarily withdraw Rely from the market in September 1980.

The disappearance of Rely, however, did not result in the disappearance of toxic shock syndrome. Although statistics from the CDC in Atlanta indicate a more than 90% decrease in the incidence of TSS in the decade after the Rely brand was removed, the disease continues to occur, most frequently in young women aged 15–24 and usually in association with tampon use. But compared with a high of 814 cases in 1980, there were only five confirmed menstrually related cases of TSS in 1997 and no deaths.

Fifteen percent of TSS cases currently being reported to the CDC are unrelated to menstruation or tampon usage. Female nonmenstruating victims of TSS have contracted the disease after childbirth, either by vaginal delivery or cesarean section. Others, both men and women, came down with TSS in association with surgical wound infections, deep and superficial abscesses, infected burns, skin abrasions, insect bites, boils, and other types of "staph" infections. Some researchers believe that the actual incidence of TSS may be underestimated as a result of underreporting by physicians and that the current frequency of the disease may be greater than it appears.

Symptoms of Toxic Shock Syndrome

One reason why the true incidence of TSS is unknown and why TSS cases may be more common than believed may result from the strict case definitions of toxic shock set up by the CDC. There is no specific diagnostic laboratory test to confirm TSS, so to qualify for reporting a case of toxic shock syndrome, the following criteria must be met:

1. Fever—temperature higher than 102°F
2. Rash—diffuse, sunburnlike rash
3. Skin peeling—usually 0–2 weeks after onset of illness, primarily on palms and soles
4. Low blood pressure—systolic BP 90 mm Hg for adults or below age-related norms, including a drastic drop in blood pressure or fainting when getting up from a lying to a sitting position
5. Involvement in three or more of the following systems:

    Gastrointestinal—vomiting or diarrhea at onset of illness

    Muscular—severe muscle aches or laboratory enzyme tests indicating muscle damage

    Mucous membranes—reddening of throat, conjunctiva of eye, or vaginal wall

    Urinary—blood urea nitrogen (BUN) levels twice normal or pus cells in the urine in the absence of urinary tract infection

    Hepatic (liver)—enzyme levels (SGOT, SGPT) twice normal

    Blood—platelet count below normal

    Central nervous system—disorientation, confusion, or alterations in consciousness when fever and hypotension are absent

6. Laboratory tests that differentiate TSS from other infectious diseases such as Rocky Mountain spotted fever, measles, or streptococcal scarlet fever

Milder cases of TSS may have some combination of the above findings but usually do not show severe low blood pressure or shock. The stringent criteria for reporting may have resulted in fewer mild, early-recognized cases being reported to state health departments with the consequence of an apparent decrease in the numbers of cases. Besides, symptoms of vomiting, fever, and muscle aches sound very much like "the flu" or "a virus" or even as "that time of the month" problems for some women. Although TSS is relatively uncommon, women should be aware that any sudden onset of fever, nausea, and vomiting during or just after a menstrual period requires immediate medical assistance, and, if a tampon is being used, it should be immediately removed.

Treatment of Toxic Shock Syndrome

The treatment of toxic shock syndrome includes massive fluid replacement and all other supportive measures for shock and heart rhythm irregularities within an intensive care environment. Because the throat and vaginal cultures will frequently show a penicillin-resistant strain of *Staphylococcus aureus,* the penicillinase-resistant semi-synthetic penicillins such as oxacillin, nafcillin, methicillin, or a cephalosporin antibiotic are used. If the TSS has occurred in a menstruating woman, sometimes local vaginal disinfectants or antibiotics may be used to reduce the number of organisms or toxins in the vagina. With early diagnosis, proper treatment, and luck, the patient is generally released from the hospital in about a week.

Causes of Toxic Shock Syndrome

There is much unknown about the pathogenesis of TSS. It has been established that specific strains of *Staphylococcus aureus* are capable of producing a unique toxin associated with symptoms of TSS. Originally, it was believed that the toxin-producing strains produced two types, enterotoxin F and exotoxin C. These were subsequently shown to be identical to each other, and the single entity is now generally referred to as toxic shock toxin, or TST. It has not been definitely proved, however, that the toxin causes TSS. Injections of TST into a number of various animals have shown that toxic shock symptoms can be produced only in rabbits and baboons.

Furthermore, not everyone who harbors *Staphylococcus aureus,* even the TSS strains, develops the disease. "Staph" bacteria are normally found in the nasal passages and on the skin of perhaps 20%–50% of the population, and an estimated 5%–15% of women have the organisms as natural constituents of their vaginal bacteria. Why relatively few women get TSS when there are so many that are potentially vulnerable is not known. It is believed that most women over 30 years of age have developed antibodies to the toxin, which may be why those who appear to be at the greatest risk for TSS are younger women, who have not as yet had an opportunity to make antibodies after exposure.

Tampon use is clearly not a necessary requirement for coming down with TSS, since menstruating women who do not use tampons contract TSS, and 15% of TSS victims are nonmenstrual. A number of studies strongly indicate, however, that if TSS is menstrually associated, it is linked to tampons, and that both the degree of absorbency and the chemical composition of the tampons are involved.

How are tampons related to the presence of *Staphylococcus aureus* or the toxins they produce? What was there about Rely that apparently carried a higher risk? For that matter, what is in a tampon anyway? There are only speculative answers to the first questions, and as for the actual composition of tampons, only the manufacturers know for certain because "grandfather clauses" and "trade secrets" provisions of the Food and Drug Administration regulations generally protect total disclosure.

Tampons came on the market in 1936, launched by Tampax as a disposable, flushable means of internal protection. They had been invented in 1933 by a Denver physician, Earle Haas, who was experimenting with wads of cotton because his wife told him that the traditional napkins were not good enough. Interviewed by the *Chicago Tribune* at the age of 96, Haas said, "I just got tired of women wearing those damned old rags and I got to thinking about it . . . it was designed so that it would absorb. It didn't block. It followed the natural contour of the vagina. Of course, after it was full, it would run over. . . ." He patented his device, called it a tampon, and sold it to a company named Tampax. For 40 years, tampons remained wads of cotton and a string packed into a cardboard tube, but then synthetic polyester and rayon fibers and materials like carboxymethylcellulose were added to tampons to make them more absorbent and avoid "running over." They became *super-absorbent* and no

longer merely soaked up menstrual flow, but expanded within the vagina to block it. Some have theorized that the superabsorbent tampons effectively occlude the vaginal canal and convert the posterior vaginal area into an anaerobic (without oxygen) environment that supports the growth of TSS bacteria (Monif, 1982). Others suggested that the insertion of tampons introduced more oxygen into the vagina, creating an aerobic environment that supports the growth of *Staphylococcus aureus* (Wagner, Bohr, Wagner, & Peterson, 1984). There is also research indicating that the oxygen normally present in the cotton and rayon fibers of the type used in the manufacture of tampons can modulate the production of the toxin produced by the staph organisms (Fischetti et al., 1989).

At any rate, evidence in a lawsuit against Procter & Gamble, manufacturers of Rely, revealed that the toxin-producing strains of *Staphylococcus aureus* produce more toxic shock toxin when the organisms were cultivated on the polyester foam cubes and cross-linked carboxymethylcellulose composition of Rely. Additional experiments showed that while toxin was produced on carboxymethylcellulose, no toxin was able to be detected when the staph was grown on plain cotton under similar conditions.

By 1985, tampons containing carboxymethylcellulose were withdrawn from the market, and they are now made with cotton or rayon fibers. Although information about the main ingredients is likely to be on the tampon box label, other substances such as the binders, lubricants, or perfumes used need not be revealed by the manufacturers.

The Centers for Disease Control estimates that the risk of TSS is still greater for women who use tampons than for those who do not and that the risk increases with each 1-gram increase in tampon absorbency. In addition to tampon composition and absorbency, other mechanisms for tampon association with TSS have been suggested. They include such possibilities as trauma or laceration of the vagina caused by the plastic or cardboard applicator tips; ulcer formation on the vaginal walls because the "supers" absorb everything, including the normal secretions within the vagina; and perhaps even an increase in the number of organisms in the vagina through introduction from the fingers when inserting a tampon. Perhaps the risk of menstrual TSS could be almost eliminated by avoiding tampons entirely; however, women who do not want to give up the convenience but are concerned about the safety should observe the following precautions:

- Women, especially young women between the ages of 15 and 24, should avoid the use of high absorbency tampons. It is better to use the lowest absorbency tampon and change more frequently than to use highly absorbent types.
- Tampons should be worn only when the flow is heavy and not throughout the entire period (*never* through the entire month). At night a pad should be used.
- Hands should be washed with soap and water before and after inserting a tampon. If the tampon accidentally falls on the floor before insertion, throw it away.
- Women who have given birth should avoid tampons for 6–8 weeks. Women who have had toxic shock should never use tampons at all.

It took nearly a decade from the time that tampons with high absorbency first were linked to TSS for a federal regulation requiring tampon packages to be labeled with absorbency information to go into effect. It also took a lawsuit by the Public Citizen Health Research Group and an order from a federal district judge against the FDA, which had acknowledged the need for uniform labeling in 1981 but had waited lethargically for the tampon industry to devise its own labeling program. Finally, in 1990 the FDA required the standardizing of the meaning of the terms used to describe tampon absorbency (junior or slender, regular, super, and super plus) and also required the display of the standards on the box. Formerly, one manufacturer's "super" may not have been as absorbent as another manufacturer's "regular." Now the label shows the number of grams of fluid absorbed in a test that simulates actual usage as follows:

Package Term	Absorbency in Grams
Junior (or slender)	6 and under
Regular	6–9
Super	9–12
Super plus	12–15

The regulation also required tampons to be labeled with information about the risk of TSS with tampon use and how to reduce the risk. The major brands of tampons have incorporated absorbency and composition information into their packaging. But now that women are able to compare brands in order to choose tampons with the minimum absorbency needed to control their flow, the manufacturers have attempted to create product differentiation by offering more options: with or without deodorant ("a delicate scent that neutralizes odor for a feeling that's fresh and very feminine"); no applicator or applicator that is flushable, nonflushable, plastic, cardboard, double-layered, or single stick; and compact or portable tampons, which means they come in a little case.

ENDOMETRIOSIS

Endometriosis is a condition in which bits of functioning endometrial tissue are aberrantly located outside of their normal site, the uterine cavity. These endometrial implants can occur deep in the uterine muscle, on the surface of the uterus, on the ovaries, on the broad ligaments, on the pouch of Douglas, or anywhere else in the pelvis. Sometimes, they are found in the vagina and on the cervix; infrequently on the vulva and perineum; and (exceedingly rarely) even on the arm, leg, and lung. The glands and arteries of these ectopic endometrial tissues respond to cyclic ovarian hormones just like the endometrial lining of the uterus; when the lining bleeds during menstruation, so may these implanted sites, right into the peritoneal cavity. Endometriosis is a common disease, but it is often without symptoms. It is experienced by an estimated 2%–4% of women during their reproductive years and is found unexpectedly in 30%–50% of women undergoing pelvic surgery for any reason.

Internal endometriosis, or adenomyosis, indicates that the endometrium of the uterus has dipped into or invaded the muscle or myometrium of the uterus. More commonly found in older women, its greatest incidence occurs between 40 and 50 years of age. External endometriosis, located anywhere in the pelvis, occurs in younger, nonparous women and is often associated with infertility, perhaps because it so frequently (50%) occurs on one or both ovaries. When the ovaries are involved, the endometrial implants become blood-filled cysts that can easily rupture, spill their contents into the peritoneal cavity, and form adhesions. The larger cysts that form as a result are often called "chocolate cysts" because of the color and consistency of their contents.

Etiology

The cause of this inordinate ability of endometrial tissue to become transplanted and grow in sites other than its regular location is not definitely known, although there are several theories. One explanation of pelvic endometriosis was proposed in 1921 by Sampson, who suggested that menstrual blood containing little fragments of endometrium was regurgitated upward through the fallopian tubes into the peritoneal cavity during menstruation. The escaped endometrial particles implant and then grow on the peritoneal surfaces. Based on this hypothesis, it was proposed that endometriosis may be encouraged to develop as a result of douching during menstruation, by strong menstrual cramping, or even by sexual intercourse during menstruation. Sampson's theory has been supported by observations that during laparoscopy in a menstruating woman, blood has been seen to flow out of the fimbriated end of the oviduct. Also in a classic experiment on

female monkeys in which their cervices were sutured so that their menstrual flow was directed out the tubes into the peritoneal cavity, the monkeys developed endometriosis.

Perhaps a more inclusive theory than Sampson's is that of "coelomic metaplasia"—that the cells of the peritoneum are embryologically derived from the same cells that give rise to the reproductive organs, the coelomic epithelium of the genital ridge. It is thought possible that some of the cells of the peritoneum may remain undifferentiated into adult life and, under hormonal or inflammatory stimulation, retain the capacity to become endometrium. This theory can account for endometriosis occurring anywhere in the pelvis, and in sites inexplicable by the Sampson theory. There are other ideas as well; probably more than one mechanism functions in the development of endometriosis. Because many women could have endometrial fragments refluxing into the peritoneal cavity at each menstrual period but not all develop endometriosis, genetic or immunological factors may influence susceptibility. It is estimated that a woman with an affected mother or sister has a greater risk of developing the problem. For the woman who has the disease, where it came from is less significant than what to do about it.

Symptoms and Diagnosis

Endometriosis is not easy to diagnose. Some of its manifestations are the same as in other conditions, such as pelvic inflammations, ovarian cysts, and even ovarian cancer. It is even possible that there may be no symptoms at all, whether the endometriosis is minimal or is extensive. On the other hand, there may be a great deal of pain, either before menstruation, during menstruation, and/or during sexual intercourse. There may also be abnormal uterine bleeding. Absolute or relative infertility very often is present in endometriosis patients. Minimal endometriosis evidently has little effect on fertility, but when it is extensive and involves the tubes and ovaries, the mechanical reasons for infertility are understandable—endometriosis could cause scarring or adhesions or interfere with ovum pickup mechanisms. Why peritoneal endometriosis should cause infertility is less clear, but when it is moderate or severe, subfertility or infertility may result. Many physicians believe that endometriosis should be suspected in any woman with infertility, especially if the infertility is accompanied by dysmenorrhea and pain on intercourse.

A pelvic examination could show signs suggestive of endometriosis. The cervix may be displaced laterally to the left or right of the midline due to shortening of one of the cardinal ligaments. Or there may be nodules felt on the uterosacral ligaments and tenderness in the posterior fornix during vaginal, rectovaginal, or rectal examination.

The only certain method of diagnosing endometriosis is by seeing it. This can be done through laparoscopy, the direct visualization of the internal organs with an optical instrument and light inserted through abdominal incision. A tissue biopsy of the suspected nodule taken at the same time and examined microscopically can confirm the diagnosis.

Treatment

The treatment of endometriosis obviously depends on the extent of the disease, the age of the woman, whether or not she wants to become pregnant and is having difficulty, and whether there is any pain. The sites do not become cancerous, and they are completely dependent on hormonal cycles during the reproductive years. If there are no distressing symptoms, and particularly if a woman is approaching menopause, no treatment is the best treatment.

Hormonal Therapy.   Oral contraceptives eliminate ovulation, prevent dysmenorrhea, and control the growth of endometriosis. Given continuously throughout the month, they completely eliminate menstruation and produce amenorrhea for long periods. In many instances, such hormonal suppression of ovulation and menstruation produces relief of symptoms of pelvic endometriosis. The anovulation and amenorrhea can persist for a long time after hormones are discontinued, however, so this is not a method for a woman who wants to become pregnant. Women who are concerned about taking hormones or who fall into the group for whom oral contraceptives are definitely contraindicated also should not choose this form of therapy.

Danazol (Danocrine) is a synthetic steroid derived from testosterone. It acts to suppress pituitary FSH and LH production, thus inhibiting ovulation. In the usual dose of 800 mg daily for 6 months, danazol causes regression and atrophy of the endometrium in the uterus and the ectopic sites, resulting in amenorrhea and relief of pain within the first month. Some doctors give 200 or 400 mg daily to decrease side effects, but it may take more time to get pain relief. The pituitary suppression is usually reversible, ovulation and menstruation return, and with luck the pain does not return for a while. The majority of women (85%–90%) experience pain relief after 4–6 months, but unfortunately the endometriosis sites slowly grow back and symptoms tend to recur within a year after discontinuation of the drug in about half of the women.

Danazol can buy time for a previously infertile woman and provide her with an opportunity for pregnancy. Approximately 50% of women treated with danazol can become pregnant in the interval before it recurs and even those who do not want a pregnancy are pain free. Danazol, however, has side effects that include hot flashes, acne, weight gain, muscle cramps, irritability, and occasionally masculinization symptoms such as growth of facial hair and voice deepening. In the high androgen, low estrogen environment created by the drug, there is a decrease in plasma levels of high-density lipoproteins (HDLs) and an increase in levels of low-density lipoproteins (LDLs). Low HDL and high LDL levels correlate with the development of coronary heart disease; whether this side effect has long-term significance is uncertain.

Oral progestin (usually Provera, or medroxyprogesterone acetate, 30 mg/day) has been as effective as danazol in treatment of endometriosis in a comparison study (Hull, Moghissi, Magyar, & Haves, 1987). Provera is cheaper and may have fewer side effects but is associated with break-through bleeding. Some physicians will recommend Provera as a first-choice treatment.

The newest drug treatments are the synthetic GnRH analogs (or agonists), which are produced by chemically altering amino acids 6 and 10 of GnRH and are usually many times more potent than naturally occurring GnRH. Originally believed to be fertility-enhancing agents (hence the term "agonists"), the synthetic derivatives turned out to be powerful inhibitors of FSH and LH, an ability called downregulation of pituitary secretion and not fully explained. Numerous GnRH agonists, which include nafarelin (Synarel), leuprolide (Lupron), buserelin, goserelin (Zoladex), histrelin, and tryptolin, have either been approved by the FDA for treating endometriosis or are being clinically evaluated in trials toward approval. Nafarelin is administered via a nasal spray; the others must be injected daily or in depot form—a monthly intramuscular injection or implant. The side effects of the GnRH agonists resemble those of menopause—hot flashes, vaginal dryness, and loss of bone density—but despite this, many women are better able to tolerate the effects of GnRH agonists than danazol. As yet, however, there is no information about the long-term effects of repeated courses of GnRH treatment on bone density.

Surgical Treatment.   Surgical treatment is used, but generally it is very conservative unless a huge cyst has formed on the ovary or the disease is widespread enough to cause bowel or ureter obstruction and acute pain. When a woman who is older than 40 or somewhat younger but does not want any more children has very severe symptoms and extensive endometriosis, a hysterectomy can be performed without removing the ovaries. Pain does not usually recur even though ovarian function remains. Some doctors, however, advocate hysterectomy plus bilateral salpingo-oophorectomy (removal of both ovaries and both fallopian tubes), believing that leaving a source of estrogen and progesterone will encourage growth of endometrial implants and recurrence of the symptoms. Some women, although only a small percentage, may continue to suffer the pain of endometriosis even after total abdominal hysterectomy and removal of the tubes and ovaries.

Sometimes a residual bit of ovarian tissue is still present and then must be surgically removed or hormonally suppressed.

A conservative surgical approach tries to remove as much of the endometriosis as possible and still preserve reproductive function. This may be accomplished by electrocautery or laser removal of the endometrial implants at the time of the diagnostic laparoscopic examination, a procedure with minimal recovery time. If the endometriosis is severe, it may require a laparotomy, or abdominal incision.

Some women with endometriosis have tried alternative treatments such as dietary changes, homeopathy, allergy management, traditional Chinese medicine, or other herbal remedies with varying success rates.

Endometriosis is a chronic condition that produces severe pain in many women. It is difficult to diagnose, its cause is unknown, the classification system used to assess its extent is arbitrary, and its treatment is often frustratingly inadequate. Founded in 1980 in Milwaukee, Wisconsin, by Mary Lou Ballweg and Carolyn Keith, the Endometriosis Association has served as a clearinghouse for information about endometriosis and offers support and help to affected women. Recognized as an authority in its field, the nonprofit association is currently a worldwide organization with chapters, groups, sponsors, and women in 66 countries and with information in 20 different languages. Information and chapter locations can be obtained from Endometriosis Association International Headquarters, 8585 North 76th Place, Milwaukee, WI 53223. A free packet of information can be obtained by calling 1-800-992-3636. The e-mail address is endo@endometriosisassn.org and the web site is www.endometriosisassn.org.

PREMENSTRUAL SYNDROME

Many women have no premonition at all that they are going to menstruate, or they have little reason to pay any attention to their impending menstrual flow. A look at the calendar or the beginning of bleeding is their only indication that the time has come again.

Other women are aware of breast tenderness, abdominal swelling, perhaps constipation, or an aggravation of acne just before menstruation or in the 10–14 days of the preceding luteal phase. Some definitely recognize increased nervousness or notice that they are less tranquil and somewhat short tempered before menstruation. Such psychological changes could be related to the physical manifestations, since it would not be unusual if puffiness, swelling, and an increase in the number of pimples on a woman's face were to make her vaguely tense and irritable. Most women who have these changes are not incapacitated by them and are able to consider them more as a nuisance than as *symptoms* or *problems.* Other women, however, do have a much greater degree of predictable and recurrent physical, psychological, or behavioral distress that is more than just annoying. Each woman is unique, and each experiences her menstrual cycle individually. Although it is possible that some of the same things that are ignored by some are considered distressing symptoms by others, it is evident that some women experience dramatic premenstrual changes that cause a disruption in their personal and professional lives and result in limitation of their usual activities. In the past few decades, these difficulties have collectively been known as **premenstrual syndrome (PMS).** In medical parlance, a syndrome is a group of symptoms that collectively indicates a disease state or at least an abnormal condition.

The existence of PMS is real. It is not an imaginary disorder produced in the minds of "neurotic" women, the way in which many women's health problems have been viewed in the past by health professionals. But the extent to which the symptoms debilitate or incapacitate a woman is highly variable, and while there is every reason to take PMS seriously, there is little consensus in the medical literature and among researchers about exactly what constitutes the disorder, what causes it, and how to treat it. Even obtaining an accurate and consistent description of the condition has been problematic. The term *premenstrual*

tension was first used in 1931 when American gynecologist Robert Frank described 15 women with a "syndrome" of irritability, anxiety, depression, and edema (swelling) in the days before menstruation or in the first 4 days of the flow. Frank attributed the syndrome to "excess circulating levels of female sex hormones." The nebulous clinical state has subsequently been referred to as *premenstrual distress, congestive dysmenorrhea, pelvic congestion syndrome, the toxemia of menstruation,* and now *premenstrual syndrome.*

In the 70-plus years that have elapsed since Frank's description, the original four symptoms have been expanded to include many more physical and emotional manifestations, such as nervousness, depression, inability to concentrate, paranoid attitudes, suicidal thoughts, insomnia, tendency to drop things, acne, greasy hair, dry hair, fatigue, exhaustion (or alternatively, greatly increased physical activity), heightened acuity in sight, smell, and hearing, increased thirst, increased appetite, craving for sweets, weight gain, breast tenderness, hot flashes, diarrhea, constipation, headache, nausea, vomiting, hand tremors, clumsiness, decreased motivation, decreased efficiency, lack of impulse control, increased (or decreased) sexual receptiveness, even asthma and epilepsy—the list goes on and on. More than 150 different cyclic changes have been included, and just a few of these have any positive aspects; all the rest are illness symptoms. The psychological symptoms have been interpreted as either instigating or resulting from the physical symptoms, depending on the investigator. The timing of the symptoms in relation to menstruation has also been expanded. Originally designated as occurring during the 8 days of the para-menstruum (4 before flow, 4 during flow), PMS symptoms can now also start at ovulation and continue through the menstrual period. They would obviously have to disappear at some time during the cycle, however, or there would be no basis for a menstrually related link.

Because there is vagueness and considerable confusion as to what should be included in PMS—some have even added dysmenorrhea to the list—it is not unexpected that the reported incidence reflects a similar inconsistency. Estimates in the scientific literature as to what percentage of women experience these symptoms are reported to be between 5% and 95% of all women, with ages of occurrence being between 10 and 60 years. Much of the difficulty in determining the exact incidence has resulted not only from indecision about which symptoms to include but also because little attention has been given to the question of severity of the symptoms. Studies have not distinguished between tolerable premenstrual changes of the nuisance type and the incapacitating variety that restricts the daily routine.

When a range of physical and emotional changes becomes that widespread, the plausibility of a single explanation, that is, PMS, becomes questionable. After all, if one were to construct a questionnaire and ask all people—men, women, and children—to assess which of the aforementioned signs they experienced at any time during a 30-day period, it would not be unrealistic to expect that 100% of them would report one or more of them. Much of the evidence for the incidence of premenstrual symptoms does come from retrospective questionnaires that ask women to report on their memory of various changes. One such comprehensive and widely used instrument was the 47-item Moos Menstrual Distress Questionnaire, first devised by Rudolph Moos in 1968. As typified by the title, primarily negative effects are measured. Psychologist Mary Jane Parlee first (1974) pointed out the questionnaire's methodological weaknesses (half of Moos's samples were taking oral contraceptives and 10% were pregnant) and suggested that because the questionnaire may really have been measuring unwarranted assumptions and stereotyped beliefs about the menstrual cycle, its results should be interpreted with caution. Nevertheless, this questionnaire remains a primary symptom-rating scale. Even better-designed self-assessment questionnaires, however, could still have problems with a built-in bias on the part of the subjects because of the pervasive negative expectations society has concerning premenstrual symptoms. Diane Ruble's classic study (1977) of women undergraduates at Princeton University demonstrated that when women were persuaded through bogus "brain-wave"

tests that they were premenstrual, they reported more negative symptoms of premenstrual tension and anxiety than women who were led to believe that they were in the middle phase of the cycle. In actuality, all the women were somewhere in between these two phases, suggesting that there is a strong tendency to attribute any bad days or negative symptoms as being menstrually related, even though such experiences could occur randomly throughout the cycle. Additional studies like Ruble's, in which the real menstrual cycle is disguised, substantiated that cyclical variations in mood and behavior may be influenced by cultural expectations (Englander-Golden, Whitmore, & Diensbier, 1977; Steege, Stout, & Rupp, 1985). And why not? The media and popular press coverage of premenstrual symptoms and premenstrual syndrome certainly supports a stereotype of an incapacitated or disturbed woman. While PMS is no longer the subject of nearly every TV and radio talk show as in the early 1980s, women's presumed menstrual mood changes are freely satirized by stand-up comedians, and articles with titles such as "PMS, One Woman's Nightmare," or "Dr. Jekyll and Ms. Hyde" appear regularly in magazines and newspapers. Chrisler and Levy (1990) did a content analysis of 78 magazine articles describing PMS. They concluded that because virtually all of them had a strong bias toward reporting *negative* menstrual cycle changes, women reading the articles are continually getting negative reinforcement of their attitudes toward the menstrual cycle. Even if women have no idea what kind of physical or emotional difficulties PMS involves, a recent investigation showed they report more severe PMS after they find out. Dr. Maria Marvan and her colleague at the Universidad de las Americas in Mexico (1999) showed a 10-minute videotape describing the negative aspects of PMS to half of a group of 86 Mexican women and showed the other half (the control group) a videotape merely describing the menstrual cycle. All the women in the study averaged 6 years of education and had no preconceptions or even knowledge about PMS. Both before and after viewing the tape, which they watched during the first week after menstruation, both groups were asked to report on symptoms they experienced in their premenstrual periods. Before viewing the videotape describing PMS, more than half of the experimental group reported no symptoms of pain, psychological distress, or other symptoms. Some reported mild symptoms, 2% reported moderate symptoms, and none reported severe symptoms. After viewing the tape, only 2% reported no symptoms, 7% reported severe symptoms, 54% reported moderate symptoms, and 37% reported mild symptoms. In contrast, in women in the control group, there were no significant differences in premenstrual symptoms reported both before and after the women watched the videotape. None reported any severe symptoms.

Etiology of PMS

Many of the physical symptoms are the ones that are inconsistently present, and it is the psychological and behavioral changes that are more frequently reported. The one physical symptom that has been classically described, however, and is most easily measured is *edema,* or swelling, as a result of water retention. Edema of the digestive tract leads to bowel and abdominal distension; edema of the breasts results in swelling and tenderness of the breasts; and edema of the cerebrum may account for premenstrual headache and could also be related to mood changes. Salt and water retention is widely accepted as one possible reason for PMS.

There is no evidence, however, that edema is actually related to premenstrual symptoms. When diuretics (to cause elimination of body water) were tested in double-blind controlled experiments in which neither the physician nor the subject knew who was getting the diuretic, there was no apparent relationship between salt and water retention and mood changes. Furthermore, when sodium and water retention occurs in those conditions associated with adrenal, heart, kidney, or liver disease, it produces no emotional mood swings or other changes that are said to occur in the premenstrual syndrome.

It has also been difficult to establish the reason for the salt and water retention. One popular theory to account for it is faulty estrogen metabolism, which causes excessive amounts of estrogen to be retained instead of metabolized relative to the amount of progesterone. Similarly, the also popular hypothesis of faulty luteinization could result in the same disordered estrogen-progesterone ratio. Estrogens have a weak action in causing water and salt retention, which might account for the edema. But although some studies have reported elevated estrogen levels or elevated estrogen/progesterone ratios in women with PMS, virtually an equal number have found normal estrogen values and no changes in the estrogen/progesterone ratios in the luteal phase of the cycle.

An abnormality or some change in the circulating levels of other hormones, such as prolactin from the anterior pituitary gland, vasopressin from the posterior pituitary gland, or aldosterone from the adrenal cortex, has also been proposed to account for water retention and subsequent premenstrual symptoms. These theories have stood up to further exploration no better than the other hypotheses. Not only is there no evidence that prolactin has water-retention effects in humans, but, in a number of studies when prolactin levels were measured in women with PMS and controls, no demonstrable differences could be shown. Neither have aldosterone nor vasopressin levels been proven as yet to be elevated in women with PMS.

Many investigations have attempted to identify a relative progesterone insufficiency as a cause of PMS, since symptoms tend to intensify late in the luteal phase as progesterone levels normally decline. But as pointed out in a review by Rubinow and Roy-Byrne (1984), out of 10 studies of progesterone in relation to PMS, 5 showed *lowered* levels in the luteal phase of women with PMS when compared with controls, one demonstrated that one-third of the PMS patients had *significantly* low progesterone, three studies found *no difference* in progesterone levels between PMS women and controls, and one revealed a *higher* level of progesterone in women with PMS. Clearly, changes in progesterone levels have not been shown to account for premenstrual symptoms.

Vitamin B_6 deficiency has also been suggested as a cause of PMS on a theoretical basis; B_6 may enhance estrogen clearance from the blood or may act as a coenzyme in the synthesis of certain brain neurotransmitters (dopamine and serotonin) that could be involved in the regulation of mood and behavior. Moreover, because some women experience symptoms premenstrually that are similar to those produced by hypoglycemia or low blood sugar (faintness, fatigue, shakiness), abnormalities in glucose metabolism have also been proposed as a reason. So have changes in endogenous opiate levels, prostaglandins, thyroid hormone, melanocyte-stimulating hormone, and adrenal corticoid hormones. None of these theories has been proven, and there is no evidence that levels of any of the hormones differ in women with or without premenstrual symptoms.

A study by Rubinow and coworkers (1988) of a variety of hormones that have been proposed as causing PMS showed no relationship between any of them and the premenstrual mood or behavioral disturbances of the women with PMS in the study group. The researchers concluded that theories ascribing PMS to abnormal secretions of the nine hormones evaluated were "simplistic and inaccurate" and questioned the value of hormonal therapy for the problem. The exact cause or causes of PMS are still unknown, but it is possible that interactions between some hormones and other of the biologically active substances mentioned may play a role.

Treatment of PMS

The wide variety of symptoms that fall under the umbrella of PMS are not likely to have a single cause. They are, therefore, not likely to be amenable to treatment with a single therapy. Because there are no diagnostic laboratory tests that can reliably determine the existence of PMS, it is a woman herself who must decide whether what she experiences cyclically is too mild in magnitude to qualify as a syndrome or disorder, is moderate and can be handled through self-help methods, or is so severe and debilitating that she requires medical treatment. But because a syndrome is an aggregate of signs and symptoms and, in the case of PMS, an unusually complex number of them, there are no quick and easy pill-or-potion solutions to the problem.

In addition to various combinations of steroids, both natural and synthetic, doctors have prescribed diuretics (water pills), painkillers, prostaglandin inhibitors, high doses of vitamins, tranquilizers and other psychoactive drugs, oral contraceptives, antiestrogen, bromocriptine (a drug capable of lowering plasma prolactin), lithium carbonate (a drug used therapeutically in psychotic or manic-depressive states), danazol, and placebo. A placebo is an inactive substance in the form of a medicine administered for suggestive effect. Danazol taken during the luteal phase only has been determined to be ineffective for general PMS symptoms but evidently is highly effective for premenstrual breast pain (O'Brien & Abukhalil, 1999).

Seritonin (5-hydroxytrypamine, 5-HT) is a neurotransmitter in the brain and other parts of the body and is believed to play an important role in pain modulation. Some antidepressants are selective seritonin reuptake inhibitors; that is, they enhance the amount of seritonin in the brain. Prozac (fluoxetine), Zoloft (sertraline), and Paxil (paroxetine) have been administered for PMS and for some have alleviated severe PMS when taken daily, as has Xanax (alprazolam), an antianxiety drug, when it is taken for a week to 2 weeks prior to menstruation. None of these is without side effects, of course.

The results of these therapies are variable and generally inconclusive. More than 50 treatments have been suggested over the years, and each of them (including placebo) has reportedly been effective for some women. During the 1980s, a very publicized and popular therapy was natural progesterone. Although oral natural progesterone is available today, at that time the hormone had to be administered by injection or vaginal or rectal suppository. For some women, as with virtually every other treatment, progesterone was the answer, but a number of researchers were unable to substantiate progesterone's alleged beneficial effects. A very convincing study, however, was that of Freeman, Rickels, Sonheimer, and Polansky in 1990. In a randomized, placebo-controlled, double-blind, crossover study (the best kind of clinical trial), using a sample size of 168 women, the researchers found no difference in symptoms between progesterone and placebo groups.

Not everyone is equally convinced that PMS is a well-defined entity that affects such large segments of the population and requires therapy. Women's health advocates are concerned about the "medicalization" of menstrually related symptoms and the labeling of PMS as another hormone-deficiency disease to be "cured" by doctors with drugs with the potential for unknown long-term adverse effects. At this point, no one has all or even some of the answers about premenstrual syndrome, and it is evident that what works for one woman may not be effective for another. If symptoms are severe enough to require therapy, there are a variety of nonmedical self-help approaches that could be tried first. They may not offer the quick-fix promise of a drug, but they may provide enough relief to avoid a possible long-term risk.

An easy, nonharmful way of alleviating PMS symptoms for some women is by taking a substance they should be ingesting anyway—calcium supplements. In research funded by SmithKline Beecham, maker of Tums, the calcium carbonate antacid/supplement, investigators found that taking 1,200 mg of calcium per day on a regular basis resulted in a reduction in overall symptoms of PMS during the 2 weeks preceding a menstrual period. Susan Thys-Jacobs and her colleagues (1998) studied 466 women with moderate to severe PMS, recruiting them from 12 outpatient facilities across the country. The women received two tablets of Tums E-X with 600 mg of elemental calcium or a calcium-free placebo for three menstrual cycles. By the third cycle, calcium takers had a 48% reduction in overall symptoms compared with a 30% reduction in placebo takers. Tums are inexpensive and widely available, but it evidently takes 2–3 months of daily ingestion before they take effect. Regular Tums have only 200 mg of elemental calcium, so it would require taking six tablets rather than two of the E-X type. Taking calcium with meals promotes better absorption.

Another study compared a daily supplement of oral magnesium with placebo and found that by the second cycle of administration, magnesium reduced mild premenstrual symptoms of fluid retention (Walker et al., 1998). Taking 360 mg of oral magnesium daily for 2 weeks prior to menstruation is said to be helpful in some cases.

Before any treatment, either self-care or medical, is instituted, however, it is essential to establish definitely the presence of PMS and the severity of the symptoms. This can be done only by charting a daily diary of distressing symptoms for at least two complete cycles. The day of the cycle, the date when bleeding occurs, and all symptoms should be noted. Any unusual changes from the regular routine or external stresses should also be recorded. Qualifying PMS symptoms should begin not more than 14 days before menstruation and should occur at almost exactly the same day of the cycle each month, disappearing on the day of, or shortly after the onset of, menstruation. If the symptoms shift around to other times of the month, they are unlikely to be related to menstruation and are probably associated with some other factor (perhaps physical, or an external stress). Once it has been established that the symptoms are cyclic, premenstrual in nature, and defined, the major ones should be selected for control. If the major symptoms are water retention and edema, salt restriction may solve the problem. If they are similar to those caused by low blood sugar, elimination of sweets and institution of frequent protein and complex carbohydrate meals (a hypoglycemia diet) could be effective. If nervousness, irritability, and short temper are prominent, caffeine should be eliminated. When depression is a major symptom, there are reports that vitamin B_6 or pyridoxine, in doses of 100–200 mg daily throughout the cycle for at least 6 weeks may alleviate it. Vitamin B_6 in higher doses (up to 800 mg) has been tried and is allegedly beneficial for depression, but, unfortunately, megadoses of pyridoxine can produce symptoms of overdose that include nausea, headache, dizziness, *and depression*. Exercise and other means of stress reduction, important for fitness and health at any time, can also be effective in alleviating PMS. The point is, because prescription drugs have not really been shown to be any more effective than some of the self-care regimens for PMS, it is worthwhile trying those regimens for a few months. Hormonal, antihormonal, antidepressant, or antianxiety medications should be reserved for the most severe situations that do not respond. As previously indicated for pyridoxine, however, the consumption of large doses of vitamins, minerals, herbs, or amino acids just because they are over the counter and "natural" may not necessarily be without risk. The amino acid L-tryptophan, for example, had been available as a supplement for years, marketed in pharmacies, supermarkets, and health food stores and reportedly a "natural" antidepressant advocated as a treatment for PMS, sleep disorders, stress, and alcohol and drug abuse. Although L-tryptophan is an amino acid that occurs naturally in many foods, ingestion in pill form was discovered in 1989 to be associated with the development of a new disease, eosinophilia-myalgia syndrome, characterized by severe muscle and joint pain and swelling, skin rash, and fever. As reported by the Centers for Disease Control, the syndrome affected more than 1,000 people by early 1990, with seven deaths. Since 84% of the cases were in women, it is reasonable to assume many of them were PMS sufferers taking L-tryptophan for relief. It was never clearly established whether it was the amino acid itself or some contaminant that caused the symptoms, but it should be understood that the word "natural" when applied to any vitamin, mineral, or herb consumed in megadoses does not mean "safe." And although the manufacturers of packaged PMS formulas and supplements can produce no evidence that their products are effective, they, as well as the drug and health food stores that sell the formulations, are making such claims as well as huge profits. *Premenstrual Dysphorias: Myths and Realities,* a 1994 book edited by psychiatrists Sally Severino and Judith Gold, is a comprehensive guide to PMS written for clinicians. It covers methodological problems of research, sociocultural issues, and directions for future research. Gynecologist Michelle Harrison's book, *Self-Help for Premenstrual Syndrome* contains monthly charts and guidelines to diagnosis and self-treatment of PMS.

The Politics of PMS

One hundred years ago, Victorian physicians warned that menstruation might cause temporary insanity and that women could go berserk, attacking friend and family and even killing their infants. Such unfortunate women are so subject to their menstrual influence, said the doctors, that they should be locked up during their menstrual years for their own good and the good of society.

In 1970, a Washington, D.C., physician made headlines with the "raging hormonal influence" theory of unequal opportunity when he asserted that women are unsuited for top executive jobs because "there just are physical and psychological inhibitants that limit a female's potential." A female president is out of the question, he said, because she could hardly make decisions affecting public life and safety when under "the raging hormonal influences at that particular time." Clearly overlooking the way that some decisions made by male chief executives have affected our lives and safety, this doctor, like his Victorian counterparts, believed that women are periodically deranged.

In 1981, in a harrowing echo of the violent menstrual insanity described by 19th-century doctors, a precedent based on women's cyclic craziness was established in the British courts. But instead of being locked up after going "berserk," the two English women involved were sent for hormone injections to quell their monthly lack of control. Both women claimed that it was premenstrual syndrome that provoked them to violence and, in separate court cases, successfully used PMS as a defense. One woman, 37 years old, was charged with murder after she drove her car into her lover, pinning him to a telephone pole. The other, a woman of 29 and already on probation for stabbing a woman to death in a brawl, threatened to stab a police sergeant for insulting her. She became a "raging animal" each month (presumably due to the raging hormones) unless treated for premenstrual syndrome with progesterone, according to her attorney. After the trials, both women were placed on probation, and the one who used her auto as a weapon was barred from driving for a year.

That there is something in a woman's physiology that allows for diminished responsibility in a murder charge is a chilling notion, but PMS is a legal defense in England and in France can be the grounds for a plea of temporary insanity. In the United States, premenstrual syndrome to this date has not been successful as a legal defense in a criminal action, but in several cases it has been considered as evidence or as a "mitigating factor." In 1991, a judge in Virginia dismissed a drunken driving charge against a woman who claimed she was suffering from premenstrual syndrome when she used vulgar language and kicked a state trooper. The woman, who was an orthopedic surgeon, had a blood-alcohol level of 0.13% at the time of arrest. Virginia considers a blood-alcohol level of 0.10% to be legally drunk. While the female prosecuting attorney called the PMS argument ridiculous and said the defendant's behavior at the scene and at the jail was consistent with intoxication, the male defense attorney brought in a gynecologist expert witness who testified that the behavior of the accused was similar to that exhibited by a woman suffering from PMS.

Clearly, the potential for acceptance of the legal status of PMS in the United States exists and many are concerned. The long- and hard-fought gains in the status of women could hardly be advanced by the idea that women's nature is prone to uncontrollable rages and uncontrollable acts. Believing in a women's monthly insanity could even justify the Victorian remedy—if she is out of control, it is necessary to control her.

Further concern about legitimizing a view of women as cyclically unstable resulted from the labeling of PMS as a mental disorder. In a highly controversial decision, PMS was included in the research appendix of the revised edition (1987) of the American Psychiatric Association's *Diagnostic and Statistical Manual III (DSM-III-R)* with the cumbersome name of late luteal phase dysphoric disorder. The 1994 edition of the *DSM (DSM-IV)* had changed the name to premen-

strual dysphoric disorder. "Dysphoric" means extreme discomfort, unpleasant, ill at ease. To qualify for premenstrual dysphoric status, a woman must have at least 5 of 10 psychological and physical symptoms. These must occur during the week before and a few days after the onset of menstruation and include one or more of the first four psychological symptoms on the list—marked mood swings, persistent anger or irritability, marked anxiety or tension, or depression and feelings of hopelessness.

The *DSM* is the bible for virtually every mental health professional in the country, and inclusion in the book has economic implications for therapists and patients. If a diagnosis is in the *DSM,* health insurance companies will pay for treatment; if it is not, the patient may not be reimbursed. But there are also political and social implications. Opponents of the psychiatric category for PMS believe that classifying it as a mental disorder could unnecessarily stigmatize women as psychiatrically disturbed, when their problems may be primarily biological. Proponents of the designation claim that now a subgroup of women with severe PMS who meet the criteria that qualify their mood disturbances as a psychiatric illness can benefit from psychiatric treatment. The dilemma for many women is that turning PMS into a mental disorder could raise again the raging hormone notion of periodic derangement and their inability to hold down jobs, let alone positions of leadership.

How much scientific evidence is there that even some women can be controlled by and at the mercy of their recurrent cycles? Women are certainly exposed to wide fluctuations of hormonal levels during the month, but, as previously indicated, attempts to correlate those varying hormone levels with symptoms that occur cyclically have produced conflicting and inconclusive data.

Katharina Dalton, a British physician, has done research for 45 years, has written extensively on what she has called "the curse of Eve." She claims that 75% of women experience some aspect of PMS and that menstruation can produce disastrous effects, having correlated with the premenstrual or the menstrual period an increase in sick days among factory workers, more emergency admissions to hospitals for accidents or psychiatric disorders, an increase in misbehavior and decrease of intellectual performance among schoolgirls, and an increased incidence of crimes of violence and convictions for alcoholism and prostitution. She has reported that more than half of the emergency admissions of children to a British hospital occurred when their mothers had or were just about to have their menstrual periods, and Dalton attributed the occurrence to the mother's inattentiveness, poor motor reactions, or general bad temper. Evidently believing that the behavioral influences of the menstrual period apply to all women, Dr. Dalton wrote a leaflet for the Royal Society for the Prevention of Accidents in Great Britain in which she advised that women should "understand, recognize and sensibly adjust their lives" around their menstrual cycles and not drive an automobile on long journeys during the 8 days before, during, and after their menstrual periods. Stating that women are 2½ times more likely to have an accident at this time, she further cautioned that women are at their "lowest ebb" and have "increased irritability and aggression, duller mental and physical ability, [are] tense, irrational, impatient and more easily tired" during the paramenstruum. Although evidence for all of these detriments may be specious and inconclusive, the benefits of such advice, if heeded, to the Royal Society are clear: getting half the population of Great Britain off the roads for 8 days a month is bound to prevent accidents.

In addition to Dalton's investigations, there are a number of other studies and large accumulations of data that apparently substantiate the assumption that women are more vulnerable to serious psychological problems premenstrually or that, at least in some women, an underlying emotional disorder may be triggered or precipitated at that time. Study after study links the time just before and during the menses with drastic negative behaviors and almost obscures the obvious: that the vast majority of women manage to live through their monthly cycles without any extreme variation in their behavior. Some of the claims that

relate the paramenstruum to great emotional upsets have been challenged by other investigators as to the methodology that was used in the studies, and the interpretations that have been placed on the data. When the relationship between the menstrual cycle and child illness, accident proneness, attempted suicide, or crime is studied, rarely has the relevance of external environmental situations been considered. Rare, too, is mention of the fact that men also have car accidents, have psychiatric admissions to hospitals, attempt suicide, and commit crime, and that their percentage is higher than it is for women. Ultimately, someone will undoubtedly attempt to correlate the incidence of great emotional upset in these men with the menstrual cycles of their wives, mothers, sisters, or lovers.

As many have noted, there has been an obvious and serious omission in the studies that have produced the speculations, suggestions, and claims concerning the effect of the menstrual cycle on behavior. *There are virtually no investigations linking positive behaviors like creativity, increased self-confidence, and optimism with the phase of the cycle.* The assumption that the menstrual cycle affects behavior in a negative fashion may indeed be a reflection of cultural bias and stereotyped beliefs in our society.

It could also be possible that the degree of difficulty that a woman has paramenstrually depends on her personality, the current environmental stresses to which she is subject, and her general physical state, which could include hormonal changes. But it is not possible at the current time to establish biological variables that would have a cause-and-effect relationship to her difficulties.

Why has it not occurred to more researchers that men, like women, are also subject to a changing internal environment? Cyclic changes in gonadotropins and steroids occur in males and may well affect mood and behavior, but these fluctuations have been extensively explored and studied only in females. If there are any behavioral effects of their internal rhythms in men, they have learned to deny them. Women have learned to accept, expect, or even exploit them. With all the emphasis on the psychological and physiological correlates of hormonal cycles in women, with all the literature both scientific and popular that described premenstrual syndrome, any depression, hostility, or anxiety that may have greater relationship to her stressful life experiences than to her hormone levels can easily be blamed on the menstrual cycle. Emotional instability is part of our culturally defined female stereotype. Some women may find that it is permitted—even expected—in our society to exhibit negative behaviors. They are supposed to be once-a-month witches and bitches.

Scientific investigation is seriously hampered in an atmosphere of unwarranted assumptions, sexual stereotyping, and cultural bias. Why should there be so much emphasis on only the menstrual cycle? The validity of data concerning the effect of biorhythmic phenomena on such things as behavior, illness, effects of medication, job performance, competency, psychiatric hospitalizations, and accident rates is obscured when it is applied to only one-half the population. When research frees itself from cultural bias and explores human rhythms in their broadest aspects, the contributions to society at large will be of greater value.

ℛEFERENCES

Abraham, S. F., Beaumont, P. J., Fraser, I. S., & Llewellyn-Jones, D. (1982). Body weight, exercise and menstrual status among ballet dancers in training. *British Journal of Obstetrics and Gynaecology, 89*(7)507–510.

Altchek, A. (1991). Dysfunctional uterine bleeding in the adolescent. *Female Patient, 16*(4), 53–58.

American Psychiatric Association. (1987). *Diagnostic and statistical manual of mental disorders* (3rd ed. rev.). Washington, D.C.: Author.

American Psychiatric Association. (1994). *Diagnostic and statistical manual of mental disorders* (4th ed.). Washington, D.C.: Author.

Chrisler, J. C., & Levy, K. B. (1990). The media construct a menstrual monster: A content analysis of PMS articles in the popular press. *Women and Health, 16*(2), 89–105.

Cumming, D. C., Vickovic, M. M., Wall, S. R., & Fluker, M. R. (1985). Defects in pulsatile LH release in normally menstruating runners. *Journal of Clinical Endocrinology and Metabolism, 60,* 810–812.

Dalton, K. (1984). *The premenstrual syndrome and progesterone therapy* (2nd ed.). Chicago: Year Book Medical Publishers.

Davis, J. P., Chesney, P. J., Wand, P. J., et al. (1980). Toxic shock syndrome. *New England Journal of Medicine, 303*(25), 1429–1435.

Drinkwater, B., Johnson, M., Loucks, A., et al. (1997). The female athlete triad. *Medical Science and Sports Exercise, 29,* 1–16.

Englander-Golden, P., Whitmore, M. R., & Diensbier, R. A. (1977). Menstrual cycle as a focus of study and self-reports of moods and behaviors. *Motivation and Emotion, 2,* 75–87.

Fischetti, V. S., Chapman, F., Kakani, R., et al. (1989). Role of air in growth and production of toxic shock syndrome toxin 1 by *Staphylococcus aureus* in experimental cotton and rayon tampons. *Review of Infectious Diseases, 11*(Suppl. 1), S176–181.

Frank, R. T. (1931). The hormonal causes of premenstrual tension. *Archives of Neurology and Psychiatry, 26,* 1053–1057.

Freeman, E., Rickels, K., Sonheimer, S. J., & Polansky, M. (1990). Ineffectiveness of progesterone suppository treatment for premenstrual syndrome. *Journal of the American Medical Association, 264,* 349–353.

Frisch, R. E. (1985). Fatness, menarche, and female fertility. *Perspectives in Biology and Medicine, 28*(4), 611–633.

Frisch, R. E. (1987). Body fat, menarche, fitness and fertility. *Human Reproduction, 2*(6), 521–522.

Frisch, R. E. (1993). Critical fat. *Science, 261*(5125), 1103–1104.

Frisch, R. E. (1994). The right weight: Body fat, menarche and fertility. *Proceedings of the Nutritional Society, 53*(1), 113–129.

Frisch, R. E. (1996). The right weight: Body fat, menarche, and fertility. *Nutrition, 12*(6), 452–453.

Frisch, R. E. (1997). Critical fatness hypothesis. *American Journal of Physiology, 273*(1 Pt. 1), E231–232.

Frisch, R. E., & Revelle, R. (1970). Height and weight at menarche and a hypothesis of critical body weights and adolescent events. *Science, 169,* 397–399.

Frisch, R. E., Wyshak, G., Albright, N. L., Albright, T. E., & Schiff, I. (1989). Lower prevalence of non-reproductive system cancers among female former college athletes. *Medical Science and Sports Exercise, 21*(3), 250–253.

Furia, J. (1999). The female athlete triad. *Medscape Orthopedics & Sports Medicine, 3*(1), 1–7.

Gold, J., & Severino, S. (eds.). 1994. Premenstrual dysphorias: Myths and realities. Washington, D.C.: American Psychiatric Press.

Harrison, M. (1999). *Self-Help for Premenstrual Syndrome* (3rd ed.), London: Random House.

Hull, M. E., Moghissi, K. S., Magyar, D. F., & Haves, M. F. (1987). Comparison of different treatment modalities of endometriosis in infertile women. *Fertility and Sterility, 47*(1), 40–44.

Marvan, M. L., & Escobedo, C. (1999). Premenstrual symptomatology: Role of prior knowledge about premenstrual syndrome. *Psychosomatic Medicine, 61*(2), 163–167.

O'Brien, P. M., & Abukhalil, I. E. (1999). Randomized controlled trial of the management of premenstrual syndrome and premenstrual mastaglia using luteal phase-only danazol. *American Journal of Obstetrics and Gynecology, 180*(1 Pt 1), 18–23.

Parlee, M. J. (1974). Stereotypic beliefs about menstruation: A methodological note on the Moos menstrual distress questionnaire and some new data. *Psychosomatic Medicine, 36*(3), 229–240.

Reame, N. E., Sauder, S. E., Case, G. D., et al. (1985). Pulsatile gonadotropin secretion in women with hypothalamic amenorrhea: Evidence that reduced frequency of gonadotropin-releasing hormone secretion is the mechanism of persistent anovulation. *Journal of Clinical Endocrinology and Metabolism, 61*(5), 851–858.

Reid, R. L., & Van Vugt, M. A. (1987). Weight-related changes in reproductive function. *Fertility and Sterility, 48*(6), 905–913.

Rubinow, D. R., Hoban, M. C., Grover, G. N., et al. (1988). Changes in plasma hormones across the menstrual cycle in patients with menstrually related mood disorder and in control subjects. *American Journal of Obstetrics and Gynecology, 158*(1), 5–11.

Rubinow, D. R., & Roy-Byrne, P. (1984). Premenstrual syndromes: Overview from a methodologic perspective. *American Journal of Psychiatry, 141*(2), 163–172.

Ruble, D. N. (1977). Menstrual symptoms: Reinterpretation. *Science, 197,* 291–292.

Sampson, J. A. (1921). Peritoneal endometriosis due to menstrual dissemination and endometrial tissue into the peritoneal cavity. *American Journal of Obstetrics and Gynecology, 14,* 442–448.

Steege, J. F., Stout, A. L., & Rupp, S. L. (1985). Relationships among premenstrual symptoms and menstrual cycle characteristics. *Obstetrics and Gynecology, 65*(3), 398–402.

The tampon controversy. *American Journal of Obstetrics and Gynecology, Chicago Tribune.*

Thys-Jacobs, S., Starkey, P., Bernstein, D., & Tian, J. (1998). Calcium carbonate and the premenstrual syndrome, effects on premenstrual and menstrual symptoms. Premenstrual Syndrome Study Group. *American Journal of Obstetrics and Gynecology, 179*(2), 444–452.

Todd, J., Fishaut, M., Kapral, F., & Welch, T. (1978). Toxic shock syndrome associated with phage-group-1 staphylococci. *Lancet, 2,* 1116–1118.

Veldhuis, J. C., Evans, W. S., Demers, L. M., Throner, M. O., Wakat, D., & Rogol, A. D. (1985). Altered neuroendocrine regulation of gonadotropin secretion in women distance runners. *Journal of Clinical Endocrinology and Metabolism, 6*(13), 557–563.

Wagner, G., Bohr, L., Wagner, P., & Peterson, L. (1984). Tampon-induced changes in the vaginal oxygen and carbon dioxide tensions. *American Journal of Obstetrics and Gynecology, 148*(2), 147–150.

Wakat, D. K., Sweeney, L. A., & Rogot, A. D. (1982). Reproductive system function in women cross-country runners. *Medical Science and Sports Exercise, 14*(4), 263–269.

Walker, A. F., De Souza, M. C., Abeyasekera S., et al. (1998). Magnesium supplementation alleviates premenstrual symptoms of fluid retention. *Journal of Women's Health, 7*(9), 1157–1165.

Warren, M. P. (1985). Effect of exercise and physical training on menarche. *Seminars in Reproductive Endocrinology, 3,* 17–25.

Warren, M. P., Voussoughian, Greer, E. B., et al. (1999). Functional hypothalamic amenorrhea: Hypoleptinemia and disordered eating. *Journal of Clinical Endocrinology and Metabolism, 84*(3), 873–877.

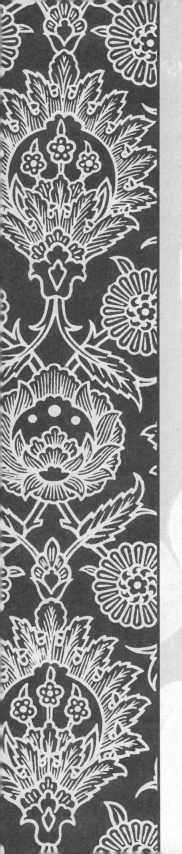

THE BASIS OF BIOLOGICAL DIFFERENCES

KEY TERMS

Amniocentesis

Barr body

Chromosomes

Deoxyribonucleic acid
  (DNA)

Genome

Genotype

Karyotype

Parturate

Zygote

*B*ack in the 1960s, when young men began to let their hair grow down below their collars, and length of hair was virtually considered a measure of how radically young people had strayed from what was considered appropriate social behavior and political thought, the older generation would say, sometimes plaintively, sometimes with amusement, but often with resentment, ". . . from the back, you can't tell 'em apart. The boys look just like the girls!" This was considered a devastating comment on the lamentable actions of young people and was voiced long before unisex hairstyles and clothing became the fashion trend for all ages.

Although the statement was not intended as an accurate morphological observation, it is quite true. Furthermore, when people are fully clothed and we are denied a look at the external genitalia, sometimes it's hard to tell 'em apart from the front as well. Physical *sexual dimorphism,* the differences in body configuration between sexually mature adult males and females, is far less marked in humans than it is in some animals, in which the differences between the sexes are so great that the males and females do not even seem to belong to the same species. Even in our close primate relatives, the orangutans, gorillas, and baboons, the sexual differences in such features as skull size, dentition, general stature, and overall physique are highly exaggerated. This is not so in humans, who are the most highly variable of all species. There are many women who are taller and larger than many men; some men have narrow shoulders and wide hips, and some women have narrow hips and are small breasted. The physical differences in size, shape, and stature that occur between two individuals of the same sex are often far greater than the degree of difference between two individuals of opposite sexes. Not too many people actually possess the cultural ideal of the typical male or the typical female form, and even that ideal changes from generation to generation.

Our lesser sexual dimorphism, as compared with other primates, may be associated with our human *paedomorphism,* or tendency to carry many childlike, or even fetal, characteristics into adulthood. Anyone who has ever made fatuous comments about a pretty little baby girl only to be informed that *she* is actually a *he* recognizes that the physical differences between male and female infants, or even children until puberty, are minimal indeed. This retention of fetal or infantile physical features into adulthood is variable, but it is particularly apparent in some women who have high foreheads, smooth skin, and very rounded contours.

Adult retention of childlike morphology is also true of males, for they also diverge far less from their own juvenile forms than do other primates. From any fossil evidence available, physical differences between the sexes in humans are now less pronounced than they once were. Millions of years of evolution appear to have produced in us lesser, rather than greater, somatic variation between males and females.

Internally as well, males and females are anatomically very much the same. No one could distinguish the human liver, kidney, heart, or other organ of a man from that of a woman. The size of these organs is more related to the size rather than the sex of the owner. The brain weight in an "average" female is about 100 g less than in the male. Much was made of this to prove the lesser intellectual capacity and ability of a woman, until it was recognized that the range in brain weights of adults is very great, and that proportionally, males and females differ less in brain weight than in total body weight. Table 5–1 shows the average weights of various human organs in adult males and females. Of the 10 trillion cells, more or less, that make up the human body, only those that are specialized into the reproductive system result in the physical differences between males and females. The functioning of all the rest of the systems is dedicated to the survival of the individual; only the reproductive system and its hormones, dedicated to the survival of the species, account for the anatomical variation between the sexes.

Of course, there are dissimilarities in the bodies of men and women. A male has a penis and a female has a vagina. These are the primary sex differences and, with their appropriate internal organs and ducts, are what make a male, *male,* and a female, *female.* But besides the gonads, ducts, and genitalia, there is little physical difference between boys and girls until sexual maturity. One exception is in the length of the forearm, which from birth is generally greater in males with respect to the length of the upper arm or the total body height, than it is in females. Girls also have somewhat more subcutaneous fat, on average, than boys.

TABLE 5–1   Average Weights of Various Human Organs (Adult in Grams)*

Organs	Females	Males	Total Adult Range
Brain and meninges	1,258	1,375	1,100–1,600
Thyroid	34	30	11–60
Thymus	14	14	1–25
Heart	250	300	240–360
Lung (right)	525	626	400–650
Lung (left)	470	600	350–625
Liver	1,500	1,600	1,200–1,700
Spleen	150	165	80–300
Kidney	140	160	120–180

*From various sources

With puberty, however, visible changes appear that are the result of the secretion of pituitary gonadotropins and the subsequent secretion of androgen by the testes in males and estrogens from the ovaries in females. As the ability to reproduce is attained, the testes in males are able to produce millions of spermatozoa, and the male is able to have erections, ejaculations, can impregnate a female, and, thus, can father a child. Females have menstrual cycles, generally produce one egg a month, can become pregnant and carry a fetus for 9 months, give birth to it, and nurse it. More succinctly, females menstruate, ovulate, gestate, **parturate,** and lactate.

The transformation from childhood to adulthood involves not only the acquisition of reproductive capacity but also certain changes in physique and physiology. These differences are the result of the action of sex steroids not only on the penis and scrotum in the male and the labia and clitoris in the female, but on many target tissues that are common to both sexes. Developmental changes in the skeleton, breasts, hair follicles, and muscles are quantitative rather than qualitative, however, and the adult differences in these *secondary sex characteristics* are merely a matter of degree.

CHANGES IN MALES AND FEMALES AT PUBERTY

The key word for the physical changes that accompany sexual maturation in both sexes is *increase*. There is a tremendous increase in the rates of growth of various body parts, and this acceleration results in changes in the skeleton; changes in the relative amounts of bone, muscle, and fat; physiological changes in the circulatory and respiratory systems; and development of the reproductive system. The age range during which the various changes occur is wide and depends on which event is being considered. James Tanner and his colleagues at the University of London Institute of Child Health did longitudinal studies of hundreds of British children, observing them and making measurements from onset to completion of puberty (1973). In girls, the first outward sign of the onset of puberty is the beginning of development, or budding, of the breasts, and it can occur anywhere from ages 8½ to 13½. The growth of pubic hair is usually the next sign; it appears approximately a year before underarm hair starts to develop. About a year after the beginning of breast development, a girl reaches the peak of her adolescent growth spurt, and menarche starts 1 to 1½ years later. Tanner's data were accumulated in Great Britain; American girls are about 6 months earlier for each stage (Zacharias, Rand, & Wurtman, 1976).

The results of several studies in the United States indicate that the average age at which girls menstruate is 12.8 years and is not significantly different from the age at which their mothers first menstruated. Recent research, however, indicates that a low percentage of girls (not boys) are showing signs of earlier onset of puberty by breast development and the growth of pubic hair between 7 and 8 years in white girls and between 6 and 8 years in African-American girls. Such early sexual maturation, which formerly was viewed as "precocious puberty"—something to be concerned about—is now seen as part of a normal variation in the timing of puberty (Herman-Giddens et al., 1997; Kaplowitz & Oberfield, 1999). The reason why earlier maturation and its accompanying racial difference occur in some girls and not in boys is unknown. The increase in childhood obesity (fatty tissue is a source of estrogen) has been speculated.

In boys, the first outward indication of the onset of sexual maturation appears at age 11 or 12, later than it does in girls. Testicular enlargement is usually first, followed by growth of pubic hair. The penis begins to grow rapidly a year or so later. Axillary and facial hair appear usually 2 years after the development of pubic hair.

Girls start and complete their growth in height 2 years before boys. The increasing amounts of estrogen produced hasten the closing of the growth plates (epiphyses) in the bones. On the average, the long bones in females stop growing at 18. At that age, according to the National Center for Health Statistics for the year 2000, the average American young woman is 5 ft, 4½ in. tall and weighs 123 lb. Her male counterpart of the same age is 5 ft, 9 in. tall and weighs 150 lb, but he will grow another quarter to half inch until his early 20s, when his long bones, under the influence of testosterone, cease growing. Males end up about 10% taller because they have had 2 years longer in which to grow.

In both sexes, the vertebral column continues to grow until age 30 but adds very minimally to the height. The velocity of growth in the shoulders and the hips increases in both sexes at about the time of the growth spurt in height. The rate of growth in the hips accelerates by approximately the same amount in males and females so that hip width ends up about the same in both sexes. The shoulders and thoracic cage grow more rapidly in males, however, so that men have wider shoulders in relation to their hips, while women have wide hips compared with their shoulders.

The relative amounts of bone, muscle, and fat are different in males and females. As boys mature, they lose fat and gain in muscle mass and bone density. Females gain less in muscle and bone, but they continue to gain in fat, which is distributed differentially on their hips and buttocks and in their breasts.

There are more physical differences that develop at puberty, and these result from the high androgen output in males and the high estrogen output relative to androgen in females, and the effect of these steroids on what are essentially the same target organs. Males, therefore, develop a larger larynx and hence a deeper voice; greater facial bone growth (leading to more prominent features); a ruddier and coarser complexion, with more hair on the face and progressively less hair on the scalp; greater blood volume; and more hemoglobin and more red blood cells, leading to a greater aerobic capacity and larger lungs and respiratory capacity. Although both sexes have the same numbers of sweat glands, males produce more sweat at a lower environmental temperature. Because sweating is a thermoregulatory mechanism that keeps body temperature down, men have a greater heat tolerance. Frye and Kamon (1983) found, however, that when men and women both exercise strenuously in a hot humid environment, the reduced sweat loss in women aids their conservation of body water and gives them the advantage.

After the first group of women cadets was admitted to the U.S. Military Academy at West Point, tests of their physical abilities compared with male cadets were performed both before and after basic training.

Before training, there were some statistically significant differences between males and females in the physical abilities tested. The greater capacities of the male cadets in upper body strength and power, leg strength and power, and hand grip strength remained after training. That males still excelled in muscular strength and power both before and after training may be related to their superior size and prior greater muscle mass, but it is also possible that specific training exercises designed to develop arm and leg strength in women cadets could have narrowed the gap. The weeks of basic training did enable the women to attain the same cardiopulmonary (heart–lung) efficiency as the men.

In the final analysis, however, physical and physiological sex differences are relative. They hold true only in terms of an average difference that occurs in a large population. Individual variation can be enormous, and the overlap between the two sexes for any particular characteristic is usually considerable. People's genetic endowments have a lot to do with their appearance, and so does their nutrition (or lack of it), physical activity, social and economic status, geographical location, climate, and many other variables of environment and culture. Males and females do not seem to have a great deal of difficulty recognizing each other's gender, but many of those signals are artificially exaggerated and emphasized by dress and behavior.

*B*ASIC GENETIC MECHANISMS

Certainly for the first 8 years or so after birth, there is more similarity than difference in physique and physiology between boys and girls. Even after large amounts of the sex-appropriate hormones are secreted, which result in the dissimilarities that become defined at puberty, there is still a wide and almost infinite range of gradations in size, shape, and appearance of men and women. We cannot get any more specific than "on the average," or "for the most part," or "generally speaking," males tend to be taller, heavier, broader, and

stronger than many females. For one basic difference, however, there is, at least 99% of the time, only an either/or possibility. For sex itself, for being born a male or being born a female, there is a determination at the moment of conception. When the sperm fertilizes the egg, genetic *sex* is established. This is the real sexual revolution—the biological phenomenon that originated several billion years ago to provide for the enormous hereditary variation on which natural selection has acted throughout evolution. Two parents, combining their genes to result in a new individual, provide the first embryonic event in a series that culminates in the birth of a baby boy or of a baby girl. But no biological process is ever 100% perfect, and some of the time there are errors in the sequence of developmental stages. Too many chromosomes, too few chromosomes, mutations of genes, hereditary metabolic defects, trauma, exposure to hormones or drugs, infections—any of these can alter the embryonic and fetal program that leads to normal sexual differentiation. An understanding of the basis of normal and abnormal sexual dimorphism requires a little medical genetics, so a discussion of cells, chromosomes, and genes is a logical place to begin.

Cells

Anyone who has ever taken a biology course has heard about how the 17th-century physicist Robert Hooke looked through the microscope at a thin piece of cork and coined the word "cells" for what he saw. The little empty squares reminded him of the small chambers in monasteries in which monks prayed. Hooke was looking at dead and dried-out plant tissue, but even now, 300 years later, when biology students examine thin, stained, and fixed samples of animal tissue on a slide, they still, for the most part, merely see the same little squares. It is sometimes difficult for them to appreciate that these are the basic units of *life*—that these can respond to being poked or prodded; take in food and utilize it to get energy; synthesize new substances for their own use or secrete the substances for functions elsewhere; in some cases, move under their own power; grow and reproduce—these things are not evident on a slide under the microscope. All those physiological properties of cells and more are based on the activities of subcellular components, or *organelles* within the cells, and of the macromolecules of which the organelles are composed.

Located in the cytoplasm of cells, all of the organelles are either made up of membranes or are closely associated with membranes. Surrounding the cell is the *cell* or *plasma membrane,* a highly invaginated complex structure, continuous with membranes inside the cell. Nutrients needed by the cell for its continued existence pass through the cell membrane, and all waste products and cell secretions or products also pass through it on their way out. Inside the cytoplasm of the cell, the *endoplasmic reticulum* (ER) forms a network of membranous, fluid-filled channels. Rough ER has tiny granules, or ribosomes, which are clustered along the channels and function in the synthesis of proteins. Smooth ER lacks ribosomes and is involved in the synthesis of lipids, steroids, and complex carbohydrates. *Peroxisomes* are small, discrete organelles that use oxygen to carry out their metabolic reactions and are thought to be responsible for detoxifying various molecules. *Mitochondria* are the larger, oval, but also membranous structures that are the site of the enzymes that catalyze the reactions called cellular respiration—the chemical reactions that derive an energy-rich molecule called adenosine triphosphate (ATP) from food and oxygen. Cells store ATP as fuel for all cellular activities. Another system of membranous channels, sacs, and vacuoles, the *Golgi apparatus,* packages the products of the ER by enveloping them with membrane before their release from the cell. The Golgi body itself is involved in lipid and mucus manufacture. *Lysosomes* are organelles that contain enzymes that act as a digestive system in healthy cells and are able to break large molecules into smaller ones. They are also believed to be responsible for the changes that occur in tissues after death. In addition to the membrane-enclosed organelles, the cytoplasm contains *microfilaments* and *microtubules,* which contribute to the supporting elements of the cell, and *centrioles* involved in cell division (see Figure 5–1).

All the work that cells do both to maintain themselves and for the general good of the body is performed by the cytoplasm and its organelles, under the control of the nucleus. When a muscle cell contracts, when a nerve cell conducts, when a cell that lines the digestive tract secretes digestive enzymes or absorbs the products of digestion—whatever a cell does at any time in its life is the responsibility of its nucleus. Even when it wears out and dies a natural death, that event, too, is programmed from its nucleus. When cells have deteriorated or have been destroyed, most of them, except for some that have become so highly specialized that they have lost the ability to reproduce, can be replaced by division of other cells. Reproduction of cells is also controlled by the nucleus.

Chromosomes and Genes

The reason that the nucleus is the controlling factor in all cellular activities, whether the cell is reproducing itself or breaking down nutrients to release ATP or synthesizing proteins to renew its enzymes, replace its organelles, or form its secretions, is that the nucleus contains **chromosomes,** and on these chromosomes are located the specific "how-to" units of instruction, the *genes.* When the cell is manufacturing a protein, the genes provide the blueprint for the synthesis of that particular molecule by transcribing the directions onto a messenger molecule that leaves the nucleus and takes the information to the cytoplasm. There, the message is translated and interpreted. When the cell is going to divide, the genes stop directing protein synthesis or their other metabolic activities and concentrate on duplicating themselves so that each of the two cells that is formed inherits exactly the same information as the original cell.

Chromosomes are composed of protein and an exceedingly long and thin filamentous molecule called **deoxyribonucleic acid (DNA)** in the form of a double thread. It has been estimated that the human

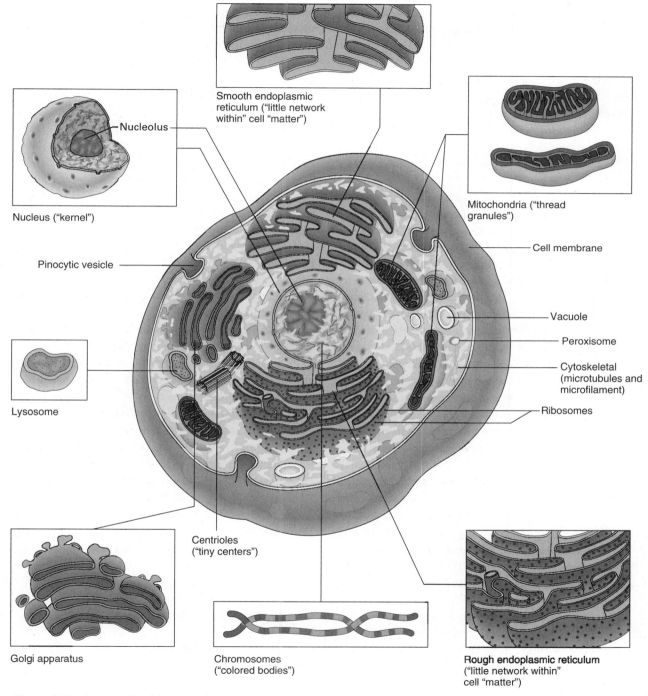

Nucleus ("kernel")

Nucleolus

Smooth endoplasmic reticulum ("little network within" cell "matter")

Mitochondria ("thread granules")

Cell membrane

Pinocytic vesicle

Vacuole

Peroxisome

Cytoskeletal (microtubules and microfilament)

Ribosomes

Lysosome

Golgi apparatus

Centrioles ("tiny centers")

Chromosomes ("colored bodies")

Rough endoplasmic reticulum ("little network within" cell "matter")

Figure 5–1   A generalized human cell.

body contains somewhere between 10 billion and 20 billion miles of DNA distributed in its trillions of cells, so one can imagine the incredible way in which it is packed into the nuclei. A nucleus does not contain only one long filament of DNA; DNA is found in the form of a number of shorter pieces or chromosomes. In a cell that is not about to divide, the pieces are highly coiled and folded so that they look like little masses or granules when they are stained and viewed under the microscope. They are then referred to as *chromatin*.

The number of chromosomes varies in different species of plants and animals, and human beings have 46 chromosomes in all the cells of the body, except for some cells that lack nuclei, or egg and sperm cells, which have only 23. Each human cell contains two of each distinguishable kind of chromosome in its total of 46, so there are actually 23 pairs. In males there are 22 matched pairs called *autosomes,* and two single, dissimilar chromosomes called the *sex chromosomes,* X and Y. Females do not have a Y chromosome; instead, the sex chromosomes are both X chromosomes. The **genotype,** or genetic constitution of normal males, then, is 44 autosomes plus X and Y and is usually written as 46,XY to designate the total number of chromosomes and to indicate that the male is normal for sex chromosomes. The genotype of normal females is 46,XX.

DNA Structure and the Genetic Code. The DNA molecule of a chromosome is in the form of a ladder that is twisted into a spiral staircase, the "double helix."★ The side pieces of the ladder, or its backbone, are made of a sugar, deoxyribose, and of phosphate, occurring in alternating groups. The cross connections or rungs of the ladder are attached to the deoxyribose

and are composed of nitrogen-containing compounds or nitrogenous bases called *purines* and *pyrimidines.* There are two kinds of purines, adenine (A) and guanine (G), and there are two kinds of pyrimidines present, cytosine (C) and thymine (T). Adenine always bonds to thymine, and cytosine is always attached to guanine so that each rung of the ladder consists of a purine loosely linked to a pyrimidine. The term *nucleotide* refers to one of the purines or pyrimidines attached to the sugar unit, which is in turn attached to the phosphate group. The deoxyribonucleic acid molecule, then, is made up of two strands of nucleotides, strung along in various sequences, but always with a purine hooked up to a pyrimidine to form a nitrogenous *base pair.* The bonds that hold one member of a base pair to the other are very weak, and they can break apart easily (Figure 5–2).

The sequence of the base pairs as they form each rung of the ladder is referred to as the *genetic code.* Although there are only four variations of the linkage (i.e., thymine—adenine, adenine—thymine, cytosine—guanine, and guanine—cytosine), the order in which they occur can provide an almost infinite variety of combinations. A *gene* is a particular *segment of sequences* that gives the instructions for the synthesis of a particular protein, which is in turn responsible for some other activity in the cytoplasm of the cell. Proteins are made up of long, linked chains of amino acids, and every sequence of three nucleotides, like AAT, or CTA, or CGC, and so forth, is a code word for a particular amino acid. Thus, genes are of different lengths, depending on the protein, and follow one another along the DNA strand. No one really knows how many genes are located on a chromosome—there may be tens or hundreds of thousands.

There are an estimated 3.3 billion base pairs coding for the genes embedded in the DNA of the human chromosomes. The **genome** is the term for all the DNA in an organism. The Human Genome Project, coordinated by the National Institutes of Health (NIH) and the Department of Energy (DOE), was started in 1990 as a 15-year project with the ambitious goal of cracking the genetic code, that is, determining

---

★James Watson and Francis Crick received the Nobel Prize in 1953 for delineating the structure of the DNA molecule. So did Maurice Wilkins, a crystallographer at Kings College in London. Students of biology should be aware that Rosalind Franklin, who worked with Wilkins and upon whose key observations Watson and Crick relied, did not receive the award.

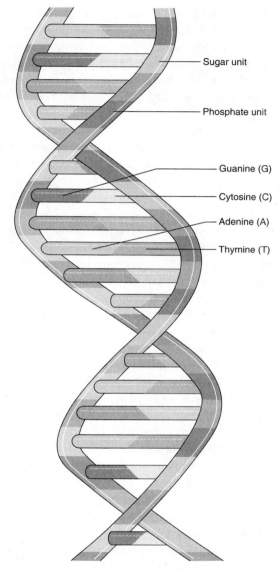

Sugar unit

Phosphate unit

Guanine (G)

Cytosine (C)

Adenine (A)

Thymine (T)

Figure 5–2 Diagrammatic representation of the DNA molecule. DNA contains the organism's hereditary material and is located in the nucleus of every cell.

by January 1999. Six major research centers in the United States and a number of international centers are coordinating the effort, which, when completed, will enable the identification and potential treatment of countless genetic diseases. The project is not without controversy regarding its cost, which many believe diverts funds from other basic research initiatives, and also the ethical, social, and legal implications of the project's outcome. Which patients should receive health care customized to their genetic constitutions? Who would get gene-replacement therapy for genetic disease? And once a person's genetic predisposition is known, how is confidentiality maintained to prevent discrimination in getting a job or obtaining health or life insurance? These are only a few of the potential questions raised by the program. Some attention is being paid to such issues by the DOE and NIH, but a mere 3%–5% of their budgets is set aside annually to address them.

Reading the Code. Although the same genes are present on the same chromosomes of all the cells, not all cells perform the same work, synthesize the same proteins, or even look the same, for that matter. But because all the body cells do have the same DNA with the same information inscribed on it, it must be that different parts of the code are translated in different cells. That is, some genes are active in some cells, while other genes are active in other cells or at different times during development. Follicle-stimulating hormone, or FSH, for example, is synthesized in the cells of the anterior pituitary gland, and even though the genetic instructions for making FSH are present in the muscle cells, it is certainly not manufactured there. The kinds of genes that actually code for the synthesis of a specific substance like FSH or any other kind of protein that is concerned with the specific functions of a cell, like growth or secretion, are called structural genes. Structural genes are switched on and off, or regulated, so that the appropriate amount of a given protein is produced at the proper time. Such gene regulation, necessary for normal function, is carried out by a class of proteins called *transcription factors.* These factors dictate which genes in the particular cell

the location and sequence of the 80,000 genes within human DNA. Technological advances accelerated the project to an expected completion date of 13 instead of 15 years, that is, 2003, although only 7,600 genes had been mapped to particular human chromosomes are to function and which are to remain inactive. Identifying transcription factors and understanding their highly complex interactions are a major focus of research in molecular genetics.

Because chromosomes exist in matching or homologous pairs, genes also exist in pairs, called *alleles.* Each chromosome of a pair carries a sequence of nucleotides, the gene, that governs a particular activity, and the other chromosome carries the gene partner at the same location. While the two gene counterparts are concerned with the same function, their arrangement of nucleotides may not be exactly the same, and the individual is then said to be *heterozygous* for that particular gene. Then, one of these genes generally is *dominant* to its *recessive* allele. If the arrangement is exactly the same between the two members of the allele, the individual is *homozygous* for that pair.

If the arrangement of nucleotides in a gene is even minutely rearranged by mutation, a specific abnormality may result, a malfunction that is then transmitted as a hereditary disease to future generations. Tay-Sachs disease, cystic fibrosis, and sickle cell anemia are examples of hereditary diseases caused by genetic mutation. Gene defects may also occur as a result of environmental factors such as x-rays, chemicals, viruses, and infections. Classical human genetics is concerned with gene defects.

Cell Division

As cells go about their metabolic business, performing their own specialized work under the control of the genes in their chromosomes, they may have to reproduce themselves, or other cells have to reproduce to replace them, in the normal course of maintenance and repair. Some cells last longer than others. Nerve cells for example, are not able to divide and must last virtually a lifetime, but every second, millions of blood cells die, and millions more must be there to take their place.

When cells do divide, it is tremendously important that all offspring cells have the identical chromosomal information as the parent cells so that the genetic code can be passed to all future generations of cells. Therefore, before a cell divides, its chromosomes must replicate themselves. The process of chromosomal replication, followed by nuclear and cytoplasmic division that ensures the preservation of the genetic code, unchanged from cell to cell, is called *mitosis.*

Mitosis.   Mitosis of a cell takes place in four consecutive stages called *prophase, metaphase, anaphase,* and *telophase,* but the actual duplication of the chromosomes occurs before prophase, during *interphase.* Each ladder of the DNA double helix "unzips" its loose bonds between the purines and pyrimidines of its rungs, and a new strand of complementary nucleotides, made up from the free phosphates, sugars, and purines and pyrimidines that are available in the nucleus, zips onto each half of the ladder. Where there was formerly one DNA double-helix molecule, there are now two double strands that are formed. Each one has one-half from the old molecule, and one-half of each is new (Figure 5–3).

The doubled chromosomes are called sister *chromatids* at this stage in mitosis, and they lie next to each other in the nucleus, attached at a point called the *centromere.* Even though each of the 46 chromosomes consists now of two chromatids, each is still considered to be only one chromosome. Later in the process, when the centromere divides, the two chromatids separate from each other, and one of them from each chromosome moves toward the opposite end of the cell. Then each chromatid is considered a chromosome in its own right.

After the chromosomes move apart, the cytoplasm also pinches apart to divide. All the organelles in the cytoplasm—the mitochondria, Golgi body, ER, and so forth—get roughly divided into equal parts, and mitosis is complete.

Meiosis.   It was noted earlier that all of the body cells with nuclei have 46 chromosomes, except for the egg cells in the female and the spermatozoa cells in the male, which have only half that many, 23 chromosomes. It should be obvious why this is so. If a sperm

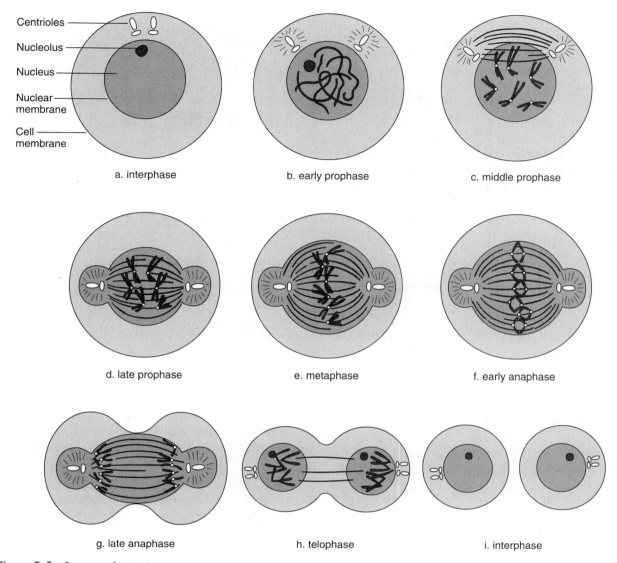

Centrioles

Nucleolus

Nucleus

Nuclear membrane

Cell membrane

a. interphase

b. early prophase

c. middle prophase

d. late prophase

e. metaphase

f. early anaphase

g. late anaphase

h. telophase

i. interphase

Figure 5–3 Process of mitosis.

had 46 chromosomes, and an egg had 46 chromosomes, when the sperm fertilized the egg, the resultant zygote would have 92 chromosomes, with further doubling of the number in each successive generation! Of course, this kind of doubling of chromosomes cannot occur, and the chromosome number of each given species must be kept constant. In the formation

of the *gametes,* or eggs and sperm, a special kind of reduction division takes place that ensures that each gamete contains only *half* of the number of chromosomes. This special division is called *meiosis.* Then, when the sperm fertilizes the egg, the resultant zygote, from which all the cells of the new individual form, contains 46 chromosomes. Because the egg contains only 23 chromosomes and the sperm contains 23 chromosomes, meiosis also ensures that in any body or *somatic* cell, half of those 46 chromosomes are of maternal origin and half of them of paternal origin. In both males and females, gametes are produced in the gonads and are derived from a cell with 46 chromosomes that undergoes two divisions to result in four cells. In males, all the cells are viable and are called spermatozoa; in females, only one is a viable egg cell. All the rest become polar bodies and fail to develop.

The chromosomes replicate themselves in meiosis the same way they do in mitosis, but after duplication the two chromatids of each chromosome seek out the two chromatids of the homologous partner and arrange themselves next to each other, with all four chromatids stretched out along their entire lengths; that is, all the chromosomes of *maternal origin* lie next to their matching partners of *paternal origin,* with all their matching genes strung along, one after the other. The two homologous chromosomes, each consisting of two chromatids, are held together by their centromeres. At this point, a very important thing happens. In each pair of four chromatids, one of the maternal chromatids reciprocally exchanges material with one of the paternal chromatids. This is called *crossing over,* and the sites of the exchanges are called *chiasmata.* The only pair of chromosomes in which this does not happen is the XY in males. There is no particular pattern to the breakages and exchanges of fragments of DNA—it occurs absolutely at random— and the reshuffling of the genes, the rearrangement of the array of genes that results, provides for the absolute uniqueness of every human being (Figure 5–4).

After crossing over is finished, each of the homologous chromosomes separates from the other and goes to the opposite pole of the cell. When the cytoplasm divides, each cell will contain 23 chromosomes, but each chromosome still consists of two chromatids. The second meiotic division resembles mitosis in that the chromatids separate, each to migrate to an opposite pole and then to become chromosomes in their own right. In females, the second meiotic division is completed only in an egg that has been fertilized by a

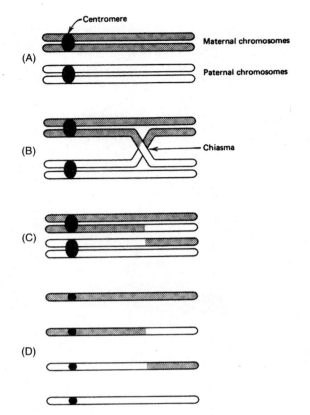

Figure 5–4 Crossing over and recombination of chromosomes. (A) Homologous chromosomes, held together by their centromeres, are paired together during metaphase of the first meiotic division. (B) Two of the chromatids undergo breakage at exactly the same point. A part of one maternal chromatid is exchanged with a corresponding part of a paternal chromatid in a process known as crossing over. The site of the exchange is a chiasma. (C) Appearance of the chromosomes following crossing over. Whatever genes were located on the original homologues are now in a new combination as a result of the exchange. (D) After separation, each gamete will contain one of the chromosomes. Note that two of the gametes will carry recombined chromosomes and two will not. In long chromosomes, several crossovers (breakages and recombinations) may occur.

sperm. Then the nucleus of the egg, containing 23 chromosomes, merges with the nucleus of the sperm, also containing 23 chromosomes, and the full set of 46 chromosomes is re-formed.

That first cell of the new individual divides (by mitosis) to form the myriad numbers of cells of the body. Within hours of fertilization, the first 2 cells form, then 4 then 8, 16, 32, 64, 128, all the while that the embryo is progressing down the fallopian tube. As the multiplications continue, the cells begin to develop along different lines, and from then on will no longer look alike. Some will become brain cells, some bone cells, some will be the eye, heart, or kidney cells, and some will even become segregated at that early stage to become future egg or sperm cells. That depends, of course, upon the sex of the embryo and was determined when the sperm fertilized the egg. Figure 5–5 contrasts mitosis and meiosis.

Sex Determination

Remember that the genotype of females is 22 pairs of autosomes and two sex chromosomes, XX, and that the genotype of males is 22 pairs of autosomes and the two sex chromosomes, XY. Since the sex chromosomes behave like members of an ordinary pair and separate during meiosis, it is apparent that while females can produce only eggs with an X chromosome, males can produce two kinds of sperm—those carrying an X and those carrying a Y. Then, if a sperm bearing an X chromosome fertilizes an egg, the resulting XX **zygote** (or fertilized egg) will be female. If a Y-carrying sperm fertilizes an egg, the XY zygote will develop into a male. Because half the sperm will carry an X and the other half will carry a Y, the chances of a male or a female baby being conceived are 50–50 (Figure 5–6). The male and his sperm solely determine the sex of the offspring. What would all the wives throughout the ages who were blamed for not being able to produce sons, and all the queens in history who were discarded or beheaded for the same reason, have given for that information! (But who would have believed them anyway?)

Although the sex ratio of males and females conceived is theoretically 50:50, in actuality, the birth sex ratio is 103 and 105 males born for every 100 females. The lower ratio occurs in nonwhites (blacks and other ethnic groups) and the higher one in whites, both in the United States and in other countries that keep records. Greater numbers of males are born relative to female births, even though more male fetuses are spontaneously aborted or stillborn, so that there probably are more males than females conceived. The reasons why male conceptions have the edge on the numbers of females conceived is unknown, although several theories have been proposed. One idea is that the X-bearing sperm, larger and of greater mass, swims more slowly and does not get to the egg as successfully or as often as the Y. Another idea is that the Y-bearing sperm finds the environment in the female reproductive tract more favorable for survival, or perhaps is more efficient at fertilizing ova than the X-bearing sperm. There is as yet no convincing evidence to substantiate any of these speculations.

Genes on the Sex Chromosomes

The human Y chromosome carries a sequence of nucleotides, or a gene, that instructs certain cells of the embryonic gonads to form testes. Those testes will then secrete hormones that will direct further differentiation into a male reproductive tract and male genitalia. In the absence of the Y chromosome, testes do not develop, and the embryo develops as a female. That a testis-determining gene called TDF (for testis-determining factor) exists on the Y has been known for more than 30 years. Exactly where this factor is located on the 30–40 million nitrogenous bases that comprise the Y chromosome has been an ongoing question, although researchers had mapped it in the 1960s to the short arm of the Y (the shorter portion above the centromere). For a number of years it was believed that H-Y antigen, a cell membrane surface protein, was the testis inducer and that the gene coding for its production was the TDF. The theory lost credibility when mice were found that had testes but lacked H-Y antigen. In 1990, the search for the definitive TDF narrowed again with the discovery of a gene termed by the researchers as SRY, for sex-determining region of the Y (Sinclair, Berta, & Palmer, 1990).

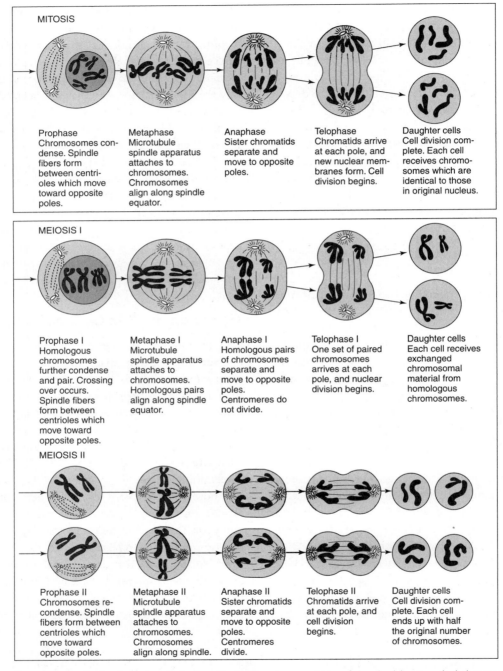

Figure 5–5 Comparison of mitosis and meiosis. In mitosis there is no pairing of the double-stranded chromosomes. They move to the spindle individually and separate to form new single-stranded chromosomes derived from one original double-stranded chromosome. In meiosis, the homologous double-stranded chromosomes form a synaptic pair and each pair separates. The new cells formed thus have half the chromosomes that were present in the parental nucleus.

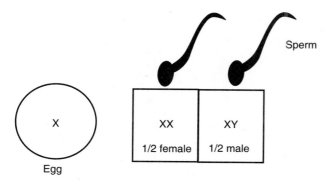

Figure 5–6 The male parent produces equal numbers of X-bearing sperm and Y-bearing sperm. It would then be expected that equal numbers of males and females will be conceived.

Although it has not been conclusively established that SRY is the testis determiner, it has been identified in all of the male mammals examined, including mice, chimpanzees, pigs, tigers, and men—making it currently the most promising candidate for the elusive TDF. The SRY gene may not act alone, and other genes, either adjacent to it or on other chromosomes, are also likely to play a role in triggering the development of maleness in XY embryos. But as far as anyone knows, there are no other genes on the Y chromosome for any other human activity or trait except for the testis-determining factor.

In contrast to the Y chromosomes, the X does have genes that influence the expression of many characteristics other than those concerned solely with reproduction. These genes are called *sex linked,* and among the most familiar are those affecting color vision, blood clotting, and muscle function. Abnormalities of these genes lead to color blindness, hemophilia, and a type of muscular dystrophy. One of the most common types of mental retardation, second only to Down syndrome, is due to a gene located on the X chromosome at a fragile site, so called because affected individuals have a constriction on the X that tends to break during laboratory tests. Called fragile X syndrome, the abnormality is caused by a sex-linked dominant gene with reduced penetrance, meaning that either sex may exhibit retardation when carrying the gene. It is expressed in about 1 of every 1,250 males and 1 of every 2,500 females. Its severity ranges from mild learning disabilities to severe retardation. The gene for the disorder was identified by Verkerk and colleagues (1991) and definitive prenatal diagnosis for the disease is now possible.

Barr Body

One of the X chromosomes in the nucleus from a cell of a female can actually be seen under the microscope, most easily in a stained smear of cells from the inner lining of her cheek, or in her white blood cells, but it is also visible in living cells with the use of phase-contrast microscopes. Originally called sex chromatin, or X-chromatin, its discovery in 1949 by two Canadian researchers, Murray Barr and Edward Bertram, led to a whole new field of study, human *cytogenetics,* the study of chromosome abnormalities. Barr and Bertram were working on stained sections of nerve cells in cats when they noticed a tiny, dark-staining blob of material that was always present only in the nucleus of the female cats and never in the males. It was subsequently determined that the little stained body was one of the X chromosomes, an inactive one that remained coiled and condensed so it could be seen, and that it was visible in human female cells as well. The **Barr body,** as it came to be known, is not seen in the nuclei of the cells of normal males. One of the two X chromosomes of a female embryo becomes inactive and, hence, visible at approximately 2 weeks of age, when the embryo consists of only a few hundred cells. From then on, it is the *invisible* X that has active functioning genes and goes about its business directing cellular activities. The X chromosome that appears as the Barr body is the inactive one, devoid of genetic duties. This inactivation of one X chromosome results in both sexes having an equal dosage of X chromosomal genes. Which of the two X chromosomes becomes a Barr body at the time of inactivation is a matter of chance. It could be the maternally derived X in some cells and the paternally derived X in other cells. From then on, interestingly enough, all those cells that are offspring of a cell in which the X chromosome from the father became active are then slightly different from all the descendants of the cell in the embryo in which the X chromosome from the mother's side became active. This is why geneticists say that a normal human female is a *mosaic*. She is composed of a mixture of two slightly different kinds of cells. The original description of the nature and significance of the physical inactivation of one of the X chromosomes was made by Mary Lyon and is referred to as the Lyon hypothesis (Figure 5–7).

Another way of identifying X chromosomes is by looking for the "drumstick," a little separate lobule that is apparent on approximately 0.5%–10% of the nuclei of white blood cells called *neutrophils* in a well-stained blood smear from females. So if large numbers (at least 500) of neutrophils are examined, it is possible to determine genetic sex in an XX individual (Figure 5–8).

The presence of Barr bodies, however, does not always mean that an individual is female, and their absence is not always conclusive evidence that an individual is male. A Barr body indicates only that the cells contain at least *two* X chromosomes. In cases of certain kinds of chromosomal abnormalities, genetic sex can be determined only by establishing whether or not the somatic cells contain a Y chromosome. This is done by examining the chromosomes, arranging them in groups, and counting them. Viewed in this manner, the chromosome complement is called a **karyotype.**

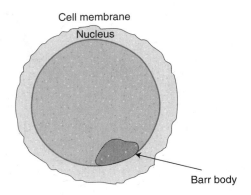

Figure 5–7 The Barr body, or one of the X chromosomes of a female as seen in the nucleus of a cell from a woman's cheek lining. A simple scraping made with a toothpick can be placed on a slide (buccal smear), stained, and examined. The percentage of Barr bodies in buccal smear surveys of normal populations varies from about 10% to 60% in normal females.

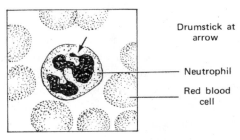

Figure 5–8 The drumstick appendage, equivalent to the sex chromatin of the Barr body, can be seen in a small percentage of certain white blood cells of a female.

Human Karyotype

The easiest way to examine chromosomes is to look at them during the metaphase stage of mitosis when they are condensed, separate from each other, and most visible. The easiest tissue to examine for cells is blood because it can be obtained from a vein with relatively little discomfort. To make a karyotype, a sample of blood is taken from an individual and incubated in a nutrient medium at body temperature for several days to encourage cell division. The culture is centrifuged to separate the red cells, which are then discarded. A nontoxic chemical derivative of colchicine, a drug that stops cell division in metaphase, is added to the white cells; after several hours, a very weak salt solution is added to swell the cells and separate the chromosomes. When a drop of the cell suspension is spread out on a slide, stained, and then viewed under the highest power of a microscope, the chromosomes can be examined. This is called a metaphase spread. The

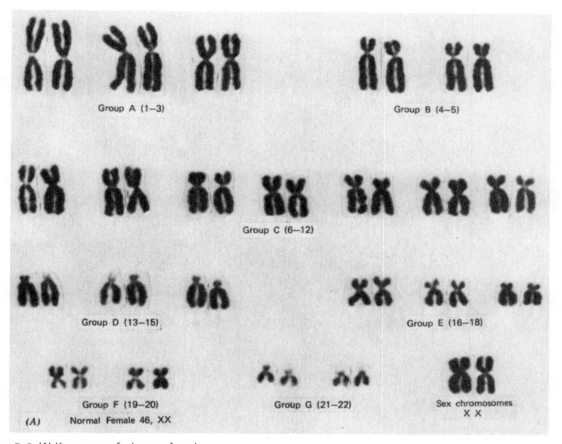

Figure 5–9 (A) Karyotype of a human female.

problem is, how is it possible to tell one chromosome from another?

Chromosomes consist of two chromatids, held together by the centromere, so all of them will have an X configuration, but they come in different sizes. For a karyotype to be described in some standardized way, an international system of chromosome nomenclature is used to divide the chromosomes into groups based upon their length and the position of the centromere. When a photograph of the view under the microscope is enlarged several thousand times, the individual chromosomes can be cut out with a scissors, matched and arranged according to their length and shape, and divided into seven groups—A through G (Figure 5–9 A,B). The only difference in the karyotypes of a male and female is that the male has one X and one Y chromosome and the female has two X chromosomes.

Preparation of the human karyotype is obviously time consuming, and analysis of the chromosomes is certainly subject to human error. Newer methods of identifying chromosomes include the use of fluorescent dyes or special stains that preferentially bind to certain segments of DNA on specific chromosomes for more precise recognition. Such techniques are called *banding* (Figure 5–10).

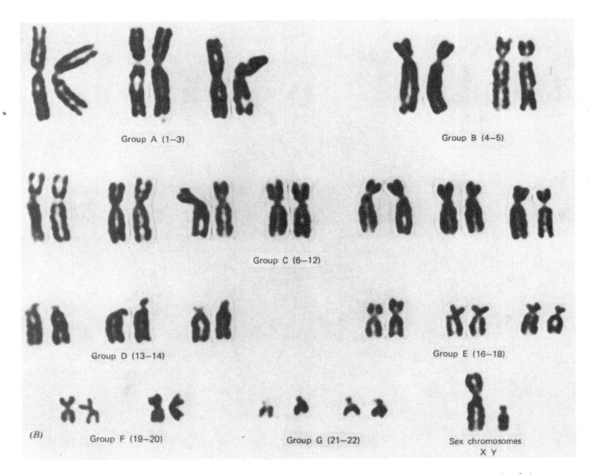

Figure 5–9 (B) Karyotype of a human male. The chromosomes are cut out of an enlarged photograph of chromosomes in metaphase, arranged in pairs, and systematically grouped. The autosomes are numbered from 1–22 on the basis of decreasing size.

CHROMOSOMAL DISORDERS

The mechanisms underlying cell division are so complex that an occasional slipup in the orderly processes is not unexpected. Chromosomal abnormalities can occur during the early stages of meiosis in the development of the gametes, but they can also arise after fertilization from faulty mitotic division of the zygote. There are two major kinds of chromosomal aberrations: either there are changes in the *number* of chromosomes, or there are *structural* changes as a result of chromosomal breakage that may be due to environmental influences, such as drugs or infections. In *nondisjunction,* there is a failure of homologous chromosomes to be distributed normally when they pull apart, and the result is a cell with too many or too few chromosomes. *Trisomy* indicates there is an extra chromosome, and *monosomy* means the absence of a chromosome. If a piece of a chromosome breaks off and is lost, it is termed a *deletion*. Sometimes the broken-off piece is not lost but is inserted improperly on another

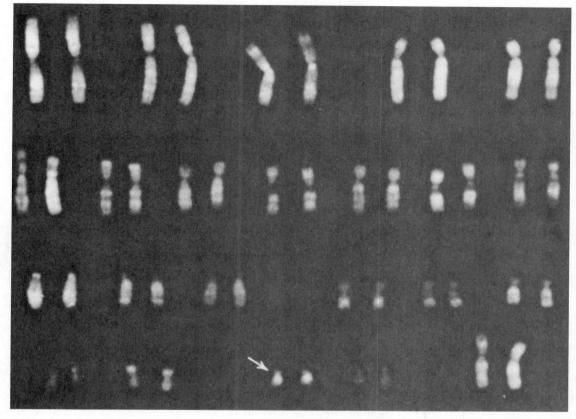

Figure 5–10 Female karyotype with quinicrine-induced fluorescence of chromosomes, believed to result from the stain's interaction with adenine-thymine-rich areas of DNA. Note that chromosome 21 (arrow) fluoresces more brightly than chromosome 22. The crosswise striations on chromosomes produced by quinicrine are called Q bands; other stains cause G bands, C bands, and R bands for detailed chromosome identification and spectacular effects.

chromosome and becomes an *addition*. When broken segments are exchanged between two chromosomes, it is called *translocation*.

No one really knows the number of fertilized eggs that carry a chromosomal abnormality, but the number of children born with a chromosomal disorder (at least one that is observable with a light microscope) is 0.5%, or 1 in 200. Most of the chromosomal defects result in such major deformities in an embryo that they are incompatible with life and are spontaneously aborted, sometimes even before the woman realizes she is pregnant. When such spontaneously aborted

fetuses (called abortuses) have been analyzed for karyotype, chromosome abnormalities have been found in 20%–30%. Because there is no way of getting data, it is impossible to estimate the number of fertilized eggs that never implant at all and are lost because of chromosomal defects.

Down Syndrome

All autosomal trisomies, in which the affected person has three rather than the normal two of a particular chromosome, for a total of 47 chromosomes instead of

46, cause severe mental and physical abnormality. The most frequent trisomy in live births, affecting perhaps 1 in 800 children, is trisomy 21, in which there are three copies of the smallest autosome, number 21. Children with this condition, also called Down syndrome and formerly known as "mongolism," are almost invariably mentally retarded, small in size, and have poor muscle tone. There are about 10 or so major symptoms present, including the "simian crease," a slight abnormality in palm and sole print patterns sufficiently different from the normal that it can be used for diagnosis.

Most cases of Down syndrome (about 95%) result from meiotic nondisjunction of the number 21 autosome. At the stage of meiosis during which the homologous pair would normally separate, with each member of the pair going to an opposite pole of the cell before cytoplasmic division, the pair instead remains together. One cell will then get both chromosomes, and the other cell will get none. An abnormal gamete with an extra chromosome is produced, which in the case of trisomy 21 is almost always the egg. If such an egg is fertilized by a normal sperm, autosome 21 will be in triplicate rather than paired (two chromosomes from the egg and one chromosome from the sperm), and the resultant embryo will have 47 chromosomes (Figure 5–11).

Although there is some evidence that paternal age, especially if the father is over 50, is also associated with an increase in Down syndrome birth, the risk of having an affected child statistically increases with the age of the mother. The incidence is about 1 in 1,700 in women aged 15–19; 1 in 1,400 in mothers aged 20–30; 1 in 750 in those aged 30–35; thereafter, the risk becomes much greater, increasing about 15% with each additional year. At the age of 40, the odds of having an afflicted child are 1 in 100; and when the maternal age is 45 or older, the chances of giving birth to a baby with Down syndrome may be as high as 1 in 16, or 6%. If a woman has already had an affected child, the risk of recurrence is 1% in younger women and also increases with maternal age. The higher incidence of meiotic nondisjunction in the ova of older women has generated a number of theories

as explanation. It may be that the increased risk is related to the age of the ova in the older woman's ovary. The oocyte in a primary follicle that has resumed meiotic division on its way to ovulation in a woman of 45 has been dormant in the ovary for about 45 years and 3 months. Cells in an arrested state of meiotic division are known to be particularly susceptible to environmental influences—viruses, x-rays, toxic chemicals—that can interfere with normal cell division. The older a woman is, the longer these damaging agents have had to affect those oocytes. It has also been suggested that because older women are usually married to older men, and it is presumed that there is less frequency of sexual intercourse in older couples, the egg remains in the female tract longer before fertilization. In animal experiments, it has been found that such delayed fertilizations result in more chromosomal anomalies in the zygote. It has not as yet been determined whether (1) intercourse is really that much less frequent in people 40 years of age or older and (2) couples aged 40 or older who have a child with trisomy 21 have had less frequency of intercourse than similarly aged couples who have produced a normal child. Thus, the delayed fertilization theory has not been substantiated. The reasons for the increased incidence of Down syndrome in children of older women are really unknown.

Despite the maternal age effect, two-thirds of the children with Down syndrome are born to mothers younger than 35 because there are so many more children born to the younger age group. A prenatal blood test, performed during the second 3 months of pregnancy and followed by amniocentesis and chromosome analysis on those women identified by the test as being at risk, assays the level of three hormones—human chorionic gonadotropin (HCG), unconjugated estriol, and alpha-fetoprotein (AFP)—whose concentration may indicate the presence of a fetus with Down syndrome. The concentration of HCG from the placenta increases in affected pregnancies while unconjugated estriol, produced by the fetal adrenals, fetal liver, and the placenta, is abnormally low in affected pregnancies. The concentration of AFP, a fetal protein produced by the liver and partly from the yolk

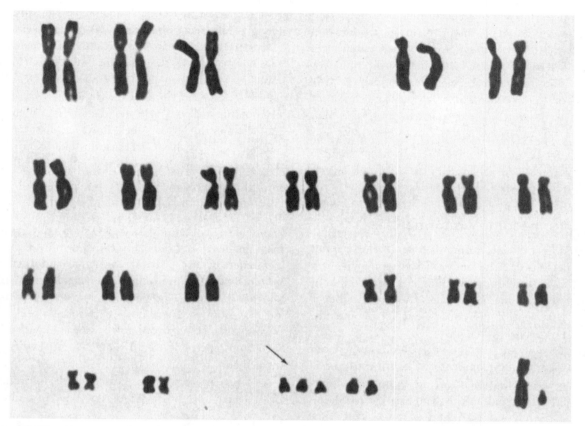

Figure 5–11   Karyotype of a male with trisomy 21, or Down syndrome. This individual has three copies of chromosome 21, which results in mental retardation as well as a number of abnormalities affecting the internal organs.

sac, increases in maternal blood in certain fetal abnormalities but decreases to abnormally low levels when a fetus is affected with Down syndrome. Researchers claim that the expansion of genetic screening to include the three biochemical tests could, if generally adopted, detect 67% of the 5,000 fetuses affected with Down syndrome in the United States each year. But without the blood tests, only 40% of all affected fetuses would be found through current screening methods, even if all older pregnant women had amniocentesis and all younger ones had an AFP screening (Randall, 1991).

Down cases due to nondisjunction are not hereditary, but there is a small percentage of Down syndrome births in which the cause is another kind of chromosomal aberration, called a translocation. In these cases, one of the parents, either male or female, carries the chromosomal rearrangement and may produce more than one affected child or pass the translocation to unaffected children, who may subsequently have offspring with Down syndrome. It is obviously important to identify such carriers, and all parents of a trisomy 21 child who shows a chromosomal translocation should have a chromosome analysis done.

There are several other kinds of autosomal abnormalities that result in multiple congenital (i.e., present at birth) defects that include both mental and physical retardation. Some are trisomies and some are deletions of a chromosome, but these occur much less frequently than Down syndrome. Among them are trisomy 18, formerly called Edwards' syndrome, which has an incidence of 1 in 6,500 live births but usually produces death within the first year. Lejeune syndrome, the *"cri-du-chat"* or *"cat-cry"* syndrome, is a very rare condition caused by a deletion of the shorter arm of one chromosome 5. Affected babies have physical deformities and are mentally retarded and, as a result of a defect in the larynx, have a characteristic high-pitched cry that sounds very much like the meowing of a kitten.

Sex Chromosome Abnormalities

The random accidents during meiotic development of the gametes that cause autosomal abnormalities can also, of course, produce trisomies and monosomies of the sex chromosomes. Sometimes the result is abnormal development of the gonads, but very frequently, there is no visible effect at all.

Nondisjunction of the sex chromosomes can occur during the development of the ovum *(oogenesis)* or during the development of the spermatozoa *(spermatogenesis)*. If such a number change has occurred, the result at fertilization can be an individual with any one of several abnormal sex chromosome complements: 45,XO or Turner's syndrome; 47,XXY or Klinefelter's syndrome; 47,XXX or trisomy X; 47,XYY or Double–Y syndrome; also XXYY, XXXY, XXXX, and even XXXXY or XXXXX! People with a Y chromosome will be male, no matter how many X chromosomes they have. A cell, however, must have at least one X to survive. Combinations like YO or YY have never been observed, and it is assumed that they are lethal, that is, incompatible with life. Table 5–2 illustrates the mating possibilities between abnormal and normal sperm and ova that produce the most frequent clinical conditions. Table 5–3 shows the approximate frequency and the major clinical symptoms.

Generally, any physical or mental abnormalities produced by sex chromosome anomalies are very mild compared with those produced by autosomal trisomies and monosomies. There does seem to be a tendency for some mental retardation to be associated with extra X chromosomes, but even if there is some intellectual impairment, it is usually borderline and minimal. Surveys of patients in schools, hospitals, and institutions for the mentally disabled indicate there is a higher

---

TABLE 5–2 Various Mating Possibilities Between Normal and Abnormal Sperm and Ova and the Genotype Produced

Normal Ovum	Abnormal Sperm	Expected Genotype
X	O	XO
X	XX	XXX
X	XY	XXY
X	YY	XYY

Abnormal Ovum	Normal Sperm	Expected Genotype
XX	X	XXX
XX	Y	XXY
O	X	XO
O	Y	YO (inviable)

TABLE 5–3 Frequent Sex Chromosome Abnormalities

Genotype	Name of Syndrome	Frequency	Symptoms
XO	Turner's syndrome (gonadal dysgenesis)	1/3,500 females	Female, is short in stature, has typical webbed neck (in 50%), poorly developed breasts, and immature external genitalia. Ovaries may be absent. The mental capacity is normal.
XXY	Klinefelter's syndrome	1/800 males	Male, is above average in height, with long arms and legs relative to the rest of the frame; has small testes and penis and is usually sterile. The breasts may be somewhat enlarged.
XYY	Double-Y syndrome	1/700 males	Male, is taller than average, normally fertile, but possibly of somewhat lower intelligence.
XXX	Trisomy X	1/1,000 females	Female, is normal physically, fertile, but possibly with greater tendency toward mental retardation.

incidence of XXX females and Klinefelter's males than in the general population. Perhaps because so many studies have been made on individuals in institutions, there may be a tendency to attribute too much of their behavior to their chromosome constitutions. A case in point is the concern that developed over XYY males when studies in Europe and the United States reported that they seemed to be overrepresented in penal and mental institutions, and the belief arose that these men were overly aggressive and had criminal tendencies. Newspapers and magazines have published lurid and sensational stories about the crime and violence committed by XYY males. It was subsequently determined that the XYY defect was not at all as rare as was supposed and that it was actually present in 1 in 1,000 newborn males, making it one of the most common chromosomal disorders. Many unsuspecting XYY males must be living among us, leading quiet, nonviolent lives. Their only consistent physical feature is excessive height, with 50% of XYY males being above the 90th percentile of normal. Studies have shown they are not overly aggressive nor do they exhibit particularly antisocial behavior, but they generally have somewhat lower intelligence than XY males (Witkin, Mednick, & Schulsinger, 1976; Owen, 1979).

PRENATAL DETERMINATION OF GENETIC DEFECTS

It is possible to detect chromosomal abnormalities and a number of hereditary metabolic defects in the fetus before birth by **amniocentesis,** which involves piercing the abdomen of the mother to remove a sample of fetal cells for analysis.

Use of the procedure is a controversial issue for those who object to abortion under any and all circumstances. Despite the recent development of techniques that increase the potential for prenatal correction of some fetal defects, when an abnormality is determined by amniocentesis the only options available in most cases are to have an abortion or to give birth to a baby with the kinds of defects that may result in a lifetime of suffering for both child and parents. For some people, this would hardly be an agonizing decision: the abortion would be performed and another pregnancy would be attempted, if desired. For those who object to abortion, this type of prenatal diagnosis is not useful.

Actually, the notion that amniocentesis invariably leads to abortion is mistaken. Most women who undergo the procedure get good news, discover that they are not carrying a fetus with the suspected disorder, and deliver a normal baby. There are indications, however, that some women elect to have amniocentesis as a method of sex selection; if the fetus they are carrying is not of the desired gender (and there is some evidence that there is a preference toward males), the pregnancy is terminated. Apart from the ethical and moral issues, the social implications of such a course have been questioned by even the most committed of those who believe in freedom of choice in abortion. Besides, any technique that is invasive (requires entering the body) is never entirely risk free, and the potential benefits of such procedures should always be weighed against the potential risks. For the vast majority of pregnant women, "I don't care what it is, so long as it's healthy!" supersedes any actual preference for a boy or a girl baby.

The method itself has been known for more than a century but has been used for prenatal diagnostic purposes only for approximately the past 25 years. During development in the uterus, the fetus floats in a fluid-filled sac, familiarly known as the "bag of waters," surrounded by two fetal membranes, the *chorion* and the *amnion*. Although some of the water and ions in this amniotic fluid may originate from the mother, the cells in the fluid have sloughed off from the fetus or from the amnion membrane and are genetically identical to those of the fetus. On an outpatient basis, an amniotic fluid tap is performed between the 14th and 16th weeks of pregnancy, when the volume of the amniotic fluid is between 175–225 ml. The procedure is done with or without a local anesthetic and is preceded or accompanied by ultrasound studies to localize the placenta and assess the age of the fetus by measurement of the diameter of the head. A long needle attached to a syringe is inserted through the abdominal wall, through two layers of the peritoneum, through the uterine muscle, and into the amniotic sac. A sample of approximately 20 ml of amniotic fluid is withdrawn and centrifuged. The sediment contains the cells, which are incubated and cultured for chromosome analysis and also for biochemical studies of various types. The supernatant is used for enzyme analysis and virus studies and to check the AFP concentration to detect neural tube disorders (Figure 5–12).

Amniocentesis in the second trimester of pregnancy makes it possible to diagnose specific chromosomal abnormalities, inborn errors of metabolism, and neural tube defects. It can replace a genetic probability with a diagnostic certainty and provide the option of therapeutic abortion and another pregnancy for particular high-risk couples whose former alternatives were refraining from childbearing or giving birth to an affected child. It cannot guarantee the absence of physical deformity or mental retardation; nutrition, drugs, and environmental pollutants are also suspect in causing birth defects. The major criterion for having the procedure would be when the probability of finding an abnormality is greater than the risk of having amniocentesis. Currently, this criterion is met in one or more of the following situations: pregnant women over age 35; any couple who has previously conceived a child with Down syndrome or other chromosomal abnormality; when either parent has a chromosomal aberration diagnosable by amniocentesis; if there is a history of genetic disease in a close relative; when a previous pregnancy has resulted in a child with multiple structural malformations and no cytogenetic studies were

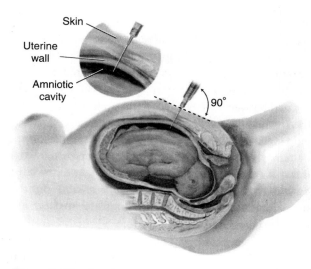

Skin

Uterine wall

Amniotic cavity

90°

Figure 5–12 Amniocentesis.

performed; or when a couple has experienced three or more miscarriages, early infant deaths, or both. When the parents have indicated a willingness to accept the possible necessity of a therapeutic abortion, amniocentesis, performed competently by experienced physicians, is an invaluable and relatively safe diagnostic tool.

A necessary adjunct to the procedure is skilled genetic counseling by trained professionals who can give accurate medical information and help couples interpret it within their own frame of reference.

In addition to the chromosomal aberrations that can be diagnosed by amniocentesis, there are more than 70 biochemical disorders for which prenatal diagnosis has been possible. These so-called "inborn errors of metabolism" are inherited defects due to a single mutant gene, generally resulting in the inability to produce a certain enzyme. Tay-Sachs disease, for example, is the failure to function or the complete absence, in nerve cells, of the enzyme hexosaminidase A. Lack of this enzyme leads to an accumulation of a carbohydrate-lipid molecule in nerve cells throughout the body, in turn causing blindness and mental retardation. Table 5–4 lists some of the best-known examples of metabolic disorders diagnosable by amniocentesis. There are also certain structural deformities known as neural tube defects (NTDs), such as spina bifida or anencephaly (in which the entire brain and spinal cord fail to form), that can be diagnosed prenatally. The test is based on the greatly increased levels of AFP that appear when the fetal central nervous system comes into direct contact with the

TABLE 5–4 Some Hereditary Metabolic Disorders Diagnosable by Amniocentesis

Disorder	Major Clinical Manifestations
Fabry's disease	Purple skin papules, renal failure, cardiac and ocular involvement
Gaucher's disease	Mental retardation from birth; skeletal changes
Tay-Sachs disease	Onset at 5–6 months, degenerative neurological disorder, profound mental and psychomotor retardation leading to death
Niemann-Pick disease	Variable skeletal and neurologic involvement; four types possible
Hunter's disease	Gargoylelike appearance, mental and physical retardation, liver and spleen enlargement, joint stiffness
Maple syrup urine disease	Mental retardation, early death
Galactosemia	Cirrhosis of liver, cataracts, mental retardation
Adrenogenital syndrome	Virilization of female, adrenal insufficiency
Lesch-Nyham disease	Self-mutilation, spasticity, mental retardation

amniotic fluid as is the case with neural tube defects. High AFP levels in the fluid are also associated with other fetal abnormalities such as intestinal obstruction, intestinal protrusion through an opening in the abdominal wall, or congenital kidney disease. Because the higher AFP levels are reflected in maternal blood, screening tests for maternal blood levels can be done early in the second trimester of pregnancy. A raised AFP level in the mother's blood can also be due to reasons other than fetal abnormality, so it is essential to make certain the result was not a "false positive" and to verify the elevated value through ultrasound and, if necessary, amniocentesis. There are also biochemical assay techniques that can differentiate among the various causes of increased AFP levels.

Risks of Amniocentesis

Although complications of the procedure are infrequent, amniocentesis is not without some danger to the fetus and to the mother. Fetal risks can include rupture of the membranes and a subsequent miscarriage, but a cause-and-effect association between amniocentesis at 16 weeks and miscarriage is difficult to analyze because a risk of spontaneous abortion is known at this gestational age anyway. The estimated increased risk of miscarriage as a result of amniocentesis is 0.08%–2.5%, based on data from a number of studies. The risk of miscarriage is greater in twin pregnancies.

Other consequences of amniocentesis for the fetus could be bleeding as a result of the needle hitting a fetal blood vessel or the placenta or punctures of the fetus leading to scars, depressions, or dimples, but these injuries are not lethal and are generally believed to be not serious complications.

Maternal risks can include puncture of the bladder, intestine, or a blood vessel, but the likelihood of serious injury is quite small, although it appears to be greater for the fetus and mother when amniocentesis is performed during the last 3 months of pregnancy.

Another method of prenatal detection of genetic defects that can be performed in the first trimester of pregnancy and yield some results within a day of the test rather than the 4-week wait required for amniocentesis is called *chorionic villi sampling* (CVS). The procedure was developed in medical schools in Milan and London and was first offered in the United States at Michael Reese Hospital in Chicago in 1983. Performed between the 8th and 10th weeks of pregnancy, the technique involves the insertion, under ultrasound guidance, of a small plastic catheter through the cervix or transabdominally into the uterus in order to withdraw about 30 mg of chorionic villi tissue, the fetal contribution to the not-yet-formed placenta. The tissue sample is processed for chromosome studies, and preliminary results of the chorionic cell analyses can be obtained within 24 hours, with completion of studies 10 days later. If the tests indicate a defect, the woman may choose to have a first-trimester abortion, a safer and simpler technique than the second trimester pregnancy interruption that could follow amniocentesis. Candidates for the procedure would be those who fit the current criteria for amniocentesis—over age 35 and/or a known carrier of chromosomal abnormalities or inborn errors of metabolism. The chorionic sampling procedure has the advantage of earlier detection over amniocentesis, but the risks have not yet been as clearly defined. The miscarriage rate, although small, currently is estimated to be greater than that associated with amniocentesis performed at 15–18 weeks of gestation, but studies have indicated that the experience of the physician performing the procedure is a major factor. Maternal risks are also not clearly defined. Cramping and vaginal bleeding may occur, and there have been some reports of uterine infection with serious complications. A comparison study of CVS and amniocentesis found that laboratory problems with cell contamination or errors in biochemical analysis were reported with a greater frequency after CVS than were those reported for amniocentesis (Canadian Collaborative CVS-Amniocentesis Clinical Trial Group, 1989).

An even newer prenatal screening technique is percutaneous umbilical blood sampling, which can take place any time after 18 weeks of gestation. The procedure involves the withdrawal of fetal blood from the umbilical cord by needle puncture under ultrasound guidance. The technique allows chromosome analysis as well as tests for certain blood disorders not apparent in placental tissue or amniotic fluid cells. The disadvantages currently include a greater miscarriage rate, increased possibility for maternal contamination of the fetal blood cells, and an inability to perform the procedure safely and accurately prior to 18 weeks.

Fetal cells also have been found to circulate in the maternal blood in very small numbers, but a consistent method for analyzing their genetic material for prenatal diagnosis is still in the early stages. A promising technique is the amplification of minute amounts of DNA, using a method called the polymerase chain reaction. Obviously, the development of a maternal blood test to replace the current risky and invasive prenatal tests would be a major accomplishment.

*N*ORMAL SEX DIFFERENTIATION

After the sex chromosomes have determined the sex in the normal course of events, the genetic constitution induces the differentiation of testes or ovaries in the embryo, and the testes and the ovaries produce hormones. In that hormonal environment, the result is the differentiation of the internal duct systems and the formation of the external genitalia and, just possibly, differentiation of the central nervous system to establish patterns of hormone secretions in the adult.

All of this happens long before birth. Actually, sexual differentiation is essentially completed by the 12th week after fertilization (as are most of the major events in human development).

During the 4th week of intrauterine life, only a few days after the first missed menstrual period and when the embryo consists of only a few hundred cells in all, there are large, round, primitive sex cells called *primordial germ cells* that become segregated from the other cells. These are visible in the wall of the yolk sac, a cavity that lies below the developing embryo. When the embryo folds during the 5th week, part of the yolk

sac is incorporated into it, and during the 6th week, the primordial germ cells migrate to what will be their permanent location, the gonads. Here they settle down, ready to be the progenitors of eggs or sperm when their time comes.

The gonads have become visible during the 5th week as a thickened area of epithelium called the gonadal ridge, which is located on the lower border of a temporary excretory organ, the mesonephros. The ridges contain numerous primordial germ cells rich in glycogen. Although the mesonephric kidney does not become the permanent organ (a role taken by the metanephros, which develops independently), the ducts of this transitory nephric system become incorporated into the genital duct system of the male.

In the 7th week of embryonic life, the gonads consist of an outer zone called the *cortex* and an inner area called the *medulla,* containing masses of cells, the primary sex cords. The primordial germ cells are incorporated into the sex cords. Two pairs of ducts are present next to the gonads at about this time. A paired *mesonephric* or *wolffian duct* forms to become a collecting duct that drains the mesonephric tubules of the primitive kidney. (Laterally, and a little lower down, the permanent kidneys and the ureters form; they open into the urinary bladder.) Alongside the mesonephric ducts, a pair of *paramesonephric* or *müllerian ducts* develop independently.

Even earlier, during the 4th week after fertilization, a small swelling or bump, called the *genital tubercle,* forms in the approximate position of the future external genitalia. Below it form the outer labioscrotal swellings, and inner urogenital folds form on either side of the cloacal opening, the common exit of the urogenital and gut tubes (Figure 5–13).

Now then, in the 7th week of life, the embryo is an "it," neither a "he" nor a "she." The only evidence of sexual organs is a bump and a swelling externally; internally, some noncommitted tissue masses and tubes exist, yet to differentiate. The embryo is 20 mm long (i.e., less than 1 in.) and looks unquestionably like a primate, although not necessarily human—that will take another week. Although the sex was determined

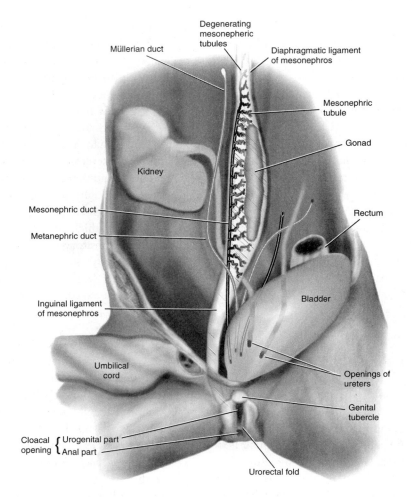

Figure 5–13 Schematic diagram showing the developing urogenital system before sexual differentiation has taken place.

at the moment of fertilization—XX or XY—those sex chromosomes have not yet had any visible effect.

Male Differentiation

The differentiation of the gonad into a testis takes place earlier than ovarian differentiation. If there is a Y chromosome in the cells, it contains the sex-determining region (SRY) or primary gene that causes testis differentiation, probably by reacting with other genes elsewhere on the Y, on the X, or on the autosomes. The medulla portion of the gonad develops while the cor-

tex deteriorates. The primary sex cords become the seminiferous tubules of the testis, and the cells that lie between the seminiferous tubules increase in size and number. These interstitial cells secrete the androgen, testosterone. Testosterone and its metabolite, dihydrotestosterone, formed by the enzymatic reduction of testosterone by 5-alpha-reductase, are responsible for the stabilization of the mesonephric or wolffian duct and cause the masculinization of the external genitalia. The mesonephric duct is incorporated into the male system as the epididymis, the vas deferens, and the ejaculatory duct, and it also gives rise to the seminal vesicle.

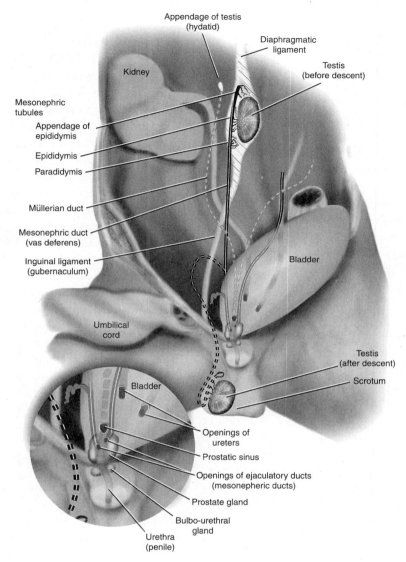

Figure 5–14 Schematic diagram showing the development of the male reproductive system.

The fetal testis also secretes a "müllerian duct inhibitor" that causes the regression of the müllerian duct. If both of these endocrine substances, the testosterone and the müllerian duct inhibitor, are secreted, and if the target tissues contain 5-alpha–reductase and have receptors for the hormones, a normal male will result (Figure 5–14).

Female Differentiation

Ovary differentiation from the undifferentiated gonad is directed by genes much as is testis differentiation. But the location of the ovary-determining gene(s) has not been determined as yet and few clues exist. The ovary inducers may or may not be on the X chromosomes, which carry many genes, and could also be anywhere else on the 44 autosomes. In contrast, the Y chromosome has been known to be necessary for testis induction in mice and human males since 1959. This narrowed the search for the gene locus among the 30–40 million bases on the Y, but it still took 31 years to identify the 35-kb (kilobase or 35,000 bases) region of the SRY, currently believed to be the major testis-determining gene. According to one hypothesis, autosomal genes for both testis and ovary determination are necessary in addition to the testis inducer on the Y. It may be that in XY individuals, the testis-determining factor, which is active prior to ovary differentiation, inactivates the ovary-determining genes. In XX individuals, who lack the repressive effect of the TDF, ovary-determining genes dominate with subsequent development of ovarian tissue (Eicher & Washburn, 1986).

About 2 weeks later than when testes develop, if there is no Y chromosome in the cells of the gonad, the medulla degenerates and the cortex develops into an ovary. The primary sex cords break up into clusters and become primordial ovarian follicles, each containing a germ cell surrounded by a layer of granulosa or follicular cells derived from the sex cords. Nothing has to be secreted, and no hormones are involved in the development of the female tract and the external genitalia. The mesonephric ducts spontaneously regress, and the upper parts of the paired müllerian ducts become the fallopian tubes, while the lower parts fuse. The upper portion of the fused müllerian ducts becomes the uterus, and the lower fused segment becomes part of the vagina. Fusion of the müllerian ducts also brings together two folds of the peritoneum, and the right and left broad ligaments as well as the pouch of Douglas and the uterovesical pouch are formed (Figure 5–15).

During the conversion of the müllerian and the wolffian ducts into the adult structures, some remnants may persist in both males and females. Unless pathological changes develop in them, these vestiges are unimportant.

External Genitalia

At 7 weeks, the external genitalia are said to be in an "indifferent stage," although Figure 5–16 illustrates that they actually appear quite femalelike. In females, the genital tubercle elongates rapidly at first, and then its rate of growth gradually slows; it becomes the clitoris. The urogenital folds become the labia minora, and the urogenital sinus outlet that they originally enclosed remains practically unchanged and constitutes the vestibule. The labioscrotal swellings become the labia majora, fusing anteriorly to form the mons pubis.

Under the influence of androgen in the male, the genital tubercle elongates to form the penis, and, as it gets longer, the penis pulls the urogenital folds forward to form the lateral walls of a urethral groove. The urogenital folds close over the urethral groove along the undersurface of the penis to form the penile urethra, and the external urethral opening in the male is caused to move from its original location at the root of the penis to its ultimate opening at the tip of the penis. The labioscrotal swellings develop and merge with each other in the midline; they become the scrotum, and later in fetal life the testes will descend from the body cavity to lie within the two scrotal sacs (Figure 5–16, Table 5–5).

Who Really Came First—Adam or Eve?

It should be obvious that the actual state of affairs in the embryology of the reproductive systems cannot be an affirmation of the Adam and Eve story. All embryos seem to be innately programmed to become females. In mammals, if the embryonic gonads are removed before differentiation occurs, the embryo goes right ahead and develops as a female—but one lacking ovaries. For the basic female pattern to be changed, the Y chromosome must be present. The gonads have to become testes, and the testes must secrete testosterone to develop the male tract and müllerian duct inhibitor so that the fallopian tubes and uterus do not develop. In contrast, no hormones from the fetal ovary are necessary to induce the differentiation of femaleness. The developing ovaries form estradiol, and perhaps it plays some role locally in

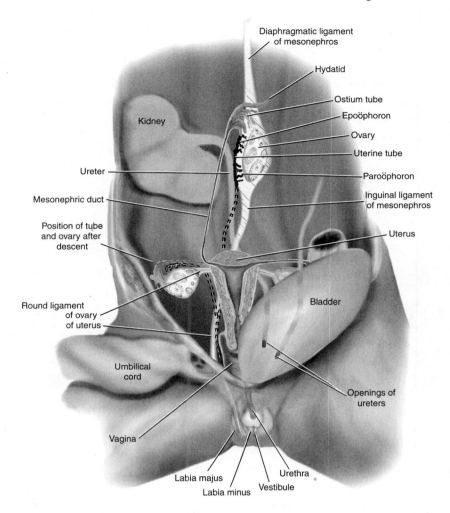

Figure 5–15 Schematic diagram showing plan of developing female reproductive system. The dotted lines indicate the position of the ovary and fallopian tube after their descent into the pelvis.

differentiating ovarian tissue, but the hormone is not essential in female development. Embryos of both sexes, of course, are exposed to levels of estrogen and progesterone from the mother, secreted both by her ovaries and the placenta, and to steroids from the fetal adrenals. Sufficient quantities of male hormones must be secreted by the male embryo's testes to overcome not only its own innate predisposition to femaleness but also the high circulating levels of maternal hormones. As a result, mammalian males, even after sexual differentiation is complete, continue to show a very high resistance to experimentally injected estrogens, requiring very large amounts before any feminization appears.

Mammalian females, whose female anatomy is genetic and innate and not determined hormonally, are, in contrast, easily masculinized and responsive to even very small quantities of androgen. The presence of endogenous (from the mother) or exogenous (administered) male hormone during the critical differentiation period in a female fetus can interfere with normal female development of the internal organs and the external genitalia.

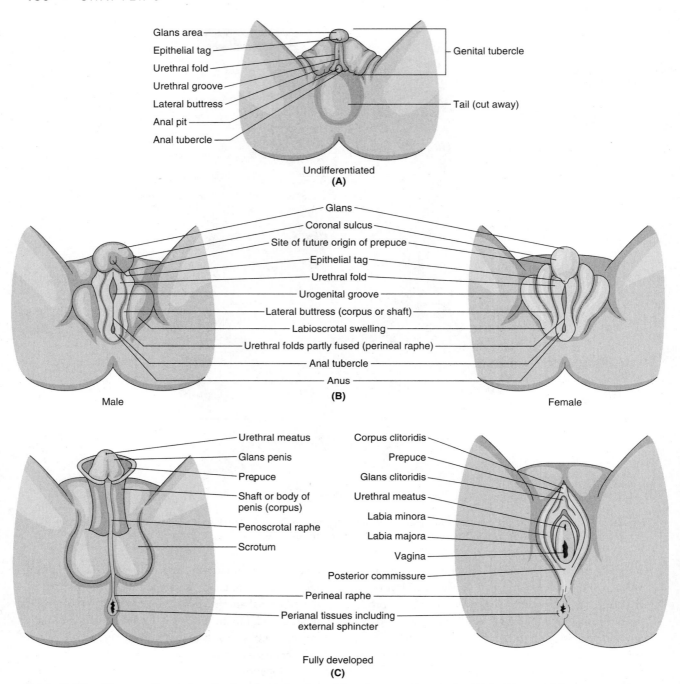

Figure 5–16 Diagrams illustrating development of male and female external genitalia. (A) At 7th week of gestation. (B) At 10th week of gestation. (C) Shortly before birth.

TABLE 5-5 Embryonic Differentiation: Gonads, Reproductive Tract, and External Genitalia

Undifferentiated Structure	Male	Female
Cortex of gonad	Regresses	Differentiates into ovary
Medula of gonad	Differentiates into testis	Regresses
Primary sex cords	Seminiferous tubules, tubuli recti, rete testis	Degenerate; follicles are derived from secondary (cortical) sex cords
Wolffian ducts	Epididymis, vas deferens, seminal vesicles	Small vestigial remnants
Müllerian ducts	Degenerate	Fallopian tubes, uterus, inner 4/5 of vagina
Inguinal ligament of mesonephros	Gubernaculum testis	Ovarian ligament, round ligament of uterus
Urogenital sinus	Urinary bladder, urethra, prostate gland, bulbourethral glands	Urinary bladder, urethra, lower vagina, Bartholin's glands
Genital tubercle	Penis	Clitoris
Urogenital folds	Underpart of penis	Labia minora
Labioscrotal swellings	Scrotum	Labia majora

SEXUAL AMBIGUITY

Within moments after the birth of a baby, there is an immediate exclamation: "It's a boy!" or "It's a girl!" This instantaneous diagnosis is based on what is easily observed. This baby has a penis and a scrotum—he must be a male. This one has a vulva and vagina—she must be a female. More than 99% of the time, babies are born unambiguously male or female, but in approximately 1 in 500 births, the sex is doubtful because of the external genitalia. The baby is evidently not male, but neither is it clearly female. This apparent intersex state of the external genitalia is the result of an error of embryonic differentiation, and the extent of the abnormality depends on why or when the error took place.

True *hermaphroditism* (from Hermaphroditus, the son of Hermes and Aphrodite, half man and half woman) occurs very rarely and is the term for individuals who have both ovarian and testicular tissue internally. The genitalia are usually ambiguous, but the male configuration generally predominates. The sex assignment as a boy or a girl is made, as it is in all intersex states, on the basis of which appears to be the dominant sex and on the ease of surgical correction.

Pseudohermaphroditism implies that there is a difference between the external genitalia and the internal gonads. Male pseudohermaphrodites have testes but external genitalia that are feminine or of doubtful gender, and female pseudohermaphrodites have ovaries but masculinized or ambiguous external genitalia.

The reasons for these developmental mistakes are varied and sometimes completely unknown. Embryonic defects can sometimes occur spontaneously and without any obvious explanation. Some of them are the result of chromosomal abnormalities, but many of the XO, XXY, XYY, and XXY variants that have been described are not even recognizable as a difficulty until puberty. Even then, the chief problem in most of them is infertility. Sex chromosome abnormalities usually produce such minimal or subtle changes in the external genitalia at birth that they are likely to be overlooked.

Ambiguous external genitalia are more usually the result of hormone imbalance during embryogenesis, either inadvertently induced by hormone administration during pregnancy or because a genetic defect of metabolism was expressed as a hormonal dysfunction. The testicular-feminization syndrome that occurs in genetic males and the adrenogenital syndrome and progestin-induced virilization that can occur in genetic females are examples of abnormal sexual differentiation caused by hormonal imbalance.

Testicular-Feminization Syndrome

Testicular-feminization syndrome is also called the androgen-insensitivity syndrome. It is an X-chromosome-linked recessive gene defect in which women carriers transmit the disorder to half their male offspring. Gene expression results in the inability of the mesonephric ducts, the genital tubercle, or any somatic cells to respond to androgen, evidently because they lack androgen receptors in their cytoplasm. The karyotype of these individuals is male, 46,XY, but their external genitalia are female, usually with a blind-ending vagina. Internally there are testes, usually undescended, although they have been occasionally found in the labia, and there may be very rudimentary fallopian tubes and a uterus without a cavity. In the embryonic development of males affected with this condition, the testes, under the influence of the Y chromosome, produce both androgen and the müllerian duct inhibitor. But because the target cells, lacking receptors, cannot respond, the wolffian ducts do not develop to any extent. The müllerian ducts respond

normally—they are inhibited. The external genitalia, also unresponsive to androgen, develop along female lines. The baby is born, is observed to be female, and is reared as a girl. Of course, the inability to respond to androgen continues throughout life. At puberty, stimulated by gonadotropic hormones, the testes release androgens and some estrogens as well. The target tissues respond only to the estrogens, so there is breast development and the body configuration is feminized. Menstruation does not occur, and this may be the first sign that something is wrong. A pelvic examination followed up by cytogenetic studies can establish that these females are actually chromosomal and gonadal males. If this knowledge is handled appropriately on both an intellectual and an emotional level (that is, if the parents are not abruptly apprised that their daughter is really their son), these girls do not necessarily have sexual identity difficulties. They have been raised as girls; they will grow up to be women and will marry and lead normal sex lives, though they will be unable, of course, to bear children. The testes of individuals affected with the testicular-feminization syndrome are known to be more likely to become malignant, and because of this risk, they are frequently removed. If such removal is done before puberty, the breasts fail to develop, indicating that it is the testicular estrogens that cause the female development.

Congenital Adrenal Hyperplasia (CAH)

In contrast to the above condition, in which the body is female but the sex chromosomes, gonads, and ducts are male, there are disorders in which the external genitalia are masculinized to a varying degree, but the sex chromosomes and internal organs are female. Because the inherent program of development is female and androgen has to be added to produce maleness, any female embryo or fetus that is exposed to androgen during sexual differentiation may be born with ambiguous virilized genitalia. There may be an elongated clitoris with an external vaginal opening, or there may be a "penoclitoris" with enough midline fusion to obliterate any vaginal orifice. Only the external genitalia are affected because androgen alone is not enough to cause development of male duct structure; müllerian duct inhibitor also has to be secreted by male testes to prevent the uterus and fallopian tubes from forming so that the wolffian ducts can be organized into male structures. These fetuses are female, however, and lack testes, so the internal ducts are not masculinized.

The most frequent cause of female fetal masculinization is congenital adrenal hyperplasia (CAH), an inherited defect (1 in 20,000 live births) in the ability of the adrenal glands to synthesize glucocorticoids. The adrenals, two small endocrine glands that are located on top of the kidneys, produce three kinds of steroids: the mineralocorticoids, which control the amounts of sodium and potassium in the body; the glucocorticoids, which affect carbohydrate metabolism; and the sex steroids, estrogen and androgen, normally produced in insignificant amounts compared to gonad production. In CAH, the fetal adrenals fail to synthesize glucocorticoids because the necessary enzyme, C-21-hydroxylase, is lacking as a result of hereditary defect. Because there is less glucocorticoid hormone circulating in the fetus, there is less inhibitory feedback to the fetal pituitary gland. The pituitary attempts to compensate for the lack by putting out increased amounts of adrenocorticotropic hormone. The fetal adrenal glands are overstimulated, and the zone of the adrenals that produces androgens undergoes hyperplasia (more cells), and greater production of androgens results. Normally, the enzymes involved in glucocorticoid synthesis by the adrenals develop in the 8th to 10th week of fetal life; if they fail to develop, the timing is such that the excessive androgens are produced at the very time of the differentiation of the external genitalia, and they are masculinized. Most of the time, the deficiency of C-21-hydroxylase is incomplete, and the only result is virilization of the genitalia. In about one-third of the clinical cases, however, lack of the enzyme results in life-threatening deficiency of adrenal corticoids, and substitution therapy must be continued throughout the life of the individual. The masculinization effects of CAH are limited to the external genitalia; once surgical alteration is made, the baby can be raised as a female, and further growth, development, and reproductive functions are normal.

Another source of virilization in a female fetus is an androgen-secreting ovarian or adrenal tumor in a pregnant woman, but this is rare because women with such preexisting tumors seldom become pregnant. More commonly, masculinization has resulted from the treatment of pregnant women with hormones to avert miscarriage. About 25 years ago, the accepted belief was that spontaneous abortion (miscarriage) was often due to insufficient production of progesterone from the placenta or corpus luteum of pregnancy. It seemed reasonable, therefore, to administer progesterone in the hope of maintaining the pregnancy. Natural progesterone is inactivated if it is taken orally, so synthetics that were orally effective were used in cases of threatened spontaneous abortion. The difficulty is that most synthetic progestins are androgenic to a varying degree. Although their masculinizing effects have been well known since 1958, and despite evidence that not only were progestins of doubtful value in preventing miscarriage but that these hormones caused other birth defects, they continued to be prescribed for pregnancy testing, prevention of miscarriage, and other complications of pregnancy well into the 1970s. The Food and Drug Administration (FDA) withdrew approval of these drugs for use during pregnancy in 1974, but several years after the warning, the drugs were still being administered (only 10% fewer prescriptions were written in 1975 than in the year before the warning had been issued). Fortunately, the number of birth defects seen has been extraordinarily low considering the total number of women who have taken prescribed hormones, suggesting that only a small part of the population is susceptible to their effects. There are few, if any, reasons to administer hormones during pregnancy, and all pregnant women should be aware of the potential hazard of taking sex steroids during the first 3 months of pregnancy.

Is THERE A MALE BRAIN AND A FEMALE BRAIN?

The male sex hormone plays the critical role in the differentiation of the male sexual anatomy. Without androgen, all fetuses would develop into anatomic females. The question that has been the subject of a great deal of attention and research and has generated considerable controversy concerning the interpretation of such research is, does androgen also play a role in the differentiation of the central nervous system? That is, is it possible that there is also a critical or sensitive period during which the brain is susceptible to male sex hormone and is organized to result in subsequent masculine behavior, and perhaps not just reproductive behavior?

The hypothalamus contains an area of steroid-sensitive neurons that are responsible for the secretion of gonadotropin-releasing hormone that, in turn, controls the release of follicle stimulating hormone (FSH) and luteinizing hormone (LH) from the anterior pituitary gland. This region, located above the optic chiasma and called the preoptic area, can be referred to as the cyclic center in mammalian females because the pattern of gonadotropic release is periodic and cyclic rather than the continuous and basal secretion that occurs in males. There is ample evidence that in rodents there are sex differences in the responsiveness of this area to steroids.

In rats, mice, hamsters, and guinea pigs, it has been shown that the sensitive area is undifferentiated and potentially female until a certain critical period. If the brain is exposed to androgen during that period, the animal is defeminized; that is, the cyclic pattern of gonadotropin release in response to estrogen is permanently suppressed. If no exposure to androgen takes place, the hypothalamus of both male and female rodents will develop a female cyclic pattern. So the hypothalamus, like the genital anatomy, is potentially *female* in both male and female rodents, unless androgen is present. That critical period during which the hypothalamus is converted from a female type to a male type is postnatal in laboratory rats and takes place within the first 10 days after birth. During that time, it is possible to administer an injection of androgen to newborn female rats and change gonadotropic release from a cyclic to a noncyclic pattern. When females like these reach sexual maturity, they will never ovulate and will remain sterile because FSH and LH are being continually (rather than periodically) released to produce cycles. Conversely, if the testes of a newborn male rat are surgically removed, the hypothalamus remains female and retains the ability to induce cyclic activity in an ovary. This can actually be observed if an ovary is grafted into the anterior chamber of the eye in such a castrated male rat.

When male and female rats are subjected to various experimental manipulations with their own gonadal hormones or with administration of injected steroids, they also undergo various changes in their mating behavior when they become sexually mature. If a female newborn rat is injected with androgens within 10 days of birth and is given no subsequent hormonal treatment, the typical female mating behavior toward male rats is inhibited, and she exhibits some male sexual behavior toward female rats. If the newborn female rat has been both androgenized and castrated—that is, had the ovaries surgically removed—her behavior at maturity will be sexually indifferent. She will exhibit disinterest to males and females alike. If such a postnatally androgenized and castrated female is treated with androgens as an adult, she displays some of the sexual behavior of a male.

Male rats castrated at birth with no hormone treatment will be sexually indifferent at adulthood—similar to the androgenized, castrated females. If such male rats are given doses of androgens during the first week after castration, a certain degree of masculine adult behavior is restored. If they are given estrogen and progesterone at maturity, they will display feminine sexual behavior.

Many of the same kinds of experiments were performed on other rodents; on other mammals such as guinea pigs, ferrets, dogs, sheep, and rhesus monkeys; and on several species of birds. In all animals studied, there is a developmental "critical period" for sexual differentiation during which the brain is sensitive to gonadal hormones. This time of increased sensitivity is postnatal in some species that are relatively less mature at birth and prenatal in those animals that are born more fully developed. The mechanism by which gonadal steroids are able to transform brain tissue to bring about particular behavioral and neuroendocrine functions remains undetermined, but there are several hypotheses. Perhaps hormonal receptor sensitivity is altered, or maybe neurotransmitter function is modified. One possibility getting a lot of investigation is that hormones may induce a change in gene expression and lead to a local alteration in cellular growth. Steroid exposure could thereby affect brain circuitry, that is, change the way neurons are hooked up so that the wiring is rearranged. In substantiation of the growth theory, there has been increasing evidence for morphological changes in the brains of some species. In some of the animals studied, the anatomical sex differences are subtle and require ultramicroscopy to see; in others, they are clearly visible with a light microscope even on gross examination.

The first study to find a structural sex difference in rat brains was done by Oxford University anatomists Geoffrey Raisman and Pauline Field in 1973. These workers found differences in the type and distribution of nerve fiber connections in male and female rat and hamster brains. Nottebohm and Arnold (1976) examined the brains of zebra finches and found that the song control centers, a chain of five discrete groups of neurons that controlled male singing patterns, were larger in male birds than in females. William Greenough and his associates (1977) saw differences in the shape of the stimulus-receiving ends of the nerve fibers (dendrites) in the brains of male and female hamsters. Roger Gorski at UCLA, a well-known name in anatomical sex difference research, found a very obvious difference in the brains of male and female rats that could be seen with an ordinary microscope (1979). Located in the preoptic area of the hypothalamus, a group of neurons the researcher called the sexually-dimorphic nucleus (SDN) was five

times greater in size in male rats than in female rats. Although the volume of the SDN was hormone dependent—the area shrank with castration in male newborn rats and became larger if female newborn rats were given testosterone—the specific function of the nucleus is still unknown. And according to other investigators, not only hormones but also prenatal environmental and social factors affecting hormones can play a role in the size of the SDN in male rats. Kerchner and Ward (1992) and Kerchner et al. (1995) found that when a rat is stressed during the last week of pregnancy by physically restraining her under bright lights for a couple of hours each day, the volume of the SDN as well as other sexually dimorphic nuclei in the brain and spinal cords of her male offspring was significantly smaller than in males whose mothers were not subjected to stress. Prenatal stress evidently suppresses testosterone and leads to incomplete masculinization of the sexually dimorphic areas of the central nervous system in rats.

In addition to the animal data, evidence of structural sex differences in the human brain has accumulated, but in most instances additional studies have produced conflicting results and the findings have not been firmly established. Allen, Gorski, and other researchers (1989) located cell groups of the preoptic hypothalamic area in the brains of 22 adult men and women and found one group of neurons they called the SDN to be almost three times larger in the male brains. Hofman and Swaab (1989) examined an ovoid, densely packed collection of neurons they called the SDN located in the preoptic area of the hypothalamus in the brains of adult men and women. Like Gorski's team, they found that in the male brains examined, the SDN was 2.5 times as large, more spherical than in the female brains, and contained twice as many cells. Neuroscientist Simon LeVay, who examined four groups of neurons in the brains of 41 people, reported in 1991 that the volume of one of the cell groups he called the interstitial nuclei of the anterior hypothalamus (INAH, the same as Allen and Gorski's SDN) was twice as large in men as in women, and also twice as large in heterosexual men as in homosexual men

(1991). LeVay's subjects were 19 homosexual men who had died of AIDS; 16 presumed heterosexuals, 6 of whom had died of AIDS and 10 of other causes; and 6 heterosexual women, 1 of whom had died of AIDS. The researcher acknowledged that his results could not determine whether the size difference was the cause or the result of the sexual orientation, and also indicated that until brain tissue from homosexual men dying of other causes than AIDS is studied, there is the possibility that the difference is a disease effect of AIDS, not of sexual preference. He predicted, however, that INAH would be larger in lesbian women (because, presumably, they have the sexual orientation of heterosexual men) than in heterosexual women. LeVay's study was the second report of a difference between the brains of homosexual and heterosexual men. The previous year (1990) Swaab and Hofman had contended that another group of neurons, the suprachiasmic nucleus (SCN) located near the area of the SDN, was twice as large in homosexual men as it is in heterosexual men.

In 1993, Dean Hamer and colleagues at the National Cancer Institute linked male homosexuality with markers at a gene location called Xq28 on the long arm of the X chromosome and published another study 2 years later that appeared to corroborate the original findings (Hu et al., 1995). Obviously, scientific studies that seem to provide biological underpinnings for homosexuality become highly political, particularly with the implication that there is a "gay gene" and that some gay men may inherit their homosexuality from their mothers. LeVay and Hamer became celebrities; both appeared on talk shows and wrote books. Subsequently, however, additional studies failed to confirm the existence of an X-linked gene underlying male homosexuality.

Other sexually dimorphic sex differences in human brains that have been studied are not in the hypothalamus. Some of the language-related areas in the cerebral cortex are reportedly larger in women (Schlaepfer et al., 1995), and some parts of structures connecting the left and right parts of the cerebral hemispheres, such as the corpus callosum, are larger in female brains (Lacoste & Holloway, 1982). The anterior commissure, a fiber tract that connects the two temporal lobes, and the massa intermedia, a tract that connects the right and left thalami, also has been found to be of slightly greater size in women (Allen & Gorski, 1991). The functional significance, if any, of the size difference between the sexes is unknown. This led media reports of studies like these to speculate that the size differences in the isthmus or the splenium cause women to outperform men on verbal tests, develop larger vocabularies, and make fewer mistakes in grammar.

The studies on sexual differentiation of the central nervous system in various animals led to the brain-organizing or brain-differentiating theory of the role of androgen: that fetal male hormone differentiates the embryonic bipotential brain into a "male" brain shortly after birth in rodents and during the prenatal period in other mammals. Because both gonadotropin release and mature mating and courtship behavior were evidently determined by this fundamental androgen influence on the developing brain, some workers further postulated a similar imprint operating for those characteristics thought to be uniquely male, such as aggressiveness, dominance, increased activity, rough-and-tumble play, and so forth.

The classic theory on the sex differentiating role of androgen on the brain has had to undergo some modification in the light of contradictory data. Different dosages of testosterone can produce different effects, and estrogen in animals is evidently just as effective in masculinizing the hypothalamus. Moreover, the biochemical pathways for testosterone action differ in various mammals. In rats, it is not testosterone that directly brings about sexual differentiation, but rather it is the brain's conversion of androgen to estrogen that causes the effects. Because estrogen rather than androgen does the differentiating, the male rat fetuses have to be protected from all the circulating maternal estrogen. This is accomplished in rats by an estrogen-binding protein called α-fetoprotein, which selectively binds estrogen and not testosterone. There is no evidence that human α-fetoprotein has a similar protective effect. Brain tissue also contains an enzyme,

5-α-reductase, that converts testosterone to another metabolite, dihydrotestosterone (DHT). It is DHT that binds to the androgen receptors in the brains of some species. Nevertheless, it is well established that in rodents, gender-specific behavior patterns are due to neuro-organization of the brain by early androgenation, whether primary or secondary in nature.

It appears, however, that rat brains are not the same as monkey or human brains. Attempts to confirm the sexual differentiation of the hypothalamus in primates for cyclic versus noncyclic gonadotropin release, or for behavior, have not been particularly successful. When androgens were given to female rhesus monkeys throughout pregnancy, their female offspring were, unsurprisingly, born with masculinized genitalia (elongated clitoris, sometimes with the labia partially fused). There was no suppression of the hypothalamic cyclic gonadotropin release, however, because when these female monkeys matured, they had normal ovulatory menstrual cycles and were normally fertile. It was reported that such androgenized females did exhibit some masculinization of behavior patterns. When the variables of aggressiveness, rough-and-tumble play, energy expenditure, and mounting behaviors usually seen in young male monkeys were used as measures, these females tended to behave more like male juveniles.

In human females, the opportunities for observing the effect of prenatal exposure to androgen are obviously very limited. The two clinical conditions described earlier, congenital adrenal hyperplasia and drug induced virilization, are virtually the only sources of clinical data. When such genetic females are exposed to androgen and are born with masculinized genitalia, their brains, too, have presumably been androgenized. Females like these nevertheless menstruate and are fertile after a normal, but in some instances delayed, puberty. As in the female monkeys, the cyclic release of gonadotropins was evidently not affected. Their behavior, however, has been reported to have been influenced by male hormones acting on their developing brains.

Money and Ehrhardt's classic study involved a group of 25 such fetally androgenized females during a period of several years starting in 1967. Their work is the most frequently cited as prototype evidence for the ability of androgen to program the brain because of the increased incidence of "masculine" behavior found in the androgenized girls compared with a control group. These 25 young women displayed behavioral characteristics that they themselves, their mothers, and Money and Ehrhardt collectively called "tomboyism."

What kinds of behavior do "tomboys" exhibit that suggest that prenatal androgen left an imprint on the fetal brain?

1. These girls were athletic. They liked team games, such as neighborhood football and baseball, and although some of them liked to play with girls as well as boys, some preferred boys exclusively as playmates.

2. They preferred clothing that was functional. Money and Ehrhardt say that these girls "chose to wear slacks or shorts" rather than "chic, pretty, or fashionably feminine dresses"—more practical, perhaps, for choice of activities. (Dressing for comfort rather than style, and pants on women were not as accepted in the late 1960s.)

3. The diagnostic group lacked interest in dolls and turned to the traditional boys' toys—cars, trucks, and guns—when they were younger. Later, they were said to be nonmaternal; they fantasized about having a career rather than, or in addition to, having babies and expressed little interest in wedding play. The researchers emphasized that even with all those indications of "tomboyism," these girls clearly had a female sexual identity. There was no evidence of homosexuality in their erotic interests as they became older.

4. There was a consistent tendency toward a higher IQ in the girls exposed to an excess of fetal androgen. But, as subsequently pointed out by Eleanor Maccoby, the intellectual levels of a group of prenatally androgenized females were elevated beyond that of the general population but were not higher than the IQs of their own normal siblings. Ruth Bleier noted that Money

and Ehrhardt's patients formed a highly select group of children from families that had sought and received sophisticated medical treatment from the day of the girls' birth, with all the concomitant implications concerning their intellectual and socioeconomic status. The general impression has remained in the literature, nevertheless, that excessive prenatal androgen enhances intelligence in females.

Studies of girls affected by CAH continued for the next several decades. These investigations consistently confirmed the findings of Money and Ehrhardt (Baker, 1980; Hines & Kaufman, 1994; Berenbaum & Resnick, 1997; Berenbaum, 1999). Conclusions of these studies were that there was masculinization of behavior, particularly that play activities of CAH girls were masculinized. There was an increase in tomboyism; the girls were aggressive; they spent more time playing with transportation toys than with "girl toys"; and they were less interested in pregnancy, infant care, and wedding play. Older girls showed more interest in male-typical careers than female-typical careers. One publication (Nass et al., 1987) supported the theory that the higher incidence of left-handedness in males was due to early androgen exposure because girls with CAH, who also had androgen exposure, are also more frequently left-handed than girls who do not have CAH.

It should be clear by now that these studies, like all scientific investigations, have both strengths and weaknesses and should be interpreted with caution. They reflect a rather traditional view of masculinity and femininity, and the behaviors characterized as tomboyism are only stereotypically masculine. The researchers conclude that children may show male behavior or female behavior, but not both. For a girl to want to play in Little League and prefer transportation toys to Barbie dolls does not indicate that male programming of the embryonic brain has taken place, however. For CAH girls, it is possible that expectations concerning their condition, known by the parents and the girls themselves, shaped their play behaviors long before the observations of them were made. Another reasonable

conclusion is that just because a girl wants to overcome sexual stereotyping at an early age does not mean she has an androgenized brain. It is more likely to mean she is athletic, spirited, and has a better time in Little League than playing with dolls. Being a tomboy as a child could also be a criterion for a successful career in later years. Women politicians, college presidents, actresses, artists, authors, and executives all have identified themselves as having been tomboys with the very same characteristics that were attributed to the diagnostic groups studied. Highly successful women at the top of their professions played basketball, baseball, and football; got themselves dirty; and generally had more *fun* while growing up. Of course this does not indicate that professional success is based on taking on male characteristics in childhood. It means merely that for some women, the world is less limited in childhood, that they enjoy activities on their own terms and not according to some rigid stereotyped role. It also offers proof that females whose embryonic brains have not been exposed to the influence of male steroid do not differ markedly in attitudes, interests, or behavior from females who have been prenatally exposed to androgen.

In summary, at a particular period of maturation of the brain in some mammals, exposure of a male fetus to his own circulating male sex hormones may result in the establishment of the adult male pattern of a constant and noncyclic secretion of gonadotropins. Also, in some mammals, androgens present before birth act on some developmental processes in the brain, which are then programmed for subsequent male social and sexual behavior. Evidence that this occurs in male humans or subhuman primates is highly tenuous and based on inference, although it is undeniably true in rats, mice, hamsters, and guinea pigs. Moreover, although sexual behaviors and activities in animals have been correlated experimentally to prenatal or postnatal changes in gonadal steroid levels, generalization from animal research cannot be extrapolated to humans. As yet, no definitive evidence has been shown that in humans, sexual behavior or sexual orientation is associated with alterations in testosterone or estrogen levels, gonadal cyclicity or non-cyclicity, being born with intersex genitalia, a gene, or having a larger volume of brain cells in one area of the hypothalamus. There are suggestions that there may be some neurological sex differentiation in the brain because there are neural and psychiatric diseases that exhibit a sex difference in incidence. For example, more females than males suffer from anorexia nervosa, bulimia, anxiety disorders, depression, and multiple sclerosis, while autism, schizophrenia, sleep apnea, Tourette's syndrome, and severe mental retardation are more prevalent in males. No structural or hormonal differences in the brain on which such sex differences are based have been found. And, of course, males also may have every one of the aforementioned neural or psychiatric disorders generally occurring more often in females, and vice versa. Despite the claims of those who believe that male and female abilities and behaviors are biologically based, there is little justification at this time for use of the terms male brain or female brain in humans, except in the sense that it is one found in a male or in a female.

GENDER IDENTITY

It has been seen that attempts to link gender-specific behavior or sexual preference in humans to a prenatal hormonal influence would at this time be purely speculative. There is more evidence that gender identity differentiation of the brain as male or female occurs postnatally and depends not on hormones but on the total environment in which a child is reared. When an error in embryogenesis has resulted in sexual ambiguity, corrective surgery can be performed to make the child unambiguously male or female to establish the morphological sex, and the gender can then be assigned to conform with the surgical alteration. When a child is called a female, looks female, and is treated as a female, she will grow up female, regardless of the genetic and gonadal sex. It is the sex of assignment and the sex of rearing, the entire postnatal psy-

chosexual environment in which a child is raised, that is evidently the most critical in the establishment of gender identity as a man or as a woman, and not the chromosomes, not the ovaries or the testes, and not even the external genitalia. Usually, the chromosome constitution, the gonad structure, the morphology of the internal ducts, and the appearance of the external genitalia coincide; when they do not, the sex of assignment and rearing can apparently override both the genotype and the phenotype.

Money and Ehrhardt described a situation that occurred in identical male twins. During circumcision on one of the boys, the surgeon accidentally and irrevocably damaged the tissue of the penis, which subsequently had to be amputated when the child was 7 months old. When sex reassignment to a female was suggested by a plastic surgeon, the parents had no other choice but to agree, and the required genital reconstruction was performed. At age 17 months, then, one of the twin sons became a daughter and was reared as a female; from then on, all clothing, hairstyles, toys, and so forth were emphatically feminine. Six years after the reassignment of sex, the two children acted, dressed, and behaved as traditionally appropriate to their gender, even though they were genetically identical twins and both male.

Another case in point is that of Ewa Klobukowska, who was 21 years old and the coholder of the world 100-meter dash record for women when doctors found she had "one chromosome too many" to be eligible as a woman for future competition. (The precise nature of the chromosomal anomaly was never made clear.) Because of this medical finding, the International Athletic Federation withdrew ratification of all the records, victories, and medals she had won. Subsequently, the Polish former athlete lived alone in Warsaw, dated men, and was not averse to the idea of marriage, although she had been advised that her ovaries and tubes were atrophied and that she could never become pregnant.

It would appear that Ewa Klobukowska continued a belief in her femaleness despite her "failure" of the sex test; she seemingly had a solid sense of her identity as a woman—she dated and wanted to get married—even though her gender identity belied her genetic sex. The totality of gender, the *being, acting, feeling* like an adult male or female, is usually a coinciding of genetic sex, gonadal sex, hormonal sex, morphological sex, sex of assignment and rearing, and behavioral sex or sex role. Even if a discrepancy exists within the first four items cited, the last two can still produce a fulfilled and functional adult. It is only when the biological sex is out of alignment with the gender identity in an *adult* that the real psychological dilemmas result. Transsexualism is the intense feeling of identification with the sex opposite to one's chromosomal, gonadal, and morphological sex. It can occur in both sexes and is usually described as a "man born in a woman's body," or vice versa. Such incongruities, sometimes called *psychic hermaphroditism* or *gender dysphoria syndromes,* occur somewhat more frequently in males than in females. Hormonal and surgical sex reassignment, a method of treatment for those individuals for whom psychiatric therapy has been unsuccessful, is currently considered a last resort for a highly select group of gender dysphorics. Some reassigned transsexuals have received considerable publicity or have published their autobiographies.

Sex Reversal at Puberty: 5-Alpha-Reductase Deficiency

The well-established tenet that biological sex can be overridden by the sex of rearing—that a genetic male, raised *unambiguously* as a female, will see herself unambiguously as a female—was challenged by the description in 1979 of evidently uncomplicated female-to-male sex identity reversals. The study, which reported an apparent change in gender identity and gender role that occurred in genetic male pseudo-hermaphrodites, raised questions concerning the importance of early psychosocial environmental influences as the primary determinants of gender identity. The subjects of the research, originally discovered by a vacationing physician and rediscovered by a Cornell Medical School endocrinologist, Julianne Imperato-McGinley, were 38 males in the Santo Domingo area of the Dominican Republic, all of whom were afflicted with a rare genetic defect called *5-alpha-reductase deficiency.* Testicular-feminization syndrome, in which the androgen receptors in target tissues are totally absent, was described earlier in this chapter. In 5-alpha-reductase deficiency, an autosomal recessive defect, the problem is not the absence of androgen receptors but rather a deficiency of the enzyme that converts testosterone to dihydrotestosterone (DHT), the form of androgen that binds to the cells of the fetal external genitalia in order for the male penis and scrotum to form. Male children with this inborn error of metabolism are pseudohermaphrodites, born with normal internal male ducts; testes in the abdomen, inguinal canal, or in the scrotum; a cleft scrotum that appears labialike; a blind-ending opening in the perineum that resembles a vagina; a phallus that is more clitoris than penis; and a perineal urethral opening under the phallus. In untreated individuals at puberty, conversion to DHT is no longer necessary for masculinizing changes to occur, and the increased levels of circulating testosterone result in the typical male secondary sex characteristics.

There were 38 subjects who were identified as being affected with the hereditary defect, and all came from 23 interrelated families in two rural villages. At the time of the study, 33 were still living. Of these, 19 had reportedly been unambiguously raised as girls. Seventeen of those evidently emerged from puberty with a reversed gender identity, and all but one not only felt but acted like men; that is, they adopted a male gender role. Of those 16, 15 had lived or were currently living as males with women. Under the influence of testosterone, these individuals had experienced voice deepening, penis growth with erections and ejaculations that were emitted from the perineal urethra, enlargement and pigmentation of the scrotum, and descent of the testes if they were not already in the scrotum. They also developed an increase in muscle mass and strength. The only usual male characteristic missing was facial hair, and none of them developed acne. Beardless they may have been, but, nonetheless, here was evidence that females, raised and treated like girls, changed at puberty into men, taking on men's roles, jobs, and sexual identities.

On the basis of these findings, Imperato-McGinley and others concluded that in males, when the sex of assignment and rearing is contrary to the chromosomal sex, the Y chromosome prevails if the normal testosterone-induced activation of puberty is allowed to occur. They further reasoned that the prenatal exposure of the brain to male hormone is a stronger determinant of male gender identity than is the sex of assignment and the sex of rearing.

This report of sex role reversal taking place at puberty is necessarily controversial, and many doubts were raised about its methodological validity and its conclusions. One criticism is that the affected children may not really have been unambiguously reared as girls. Individuals with the defect had been known in the society for four generations, and such children were referred to by other inhabitants of the villages as either "machihembra" (first woman, then man), or "huevodoce," which translates as eggs-at-twelve, but is actually slang for testicles or "balls" at twelve. The affected children were likely to have been confused about their identity as normal girls. Their genitalia before puberty were not completely masculine, but they were surely not normally feminine and must have looked peculiar to them. As John Money has said, ". . . if you're a girl who is not sure that you're supposed to be a girl because of your funny-looking genitals, you have an alternate choice . . . if you feel everything is wrong the way you are, maybe the correct way is the other way."

Perhaps Imperato-McGinley and her coworkers' study illustrated merely that in some societies, some pseudohermaphrodites who may be confused about their proper gender can undergo a psychological and social sex reversal after experiencing a masculinizing puberty, but the study has not demonstrated that a true gender reversal takes place. Neither has it presented conclusive evidence that prenatal androgen exposure is the primary determinant that programs the brain for gender identity in males.

THE OLD NATURE–NURTURE ARGUMENT

The very terms "gender identity" and "gender role" are confusing and unclear. What does it mean, to feel and act like a woman, or to feel and act like a man? Perhaps the feelings of identity as a male or as a female involve the personal view, the psychological awareness, the self-recognition, the intense conviction that one belongs to a particular gender. Then, the gender role that one takes in society is the way that gender identity is acted out—the countless numbers of behaviors, habits, preferences, expectancies, and attitudes that are recognized as sex-specific to that particular gender in one's sociocultural environment.

The behavioral sex differences that are perceived to exist between males and females have been examined, investigated, explored, and studied as the subject of scientific writings for centuries. Psychologists, anthropologists, sociologists, biologists, economists, and political scientists all have attempted to understand what those sex differences are, how they originated, developed, and are manifested. A major question has been, how important is biology in the determination of one's behavior as a male or as a female? What are the sex differences in personality traits, abilities, interests, and values? Do these differences really exist, and if so, are they preordained by genes and hormones? Or are behavioral sex differences psychological and social in origin and culturally determined?

The controversy surrounding these questions is very old: which contributes more to behavior, nature or biology, or nurture or environment? This kind of dispute could be dismissed as overly simplistic, irrelevant, and totally unproductive, except that it is still frequently resurrected to justify the alleged superiority of one group of humans of a different race or sex over another. If it is believed, for example, that one race or sex is genetically superior in intelligence to another, there is certainly nothing to be gained by providing equal educational opportunity to the inferior group. If it is considered that gender-appropriate stereotypes of feminine or masculine behavior are innate, natural, and biologically based, it can justify discriminating against women in lower-paying, lower-status jobs. If a woman's place is meant to be in the home, why pass legislation for her equal employment opportunity?

A traditional view, unrelinquished by many scientists, is that physical, psychological, and behavioral sex differences are of biological origin. Behavior is then viewed as a natural consequence of biological differences in size, strength, and reproductive capacities. A woman's reproductive system gives her the ability to conceive, bear, and deliver children; her body, therefore, confines her to a maternal and nurturing role. It is her nature to behave in a "feminine" way—dependent, passive, and less active. Physically, a male is stronger—he is the hunter. He has always been characterized by aggressive behavior; it is in his biology—his nature—to be dominant. This perspective, the biologic immutability of male/female differences, was expressed in the 1972 edition of *Reproduction in Mammals* edited by British biologists Austin and Short: "In all the systems that we have considered, maleness means mastery: the Y-chromosome over the X, the medulla over the cortex, androgen over estrogen. So physiologically speaking, there is no justification for believing in the equality of the sexes; vive le difference!" The authors evidently developed some sensitivity to blatant sexism in the 1982 second edition—the above statement was missing, and nothing like it has appeared in subsequent editions, the last being in 1987. But current proponents of biological determinism continue to argue that behavioral sex differences are genetic and innate. A 1991 book by Moir and Jessel, *Brain Sex,* purports that male and female behavioral patterns are dictated by differences in brain physiology established prenatally. As a result of these differences in neurological pathways, brain anatomy, and their respective hormones, men and women act as they typically do, and little can be done to change their behaviors.

Men have superior spatial ability and superior hand-eye coordination . . . Men are better than women at reading maps . . . Men's brains are more specialized. The female brain is organized to respond more sensitively to all sensor stimuli . . . to place a primacy on personal relations and to communicate . . . Women do better on tests of verbal ability . . . Women tend to be better judges of character.

There are many who challenge the preceding opinions, believing that much of the research that attempts to prove a biological basis for the social roles of males and females from animal studies, observations on the newborn, hormone experiments, or from anthropological studies is frequently inconclusive and contradictory. The relevance of a research tradition that emphasizes the biological limitations and differences between the sexes rather than the similarities is debatable. We might also question the existence of only innate biological factors that determine the traits stereotyped as male qualities (those of aggressiveness, leadership, dominance, competence, independence), when those traits are highly valued and rewarded socioeconomically and directly opposite to those traits associated with women and femininity (submission, nurturance behavior, weakness, passivity, incompetence, emotionality).

Another approach to the nature and origin of behavioral sex differences is the assumption that biological and social forces both interact. Neither can be solely responsible in the determination of personality and behavior, but postnatal influences very likely have the greater importance. There is now a substantial body of research to uphold the contention that concepts of the "typical male" and the "typical female"—that is, behavior that is stereotypically masculine or feminine—are the result of socialization and are conditioned by cultural attitudes and expectancies.

In this view, acculturation to sex roles begins in infancy when parental attitudes toward male and female children differ to reflect society's perceptions of what is deemed appropriate for each sex. As the child grows, the sex role assignments continue to be reinforced by social pressure, and the gender identity, or awareness of self as male or female, develops within this context of gender-specific behaviors. There is ample evidence from the clinical cases of ambiguous sex that gender identity is firmly imprinted by between 18 months and 3 years of age. By that time, a child has a pretty strong awareness of "I am a boy, so I will behave like a boy," or "I am a girl, so I will behave like a girl." The behaviors become quite rigidly polarized into stereotypes of masculine and feminine qualities, personality traits, and activities. Behaviors allowed to a particular sex are reinforced and rewarded, and those that overstep role boundaries are subject to social sanctions. Children are conditioned by their parents, their teachers, their textbooks, TV, the movies, and society in general to accept the traditional sex roles, and value is placed on strict adherence to the masculine or feminine image. Although little girls are generally allowed a somewhat greater leeway in displaying masculine-type behavior, at least until puberty, little boys are denied any behavior perceived as feminine, and their gender role is defined within much narrower limits. Even those parents, enlightened to a nonsexist child rearing that encourages giving trucks, erector sets, and tool kits to their daughters, have a little more trouble giving dolls to their sons.

Rigid polarization of sex roles into stereotypes of masculinity and femininity tends to further the notions of a natural male superiority, since only the "masculine" characteristics are those that are necessary for success in society. "Feminine" qualities are also valued, but they are seen as those characteristics necessary for successful homemaking and child rearing. If a woman works, it is at a job for which she is suited—being a nurse, teacher, librarian, or laboratory assistant. A young woman who wants to become a doctor, scientist, or engineer may then be regarded as deviating from her normal role, and she receives strong cultural messages that she is compromising her femininity by attempting to enter a man's world. Sex role stereotyping thus limits the full potential of all human beings by freezing them into traditional behaviors and attitudes.

The recognition that stereotyped generalizations about males and females are actually dysfunctional in our present world is a recent awareness, and it owes much to the women's movement. The roles of both men and women today have changed rapidly in response to the enormous social and economic pressures of a society that is overpopulated, inflationary, environmentally polluted, and rapidly running out of resources. A woman's place is not only in the home and has not been for many years. The traditional arrangement of homemaker wife and breadwinner husband occurs in only a very tiny percentage of American families. According to the Department of Labor, 99 out of every 100 women will work for pay at some point in their lives. More than 70%–80% of women, even those with children under a year old, currently work full time (although overall, they are paid 76 cents for every dollar men receive, a wage gap that costs working families $200 billion of income annually). Many occupy jobs that always have been perceived as "male." In the past 30 years women have made dramatic gains in male-dominated fields such as business, science, medicine, and law, and the number of women engineers increased more than twentyfold. Women are also working as electricians, carpenters, plumbers, or roofers in the construction trades—jobs that command good pay and benefits and require a high school diploma and an apprenticeship. There are even some barrier-breaking women in the good-paying jobs that require strength and little education, like the longshorewomen in New York licensed to work on the male-dominated docks. These women lift and stow boxes of bananas and 130-pound bags of coffee. And until they were laid off (last hired, first fired), there was a growing number of women coal miners in West Virginia using a pickax alongside men and doing a "man's job." Not every woman (nor every man) has the strength or the inclination to be a dockworker, coal miner, or piano mover. Not every woman wants to be a research scientist or an Army general. But those who do would agree with women's activist Florynce Kennedy: "There are only three jobs for which gender is a bona fide qualification: sperm donor, wet nurse, and human incubator."

Not everyone is ready to believe that. There are many who see such challenges to our traditional attitudes about the roles of men and women in society as highly threatening and an attack on the home and family. They blame everything on the women's movement—increasing divorce and crime rates, homosexuality, acceptance of abortion—and are convinced that a "reverse discrimination" now exists against white males. They see the traditional behavior of males and females as promoting stability and security, and they find it more comforting to cling to the stereotypes. Even if the result is the continued denial of equal opportunity to women, it is particularly appealing for some to still believe that behavioral sex differences are solely ordained by natural law, biologically determined, and that anatomy really is destiny.

While there are some scientists who contend that either nature or nurture alone is responsible for all sex differences, most contemporary researchers are more interested in assessing the relative importance of each. There have been thousands of studies of the differences in intellectual and cognitive abilities and in social and psychological behavior that exists between males and females. Some studies are designed to assess the effect of socialization processes in the development of sex differences. Other investigations continue to examine the importance of hormones on aggression or on nurturing behavior, to study the relationship between brain lateralization and sex differences, or identify gender differences in fine motor skills, response to odors, prevalence of depression, metabolism of alcohol, action of the hamstring muscles, and on and on. With all the research, however, *no measured behavior or ability has as yet been found to be unique to either males or females.* The differences are always quantitative, that is, they vary in degree and not in kind. Also, given the extreme variability of humans, the differences within one gender are always far larger than the differences between genders.

One of the side effects of research on gender differences in performance and behavior is that the conclusions of particular studies become codified in the literature, are taught to undergraduates in basic courses, and become accepted without question. For example, major research studies in the 1970s led almost everyone to believe that as fundamental sex dif-

ferences, females have superiority in verbal ability and males have superiority in visual-spatial ability and mathematics. Since beliefs can become self-fulfilling prophesies, many female students, their teachers, and most of society have had lower expectations for females when compared to males for spatial ability and mathematical performance or, by extension, for becoming scientists or mathematicians. Studies of the sex-related differences in visual-spatial ability favoring males, however, point to a trend in convergence of the scores of men and women on spatial tests and a distinct narrowing of the presumed gap (Stumpf & Klieme, 1989). Janet Shibley Hyde (1990) used a statistical technique called meta-analysis to combine data from many different studies, including those done in the 1970s, to show overall patterns and trends. Her research revealed that in the studies analyzed, there was no gender difference in verbal ability, there was a moderate gender difference in mathematical performance, and the largest difference was for one kind of spatial ability, mental rotation.

Although the gap between male and female performance on standardized tests such as the Scholastic Aptitude Test (SAT), the College Board Achievement Tests, and various graduate school admission tests, currently has disappeared for verbal ability, it has persisted in favor of male students in mathematics ability and achievement. The score disparity does not mean that men are innately superior to women in math, that their brains have been prenatally wired differently by testosterone, or, as some critics have suggested, that the tests are sex biased in favor of males. Among the many factors that could cause the difference in math SAT scores that has persisted since the 1960s is the fact that young women take fewer math and physical science courses in high school. Performance on the SAT-Math is related to high school course work; the more math taken, the better the students do. According to a report by the National Academy of Sciences called "Everybody Counts," in countries with a mandatory, rigid curriculum in math and science for both sexes in high school, no gender difference in math and science performance exists on standardized tests. When many girls, as well as many minority and disadvantaged students, no longer have unequal academic preparation, the sex differences on standardized tests may be wiped out.

In another example of how conclusions from studies on gender differences can bias societal perceptions and be detrimental to either gender but usually to females, it has been widely believed that the reading disability called dyslexia, affecting 10%–15% of the population, is more prevalent in boys. For years, educators and psychologists have assumed a biological, innate basis for the presumed gender difference in dyslexia, even linking it to prenatal androgenizing of the brain and to left-handedness. Most dyslexia research has been on the boys identified by teachers in school systems as having the impairment. Once children with dyslexia are recognized as having the disorder, they can be taught to read and, traditionally, boys with dyslexia typically account for 80% of the children treated in special education classes. Recent evidence, however, has revealed that, despite beliefs to the contrary, girls are just as likely as boys to have the reading problem (Shaywitz, Shaywitz, Fletcher, & Escobar, 1990). In a sample of 215 girls and 199 boys, the researchers found two groups of reading-disabled children: those identified through research and those identified by the school. While there was no difference in reading disability between research-identified boys and research-identified girls, when it was the school that identified the children with dyslexia, significantly more boys than girls were classified as having the disorder. According to the researchers, the children's teachers have a referral bias; that is, expecting that boys are affected, they frequently diagnose the condition in boys and fail to recognize dyslexia in girls. The unfortunate result is that the girls are left untreated and must struggle alone with their reading problems.

It is hardly realistic to raise children in an atmosphere totally free of generalizations, stereotypes, and expectancies about their behaviors, but only in this way can the relative importance of innate factors actually be determined. Perhaps biology does create a predisposition for the development of certain behaviors that are masculine or feminine, or perhaps it does not. And perhaps the answer is irrelevant. Of course, males and females exhibit differences in behavior, but so what? Our major concern should be that there are no sex differences, whatever their basis, that are able to justify sexist discrimination, that can imply male supremacy or female inferiority, or that can prevent individuals of both sexes from the realization of their full human potentials.

That sex differences exist is really not that important. It is that insistence—that demand—of society that they have to exist that can be stifling for both males and females. An inflexible categorization of masculine–feminine limits freedom of choice for women and cheats them of the opportunity to make their maximal contribution to all humanity. To set up limitations on some humans, to concentrate on the differences instead of the similarities between the sexes, not to integrate and prize the positive traits of both, is of little value. We are all people, capable of behaving in both masculine and feminine ways, whatever our sex. Such balance provides for the truly whole and integrated personality.

ℛEFERENCES

Allen, L. S., & Gorski, R. A. (1991). Sexual dimorphism of the anterior commissure and massa intermedia of the human brain. *Journal of Comparative Neurology, 312*(1), 97–104.

Allen, L. S., Hines, M., Shryne, J. E., & Gorski, R. A. (1989). Two sexually dimorphic cell groups in the human brain. *Journal of Neuroscience 9*(2), 497–506.

Austin, C. R., & Short, R. V. (Eds.). (1972). *Reproduction in mammals* (Vol. 2). *Embryonic and fetal development.* Cambridge: Cambridge University Press.

Austin, C. R., & Short, R. V. (Eds.). (1982). *Reproduction of mammals* (2nd ed., Vol. 2). *Embryonic and fetal development.* Cambridge: Cambridge University Press.

Baker, S. (1980). Psychosexual differentiation in the human. *Biology of Reproduction, 22,* 61–72.

Berenbaum, S. A. (1999). Effects of early androgens on sex-typed activities and interests in adolescents with congenital adrenal hyperplasia. *Hormones and Behavior, 35*(1), 102–110.

Berenbaum, S. A., & Resnick, S. M. (1997). Early androgen effects on aggression in children and adults with congenital adrenal hyperplasia. *Psychoneuroendocrinology, 22*(7), 505–515.

Bleier, R. (1976). Brain, body and behavior. In J. Roberts (Ed.), *Women scholars on women.* New York: McKay.

Canadian Collaborative CVS-Amniocentesis Clinical Trial Group. (1989). Multicentre randomised clinical trial of chorion villus sampling and amniocentesis. *Lancet, 1,*(8633), 334–335.

Eicher, E. M., & Washburn, L. L. (1986). Genetic control of primary sex determination in mice. *Annual Review of Genetics, 20,* 327–360.

Frye, A. J., & Kamon, E. (1983). Sweating efficiency in acclimated men and women exercising in humid and dry heat. *Journal of Applied Physiology, 54*(4), 972–977.

Gorski, R. (1979). The neuroendocrinology of reproduction: An overview. *Biology of Reproduction, 20,* 111–127.

Greenough, W. T., Carter, C. S., Steerman, C., & DeVoogd, T. J. (1977). Sex differences in dendritic patterns in hamster preoptic area. *Brain Research, 126,* 63–72.

Hamer, D. A., Hu, S., Magnuson, V. L., et al. (1993). A linkage between DNA markers on the X chromosome and the male sexual orientation. *Science, 261*(5119), 321–327.

Herman-Giddens, M. E., Slora, E. J., Wasserman, R. C., et al. (1997). Secondary sexual characteristics and menses in young girls seen in office practice: A study from the Pediatric Research in Office Settings network. *Pediatrics, 99*(4), 505–512.

Hines, M., & Kaufman, F. R. (1994). Androgen and the development of human sex-typical behavior: Rough-and-tumble play and sex of preferred playmates in children with congenital adrenal hyperplasia (CAH). *Child Development, 65*(4), 1042–1053.

Hofman, M. A., & Swaab, D. F. (1989). The sexual dimorphic nucleus of the preoptic area in the human brain: A comparative morphometric study. *Journal of Anatomy, 164,* 55–72.

Hu, S., Pattatucci, A. M., Patterson, C., et al. (1995). Linkage between sexual orientation and chromosome Xq28 in males but not in females. *Nature Genetics, 11*(3), 248–256.

Hyde, J. S. (1990). Meta-analysis and the psychology of gender differences. *Signs: Journal of Women in Culture and Society, 16*(11), 55–73.

Imperato-McGinley, J., Terson, R. E., Gautier, T., & Sturla, E. (1979). Androgen and the evolution of male-gender identity among male pseudohermaprodites with 5 a-reductase deficiency. *New England Journal of Medicine, 300,* 1233–1237.

Kaplowitz, P. B., & Oberfield, S. E. (1999). Reexamination of the age limit for defining when puberty is precocious in girls in the United States: Implications for evaluation and treatment. Drug and Therapeutics and Executive Committees of the Lawson Wilkins Pediatric Endocrine Society. *Pediatrics, 104*(4 Pt. 1), 936–941.

Kerchner, M., Malsbury, C. W., Ward, O. B., et al. (1995). Sexually dimorphic areas in the rat medial amygdala: Resistance to the demasculinizing effect of prenatal stress. *Brain Research, 672*(1–2), 251–260.

Kerchner, M., & Ward, I. L. (1992). SDN-MPOA volume in male rats is decreased by prenatal stress, but is not related to ejaculatory behavior. *Brain Research, 581*(2), 244–251.

Lacoste, U. de C., & Holloway, R. L. (1982). Sexual dimorphism in the human corpus callosum. *Science, 216,* 1431–1432.

LeVay, S. (1991). A difference in hypothalamic structure between heterosexual and homosexual men. *Science, 253,* 1034–1037.

Maccoby, E. E., & Jackoin, C. N. (1974). *The psychology of sex differences.* Stanford, CA: Stanford University Press.

Moir, A., & Jessel, D. (1991). *Brain sex: The real differences between men and women.* London: Lyle Stuart.

Money J., & Ehrhardt, A. (1972). *Man & woman, boy & girl.* Baltimore: Johns Hopkins University Press.

Nass, R., Baker, S., Speiser, P., et al. (1987). Hormones and handedness: Left hand bias in female congenital adrenal hyperplasia patients. *Neurology, 37*(4), 711–715.

Nottebohm, T., & Arnold, A. (1976). Sexual dimorphism in vocal control areas of the songbird brain. *Science, 184,* 211–213.

Owen, D. R. (1979). Psychological studies in XYY males. In H. L. Vallet & I. H. Porter (Eds.), *Genetic mechanisms of sexual development* (pp. 465–471). New York: Academic Press.

Raisman, G., & Field, P. M. (1973). Sexual dimorphism in the neuropid of the preoptic area of the rat and its independence on neonatal androgen. *Brain Research, 54,* 1–29.

Randall, T. (1991). Pregnancy hormone levels signal trisomy 21, improved screening, lower costs possible. *Journal of the American Medical Association, 265*(14), 1797–1798.

Schlaepfer, T. E., Harris, G. J., Tien, A. Y., et al. (1995). Structural differences in the cerebral cortex of healthy female and male subjects: A magnetic resonance imaging study. *Psychiatry Research, 61*(3), 129–135.

Shaywitz, S. E., Shaywitz, B. A., Fletcher, J. M., & Escobar, M. D. (1990). Prevalence of reading disability in boys and girls. *Journal of the American Medical Association, 264*(8), 998–1002.

Sinclair, A. H., Berta, P., & Palmer, M. S. (1990). A gene from the human sex-determining region encodes a protein with homology to a conserved DNA-binding motif. *Nature, 346,* 240–245.

Stumpf, H., & Klieme, E. (1989). Sex-related differences in spatial ability: More evidence for convergence. *Perceptual and Motor Skills, 69*(3 Pt. 1), 915–921.

Swaab, D. F., & Hofman, M. A. (1990). An enlarged suprachiasmic nucleus in homosexual men. *Brain Research, 537,* 141–145.

Tanner, J. M. (1973). Growing up. *Scientific American, 229*(3), 34–43.

U.S. Department of Labor. (1998). *Employment Characteristics of Families in 1997,* Washington, D.C.: United States Department of Labor, Bureau of Labor Statistics.

Verkerk, A. J., Pieretti, M., & Sutcliffe, J. S. (1991). Identification of a gene (FMR-1) containing a CGG repeat coincident with a breakpoint cluster region exhibiting length variation in fragile X syndrome. *Cell, 65,* 905–914.

Witkin, H. A., Mednick, S. A., & Schulsinger, F. (1976). Criminality in XYY and XXY men. *Science, 193,* 547–555.

Zacharias, L., Rand, W. M., & Wurtman, R. J. (1976). A prospective study of sexual development and growth in American girls: The statistics of menarche. *Obstetrical and Gynecological Survey, 31,* 325–337.

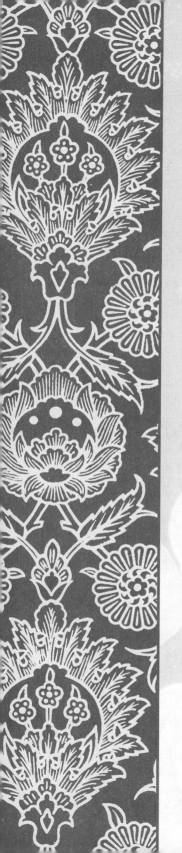

6

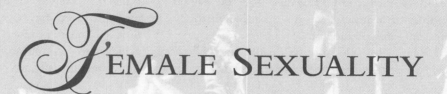

FEMALE SEXUALITY

KEY TERMS

Aphrodisiacs

Bartholin's glands

Coitus

Impotence

Orgasm

Orgasmic platform

Premature ejaculation

Vasocongestion

$\mathcal{A}$n old joke, which appeared as a bit of dialogue in a Woody Allen movie, has a couple going to a psychiatrist. The psychiatrist asks, "How often do you have sex?" The man answers, "Hardly ever—three times a week!" The woman answers, "All the time—three times a week!" The joke is funny because of our instant, if somewhat rueful, recognition of its underlying and universal assumption. For centuries, women had been conditioned by society to suppress their sexual urges and told that their role was to satisfy the physical needs of their husbands without expecting any gratification for themselves. To bear the burden of sex was as much a duty for a woman as to bear infant after infant—it was accepted that she would bear all the obligations of her life. A modest woman, a "nice girl," "a lady" may have felt *something,* but it was separate and in no way equal to what men felt and certainly not enjoyable without love. Currently, however, after several decades of research into the nature of human sexuality, women are told that they are in no way sexually inferior to males, that they have the anatomical equipment and physiological capacity for equal, if not greater sexual pleasure than males, and they are realizing that they are entitled to experience it. The research of Kinsey and Masters and Johnson should have laid to rest once and for all the myth that women obtain little satisfaction from sex. Women in today's society should feel free to express their feelings and desires more openly, without guilt or anxiety. Yet this is still a struggle.

Perhaps some of the old myths were dispelled only to be replaced by new ones. Some of the traditional and puritanical ideas about female sexuality have been at least partially discarded, but for many women, even those confident about their sex lives, the presumed sexual revolution created additional confusion and conflict about the expression of their own sexuality and the expected sexual behavior of others. The publication of data that indicate what other people are doing, and the sexually explicit movies, cable television, and magazines that show how they are doing it, may not be necessarily reassuring after years of social conditioning. Some of the changed standards of sexuality are seen by many women as goals that must be achieved: I must not be a virgin at the age of 15, or 19, or 21. I must want sex all the time, and in all ways. Today's woman, in the all-sex all-the-time media image is a supersexual superwoman. She is seen in the media as slim, gorgeous, big breasted, omnipresent, and bigger than life. And that is a most difficult burden to carry. Today's new sexuality sometimes offers women as few alternatives as yesterday's Victorian standards. The inability, unwillingness, or failure to be as "sexy" as women believe they should be can produce guilt and mental anguish in them. Has the revolution allowed women to make a choice about their sexuality, or has more openness about sex and more sex for more

people, and more kinds of sex, only dictated a different kind of exploitation of womankind?

Word has it that the negative feelings toward premarital sex have changed for most people. The old idea that males could and were expected to do anything they wanted but that females had to bring virginity to their marriage is no longer tenable. The double standard is dead. Or is it? Perhaps women have achieved freedom in sexuality in the *philosophy* of our times, but in daily reality, many young women evidently do not feel increasingly free to decide for themselves the nature and the extent of their sexual behavior. They claim that while their mothers were told that they had to say "no," they are being told that they have to say "yes," and if they are reluctant, there is something wrong with them. They feel they are being pressured into sexual activity in order to maintain a close relationship ("If you really loved me, you would. . . ."), only to discover that their expectations for the results of such relationships were unrealistic. They may find that casual and spontaneous sex can also be exploitive sex, but they are told by males that they are missing all the fun or that they are abnormal. A society that gives women little or no choice in their sexuality has not been very revolutionized. That kind of sex is as old as civilization.

The point is this: if some women are having as much fun playing the field as men used to, then perhaps a sexual milestone *has* been reached. But no milestone for all womankind has been gained when today's sexuality is in danger of offering women as few options as before. True sexual liberation should include the right to say "no" to certain kinds of sexual relationships without guilt or anxiety. In particular, young people should not have to agonize over their supposed abnormality if they are still virgins past a certain arbitrary age.

That there is enormous peer pressure to narrow the gap between the onset of puberty and the onset of sexual activity is illustrated by surveys by the National Center for Health Statistics. In 1995, the last survey date available, 50% of teenage girls between 15 and 19 say they are having premarital sex, and the proportion of girls having sex before age 15 is 19%. Even with the recognition that all this sex may not be voluntary and the number of girls having sex has declined from 55% in 1990, undeniably teen girls have sex early. There has been an increasing incidence of sexually transmitted diseases among adolescents as well. The good news, however, is that the birth rate among girls 15–19 has dropped 18% from 1991 to 1998, a statistic that has put the overall birth rate in the United States at its lowest point since records began to be kept in 1909. The teenage pregnancy rate also declined 15% from 1991 to 1996, reflecting current declines in birth and abortion rates, as recorded by the National Vital Statistics System in 2000. Whether sex education in the schools could alleviate problems of early sexual activity is an unanswered question, mainly because there is so little good sex education available. Although polls indicate that an overwhelming majority of the American public favors sex education being taught to schoolchildren, half the states require it, and the remainder officially encourage sex education in the curriculum, many programs are superficial and brief, and many teachers have had no training in the subject. According to the Sex Information and Education Council of the United States (SIECUS), fewer than 10% of American schools teach comprehensive sex education. Moreover, when the issue of sex education gets to a particular community, there is often strong and organized opposition to such instruction. People still stubbornly believe that formal sexual education equals sexual permission, and the leading sex educators of children in the country continue to be other children. Sexual myths and misinformation are easily transmitted; attitudes of sexual rights and responsibilities and the fact that sexual activity is a choice are unlikely to be conveyed. Even when sex education is included in a school curriculum, the students may learn a lot about reproductive physiology but not nearly enough about minimizing their chances of contracting a sexually transmitted disease, avoiding pregnancy, or the necessity for respect and caring for other people in all their relationships. Whether parents or schools are the source of sex education, telling youngsters about sex also has to include the reassurance that choosing *not* to enter into sexual relationships is just as healthy and appropriate as choosing to.

Another source of self-doubt and anxiety in women may be the result of the emphasis on the frequency and intensity of the **orgasm.** There is pressure for women to achieve multiple and wondrous orgasms. It is supposed to just happen. Books that have mass-market appeal allow their heroines to have skyrocket orgasms in poetic language, and films show the same event, larger than life. But it may not just happen. Merely because women have been told that they *can* reach orgasm as easily as men does not mean that they do, at least in the way they believe they are supposed to—solely through vaginal intercourse. Many women, believing that the earth should move for them every time they have intercourse, think that they are "frigid" and incapable of response, either because the earth does *not* move for them in orgasm, or because they do not achieve orgasm at all. Women may be placing a huge burden on themselves and on their sexual partners by expecting "The Big O" to happen every time, on schedule, with the same intensity, from the same formula, and simultaneously with the male orgasm.

When a male ejaculates, he has had an orgasm. Male orgasm, producing spermatozoa-containing semen, is necessary to human reproduction. In contrast, the human race could continue to survive if no woman ever had an orgasm. Although the mechanism is the same in both males and females, a reflex consisting of sensory stimulation leading to motor muscular contractions, the focal point for female sexual stimulation is in the glans and shaft of the clitoris, an organ separate from the organs that function in conception, gestation, and delivery. In women, an orgasm is a purely pleasurable experience, a natural physiological phenomenon that provides enhancement and satisfaction in sexual activity. There is nothing mysterious about an orgasm; it is a reflex, a physical manifestation, and it is a good feeling. So why is it so frequently missing in the sexual functioning of so many women? And why all the anxiety?

PHYSIOLOGY OF THE FEMALE SEXUAL RESPONSE

The actual nature of the female sexual response or any kind of sex research at all was largely a taboo subject in science until a zoologist at Indiana University, Alfred C. Kinsey, started to teach a marriage course in 1937. Dr. Kinsey was an entomologist, a specialist on insects, when he took over the course. Kinsey discovered that so little was known about human sexual behavior that, in order to provide his students with the facts, he decided he would have to gather them himself. He approached his task with the same meticulous precision with which he studied his insects. With the publication of his observations in 1948 and 1953, popularly known as *The Kinsey Report,* he opened up the field of sex research as a valid scientific discipline and foreshadowed the laboratory studies of human sexual responses observed by gynecologist William Masters and his associate, Virginia Johnson, at Washington University in St. Louis. There has been very little, if any, research on the physiology of female sexual response since the publication of their studies, primarily because of the lack of funding for laboratory sex research during the 1980s. But currently, with sales of the male impotence drug Viagra soaring, there is renewed interest in women's genital physiology because pharmaceutical companies are eager to tap the women's market as well.

Masters and Johnson, under controlled laboratory conditions, reported on the physiological responses of 382 women and 312 men between the ages of 18 and 89 during more than 10,000 "sexual response cycles," as they called them. They made observations during manual masturbation, during masturbation with a vibrator, during intercourse in several positions, while the breasts alone were stimulated without genital contact, and also during "artificial coitus" with a plastic penis containing a movie camera to record internal changes. The last method was the target for a number of attacks; the researchers were said to have mechanized and dehumanized sex. Sex in the laboratory was criticized and satirized, and many strongly objected to the approach. It was bad enough that Kinsey asked about what people did, but Masters and Johnson were *watching*!

While there may be some justification in the objections that Masters and Johnson's data missed the emotional aspects of sex by concentrating on the anatomy and physiology, until they published their research findings, there was little knowledge of the female sexual response because most of the genital response takes place *internally.* Vaginal lubrication, the distension of the inner two-thirds of the vagina, the gaping of the cervical os, the elevation of the uterus—all had been previously hidden from view. In contrast, no internal motion picture is needed to observe the male genital response; essentially, first the penis is erect, and then it is flaccid. Use of the artificial penis also made possible observations that had clinical value in infertility problems and contraceptive research.

For purposes of description, Masters and Johnson divided the female and male sexual response cycle into four phases: excitement, plateau, orgasm, and resolution. Those stages are successive; one follows the other along a continuum, and they are the same in both sexes.

During the four phases, there are two basic kinds of physiological mechanisms that cause the sexual response. One is *congestion* or an increased flow of blood into the organs so that the tissues become engorged (swollen) and usually undergo a color change. The other main physiological phenomenon is *myotonia,* the increased muscular tension that occurs both in voluntary (skeletal) muscles and in involuntary smooth muscles. Vasocongestion and myotonia result in the physical manifestations that are visible in the genitalia and also appear as extragenital responses such as changes in heart rate, breathing rate, blood pressure, and perspiration.

THE EXCITEMENT PHASE OF THE SEXUAL CYCLE

Genital Responses

Vagina. The first sign of physiological response occurs in the vagina within 10–30 seconds of the initiation of sexual stimulation. The "sweating" of the vaginal walls as a result of the **vasocongestion** of the vaginal blood vessels results in the lubrication of the entire vagina. Almost simultaneously with lubrication, and as a result of vasocongestion, the entire vagina dilates in preparation for accommodation of the erect penis. The increased flow of blood also produces a color change in the vaginal wall, and it becomes darker, turning almost a deep purple.

Uterus. As the uterus, too, becomes engorged with blood, it moves up out of its regular position, rising in the body cavity into the false pelvis. The lifting up and back of the uterus and cervix, along with the expansion of the vaginal walls, produces a tenting or ballooning out of the inner two-thirds of the vaginal barrel (Figure 6–1). This happens only if the uterus is in the typical anteverted position; it does not occur in a retroverted uterus.

Clitoris. Vasocongestion is the cause of the changes that occur in the clitoris as well, and the way in which the ischiocavernosus and bulbocavernosus muscles contribute to clitoral enlargement was described in Chapter 2. In approximately 50% of the women observed by Masters and Johnson, the glans of the clitoris doubled in diameter; in the other half of the subjects, however, there was no visible difference in the size of the glans, although swelling could be seen if the glans were observed with a culdoscope. The blood pouring into the corpora cavernosa of the shaft of the clitoris causes the shaft to increase in diameter, but only in about 10% of the women does the clitoral shaft visibly elongate.

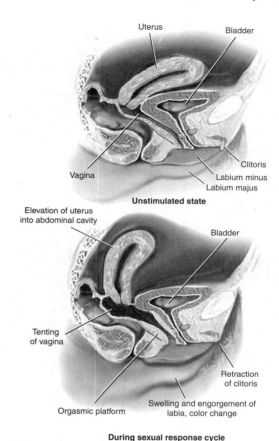

Unstimulated state

During sexual response cycle

Figure 6–1 Changes that occur in the pelvic area during the excitement and the orgasmic phases of the sexual response cycle.

Labia. As part of the whole vasocongestive reaction, the labia minora swell, and their color darkens. The labia majora also undergo congestive changes, and the extent depends on whether the woman has delivered children or not. Evidently, pregnancy results in a general increase in pelvic vascularity that results in the differences. In a nonexcited state, the major lips meet in the midline of the vaginal orifice. During the excitement phase in nulliparous women, the labia majora thin out and flatten themselves against the perineum, elevated away from and opening up the entrance to the vagina. In a multiparous woman, particularly if she has developed varicose veins, the major lips do not flatten but become swollen and distended.

Bartholin's Glands. Very late in the excitement phase, or early in plateau, **Bartholin's glands** may secrete an insignificant amount of fluid, but this is after the vagina is well lubricated. The glands play, therefore, very little part in easing penetration.

Extragenital Responses

Breasts. Nipple erection occurs in many women early in the excitement phase. Sometimes one nipple becomes erect before the other. There may be an increase in nipple length of 0.5–1.5 cm and in diameter of the nipple base of 0.25–1.0 cm. The dark area surrounding the nipple (areola) enlarges and swells later in the excitement phase; by the end of this phase, the entire breasts have increased in size by 20%–25%, more noticeably in women who have not breast-fed. The veins of the breasts become more apparent because of engorgement with blood.

Skin. Another vascular change that occurred in the laboratory in approximately 75% of the women and 25% of the men at least sometimes during the sexual cycle was the "sex flush." Beginning on the upper part of the abdomen and spreading up to the chest, throat, and neck, a pink mottling appears on the skin. It is especially obvious in fair-skinned people and looks like a measles rash.

Muscle Tension. There is increased tension in the voluntary muscles of the arms and legs, the rectal muscles, some of the abdominal muscles, and the intercostal muscles of the ribs.

Cardiovascular, Respiratory, and Sweat Gland Responses

As sexual excitement increases, heart rate and blood pressure increase. There is no observable change in respiration or perspiration at this point.

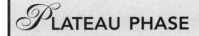
PLATEAU PHASE

Genital Responses

Vagina. The bulbocavernosus muscles (so called because they arise on the *bulbs* of the vestibule and insert anteriorly on each corpus *cavernosum* of the clitoris) are the sphincter muscles that encircle the vaginal entrance. As they contract, they compress the veins in the bulbs of the vestibule, the highly vascular tissue that is equivalent to the corpus spongiosum in the male and which lie deep within the substance of the labia majora. The bulbs become turgid and swollen, producing a vulvar erection that reduces the diameter of the outer third of the vaginal barrel by approximately 50%. This is what Masters and Johnson called the **orgasmic platform,** and it actually produces a gripping clasp around the erect penis.

Uterus. More vasocongestion produces an increase in size, and the uterus elevates more fully into the abdominal cavity and causes more tenting and ballooning of the inner two-thirds of the vagina. The complete elevation and vasocongestion produce an increasing uterine muscle irritability, and late in the plateau phase, uterine contractions may start (Figure 6–1).

Clitoris. The clitoris also elevates in the plateau phase. Its normal position is overhanging the lower border of the pubic bone. In this stage of the cycle, the body and glans of the clitoris retract from that overhanging position and withdraw deep under the prepuce, carrying the labia minora and the suspensory ligament along to end up high on the anterior border of the pubic symphysis. It is no longer externally visible after this elevation, but it still responds to stimulation by pressure on the mons veneris over the pubic bone and/or by the penile thrusting that pulls on the labia minora, producing traction on the prepuce. A finger or a vibrator or any other kind of tactile friction will have the same effect. Unless clitoral stimulation continues, orgasm is not triggered.

Labia Majora and Minora. The labia majora continues to show more of the changes that started in the first stage. In a nullipara, they flatten out even more; in multiparous women, they become more swollen and engorged. Late in the plateau phase, the labia minora experience more of a vivid color change—a sure sign that orgasm will occur within a few minutes if clitoral stimulation is continued.

Extragenital Responses

Breasts. More turgidity of the nipples occurs, and there is further swelling of the areola and entire breasts.

Skin. If a sex flush has occurred, it spreads over the shoulders, down the inner surface of the arms, and perhaps onto the abdomen, thighs, buttocks, and back.

Muscle Tension. There is a further increase in the tightening of both voluntary and involuntary muscles, and intercostals of the ribs, and there may also be voluntary tightening of the rectal sphincter and the buttock and thigh muscles.

Cardiovascular, Respiratory, and Sweat Gland Responses

The heart rate increases from a normal 70 beats per minute to 100–175 per minute. There is an elevation in systolic blood pressure of 20–60 mm Hg above resting pressure and 10–20 mm above diastolic. Late in plateau, there is an increase in respiratory rate. The actual perspiratory reaction of the sexual cycle does not occur until after orgasm, but of course if a sexual encounter is taking place in a warm atmosphere, there will be sweating throughout the phases.

ORGASM

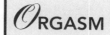

Genital Responses

Vagina. The major response is that the orgasmic platform—that is, the muscles that make up the outer third of the vaginal wall and those surrounding the turgid tissues of the vulva—undergoes rhythmic contractions that occur at 0.8-second intervals. In a mild orgasm, there may be 3 or 5 such contractions; a more intense orgasm results in perhaps as many as 12.

Uterus. Along with the throbbing sensation in the vagina, the uterus also undergoes contractions; each begins at the top (fundus) of the uterus and works its way down to the middle and then to the cervix. There are indications that these contractions are greater in intensity after self-stimulation than after intercourse. This may be why many women find masturbation helpful for dysmenorrhea, especially since the external os of the cervix remains dilated for about 30 minutes afterward.

Labia. There are no observable changes in the labia majora or minora during orgasm.

Extragenital Responses

Breasts. There are no further noticeable changes in the breasts during orgasm.

Skin. If sex flush is present, it reaches a peak of intensity with the onset of orgasm and is most pronounced.

Muscle Tension. The entire body is so involved in the experience of orgasm that voluntary muscular ontrol is mainly lost as involuntary contraction of many muscle groups takes place. The spontaneous involuntary reflex contractions of the perineal muscle and the pubococcygeus not only cause the throbbing of the orgasmic platform but also may result in the same 0.8-second contractions of the external rectal sphincter. If they occur, the anal contractions do not last as long and usually involve only two to four spasms. Both superficial and deep muscles of the arms, legs, neck, abdomen, and buttocks are often contracted to cause stiffening and rigidity. The hands and feet are extended while the fingers and toes curl under, appearing grasping or clawlike; this spastic posture is called carpopedal spasm. The amount of myotonia or muscle contraction that occurs with orgasm is an individual response. It may be so mild as to barely be visible, or it may be uncontrollably convulsive.

RESOLUTION

Within a few seconds of orgasm, the two physiological mechanisms that created the sexual responses, vasocongestion and myotonia, are rapidly dissipated.

Genital Responses

Vagina.   The blood rapidly drains out of the engorged tissues, and the orgasmic platform disappears. The anterior wall of the vagina returns to meet the posterior wall, and the deep color change fades, although the complete return to normal coloring may take as long as 10–15 minutes.

Uterus.   The elevated uterus returns to its normal unstimulated position. The cervix then dips into the "seminal pool" that has formed in the posterior fornix as a result of male ejaculation, if the woman has been on her back during intercourse. The external os of the cervix remains slightly dilated for approximately 20–30 minutes. If orgasm does not occur after a progression through the plateau phase, the vasocongestion that produced the enlargement of the uterus takes much longer to resolve, and engorgement may persist

for as long as an hour—even longer in multiparous women.

Clitoris.   Ten seconds after the last vaginal contraction, the clitoris returns to its normal position overhanging the pubic symphysis, but the engorgement with blood that produced the size increase takes longer to dissipate. The glans remains very sensitive for several minutes; in some women it is actually painful to the touch.

Labia.   The labia minora return to their ordinary color within 10–15 seconds, and they return to their ordinary size. The labia majora return to the normal midline position and size more quickly in nulliparous women. In a woman who has had several children, the labia majora may retain their engorgement for several hours. The reason for the difference is the normal increase in the number and size of the blood vessels in the genitalia and reproductive organs that takes place with pregnancy.

All extragenital responses—that is, muscle tension, heart rate, blood pressure, and respiratory rate—show a rapid decline unless there is further sexual stimulation. The sex flush disappears in reverse order of its appearance, and in approximately one-third of the women subjects there is the appearance of a widespread film of perspiration over the chest, back, and thighs. Heavier sweating occurs on the forehead, upper lip, and under the arms.

The swelling of the areolae of the breasts promptly disappears. The nipple erection remains longer than the areolar swelling; last to disappear is the swelling of the entire breast lines.

In males, the resolution phase after orgasm and ejaculation is followed by a refractory period during which the man cannot respond to sexual stimulation by another sexual cycle. The duration of the period is generally directly related to the age of the male; the younger he is, the sooner he is able to have another erection, ejaculation, and orgasm. In women, there is no such refractory period, and they are said to be multiorgasmic, having the capacity to reach repeated orgasms if they want to. It is not unusual in some women to have multiple orgasms in rapid succession with no intervening resolution phase.

WHAT DOES ORGASM FEEL LIKE?

Physiologically, the term orgasm refers to the spasmodic and involuntary contractions of the muscles in the region of the vulva and the vagina. Subjectively, the experience can be perceived in the range from "OK, nice . . ." all the way to ecstasy and "skyrockets," depending on the incredibly wide individual variation that exists and the ease with which a woman can verbalize her sensations.

The Hite Report (Hite, 1976), a questionnaire survey of 3,019 women aged 14–78, indicates that some words used in describing the subjective characteristics of arousal and orgasm are frequently repeated by many women—"tingling," "buzzing," "warmth," "pulsating"—with the focus of the sensations in the area of the clitoris. Other descriptions fairly consistently mentioned a prickling and tingling, heat, and throbbing sensations in the pelvic area. It has generally been assumed that a male's experience of orgasm—more sudden and explosive—is different from a female's experience. When a series of 48 descriptions of orgasm (24 male and 24 female) were submitted to 70 obstetrician-gynecologists, clinical psychologists, and medical students, however, they were unable to correctly identify the sex of the person describing the orgasm. There was also no ability to recognize any described characteristics of orgasm that would indicate a basis for sex differences in the subjective awareness of sensations (Vance & Wagner, 1976).

The findings in the above study suggest that the experience of orgasm for males and females is essentially the same, at least on the basis of their written descriptions of the event. But there are great differences in the way that women are able to interpret their feelings, and many psychological and cultural determinants of those differences. Some women may have orgasms and not be aware of them. The widely held assumption, "If you don't know if you've had an orgasm, you haven't!" is not necessarily true. Some women who think they never had an orgasm may recall having good feelings, fluttering or pulsations, waves, and then a sense of peacefulness afterward but never labeled their sensations as an orgasm. Such women may be suppressing many of the sensations, too inhibited, perhaps, to permit themselves to feel them. Alternatively, a good feeling about sex with a low intensity of response could be completely normal in a given individual. Usually, a feeling of warmth and some pelvic contractions are indications that orgasm has occurred.

Vaginal and Clitoral Orgasm

In his *Three Essays on the Theory of Sexuality,* Freud hypothesized his ideas about the "leading zones" of eroticism in the bodies of men and women. Based on his observations in his psychiatric practice, he said that the main erogenous area in little girls was located at the clitoris, homologous to the glans of the penis, and was thus "masculine." In the transition to womanhood, girls had to transfer this childish masculinity in their sexual sensations to the vagina. With this transfer, a mature woman then abandoned her early clitoral eroticism and replaced it with a new and superior erotic zone. If this transition from the clitoral zone to the vaginal zone is not made or is incomplete, women remain infantile and immature. Without any knowledge of the physiological mechanisms involved in orgasm, this theory is not illogical in Freud's context of women as imperfect men, that is, lacking and envying a penis. The clitoris in childhood is the substitute for the penis; it must be given up and transferred when at last the sexual act is permitted. Males, on the other hand, retain their leading erogenous zones unchanged from childhood. The fact that women have to make the transfer, putting aside their "childish masculinity," makes them more prone to "neurosis and especially to hysteria" and creates the basis for their inevitable sexual inferiority.

Freud's opinions were enthusiastically codified by later psychoanalysts and psychiatrists. Like fundamentalists interpreting the Bible, orthodox Freudians and neo-Freudians proclaimed the Word—that vaginal orgasms were superior to clitoral orgasms. Women who had vaginal orgasms were feminine, mature, and normal; women who preferred clitoral stimulation were masculine, immature, and even frigid (although the latter term logically should be reserved for an inability to feel any sexual sensations at all).

The laboratory observations of Masters and Johnson proved that these assertions are nonsense. Orgasm is orgasm—the result, apparently, of primarily clitoral stimulation. Whether such stimulation takes place through direct friction of the clitoris by manual stroking during intercourse, by masturbation, or through homosexual activity with another woman, or whether it occurs indirectly by traction on the prepuce or clitoral hood when the male penis thrusts into the vagina, the mechanism of orgasm is the same. In some women, the quality of the orgasm may be enhanced by the repetitive pressure of the penis on the cervix, resulting in movements of the uterus and its associated ligaments. This may be the basis for the sensation of a deep, inner or "vaginal" orgasm. The percentage of women for whom such thrusting on the cervix is sexually important is unknown, but it may be related to evidence that some women who have had a hysterectomy experience lesser intensity of orgasm and hence greater sexual dissatisfaction after the uterus and cervix have been removed.

Compared with the male, there has been relatively little work done on the neurophysiological and neuroanatomical bases of the female orgasm, but available evidence indicates that innervation of the clitoris is similar to that of the penis. Sexual stimulation causes sensory nerve impulses from the clitoris especially and from the vulva to travel along the pudendal nerve. The sensory signals enter the spinal cord through the lumbosacral plexus into the spinal cord and are transmitted up to the brain. Reflexes in the spinal cord result in parasympathetic nerve impulses that cause arteries to dilate in the tissues of the genitalia, and the subsequent vasocongestion is then responsible for the other changes already described. If the sexual stimulation is continued, the continued sensory input to the spinal reflex center, which can be inhibited or facilitated by the higher brain centers, results in motor impulses to the pelvic area. The sympathetic discharge results in the changes in heart rate, respiration, blood pressure, perspiration, and so forth. The onset of approximately 10 rhythmic muscle contractions around and in the vagina causes most of the blood and fluid to then empty from the pelvis. Both the clitoris and the vagina form an integral part of the orgasmic reaction, and as psychoanalyst Helen Kaplan pointed out, to ascribe more prominence to one or to the other is as senseless as trying to distinguish between the sensory and the motor components of any reflex—blink, gag, startle, and so forth.

Put that way, orgasm sounds like a simple reflex: tactile stimulation causes sensory impulses to travel to a center in the spinal cord and results in a motor response, the contraction of muscles. Reflex it may be, but in most women it is far from simple. A reflex conditioned as much by psychology and sociology as by physiology is not really comparable to the knee jerk. The entire life experience of a woman is involved in her sexual response. If the brain says "go," then the appropriate reflexes are initiated from the spinal cord, and the throbbing sensations are transmitted back to the brain for the awareness of pleasure and for the peace and relaxation that follow. But if psychological inhibition prevents cerebral "letting go," the orgasm and its intensely pleasurable fulfillment are also inhibited, even in the presence of adequate local stimulation. Although every woman, unless there is some organic pathology or anatomical reason that prevents it, has the physiological capability to have an orgasm, she may not, for multiple reasons, have the psychological capability to function orgasmically.

SEXUAL PROBLEMS IN WOMEN

When men have problems with sex, it is related to performance. They are unable to get an erection (**impotence**), or they cannot exert enough voluntary control to delay ejaculation, and they reach orgasm too rapidly (**premature ejaculation**). What is called sexual dysfunction in males results in their inability to have intercourse. The sexual problems of women, on the other hand, assuming that vaginismus is not the trouble, are a matter of satisfaction rather than performance. All that women need to successfully engage in intercourse is a moderate amount of vaginal lubrication. Even if orgasms are lacking or infrequent, a woman still may have what is apparently a successful sexual relationship. If a woman wants to pretend to have sexual pleasure, only a minicamera and vaginal transducers could deduce the truth.

There are millions of women (estimates are 10%) who never consciously experience orgasm at all by any means—**coitus,** stimulation, or masturbation. Orgasm may not be the sole measure of sexual satisfaction or happiness in a sexual relationship, and an inability to achieve orgasm is certainly no criterion of inadequacy or abnormality. But there is no reason to suppose that it does not enrich and enhance the sexual act, or that sexual activity is better or to be preferred without orgasm.

There is evidence, however, that contrary to previously held opinions, a majority of women are unable to reach orgasms solely through intercourse without additional clitoral stimulation. Shere Hite's 1976 survey revealed that only 30% of the 3,000 women who replied to her questionnaire were regularly able to climax through coitus. For many of that group, penile thrusting alone was not sufficient, and they had to use specific positions to obtain clitoral contraction. Because 82% of the women surveyed masturbated, and 95% of those women could always reach orgasm by self-stimulation, it would appear that the model described by Masters and Johnson for clitoral contact during intercourse may not always work. That is, for the vast majority of Hite's respondents, in-and-out movement of the penis did not necessarily produce labial traction on the clitoral hood for indirect clitoral stimulation. Women who are not able to achieve orgasm through intercourse but can through masturbation are, Hite believes, in no way dysfunctional, but they may have to take a more active responsibility toward their orgasm. The women surveyed were gen-

erally reluctant to express their need for manual stimulation of the clitoris to their partners, fearing to "put down" the male concerning the effectiveness of his penis. Even fewer were willing to stimulate themselves to orgasm while in the presence of their male partner. Most of them did, however, express great concern that something was wrong with them because they were unable to have an orgasm in the "right" way. The pervasive influence of Freudian theory, even if demolished in the laboratory by Masters and Johnson, cannot be underestimated.

Hite's questionnaire was distributed to a particular segment of American women, that is, to those belonging to feminist groups and to readers of only certain magazines and newsletters. They tended to be relatively well educated and lived primarily in urban areas. Her findings, therefore, may not be representative of the feelings and experiences of all women, although they do tend to concur with the reports of other researchers, such as Kinsey and Kaplan.

The fact that many women can masturbate to orgasm but cannot achieve orgasm through coitus alone carries no implication that masturbation is "better" or represents a dire forewarning concerning the future of intercourse. Although the physiological orgasmic response is the same no matter how it is produced and brings with it the relief of sexual tensions, a climax reached through self-stimulation is essentially a solitary act. For a majority of women, orgasm that is reached with a loving and loved partner is likely to have more emotional meaning and greater satisfying significance than one that is self-induced. This is as true for women whose sexual preference is for other women as it is for heterosexuals. Desires and feelings based on mutual and warm understanding between two people are the primary factors for women in achieving sexual gratification.

Most women, however, are heterosexual. For them, given the knowledge concerning the anatomy and physiology of the female orgasm, it is unrealistic to always expect the male to "bring" a woman to climax without effective clitoral stimulation. The focus of male sexual excitement is penetration and thrusting movement; the basic mechanism for females is pressure and friction on the clitoris. Different couples are built differently. What is pleasurable for the male may not always be the specific technique for every female. Her own activities and movements, together with a communication of her needs for manual stimulation, may prove a more successful combination. In some couples, the touching and movement of the male pubic bone against the female mons pubis, for example, may provide the right contact for the clitoral area. Because of the individual variation in the prominence of the pubic bone, getting this contact may require a change from the usual man-on-top position, or perhaps some other accommodation.

Time is also a very important factor in female eroticism and ability to have an orgasm—not only the time involved in the actual sexual encounter, but the total time of a woman's accumulated sexual experience. As with most other activities, practice helps, and many women find that physical sex improves with age. In interviews with married women, Kinsey found that nearly 30% of women had not experienced an orgasm by any means when they were first married, but after 15 years of marriage, there were only 10% who were still nonorgasmic. It is possible to learn to have orgasms, and once learned, the response and letting go become easier as one becomes more adept at knowing what to do to produce them. One of the best ways to teach oneself to have an orgasm is by masturbating, but even knowing how to masturbate may not come naturally to women who have been taught since childhood that touching oneself is wrong and shameful. The very intense local stimulation that is delivered by an electric vibrator may help to achieve orgasm initially. Even with a vibrator, erotic sensations can be delayed by very strong cerebral inhibition, but persistence and a real effort to release the orgasmic reflex will result in success in most women.

Sex Therapy

Therapy is no way to generalize about something as subjective as sexual satisfaction, but that does not pre-

vent a lot of people from trying. The only generalization that can be made about human sexuality without qualm is that it is incredibly, infinitely varied. There is no normal or abnormal in the capacity to respond to sexual activity or in the desire for the frequency of sexual activity. A woman could be labeled as "frigid" because her eagerness for sex is less than that of her partner. Another could be called a "nymphomaniac" because she experienced frequent desire or because her sexual excitement and need for a second coitus continued after her partner's orgasm. The persistence of such pejorative terms illustrates that many of us still have the illusion that there is some appropriate measure by which to gauge a woman's sexual desire. But in common with every other human behavior, sex cannot always be 100% emotionally and physically satisfying, and the desire for or the pleasure derived from sex may change with time, opportunity, locale, sexual partners, and a variety of situational factors.

A woman is always being advised, however, on how she should be feeling about sex. Bombarded from all sides with information concerning statistical norms, orgasmic potential, multiorgasmic potential, sexual dysfunction, her total womanhood, and of all the joy she should be having in sex, it is easy to lose sight of the fact that *her* perceptions—what *she* finds satisfying, what *she* enjoys—are the only definitions of what is right for her. She should allow no one to decide these things for her. Neither her physician, her sexual partner, a magazine article, a book, nor a movie should tell her that she has a problem or is inadequate because she does not meet some presumed standard of sexual behavior.

But there are women for whom the expression of sexuality is tied up in knots because of the whole range of sociocultural attitudes and values they have had about sex. Their feelings of guilt or fear, their reluctance to lose control, their inability to communicate their need and desires to their partners, their possible low esteem and low expectations for themselves—some or all of these may result in patterns of behavior for them that limit or prevent their appreciation of sexual activity. Where there is total lack of interest in sex, or complete absence of response to erotic stimulation (or perhaps when vaginismus is a recurrent problem), or the woman perceives a difficulty that is serious enough for her to warrant treatment, formal sex therapy in a clinical atmosphere may be helpful.

Sex therapists believe that because attitudes are conditioned and learned, they can be unlearned. Their goal is to relieve the problem, usually without treating the underlying causes, although some do use psychotherapy as an adjunct. Most therapists employ a form of behavior modification, attempting to decrease sexual anxiety and encourage communication. They prefer to work with the couple if possible, rather than with the individual patient. When no partner is available, Masters and Johnson have used surrogate sex partners. Techniques among therapists vary: some use hypnosis; some may prescribe a series of specific instructions and exercises that the patient and her partner are to follow; some may perform surgery to improve body image, such as breast augmentation or facial surgery. Some doctors have performed a kind of clitoral circumcision to remove "adhesions" between the clitoral hood or prepuce and the glans of the clitoris. This is claimed to increase the sensitivity and provide for more direct contact with the clitoris, although efficacy of the procedure is still in question.★

Another therapeutic technique, used in conjunction with other methods, is "flooding" the patients with explicit graphic materials (most people would call it pornography) in order to desensitize their anxiety about the subject matter and permit themselves to be "turned on."

It should be recognized that along with the legitimate clinics that are usually associated with a medical school or hospital, there has been a virtual explosion of treatment centers, sex clinics, marriage counselors,

★There is a very rare condition in some women in which the clitoral hood actually adheres to the clitoris. For them, clitoral stimulation and the resulting vasocongestion produces great pain, and the prepuce must be surgically separated, a much more complicated surgical procedure than freeing adhesions.

and sex therapists throughout the country. Some of these centers are staffed by incompetents, charlatans, and quacks who charge exorbitant fees. At the very least, these self-styled "sex therapists" may dispense misinformation, but some may also cause reactions in their patients that compound the original problem.

Even accredited health professionals, lacking appropriate training and having their own anxieties about sex, may be no more sophisticated than the general public and no better able to deal with intimate sexual problems. One's family physician or obstetrician-gynecologist may not be the best person to seek out for counseling. With the growing awareness that total health care includes sexual health care, more medical and nursing schools are including sex education in their curricula and holding institutes and workshops for the postgraduate education of health professionals. Although this trains personnel to provide counseling and be better equipped to deal with sexual problems, it is necessary that such sex education extend beyond medical schools, hospitals and universities to reach the general public through public schools and the mass media. The recognition that human sexuality is not just performance and satisfaction in intercourse, but is a lifelong human quality that encompasses love, warmth, and respect between human beings in their relationships, and that it can be expressed in a variety of ways, may eventually decrease the need for formal sex therapy. The realization that sex is important to *all* people as a basis for self-esteem and security will be an important step toward this goal.

LESBIAN SEXUALITY

What gay women "do," sexually, is frequently the source of curiosity (and even prurient interest) among nonhomosexuals, but what they do together is not substantially different from what heterosexual couples do or what a woman can do alone through self-stimulation. As indicated previously, the body responds to psychosexual stimulation with physiological effects, but the psychological part has as much or more to do with sexual arousal as the physical means of sexual expression. Lesbians may concentrate more on particular erogenous areas of the body and may have greater awareness of the role of the clitoris in achieving sexual gratification, but so may couples who are not of the same sex.

The Institute of Medicine, a division of the prestigious National Academy of Sciences, in a report on the health status and health care of lesbians (Solarz, 1999), recognized that there is no standard definition of what constitutes a lesbian. As with that of gay men, the sexual orientation of a woman is likely to occur along a continuum that may include three dimensions: current or past same-sex sexual behavior, same-sex desire or attraction, or self-identification as a homosexual or bisexual woman. Women may exhibit combinations of all three dimensions or may have only one, that is, the desire to have sex with other women or have primary emotional partnerships with women. What lesbian women want in a sexual relationship is no different from what heterosexual couples want—love, commitment, sharing, and meaning. But what heterosexual couples take for granted in society is what homosexual couples often lack and need from society—public acceptance and better understanding of their sexual preference.

The usually quoted statistics indicate that 10% of individuals in the United States are or will become exclusively or predominantly homosexual. If the rest of the world allows it, most gay people can live satisfied, well-adjusted, fulfilled lives and be as happy as their nonhomosexual counterparts. Unfortunately, society as a whole is unaccepting of alternative lifestyles, and the threat of disclosure, particularly for people in public life, places an enormous burden on most individuals with a homosexual orientation. Rabid antigay sentiments, exacerbated by the fear of AIDs, continue to exist in most communities. Many of the cities and states that passed specific legislation prohibiting discrimination against gays in jobs and housing during the 1980s moved toward repealing those laws in the 1990s.

It is unsurprising that the majority of homosexual men and women are keeping it a secret. But the decision to "come out of the closet" and declare their sexual orientation has been a source of great pride and enthusiasm for many gay individuals.

SEXUALITY IN THE OLDER WOMAN

In 1959, Golde and Kogan conducted a study in which a group of university undergraduates was asked to complete this sentence: "Sex for most old people is. . . ." Almost all of them replied, "past," "negligible," or "unimportant," reflecting the belief that after a certain age, people are, or should be, sexless.

Now that the most rapidly growing segment of the United States population is people over 65, that attitude may be changing, even among the younger generation. There is a growing popular acceptance of relationships between women over 50 and younger men, particularly if the women are sexy movie and TV celebrities. Such liaisons always were possible for older men with money and power, but only recently has society, encouraged by the media, begun to condone May-December romances for older women.

There are many people, however, who do find the notion of sexuality in seniors distasteful, disgraceful, or just plain ridiculous. When elderly people marry, they do so for "companionship," and they are presumed to have no interest or capability for sexual activity. With these societal expectations, it is not surprising that a self-fulfilling prophecy takes place. Many older men and women do feel asexual and suppress any erotic interest they may have as being unsuitable or wrong.

All available evidence indicates that given reasonably good health, sexual function continues throughout life. Masters and Johnson, who studied women aged 40–73 and men aged 51–89, found that while there are decreases in the durability and intensity of the physical responses in the sexual cycle with increasing age, "the aging human female is fully capable of sexual performance at orgasmic response levels, particularly if she is exposed to regularity of effective sexual stimulation." The first *Hite Report* quotes some older women who felt that sex was not that important to them anymore, but the majority indicated that their sexual pleasure had actually increased with age and that they were now enjoying more new and gratifying experiences. Postmenopausal women, free for the first time in their lives from the fear of any unwanted pregnancy and with fewer family responsibilities, may have an increase in their desire for sexual activity, particularly if they disregard the myths concerning how menopause is supposed to affect their sex lives.

Continuing to be sexually active may be one way to help remain sexually active. After menopause, there are sometimes vaginal changes that result from the decrease in estrogen levels. These changes may decrease the ability of the vagina to undergo adequate lubrication in preparation for intercourse. It is known that women who maintain regular intercourse or masturbation during their entire adult lives have much less difficulty in vaginal lubrication and expansion of the vagina than women who are sexually inactive. There are also fewer problems with atrophic vaginitis. The mechanism by which sexual activity helps to prevent vaginal changes secondary to estrogen decline is unknown. It may be that the principle of disuse atrophy, more commonly known as "use it or lose it," is playing a role.

Many older women, of course, lack the opportunity for the continuance of sexual involvement because they are widowed, divorced, or single, and many have never masturbated. It may be very difficult for those for whom self-stimulation has never been a part of their sexual value system to begin to masturbate in old age, even as a health measure. It is also curious that many people who have become accustomed to accepting childhood masturbation as almost mandatory for a functionally healthy sexuality in adulthood may still stigmatize masturbation in the elderly as a childish activity, or "sick," or sad.

SEXUALITY IN THE PHYSICALLY DISABLED

In the same manner that feelings of sexuality in the aged are sometimes regarded as inappropriate or even bizarre, society tends to regard those who are unfortunate enough to suffer from a congenital or acquired physical disability as nonsexual beings, lacking both desire and capability. We seem to harbor this universal fantasy, encouraged by the mass media, that ideal sexual activity takes place between young, beautiful people, all of whom are able bodied and active. When we see them on television commercials, it is obvious that any defects they may have are easily remedied by a different deodorant, a new shampoo, or a better toothpaste, and then they are again lovable and alluring. We have been programmed to think that vigor and physical appearance are of major importance in sexuality, and we have difficulty believing that people who are crippled by arthritis, who have cerebral palsy, who are confined to a wheelchair have any interest in sex. But sexuality is a human, lifelong characteristic, and this is equally true of an individual with chronic illness or a disabling injury as it is of any able-bodied person. The sex drive is rarely affected by disability, any more than physical handicap curtails hunger or thirst.

Approximately 1 out of 10 adult people has a physical impairment that was either present at birth, developed later as a result of illness, or was suddenly acquired through accident or injury. The sexuality of the physically disabled is a reality that has been largely ignored by the medical profession as well as by the general public. Many of the disabled, too, just like the elderly, have come to accept the prevailing belief that sex is unimportant to them. A few physicians, specialists in rehabilitation medicine, like Walsh in Great Britain and Cole in the United States, have written extensively on the need for sexual counseling, emphasizing that health professionals should expect to teach disabled patients about sexual behaviors in the same way they help them to deal with other activities of daily living. Cole very pragmatically pointed out that sexuality is so related to the self-esteem of the physically disabled that sexual activity not only leads to a better adaptation to the disability but also results in fewer medical complaints and less need for medical or social support, thus decreasing society's cost in dealing with the disabled. It does seem evident that those who have already lost their independence, their earning power, and their mobility should not have to cope with the additional loss of their sexuality.

Problems of sexuality, which certainly can exist in the physically able, are usually compounded in the physically disabled. Sexual problems in the disabled generally fall into several broad categories. Some of the difficulties may be in the realm of the psychological and social aspects of sexual relationships, in which feelings of hopelessness or depression lessen sexual drive, or where unfounded fears concerning the inheritance of the physical defect decrease sexual activity. Other problems are physical or physiological, concerned with such things as physical comfort and safety during the sex act and with the loss of sexual capability as a result of paralysis or lack of sensation. People want to know what to do when stiff joints or muscles make sexual positions difficult or painful, or when dizziness or muscle spasms occur during intercourse. They are concerned about heart palpitations or breathlessness that may occur during sexual activity and whether it is safe for them to participate. They want advice on what to do about urinary catheters or other appliances or dressings that make sex uncomfortable or unaesthetic. They want reassurance that alternatives to penile-vaginal intercourse are possible, and that other modes of sexual expression in a loving relationship exist that can be equally fulfilling. They also have a critical need for the compassionate and understanding attitudes of the people around them. Regrettably, their questions tend to remain unanswered. Sexual counseling is still taboo at many hospitals and rehabilitation centers, and too few health professionals or social workers have the training and expertise to deal with sexual problems in the disabled. After a heart attack or bypass surgery, for example, a

man frequently is told, even without his asking, that he usually can resume minimal or nondemanding sexual activity (kissing, nongenital contact, cuddling) safely within 3–6 weeks once he is stabilized and has no symptoms of chest pains, palpitations, or shortness of breath. After he regains his strength and full physical fitness as measured by a stress test, sexual intercourse does not make excessive demands on the heart. The same instructions apply to women cardiac patients, but often the physician is reluctant to discuss the topic, perhaps because the woman does not ask about the effects of heart disease or surgery on her sex life, or because the doctor thinks it is not important to her, especially if she is elderly. Steinke and Patterson-Midgley (1996) found that nurses, too, often overlook sex counseling needs in women who have had a heart attack. Seventy-one of the 96 patients that the investigators studied, however, believe that the staff should provide information on sexuality in the hospital setting. Another study by Muller et al. (1996) found that the risk of triggering the onset of a heart attack in patients with prior heart disease is *very* low, that regular exercise appears to prevent sex activity from contributing to an attack, and that the absolute risk of increasing the likelihood of a heart attack is one chance in a million for healthy individuals and that risk is not increased in patients who have a prior history of cardiac disease. In actuality, the energy required for making love is about the same as that needed for briskly climbing a flight of stairs—easily handled by most people with cardiovascular disease.

Part of the difficulty is that the subject of sexual functioning and dysfunctioning in the physically disabled is such a new area. There is relatively little in medical literature concerning patients with progressive chronic illnesses such as heart, pulmonary, or kidney disease, or who have arthritis, surgical problems that impair sexual function, or a developmental disability. What information there is deals primarily with sexual function in spinal cord-injured males.

Spinal cord injury results in *paraplegia,* which is paralysis and the loss of most or all sensation in the lower part of the body and the legs, and if the injury is higher in the spinal cord, *quadriplegia,* the loss of voluntary muscular activity (paralysis) and some or all sensation from the neck down. The extent of the denervation depends on whether the spinal cord was completely or partially cut.

Because of war, athletic injuries, and their greater numbers of auto accidents and civilian gunshot wounds, four out of five spinal cord–injured adults are male. It is generally accepted that males have a much more difficult time in sexual readjustment after spinal cord injury because of their increased difficulty in erections and their loss of fertility. Although 50%–70% of spinal cord–injured men are capable of having an erection, almost all lose the ability to ejaculate, and the ability to produce spermatozoa is lost within a few weeks or months of injury. With the high value placed on male performance and activity in sex, it is evident that loss of some sexual function can be particularly devastating.

The medical literature pertaining to sexuality in spinal cord–injured females is scant, and what there is emphasizes that female sexuality is less affected. "In fact," as one physician cheerfully observed, "the picture is much brighter for the female paraplegic than for the male." Presumably, paralysis and loss of sensation below the waist are not viewed as being very different from the ordinary state of affairs in women; they can just lie there and be more passive. In contrast to males, women do retain full reproductive ability. They experience a temporary amenorrhea after injury, but normal cycles resume after 6–8 months, and they are completely capable of becoming pregnant and delivering a child. Contraception is as necessary for a paraplegic or quadriplegic woman as it is for any woman who does not want to become pregnant. Blood clots have a greater tendency to form in paralyzed limbs, however, and spinal cord–injured women are rarely given oral contraceptives because of their link with blood–clotting disorders.

As additional evidence that there is probably more sexuality that exists between the ears than between the legs, both men and women with spinal cord injuries have reported that, given the opportunity, they can experience full sexual satisfaction psychologically even if a physical sensation is lacking. For some, the areas of the body that are still innervated become new erogenous zones to compensate for those parts that no longer respond to touch, and many individuals have the ability to produce fantasized orgasms by concentrating on the sensations received from those areas. Others derive great satisfaction from the ability to give joy and pleasure to their partners. The actual physiological manifestations of the sexual response cycle in paraplegic and quadriplegic males and females differ little from those in neurologically intact individuals. According to Cole, the vasocongestion responses are consistently present, but muscle responses in the genitalia may be absent. For example, in males, the only responses missing are those involved in emission and ejaculation. In females, the clitoris and labia become engorged with blood and swell, but the uterine and vaginal responses during the orgasmic platform are missing. All extragenital responses—heart, respiration, pulse, blood pressure, skin flush, and so on—are present in both men and women.

There is ample evidence that with a loving and caring partner and given the appropriate counseling, the reassurance concerning their sexual potential, and the technical advice about coping with physical problems during sexual activity, men and women who are physically disabled can accept themselves as total sexual human beings. We must not permit the narrow view that prizes youth and physical appearance as criteria for sexual activity to devalue this concept.

SEXUALITY DURING PREGNANCY

Masters and Johnson observed the sexual response cycles of six women throughout their pregnancies. They concluded that the physiological sexual responses during pregnancy were very similar to those of nonpregnant women, although some women complained of increased breast tenderness, especially in the nipples and areolae, during the excitement phase of sexual response. Four of the six had occasional cramping and aching in the pelvis after orgasm, and two of those four said they had subsequent lower back pain. All six women reported a heightening of sexual arousal in the second 3 months of pregnancy, which continued well into the final 3 months. Masters monitored the fetal heartbeat during orgasm and reported that, although it sometimes slowed down temporarily, it very rapidly resumed its normal rate. It was also discovered that the resolution phase after orgasm took longer and was less complete, in the sense that the women stated that orgasmic experience "did not relieve their sexual tensions for any significant length of time."

Masters and Johnson also supplemented their direct observation of the six with the subjective responses of 111 women who regularly reported their sexual feelings, behavior, and responses as their pregnancies progressed. Other investigators (Solberg, Butler, & Wagner, 1973; Kenny, 1973; Tolor & DiGrazia, 1976; Reamy, White, Daniell, & LeVine, 1982) used a similar technique of regular oral interviews or used a retrospective questionnaire to determine sexual attitudes of women during and after pregnancy. In general, the conclusions drawn from these studies indicate that the usual wide range of individual response exists but that sexual interests, frequency, and the enjoyment derived from activity was essentially the same as it is in nonpregnant women—until the last trimester of pregnancy, when a progressive decline in desire and frequency occurred.

Medical opinion concerning the advisability of sexual activity during pregnancy varies. There are still a few doctors who believe that intercourse during the first 3 months is contraindicated because of the fear of spontaneous abortion. There is the possibility that in a small group of women who have already miscarried several times and who obviously have difficulty in maintaining a pregnancy, it would be prudent to avoid all sexual activity, including masturbation, because of the uterine contractions. There is very little evidence, however, that intercourse causes spontaneous abortion. Women in the first trimester do have an increased

pelvic awareness that accompanies the uterine changes; if they are concerned that the thrusting and movement during intercourse may be damaging to the fetus, it will tend to decrease the satisfaction derived from stimulation, and orgasm may not be as frequent. The sensations during intercourse may be different from those usually experienced, but they are in no way harmful.

By the second 3 months, a woman is usually used to the different kind of feeling in the pelvic area. Masters and Johnson report an increase in sexual functioning at this time, but other researchers have not confirmed the heightened arousal, reporting only approximately the same desire and frequency as before. There is no reason to abstain from intercourse during the second trimester.

The question of abstinence during the last 4–6 weeks of pregnancy is more "iffy." Many physicians are convinced that the uterine contractions during orgasm can trigger the onset of labor or that there is more possibility of infection. There is no proof of detrimental effects of intercourse right up until the time of delivery if the pregnancy is proceeding normally. Sometimes, the glans of the penis hitting the very vascular cervix may result in a little spotting; this need not discourage sexual relations if they are desired. The woman herself knows how she feels about sexual activity in the last weeks of pregnancy; if she wants to continue intercourse, there is no reason not to. If all she is interested in is being held and loved, that is certainly another way of maintaining sexual activity.

After delivery, Masters and Johnson reported that sexual desire returned after anywhere between 2 weeks and 3 months, reappearing earlier in women who were breast-feeding. By the 3rd week after delivery, the uterine discharge had stopped and the episiotomy incision, if present, had healed sufficiently to make resumption of sexual relations comfortable. Obstetrician-gynecologist Kenneth Reamy, who has written extensively concerning sex during pregnancy and the postpartum period (1991), advises that episiotomy sutures will not be affected by the resumption of sexual intercourse even if the site is not completely healed. Coitus is safe 3 weeks postpartum unless a woman has had extensive lacerations during delivery. Before having intercourse for the first time after delivery, however, a woman should inspect the episiotomy site with a mirror to check for swelling or irritation and insert a finger or tampon into the vagina to test for soreness. Any pressure on the episiotomy site during intercourse can be reduced by putting a pillow under the woman's buttocks to direct the penis anteriorly. Also, because the significant drop in estrogen and progesterone levels after delivery may cause a temporary vaginal dryness and decrease in lubrication, a water-based lubricant (such as K-Y Jelly or Replens) could be used.

EFFECTS OF DRUGS ON SEXUALITY

Relatively few controlled, systematic studies of the effects of chemical agents on sexual activity ever appear in scientific journals. People take a very dim view of mind control, and experiments that attempt to assess the effect of psychotropic or mood-altering drugs on human behavior are so fraught with ethical and moral problems that even the most respected and intrepid sex researchers have shied away. Many of the drugs that are presumed to have a relationship to sexual function are illicit, making direct laboratory evidence even more difficult to come by. Most of what is known is, therefore, primarily based on patients' reports on the side effects of medical drugs taken for other purposes, or on the subjective and anecdotal responses of individuals who have taken hallucinogens to enhance sexual pleasure—hardly the way to obtain solid objective data.

Another major difficulty in attempting to investigate the interaction of drugs and sex is in part due to the nature of drugs and the nature of sex. No given drug ever affects everyone in the same way or even affects one person the same way at different times. The pharmacological action depends on the dosage, the size and weight of the person taking the drug, and the length of time the drug is used. Other drugs, either taken deliberately as medication or inadvertently as food additives or environmental pollutants, may interact with the original agent, or perhaps there may be an individual sensitivity, allergy, or difference in metabolism that influences the reaction. Even the time of day the drug is taken is important. But probably the prime ingredients in the effect of a mood-altering or psychoactive drug are the mood, attitude, and expectations of the taker and the belief or faith one has in the prescriber of the drug.

By now, it should also be obvious that what one obtains or finds in a sexual experience also profoundly depends on what one brings to it. The entire cultural, sociological, ecological, and psychological aspects of the individual personality, the expectations, the conscious and unconscious needs, yearnings, fantasies, and attitudes of the moment are the determinant of the total emotional effect. There are so many psychological and biological variables in both drug action and sexual behavior that to attempt to measure the pharmacological effects of the one on the other is almost impossible. There is no known drug that has been found to have uniformly consistent sexual effects. Even with that caveat, it would still be interesting to look at some chemical agents for which there have been claims of either adverse effects or increase of sexual pleasure and capacity.

Drugs That Allegedly Enhance Sexual Pleasure

Aphrodisiacs. **Aphrodisiacs** are substances that arouse an individual to increased desire and ability to engage in sexual activity. For thousands of years, males have been looking for the perfect love potion to prop up a faltering phallus. Many of the earliest substances used to increase sex drive were plants or parts of plants that resembled the human form or, in particular, the genitalia. Certain foods, like oysters or truffles, have also had aphrodisiac properties attributed to them, probably because of their presumed resemblance to testes. There is no scientifically documented evidence that any of these are effective, except as placebos. Believing that they work may make them work.

There are almost no historical references to women voluntarily taking substances that stimulated their desire for sexual activity, but only instances of their being given various agents that might improve their fertility or for enhancement of male pleasure with them. Even today, there are few reports of drug effects on female sexual responses. Several investigators have pointed out that although erection may be more visible and easily studied, the response is under the control of the same parasympathetic nerves that result in the labial swelling and vaginal lubrication in the female. Thus, penile erection is neurologically analogous to lubrication and swelling in the female, and it can be assumed that what affects the former may also affect the latter.

The supposed aphrodisiac with which most people are familiar is "Spanish fly," an extract from the pulverized wing parts of a beetle, *Cantharis vesicatoris,* which has been used for centuries. Cases of self-poisoning by men or poisoning of women by men in anticipation of producing sexual arousal still occur. The active ingredient, cantharides, is a toxic substance that produces bladder and urethral inflammation. The irritation may be severe enough to produce priapism, an extremely painful persistent penile erection with no associated sexual excitement. Permanent impotence, bloody and painful urination, and even death have resulted from its ingestion.

Poppers. Amyl nitrite, popularly known as "poppers," has more recently been touted as an enhancer of sexual enjoyment. Medically, the drug has been prescribed for the heart pain that results from blocked coronary arteries; it causes vasodilation and increases the diameter of the arteries resulting in a drop in peripheral blood pressure. The highly volatile substance is usually administered by breaking the capsule in which it is contained (hence the popping noise) and inhaling the drug, which then enters the bloodstream from the lungs. As a sexual stimulant, amyl nitrite is sniffed from an inhaler or "popped" just before orgasm. Subjectively, the drug produces a "flash" or "high" that is said to intensify or prolong orgasm. Not

only does the drug have a very unpleasant odor, it can also have most unpleasant side effects that on occasion are dangerous or even life threatening. Some users have reported headache and aching eyes, but cardiovascular distress and even death have occurred. Amyl nitrite users who are simultaneously taking other drugs could experience potentially disastrous effects. Isobutyl nitrite, a chemical relative of amyl nitrite but a nonprescription drug, is an easier "popper" to obtain. Marketed as "liquid incense" under such trade names as Rush, Bolt, Locker Room, and Bullet, isobutyl nitrite has the same side effects and a similar capability for harm.

Quaaludes. Methaqualone (Quaalude) is a sedative-hypnotic that is chemically unrelated to the barbiturates (Nembutal, Seconal, Tuinal) and glutehimide (Doriden) and is believed to act on a different brain site than the other sedatives. "Ludes" are called the "love drug" by recreational drug users, and there are claims that it causes great increase in sexual feelings and multiple orgasmic potential, but there is no known pharmacological reason for the alleged increase in desire and performance.

Marijuana. Marijuana has a strong reputation as a sexual stimulant, but its actual impact on eroticism is not clear. For many people, "pot" or "grass" decreases sexual inhibitions; it may also alter sensory awareness and distort time and in that way enhance a sexual experience. Like many supposed aphrodisiacs, if marijuana is taken with the expectation of obtaining a desired effect, it is more likely to produce that effect.

Ecstasy. Other, more powerful hallucinogens such as LSD, STP, mescaline, and psilocybin were more commonly taken in the 1960s and early 1970s, but there is a reported recent resurgence of use, especially among high-school and college students. These drugs are usually reported to be too "heavy," too "mind-blowing" to have an aphrodisiac effect. A psychedelic drug named "ecstasy," also called MDMA (3,4-methylenedioxy-methamphetamine), is a combination of synthetic mescaline and an amphetamine ("speed") in capsule form. Ecstasy became popular during the mid-1980s in the gay community, on college campuses, and particularly among the young and affluent. After taking the drug, users claim that it produces hours of intense euphoria without harming mind or body. In animal tests, however, the drug has been shown to destroy nerve endings in that part of the hypothalamus that regulates sexual arousal, mood, and emotions. According to pharmacologists, the drug is psychologically addictive, can cause paranoia and psychosis, and has been linked to several dozen deaths (Foderaro, 1988).

Crystalline meth. Methamphetamine abuse has reemerged in the United States as a significant drug problem. The smoking of methamphetamine in crystalline form, or "ice," also allegedly produces an intense sensation of euphoria. After absorption, methamphetamine is metabolized to amphetamine, which is known to induce a number of lethal and potentially lethal effects when taken orally or intravenously. Although not much has been documented concerning the adverse consequences of smoking "ice," several physicians in Hawaii described fatal toxic cardiovascular effects associated with its use (Hong, Matsuyama, & Nur, 1991).

Cocaine and Crack Cocaine. Cocaine is the psychoactive drug historically associated with sexual arousal. An alkaloid derived from the leaves of the coca plant, which grows in the Andes mountains of Peru and Bolivia, its euphoric properties have been known for thousands of years. When the drug is inhaled or "snorted," users report that they experience an intense "rush" that some have compared to an orgasmic experience. The physiological effects include increased heart rate and blood pressure, dilated pupils, and anesthesia of the nasal passages. Cocaine may be partially effective in enhancing sexual pleasure—at least initially—although the action may vary with the mode of administration and the situation in which the drug is used. The most systematic studies of cocaine and its association with sexuality were conducted at the Haight-Ashbury Free Medical Clinic in San Francisco (Gay & Sheppard, 1972; Gay et al., 1982). The researchers reported that a number of the male patients they saw in their clinic said they saved cocaine for sexual situations and half of the respondents interviewed reported spontaneous erections upon intravenous injection of the drug. Some users liked the anesthetic properties of the drug. When applied to the male genitalia, for example, cocaine allegedly delays ejaculation. Women have used the drug as a douche to obtain vaginal mucosal contractions and, as absorption slowly occurs, a systemic euphoria. According to Abel (1985), cocaine's reputation as an aphrodisiac has never been disproved, but with continued usage and as the dose increases, all enhancement of sexual pleasure disappears and the desire for the rush and the associated effects eventually replaces the desire for sex.

Like marijuana, cocaine was viewed as a soft, recreational drug during the 1960s and 1970s—non-addictive, short acting, and safe—and any information on the adverse effects of chronic cocaine abuse was downplayed. But in the 1980s, a new form of cocaine appeared. The free-base form, called "crack" because of the cracking or popping noise made in its preparation, was less expensive, easily made, and smokable. Cocaine is a powerful vasoconstrictor; when sniffed into the mucous membranes of the nose, it retards its own absorption, thus delaying the attainment of peak levels in the blood and brain. But because of the ease of absorption of the drug via smoking, peak levels are much more rapidly achieved, leading to an extremely intense "high" followed by a "crash." The severe post-euphoria crash increases the craving for more of the drug and leads to a rapid dependence on it. Crack abuse has had a major impact on almost every aspect of American society. The effects of cocaine on pregnant women and their fetuses are described in Chapter 11.

Alcohol. Ogden Nash said, "Candy is dandy but liquor is quicker!" Alcohol has traditionally been thought of as a sexual stimulant—it relaxes inhibitions and decreases anxiety and perhaps guilt. In many individuals, however, released inhibition is replaced quickly by a depression of the central nervous system. The release-of-inhibition stage proceeds very rapidly to the central nervous system depressant or totally-zonked-out stage, resulting in impotence in the male and complete passivity in the female. Shakespeare recognized the antiaphrodisiac properties of alcohol when he said in *Macbeth,* "drink . . . provokes the desire, but it takes away the performance." But increasing the possibility of sexual dysfunction is not the only risk of alcohol and sex. If alcohol decreases inhibition, it also decreases a woman's good judgment about using a condom and protecting herself against the transmission of HIV (human immunodeficiency virus) and other sexually transmitted diseases. Alcohol could also contribute to an increased risk of sexual assault by incapacitating a woman and influencing her perceptions of what is actually going on.

Date-Rape Drugs

Three dangerous drugs that have become associated with date-rape scenarios are Rohypnol, known on the street as "roofies"; ketamine hydrochloride, a veterinary anesthetic also known as "Special K"; and a drug known as GHB, or gamma hydroxybutyrate, called "liquid ecstasy." These drugs in small quantities are easily dissolvable when slipped into a drink and can render the unwitting victim unconscious and subject to sexual assault. In larger amounts, coma and death can result. Rohypnol is 10 times more powerful than Valium and, when combined with alcohol, causes disinhibition and blackouts within 15–30 minutes of consumption. GHB, which allegedly can be made easily from recipes available on the Internet using over-the-counter supplements from health food stores and drug stores (GBL or gamma-butyrolactone, GABA or gamma-aminobutyric acid), tastes somewhat salty and its use is usually masked in bizarre drink mixtures. It can cause death by inhibiting breathing, sending the body into convulsions and coma (Naylor & Cohen, 1999). The idea of stupefying unsuspecting women and raping them is a sexual predator's dream. Police suggest that a woman should safeguard herself by

ordering bottled drinks with caps or closed cans. One law enforcement officer offered this sage advice, "As a child you were taught not to accept candy from strangers. As a teenager you were taught not to accept rides from strangers. As an adult, don't accept drinks from strangers" (Teel, 1997).

Drugs That Enhance Sexual Prowess

Viagra. Perhaps no drug in recent years has captured the headlines and media attention as has Viagra, a therapy in pill form for both physical or psychogenic erectile dysfunction (ED), formerly called male impotence, that originally was developed for high blood pressure. Approved after 6 months of clinical trials by the Food and Drug Administration in March 1998, more than 6 million prescriptions were written for Viagra (sildenafil) and the drug racked up $788 million in sales for its manufacturer, Pfizer, within the first 9 months on the market. Until the introduction of Viagra, previously available therapies for impotence involved injections into the opening at the end of the penis or the implantation of pumps or other kinds of prostheses.

The physiological mechanism of erection of the penis involves the release of nitric oxide in the corpora cavernosa of the penis during sexual stimulation. At recommended doses and in the presence of sexual stimulation, Viagra enhances smooth muscle relaxation and an increased flow of blood into the corpora cavernosa by inhibiting an enzyme that diminishes the effect of nitric oxide and thus results in an erectile response approximately 60 minutes after taking the pill. Viagra is not effective in the absence of sexual arousal.

The fanfare that greeted the introduction of Viagra lost some luster after the reports of some deaths among men who were also taking nitrate-based heart medications such as nitroglycerin, isosorbide dinatrate, and isosorbide mononitrate—general names for many different brands. (Obviously another source of nitrates that should never be used with Viagra is illicit "poppers," inhaled amyl nitrates.) Because Viagra itself lowers blood pressure, it is unknown when necessary nitrates could be safely administered, and physicians now receive warnings to prescribe the drug with care.

Some adverse reactions to Viagra have included headache; flushing; indigestion; nasal congestion; and instances of transient abnormal vision with increased sensitivity to light, blurring, and a temporary blue-green color blindness. Also, there have been infrequent reports of priapism—prolonged and painful erections greater than 4–6 hours. Men are warned to seek medical attention immediately if an erection persists longer than 4 hours to avoid potential penile tissue damage.

Despite reports of potential adverse effects, Viagra dominates the male market treatment of sexual dysfunction. Pfizer could double that market if its product could work the same wonders for women. Shortly after the introduction of Viagra, physicians began to prescribe the drug to women (Rosen, 1998). The first small pilot study of the effects of Viagra on women were reported by a research team led by Steven Kaplan in 1999. Thirty-three postmenopausal women with self-described sexual dysfunction were treated with Viagra at a dose of 50 mg for 3 months. With acknowledgment that the number of women in the study was small and that 12 weeks was a short time for follow-up, the investigation concluded that overall sexual function in the women was not significantly improved by treatment with Viagra and that although the drug was well tolerated, some of the same side effects occurred in women as occurred in men.

A major difficulty with sexual problems in women is their complexity; there is also little consensus on their definition or classification. Although the clitoris in women has the same number of sensory nerve endings as the penis, becomes erect with sexual arousal as does the penis, and has the same embryological origin as the penis, dysfunction in women can also include such things as lack of desire, trouble with lubrication causing vaginal dryness and pain, or inability to attain orgasm. Despite these differences, Pfizer and a number of small pharmaceutical companies are forging ahead in the financial race for treatment of women's sexual hindrances. Creams and gels to enhance the flow of

blood to the genitalia, oral female hormones, and testosterone patches are being tested. Herbal remedies that aim to increase the libido are available.

Drugs That Impair Sexuality

The vasocongestion and muscle responses that are a part of the sexual response cycle are under the control of the parasympathetic and sympathetic divisions of the autonomic nervous system. Anything that interferes with parasympathetic and sympathetic impulses may, therefore, inhibit some aspect of the sexual response.

Anticholinergic drugs are those that block the action of the parasympathetic fibers, and they are frequently used in the treatment of gastrointestinal disturbances because they decrease muscle spasm of the digestive tract and inhibit acid secretion in the stomach. It is possible that high doses of anticholinergics may result in erection difficulties in the male and, by extrapolation to the female, swelling and lubrication difficulties. Drugs that inhibit the sympathetic nerve impulses are antiadrenergic and are often used to lower high blood pressure. Men who take antiadrenergic drugs for hypertension have reported difficulty with ejaculation since the reflex muscular contractions that result in emission and ejaculation of semen are controlled by adrenergic or sympathetic fibers. Men have also claimed decreased libido while on antihypertensive medication. Women have no muscle response corresponding to emission and ejaculation, but the absence of specific reports from females should not be interpreted to mean that drugs taken to decrease high blood pressure could not affect their sexual function as well.

Some women have reported lessening of desire for sexual activity while on oral contraceptives, but some women have claimed an increased interest in sex occurs while on the pill. There have been indications from both men and women that tranquilizers and other kinds of antianxiety, antidepressant drugs result in decreases in sexual interest, and some men have reported potency difficulties while on thiazide diuretics. Although effects of drugs on sexual function can occur at any age, they are more frequent and troublesome after age 50. Men obviously have a more visible and easier gauge by which to measure sexual dysfunction, but there is no reason why women should not also be alert to the possibility of disturbance while taking drugs with the potential of affecting some aspect of their sexuality.

REFERENCES

Abel, E. L. (1985). *Psychoactive drugs and sex.* New York and London: Plenum Press.

Cole, T. M. (1975). Sexuality and physical disabilities. *Archives of Sexual Behavior, 4*(4), 389–403.

Foderaro, L. (1988, December 11). A drug called ecstasy emerges in nightclubs. *The New York Times.*

Freud, S. (1905). *Three essays on the theory of sexuality.* New York: Avon Books.

Gay, G. R., & Sheppard, C. W. (1972). Sex in the drug culture. *Medical Aspects of Human Sexuality, 6*(10), 28–50.

Gay, G. R., Newmeyer, J. A., Perry, M., et al. (1982). Love and Haight: The sensuous hippie revisited, drug/sex practices in San Francisco, 1980–81. *Journal of Psychoactive Drugs, 14,* 111–123.

Golde, P., & Kogan, N. (1959). A sentence completion procedure for assessing attitudes towards old people. *Journal of Gerontology, 14,* 355–359.

Hite, S. (1976). *The Hite Report.* New York: Macmillan.

Hong, R., Matsuyama, E., & Nur, K. (1991). Cardiomyopathy associated with the smoking of crystal methamphetamine. *Journal of the American Medical Association, 265*(9), 1152–1154.

Kaplan, H. S. (1983). *The evolution of sexual disorders: Psychological and medical aspects.* New York: Bunner/Mazel.

Kaplan, S. A., Reis, R. B., Kohn, I. J., et al. (1999). Safety and efficacy of sildenafil in postmenopausal women with sexual dysfunction. *Urology, 53*(3), 481–486.

Kenny, J. A. (1973). Sexuality of pregnant and breast-feeding women. *Archives of Sexual Behavior, 2*(3), 201–203.

Kinsey, A., Pomeroy, W. B., Martin, C. E., & Gebhard, P. H. (1953). *Sexual behavior in the human female.* New York: Saunders.

Masters, W. H., & Johnson, V. E. (1966). *Human sexual response.* Boston: Little, Brown.

Muller, J. E., Mittleman, A., Maclure, M., et al. (1996). Triggering myocardial infarction by sexual activity. Low absolute risk and prevention by regular physical exertion. *Journal of the American Medical Association, 275*(18), 1405–1409.

Naylor, J., & Cohen, J. S. (1999, March 17). Elixir becomes date-rape killer. *Detroit News,* p. A1.

Reamy, K., White, S., Daniell, W. C., & LeVine, E. (1982). Sexuality and pregnancy. *Journal of Reproductive Medicine, 27*(6), 321–327.

Reamy, K. J. (1991). A management guide to postpartum problems. *Medical Aspects of Human Sexuality,* 20–25.

Rosen, R. C. (1998). Medical advance or media event. *Lancet,* 353, 1599–1600.

Solberg, D. A., Butler, J., & Wagner, N. N. (1973). Sexual behavior in pregnancy. *New England Journal of Medicine, 288,* 1098–1103.

Solarz, A. (1999, October/November). Lesbian healthcare issues. Exploring options for expanding research and delivering care. *AWHONN Lifelines, 3*(5), 13–14.

Steinke, E., & Patterson-Midgley, P. (1996). Sexual counseling following acute myocardial infarction. *Clinical Nursing Research, 5*(4), 462–472.

Teel, G. (1997, December 1). *Alberta Report, 24*(51), 36–37.

Tolor, A., & DiGrazia, P. V. (1976). Sexual attitudes and behavior patterns during and following pregnancy. *Archives of Sexual Behavior, 5*(6), 539–551.

Vance, E. B., & Wagner, N. N. (1976). Written descriptions of orgasm: A study of sex differences. *Archives of Sexual Behavior, 5*(1), 87–98.

Walsh, J. J. (1976). The spinal cord disabled. *Nursing Mirror, 142*(5), 53–54.

THE MAMMARY GLANDS

KEY TERMS

Areola
Axillary nodes
Colostrum
Cooper's ligaments
Ductal carcinoma in situ
  (DCIS)
Fibrocystic disease

Hyperplasia
Lactiferous duct
Lobular carcinoma in situ
  (LCIS)
Mastectomy
Oncogenes
Pectoral nodes

*A*long with warm blood and skin covered with hair, the mammary glands are such a distinguishing characteristic of our taxonomic class that it is named Mammalia because of them. Mice, monkeys, whales, elephants, lions, tigers, and human beings are all mammals, and all have in common these specialized skin glands that secrete milk to nourish their offspring. Baby mammals are born in a relatively immature and highly dependent state, unable to forage for their own food or even to digest and assimilate an adult diet. Newborns completely subsist on the secretions of the mammary glands of their mothers. Sensibly enough, the number of pairs of glands has a general relationship to the number of young in the litter. An animal like the mouse, which regularly produces large families, may have six or seven pairs of breasts; humans, fortunately, normally have only a single pair. Considering the cultural fervor with which we humans view the female breasts, it is probably just as well we have only two of them about which to be concerned.

Sexual interest in breasts is peculiar to humans; in other species the males are totally unimpressed by them. One has only to look at the paintings and sculptures in any art museum in the world to recognize that our preoccupation with breasts, our almost mystical veneration of the mammary glands, is not merely a current cultural phenomenon. The female breast as a source of eroticism, as a symbol of femininity, as a determinant of fashion, and as a measure of beauty has for centuries assumed an importance far out of proportion to the natural purpose of the glands—the nourishment of an infant.

Whatever they are called—"boobs," "bazooms," or "tits"—women know that by most male definitions, the breasts should be protuberant, conical, and large; the bigger the better. It is this *Playboy* centerfold ideal of beauty, the large-breasted, long-legged, narrow-waisted standard, that women, too, have accepted, and that has led them in many instances to dislike their own bodies. Some of them seek "remedies" such as breast implants for their presumed inadequacies, which can result in disfigurement and illness. Sometimes they delay or refuse to see a doctor when they discover a breast lump for fear of losing what they have been socialized to believe is their major badge of femininity.

Of course a woman is concerned about her breasts. As a major secondary sex characteristic that appears at puberty, the breasts are a symbol of feminine identity, forming a part of the body image and important to self-esteem. Breasts are a source of erotic stimulation, and they play a role in the expression of a woman's sexuality. Their size, shape, and appearance are unique to each woman, however, and there is no reason why they should conform to some idealized stereotype. They should not be viewed as a woman's most cherished assets, on which her "wholeness" as a real and complete woman depend. Perhaps as more women regain more control over their bodies and their lives, they will gain the self-confidence to increasingly reject the disproportionate glorification of breasts and of themselves as exclusively sexual objects. The strong pressure placed on women by our breast culture may diminish in time.

MORPHOLOGY OF THE BREASTS

Unlike other mammals, the breasts of humans, monkeys, and apes are located on the thorax and not the abdomen. Unlike other primates, who have flat breasts even during pregnancy and lactation, the human female has comparatively large and dome-shaped mammary glands. Generally speaking, the taller the woman, the higher up on the thorax the breasts are located. Differences in breast size and shape are completely determined by the relative amounts of fatty and connective tissue, dependent on genetic and endocrine factors, or as a result of how much body fat the woman has (Figure 7–1). As women gain weight, their breasts become more pendulous and larger. All women have the same amount of actual mammary gland tissue—about a spoonful. The actual size of the breasts, whether 32AA or 38D, has, therefore, no relationship to a woman's ability to nurse a baby.

The breast is a modified skin (sweat) gland, lying over the pectoralis major muscles of the chest wall and attached to them by a layer of fascia, or connective tissue (Figure 7–2). Each breast extends approximately from the second to the sixth or seventh rib and from the lateral border of the sternum to the axilla, or armpit. The upper, outer portion of the breast is thicker and primarily composed of glandular tissue. It extends to a variable degree as the "axillary tail" into

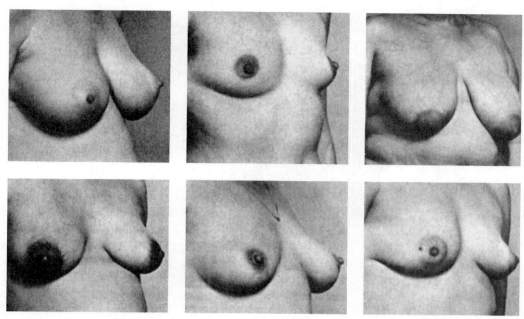

Figure 7–1 Differences in sizes and shapes of breasts in women who vary in age and weight.

the armpit—an anatomical feature significant in the spread of breast cancer. The longitudinal diameter of the breast, 10–12 cm on the average, is less than the transverse diameter, and the average weight of each breast is 150–200 g but increases to 400–500 g during lactation. The right breast is usually somewhat smaller in size than the left breast.

The glandular tissue itself consists of up to 15 lobes, each with its own **lactiferous duct,** which all converge like the spokes of a wheel on the nipple. The lactiferous ducts enlarge slightly into a lactiferous sinus before emerging, and the nipple is then perforated by tiny openings. The characteristic wrinkled and pigmented skin of the nipple extends out onto the breast for approximately 1–2 cm to form the **areola.** In prepubertal girls with light complexions and in blondes before pregnancy, the capillaries filled with blood under the areolar skin show through to impart a rosy pink color. The skin becomes more pigmented at puberty and darkens even more during pregnancy in fair-skinned women. This pigmentation never completely disappears and, to a certain extent, can distin-

guish a nulliparous woman from a parous one. In darker-skinned women, there is no noticeable change during pregnancy.

The areolae contain large modified sweat glands, Montgomery's glands, which increase in size and number during pregnancy and lactation and which may be important in lubrication of the nipple. Montgomery's glands become larger at puberty and also respond to monthly hormonal stimulation; they shrink and involute after menopause. Along the margin of the areolae are other large sweat and sebaceous glands, some associated with hair follicles, and many women are aware of the cyclic growth and recession of individual areolar hairs. The skin of the areolae and the nipples contain numerous longitudinally and circularly arranged smooth muscle fibers that are responsible for erection of the nipples when they are stimulated tactilely or by exposure to cold.

The major lobes of glandular tissue in each breast are further subdivided into 20–40 lobules. In a pregnant woman, each lobule, branching like a tree, sprouts little ducts that terminate in evaginated sacs called alveoli.

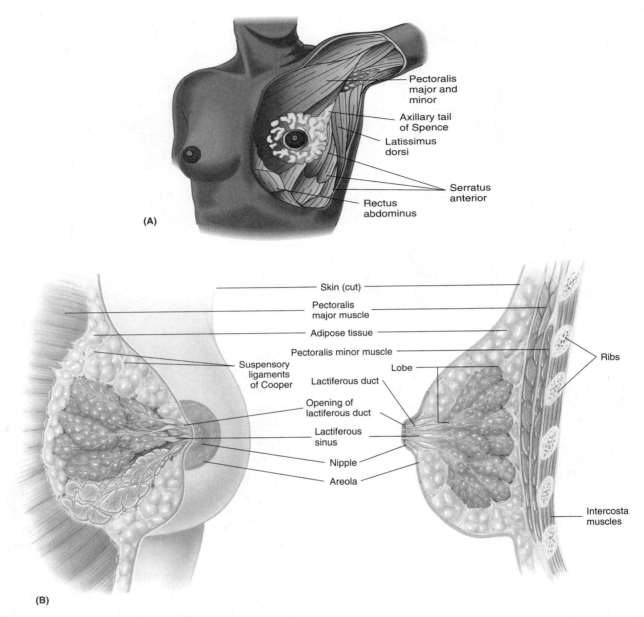

(A)

- Pectoralis major and minor
- Axillary tail of Spence
- Latissimus dorsi
- Serratus anterior
- Rectus abdominus

(B)

- Skin (cut)
- Pectoralis major muscle
- Adipose tissue
- Pectoralis minor muscle
- Suspensory ligaments of Cooper
- Lobe
- Lactiferous duct
- Opening of lactiferous duct
- Lactiferous sinus
- Nipple
- Areola
- Ribs
- Intercosta muscles

Figure 7–2   (A) Position of the breast in relation to the superficial thoracic muscles. (B) Sagittal section through the breast.

The alveolar cells, under hormonal influence, are the actual glandular units that synthesize and secrete milk. The breast of a nonpregnant woman contains just a few alveoli that have budded off from the ends of the ducts. During pregnancy, the abundant ovarian and placental steroids produced by the mother cross over into the fetal circulation and are able to stimulate the fetal mammary tissue. Eighty to 90% of all newborn babies of either sex have slightly enlarged breasts that actually secrete milky fluid ("witches' milk") for several days.

The lobes, lobules, and their ducts are surrounded and separated from each other by bundles of connective tissue. The largest of these partitions are called the suspensory ligaments of Cooper, and they extend from the layer of connective tissue or deep fascia over the muscles of the chest wall to the layer of superficial fascia just under the skin. Fat accumulates in these ligaments and in all the connective tissue of the breast, and so there is a fat layer overlying the breast just under the breast skin. Except for the smooth muscle of the areola-nipple complex, there is no muscle in the breast itself. It consists of the ducts, lobules, and alveoli of the gland tissue, a lot of fatty tissue, and connective tissue. Those amazing ads in the back pages of magazines that promise to increase the size of the breasts by "bust developers" describe an anatomical impossibility. Certain exercises are able to increase the size and strength of the pectoral muscles and can result in a small apparent elevation of the breasts, but no dramatic increase in size is possible. Better posture also raises the breasts, but there is nothing other than breast implant surgery that can change small breasts into large breasts.

Blood Supply of the Breasts

The major blood supply to the breasts is from a branch of the subclavian artery called the internal mammary, with additional contributions from the thoracic branch of the axillary artery. The veins that drain the blood from the breasts follow a pathway that quickly leads into the large vein, the superior vena cava, that enters the right side of the heart. From there the blood is pumped directly to the lungs to be oxygenated before it is returned to the left side of the heart for distribution throughout the body. The rather direct route from the breasts to the lung capillaries may be significant in the metastasis (spread) of breast cancer.

Lymphatic Drainage of the Breasts

All the cells of the body are bathed in a watery solution called tissue fluid, which contains nutrients and gases. Tissue fluid, bringing essential food and oxygen to the cells, is produced from blood plasma at the arterial ends of the blood capillaries and is reabsorbed at the venous ends of the blood capillaries. A little more tissue fluid is produced than is absorbed, and the excess passes into tiny lymphatic capillaries that are also found in the tissues. Called lymph, the tissue fluid is drained from these lymphatic capillaries into progressively larger lymphatic vessels, eventually to empty into a major vein near the heart. If it were not for this lymphatic drainage, the tissues of the body would become swollen with excess tissue fluid, a condition called edema. There are several basic causes for edema, and one of them is obstruction of the lymphatic channels.

The lymphatic vessels are interrupted in their pathway by groups of small bean-shaped lymph nodes, an accumulation of cells called lymphocytes held together by connective tissue, sometimes called lymph glands. Clusters of lymph nodes in the neck, the armpit, and the groin are of particular importance clinically; they can be palpated, and the expression "swollen glands" really refers to enlarged lymph nodes, which not only play a predominant role in immunity but also act as a filter, screening out harmful particles such as microorganisms, debris, or cancer cells.

In the breast, most of the lymph from the central part of the mammary gland, the skin, nipple, and areola drains laterally toward the axilla. The first nodes encountered are the four to six anterior **pectoral nodes,** also called the low **axillary nodes.** From there the lymph passes to the central axillary nodes embedded in a fat pad in the center of the armpit. The flow then proceeds to the upper part of the axilla to the lateral nodes along the axillary vein and then to the deep axillary or subclavicular nodes. From the back of the breast, the lymph is drained to several interpectoral (subscapular) nodes located between the pectoralis major and pectoralis minor muscles. The internal mammary nodes that lie along the sternum lie in the pathway of the lymph channels that drain from the inside or medial part of the breast (Figure 7–3).

When breast cancer cells invade the lymph system, a process known as metastasis, they first reach lymph nodes, which retain the tumor cells and try to destroy

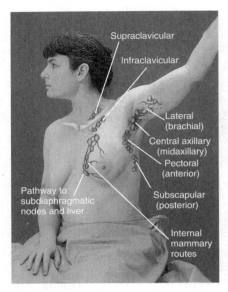

Supraclavicular

Infraclavicular

Lateral
(brachial)

Central axillary
(midaxillary)

Pectoral
(anterior)

Subscapular
(posterior)

Internal
mammary
routes

Pathway to
subdiaphragmatic
nodes and liver

Figure 7–3   Pathways of lymphatic drainage from the breast.

them. The malignant cells grow rapidly and, eventually, they overcome the nodes' capacity for destruction. Then the cancer travels on to other nodes. Because most of the breast lymph (75%) drains into the axillary nodes, it is believed that the removal of the primary tumor in the breast and the axillary nodes can frequently completely eradicate the cancer. This may not always be successful because the secondary lymph channels that pass to the internal mammary nodes or, indirectly, to the subdiaphragmatic nodes that lead to the liver, or those channels that cross over to the opposite breast may play an equal role in the spread of breast cancer. When lymph nodes have been invaded by cancer cells, they are said to be "positive" nodes.

*C*YCLIC CHANGES IN THE BREASTS

Before menarche, the mammary glands of both males and females consist only of a few ducts surrounded by a lot of connective tissue. This is the way they remain in males. With the onset of puberty in females, however, the duct tissue, stimulated by estrogen, elongates and branches, forming the buds of the future lobules and alveoli. The connective tissue also proliferates and becomes infiltrated with fat, and the breast begins to assume the shape of the mature female gland. When ovulatory cycles begin to occur and the corpus luteum secretes progesterone, the characteristic duct–lobular–alveolar structure of the breast during the childbearing years is developed. Like the uterus, the breast prepares each month for the possibility of conception. During each menstrual cycle, there is a little increase in mammary development, but the major growth takes place during pregnancy, when the increase in size, volume, and density of the breasts is very great.

During the first half, or proliferative phase, of the cycle, the high levels of ovarian estrogens in the blood stimulate the reproduction of cells in the glandular ducts and their terminal buds, the alveoli. This increase in the number of cells continues into the postovulatory or secretory phase of the cycle, when the increasing amounts of progesterone result in the dilation of the ducts and the differentiation of the alveolar cells into the actual secretory cells. After ovulation, there is also an increased blood flow to the breasts and, in the week before menstruation, some women experience fluid retention. The resultant swelling, or edema, in the mammary connective tissue causes feelings of fullness and heaviness, and the breasts get larger. The enlarged duct diameters, the increased cellular growth, and possibly some newly formed alveoli all contribute to the engorgement and the increased lumpiness or nodularity of the breasts. When menstruation starts, there is actually some secretion of droplets by alveolar cells into the alveolar lumens, but toward the end of menstruation, all the proliferated tissue begins to regress and must be reabsorbed. The ducts become narrower, the lobules and alveoli become smaller, and the tissue edema disappears. But before the tissue can totally regress, a new cycle has started and the estrogen again induces more proliferation. The ducts and alveoli never have a chance to completely return to the way they were before the preceding cycle, and each additional ovulatory cycle therefore results in a little more mammary development. This continues until approximately age 35.

Fibrocystic Disease

Most women are aware of some feelings of fullness and lumpiness in their breasts just before menstruation. This is so common that women are told not to examine their breasts for lumps until after their periods. Some women have very painfully engorged breasts, with a large number of tender nodules in the weeks before and during menstruation. This is physiological lumpiness and is not a disease, although the dividing line between such changes and the clinical entity known as "fibrocystic disease" is arbitrary and a matter of degree. The increased nodularity usually appears in both breasts in approximately the same location and disappears after menstruation. A woman who regularly performs monthly breast self-examination learns to distinguish her own normal thickenings and lumpiness from something new. Any one lump, however, that begins to grow out of line with the rest is suspicious.

There are several kinds of benign tumors that may be related to hormonal stimulation, although the cause is really unknown. One, the most frequent, is cystic disease of the breast. In cystic disease, small fluid-filled, palpable cysts, which may or may not be painful, develop rather quickly in one or both breasts. They are treated by withdrawing or aspirating the fluid with a needle and syringe or by surgical removal. Another kind of nonmalignant growth in the breast is a solid tumor commonly called adenofibroma or fibroadenoma. These tumors develop most frequently in women younger than 25 years of age and are removed surgically.

Both of these disorders fall under the catchall term **fibrocystic disease,** which is further complicated by being also named "chronic cystic mastitis," "mammary dysplasia," "cystic mastalgia," "benign breast disease," and a host of other designations. The number of variants of this benign condition is equaled only by the morass of terms used to describe all of them—around 40 at last count. The symptoms of cyclic pain; tenderness; a feeling of heaviness; and breasts that feel diffusely nodular, granular, or just generally "lumpy" occur in an estimated 50% of all women at one time or another in their reproductive lives, and microscopic examination of the breasts of women at autopsy has revealed that 90% have the histological signs. Such widespread occurrence has led surgeon and researcher Susan Love, in her *Dr. Susan Love's Breast Book* (1995), to call the condition a nonexistent disease—"a wastebasket into which doctors throw every breast problem that isn't cancerous." She suggests "mastalgia" (breast pain), "lumpy breasts," or "physiologic nodularity" as alternatives. Others have suggested replacing the term with "fibrocystic changes" or "fibrocystic complex." By whatever name, however, benign growths of the mammary gland have clinical significance for several reasons. First, it is important to distinguish these from cancer. Not only can the nodules imitate a malignant growth, but they possibly can hide a cancer present among all the lumpy changes. Second, there may be a relationship between some kinds of breast lumps and cancer. There is some evidence that the risk of developing cancer is slightly greater (between 1.5 and 5 times, depending on the study) for a woman with certain types of benign breast lumps, and a small proportion of women, only about 5%, who have breast cancer have also had fibrocystic changes. Dupont and Page (1985) reviewed the records of more than 10,000 breast biopsies performed on women with fibrocystic "disease" to check whether any of the pathologists' classifications of the tissue were associated with the eventual development of breast cancer. After distinguishing between the various types of breast lumps in fibrocystic disease, they found that 70% of the women who had biopsies had no increased risk for breast cancer. Only women who had the designation of atypical **hyperplasia** (an excessive proliferation of epithelial cells) had an increased risk for cancer 4.4 times that of women without that classification of their breast biopsy tissue. A committee of 30 breast pathology experts, convened in 1985 to assess the relationship of fibrocystic disease to breast cancer, established a histological classification of the various kinds of fibrocystic diagnoses and agreed that, of the 13 types classified, only 3, including atypical hyperplasia, had any risk of subsequent breast cancer. The conclusion that atypical hyperplasia results in a higher risk was again confirmed by London and her colleagues (1992). It appears that the potential of fibrocystic disease for subsequent malignancy has been overestimated and is, therefore, overrated. The condition is so common that if it were really strongly related to the development of breast cancer, the incidence of cancer would be greater than it is. Many physicians have said that the term is needlessly frightening and should be changed, but almost all current obstetrics and gynecology textbooks still use the name "fibrocystic disease."

But even if a woman could be reassured that the diagnosis of fibrocystic "disease" does not place her in a higher risk category for breast cancer, swollen lumpy breasts *hurt,* with discomfort that can range from merely being a nuisance helped by a brassiere with greater support to tenderness severe enough to make even turning over in bed a problem.

There is considerable controversy among physicians concerning the treatment of the condition. Almost every kind of hormonal treatment has been tried with varying success, but because the reasons for benign breast changes are not completely understood, the reasons why various hormones or hormonal inhibitors alleviate the condition are also not clear. Estrogen causes mammary duct growth, and progesterone results in alveolar growth and duct dilation, but prolactin, growth hormone, ACTH, thyroxin, and androgen are also concerned with breast function at various times. One current theory hypothesizes that the primary factors in benign breast disease are absolute estrogen excess or absolute or relative progesterone deficiency resulting in an imbalanced estrogen/progesterone ratio. Another theory blames an inappropriate or exaggerated breast tissue response to the normal variations in ovarian hormones. An underfunctioning thyroid gland has been associated with fibrocystic changes, and, possibly, hypothyroidism should be investigated in women who suffer from breast lumps.

That an alteration in the estrogen/progesterone ratio may play a role appears to be substantiated by the reduced incidence of painful nodules when a woman is on oral contraceptives that provide a balanced source of estrogen and progesterone.

Oral progestin in the form of medroxyprogesterone acetate (Provera) has been used with some benefit, and in the past, injected androgens were given, but the masculinizing side effects of hair growth and acne outweighed the pain relief. The big breakthrough in steroid treatment of fibrocystic disease, however, came with the approval in 1980 by the Food and Drug Administration (FDA) of Danazol for fibrocystic disease as well as for endometriosis. Danazol, the androgenlike antigonadotropin, is said to have response rates for severe fibrocystic disease in the 80%–90% range, depending on the dosage and the duration of treatment. The subjects of a 1983 clinical trial by Leis were 42 women with cystic disease severe enough to have required 10–28 needle aspirations in the previous year and a half. After 400 mg of oral Danazol daily for 6 months, 18 women had no further cyst formation in the 2-year follow-up period, 21 developed between one and four cysts, and only three women had more than four cysts. As previously indicated, Danazol is expensive and it should be reserved for women who are virtually incapacitated by discomfort.

Several small clinical trials, with few women as participants and unconfirmed by additional studies, have demonstrated that fibrocystic disease can be treated with dietary changes and/or vitamin supplementation. Women may want to try these measures before choosing hormonal or antihormonal therapies. John P. Minton, of Ohio State University Medical School, reported that fibrocystic disease disappears when women with the condition avoid caffeine. Because studies have shown that cellular levels of the intracellular messenger cyclic AMP are elevated in fibrocystic disease but not in normal breast tissue, and that caffeine, theophylline, and theobromine, all known chemically as methylated xanthines, inhibit the enzyme that destroys cyclic AMP, Minton and associates (1979a, 1979b) reasoned that eliminating methylxanthines from the diet should improve the symptoms of fibrocystic disease. They persuaded 20 out of 47 women, who had long-standing benign breast nodules and who were consuming a daily average of methylxanthines equivalent to that in four cups of coffee, to abstain from coffee; tea; cola; cocoa; and caffeine-containing soft drinks, cold remedies, and painkillers. Thirteen of the 20 women had complete resolution of their breast lumps in 1–6 months. In the remaining group of 27 women who refused to avoid caffeine, only one experienced a spontaneous disappearance of her nodular condition, and the rest subsequently had to have surgical biopsies. Minton also advocates a diet high in fish, chicken, veal, and grains and low in red meat, salt, and fats.

Another trial was reported by London and colleagues in 1978. In 12 women with a diagnosis of fibrocystic disease, 9 obtained good results with no side effects by taking 600 units of vitamin E daily, and several additional studies by the same researchers over the next few years produced similar response rates (1982). In 1985, London and coworkers performed a better-controlled study—randomized and double blind—that indicated that vitamin E had no effect on breast pain. Some women have found that it works for them, however. As long as daily doses beyond the 400–600 unit range are not exceeded, it may be worth trying.

Vitamin B complex in daily doses of 100 mg may possibly enhance liver deactivation of estrogen and is reportedly helpful. According to some women, vitamins C and B_6 have provided symptom relief. In mild fibrocystic disease, merely restricting intake of salt to avoid swelling could be sufficient to alleviate breast tenderness.

The former approach to fibrocystic disease was primarily surgical, with frequent breast biopsies and cyst removals. Current medical journals advocate treatment that attempts to circumvent a need for surgery: abstention from methylxanthines, other dietary changes, perhaps a diuretic taken premenstrually, and cyst aspiration for diagnosis rather than surgical removal. If the above measures are ineffective after an adequate trial, Danazol is prescribed for severe fibro-cystic disease. There are still, however, some doctors who recommend prophylactic surgery for women whom they believe are at high risk for breast cancer because of their severe fibrocystic disease or who have intractable pain. According to Susan Love, an increasing number of simple or subcutaneous mastectomies (removal of the breast tissue below the skin and replacement with an implant) are being performed throughout the country for fibrocystic disease. Although the logic of "if you don't have a breast, you can't get breast cancer" appears incontrovertible, there are other organs of the body equally subject to malignancy, and no one is advocating prophylactic removal of a lung or the testis. Moreover, the reasoning is substantially flawed. Not only is the risk of cancer in the presence of fibrocystic disease probably overestimated, but anything short of a total mastectomy is unlikely to offer complete protection because all mammary gland tissue is not removed by a subcutaneous mastectomy, and a cancer could develop in the remaining tissue.

BREAST CHANGES DURING PREGNANCY

After a number of Joe's organs had dramatically told their stories in *Reader's Digest* ("I Am Joe's Kidney," "I Am Joe's Liver," etc.), the magazine carried an article called "I Am Jane's Breast." In it, Jane's breast rather smugly declares, ". . . I am capable of baffling, almost miraculous, chemical conversions. I change blood into milk."

Actually Jane's breast is guilty of a bit of overstatement. The mammary gland does not change blood into milk any more than the salivary gland changes blood into saliva, the stomach changes blood into gastric juice, or the kidney, blood to urine. The cells of the glandular alveoli of the breasts utilize the nutrients brought to the gland in the circulating blood—the plasma amino acids, fatty acids, and glucose. From those building blocks, the gland synthesizes milk protein, milk fat, and milk sugar; adds ions, vitamins, and water; and secretes them as milk. Throughout the 9 months of pregnancy, the breasts are preparing for nursing.

Within the first 3–4 weeks of gestation, the ducts of the mammary glands sprout branches, and more lobules and alveoli are formed. These changes are much greater than those that occur premenstrually, and the breasts become definitely larger and feel tender and heavy. Each breast gains nearly a pound in weight by the end of pregnancy; the glandular cells, partially filled with secretion, the increased number of blood vessels, and the increased amounts of connective tissue and fat result in the enhanced size.

The hormones that are involved in stimulating and preparing the breasts during pregnancy are the sex steroids from the ovaries and placenta. Prolactin and growth hormone from the anterior pituitary, human placental lactogen and human chorionic gonadotropin from the placenta, adrenal corticosteroids, insulin from the pancreas, and thyroid and parathyroid hormones also all contribute to the duct and alveolar growth and differentiation into secreting cells.

Anterior pituitary prolactin, secreted in increasing levels throughout pregnancy, triggers the actual synthesis and secretion of milk after the birth of a baby. During pregnancy, prolactin, in the presence of large amounts of estrogens and progesterone from the ovaries and placenta (and the other hormones mentioned), causes some synthesis and secretion of **colostrum.** Colostrum is a milklike fluid containing protein and carbohydrate but lacking milk fat. It is only after birth, however, when the high levels of sex steroids are abruptly withdrawn, that prolactin is able to cause the glandular cells to secrete large quantities of milk instead of colostrum. This takes place within 2–3 days of birth. Development of the glandular tissue, then, is stimulated mostly by sex steroids in the presence of the other placental, pituitary, and metabolic hormones mentioned. The actual milk synthesis and milk release into the lumens of the alveoli are caused by prolactin. The milk "comes in" after several days of colostrum secretion, but before the baby can get it, another hormone, *oxytocin,* must act so that the milk can be ejected from the alveoli to the nipples. The stimulus of sucking on the nipple causes oxytocin to be released from the posterior pituitary gland.* Oxytocin gets into the bloodstream, travels to the mammary gland, and induces *myoepithelial cells* surrounding the alveoli to contract. The milk enters the ducts and begins to flow easily from the breast that was sucked and also from the other breast. As long as the mother continues to nurse, the milk will continue to flow, even for several years. Prolactin and oxytocin result in milk production under the stimulus of sucking. When the baby is weaned, the prolactin and oxytocin secretion stops, and milk is no longer synthesized and released. (A further discussion of breast-feeding can be found in Chapter 11.)

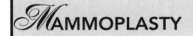

Mammoplasty

Breast Augmentation

No matter how it looks to the rest of the world, if an individual thinks that a body part is ugly or inadequate, it can become the focus of a sense of body-image deformity and produce anxiety and concern that interfere with his or her life. Small breasts in a woman do not have to impair her sex life, her activities, or her attractiveness. But if the small-breasted woman is convinced, and certainly our society helps her in her perception, that such smallness is at the root of all her difficulties, her self-image may be impaired, and she can never be truly comfortable with her body. Even though the usual method of enhancing the size of small breasts is by wearing "falsies," a woman may consider that it is more real to surgically implant the falsies. Essentially, this is the method that is used in augmentation mammoplasty.

Early operations to increase breast size used homografts of the woman's own subcutaneous fat tissue

---

*In a nursing mother, milk flow can also often be elicited merely by hearing another baby cry, or even by thinking about a baby.

transplanted from her buttock. In some countries of the world, this method is still used, but the results frequently are unpredictable and usually asymmetrical because of the tendency of fat to be reabsorbed. Another inexpensive but dangerous method of breast-size enhancement that is no longer used is the injection of free silicone fluid. The silicone, in the large quantity of fluid required, generally disperses away from the injection site and causes an infection or inflammatory response. Silicone liquid has been banned for breast augmentation since 1965.

The original types of alloplastic (nonhuman, manufactured) implants were plastic sponges. These were unsatisfactory because they became infiltrated with scar tissue that hardened and flattened them out to pancakes. But 40 years ago, researchers at the Dow Corning Corporation invented the silicone gel breast implant—silicone encased in a silicone envelope. This became the most widely used prosthetic device for breast augmentation in the United States and somewhere between 1 million and 2 million American women received these implants. Until a moratorium on their use because of safety concerns was imposed by the FDA in late 1991, about 300 women daily were having the devices implanted by plastic surgeons at a cost of about $3,000 for surgery and anesthesia. Eighty percent of breast implants were done for cosmetic reasons; the rest were for breast reconstruction after cancer surgery.

Different models of the prosthesis included solid gel-filled implants, gel-filled implants with a polyurethane coating, and the inflatables. The saline inflatable implants are hollow with a silicone shell. After placement, saline solution is injected into the shell by the surgeon until the desired volumetric breast size is reached. Inflatables feel softer than the gels and require a smaller incision for insertion. The disadvantage of inflatables is a tendency to rupture or leak, but all that would be released is the allegedly harmless saline. The skill and experience of the surgeon is important to the successful implantation of the inflatables. Too much fluid injected can cause bulging; too little fluid can cause wrinkling. If all the air is not

removed before inflation, the breasts may "squish" on palpation.

The more popular silicone gel implant was essentially a thin-walled silicone plastic bag containing semisolid silicone, a material closely related chemically to Silly Putty. The gel implant feels firm but has a certain amount of elasticity and "give." The solid gel implants have always had more of a tendency to become hard with time because of scar tissue formation.

Breast augmentation by implants is not without documented risks. Even when the surgery is performed by a competent plastic surgeon whose standards for quality medical and surgical procedures are high, the operation can still be unpredictable and subject to several kinds of complications. The contour and the feel of the breasts may be aesthetically unsatisfactory, and the surgery may have to be performed again. Women vary in the amount of scar tissue they produce, which can cause a problem with hardness of the breasts or with appearance of the scar. Some women with implants have lost sensation in the nipples and areolae, but others have felt an enhancement of sensitivity. Infection is always a possibility, but it occurs less frequently than hematoma, the accumulation of a mass of partially clotted blood within the tissue. Early detection of breast cancer is somewhat more difficult when there are breast implants, so women who have had augmentation mammoplasty should, like all other women, perform regular monthly breast self-examination and have frequent periodic clinical examinations by their physicians.

Silicone breast implants have been available for four decades, but only since 1991 has their safety become a major concern. Women who chose to have augmentation knew only that the procedure was easy and relatively affordable and had assumed that the implants were harmless. After the FDA's moratorium, however, it was learned that there was an amazing lack of directly relevant studies on the safety of implants. There was no documented scientific evidence that they are unsafe, but neither was there evidence that they are safe. Clinical testing by the manufacturer took place in women before the first results from animal tests were completed, and almost none of the studies had actually tested free silicone in the breast tissue of the animals. It also became evident that Dow Corning, which is the largest maker of implants and has dominated the market since 1960, actually had its own safety concerns about the gel implants that were neither reported nor followed up. Moreover, the federal government did not mandate that the implants meet restrictive safety standards until 1988. Breast implants had been marketed for years with virtually no regulation.

In 1976, Congress passed a law requiring proof of safety and effectiveness for all medical devices. The most rigorous standards were for Class III products, but breast implants were exempted from the stringent standards because they were already on the market. Although the FDA subsequently tried several times to put breast implants in the Class III category, the effort, opposed by manufacturers and plastic surgeons, failed. After it became apparent that numerous adverse effects and the possibility of an increased cancer risk were associated with breast implants, they finally were reclassified as a Class III medical device, and implant makers were told that they had to provide data on safety within 30 months. In November 1991, an FDA panel and Commissioner David D. Kessler held that the safety data were inadequate and asked manufacturers to stop selling them and plastic surgeons to stop inserting them.

That some side effects or harmful complications were associated with the silicone gel implants was not news to many of the women who had them inserted. Three-quarters of women experience some degree of "capsular contracture." The term refers to the natural response of the body to any foreign material, that is, a walling off of the area by scar tissue. The scar tissue, called a capsule, remains soft and pliable and presents no problem to many women. For unknown reasons, probably having to do with an individual response to collagen (fibrous connective tissue) formation, severe capsular contracture takes place in a small percentage of women. The scar tissue becomes hard and painfully contracts around the implant. Instead of two natural-looking and natural-feeling breasts, some women

develop the equivalent of two painful baseballs. The fibrous capsule may then have to be split or released, which requires a second operation. In very severe cases, it may be necessary to reopen the breasts, remove the implants, scrape out the scar tissue, and insert other implants. Additional surgery is not uncommon. An estimated one of every five women with breast implants needs another operation for a variety of complications such as painful capsular contracture, implant rupture, infection, hematoma, or asymmetrical breasts.

Leakage and rupture can occur. Almost all the silicone gel implants tend to "bleed" or leak very tiny amounts of fluid silicone, which seeps into the lymph and blood circulation to migrate to other parts of the body with unknown long-term effects. It is suspected, although there is no proof, that certain autoimmune diseases such as lupus, scleroderma, or rheumatoid arthritis may be associated with the inflammatory reaction to silicone. Although silicone is allegedly harmless, there is no real proof of its benign nature. A report in 1998 issued by a panel of four scientists appointed by a federal court judge overseeing implant liability litigation concluded that scientific evidence thus far has failed to prove that silicone breast implants cause disease but did not rule out the possibility that implants may increase the risk of those diseases in the long term. Diana Zuckerman, the scientist who initiated the congressional investigation of silicone in 1991, pointed out that "after more than 35 years of human experimentation on about a million women, we still don't know how many implant patients will have serious problems that harm their health or the quality of their lives. The story isn't over yet" (1999). The impact of the four-person scientific panel report was significant, however. In 1994, Dow Corning was going to establish a $4.2 billion fund to compensate women who could demonstrate damage from the gel implants. In 1999 settlement discussions, Dow Corning offered $1.8 billion less than the 1994 amount. In 1999, another independent panel of 13 scientists convened at the request of Congress by the Institute of Medicine, the medical arm of the prestigious National Academy of Sciences, reviewed more than a thousand research studies and held public hearings. Its conclusions were similar to those of the earlier panel—that while localized problems such as rupture, deflations, scarring, and hardening are primary safety issues with implants, there was no evidence that they caused any systemic diseases. Their report is expected to encourage women to accept settlements from implant manufacturers (Dow Corning, Baxter International, Bristol-Myers Squibb, and Minnesota Mining and Manufacturing) amounting to a combined $6.2 billion rather than sue in court.

Fortunately, after 40 years of augmentation mammoplasty with the devices, there is no actual proof that silicone breast implants cause cancer in humans. There are, however, studies that link silicone to cancer in laboratory animals, some of them done by Dow Corning. The only large clinical study to assess the cancer risk of breast implants to women reviewed the records of 3,111 women with implants in the Los Angeles area for an average of 11 years and reported no increase in breast cancer rate (Deapen et al., 1986). Because the time between exposure to a carcinogen and the development of cancer is known to be far in excess of 11 years, the data at this point could be viewed as inconclusive. Brinton and Brown (1997) maintain that the risk of cancer has not yet been addressed in epidemiological studies and that special attention be given to women who have implants with a polyurethane foam coating, which was designed to prevent capsular contracture. This type, estimated to have been implanted in 70,000 women, was found to be associated with liver cancer in laboratory rats and is no longer on the market, although how many of those women still have them is unknown. Plastic surgeons who removed this type of implant from patients for one problem or another discovered what happens to the polyurethane after implantation. After insertion, the foam-coated shell on the implant remains intact for about a week and then begins to break down into billions of polyurethane particles, some of which release a degradation product called 2-toluene diamine, which is a known carcinogen in animals. After 2–5 years, all the polyurethane foam particles are gone (to somewhere in the body), and the smooth silicone bag is subject to the excessive hardening the polyurethane coating was supposed to prevent.

Currently, silicone gel-filled breast implants are available only in a clinical study conducted by a manufacturer under an Investigational Device Exception approved by the FDA, in an adjunct clinical trial conducted by a researcher approved by the FDA, or for a woman having reconstruction as a result of breast cancer surgery for whom a saline-filled implant is deemed inappropriate. Gel-filled implants are unavailable to women who want them for breast enlargement. Saline-filled silicone breast implants are available to anyone who wants them. Since 1994, the FDA has required that companies marketing them must report laboratory, animal, and clinical data to assess their safety and effectiveness. The clinical studies are monitoring adverse effects such as rupture, infection, capsular contracture, and systemic effects. These investigations are, of course, industry supported. Although saline implants are generally assumed to be safer, there is little independent research to confirm that assumption.

In a March 2000 interview on the NBC *Today* show, Dr. Judith Reichman noted that since 1992, there has been a 300% increase in breast augmentations each year. Of the 130,000 women who had breast augmentations in 1999, most had saline implants. Sixty percent were aged 19–34; 35% were 35–50. Approximately 1,500 girls under the age of 18 received breast implants in 1999. Surgery usually costs between $5,000 and $7,000 and, like most cosmetic surgery, is not covered by insurance.

Breast Reconstruction After Mastectomy

Until very recently, the primary treatment for breast cancer has been **mastectomy,** complete removal of the breast. The response of a woman to mastectomy is intensely personal, and probably no woman really knows how she feels about losing a breast until it happens to her. To most of us, cancer is our greatest health fear. To find out that one has breast cancer is enough to produce the initial emotions of shock, fear, resentment, denial, and perhaps panic in all women, but when that knowledge is accompanied by the surgical loss of a highly visible part of the body, the psychological effects can be tremendously magnified. Some women may be as devastated by the mastectomy as they are by the diagnosis of cancer. For others, survival is their main priority. They can say, "Take my one breast, take the other one, do whatever you have to, but leave me my life," and they mean every word, particularly if it has been determined that the cancer has already spread to the lymph nodes.

Women should discuss the possibility of reconstruction with their surgeons before surgery if mastectomy is to be the treatment for their cancer (there are other available alternatives). If the medical opinion is that the reconstruction will not compromise the best chance for curing the cancer, the realization that something can be done to restore the breast may help a woman through the ordeal. Reconstruction is also an option for women who had their mastectomies 20–30 years ago, but because a radical mastectomy was more frequent then, the technique of creating a new breast contour is more technically complicated.

The two breast reconstruction techniques used most frequently are (1) the subpectoral prosthesis method, in which an implant is placed under the chest muscle, and (2) the musculocutaneous skin flap technique, in which a section of skin, muscle, and fat is removed from the abdomen or back, leaving the blood vessels attached. The section of skin and muscle, still connected to its original blood supply, is moved up under the skin to the mastectomy site. A newer method, called free flap surgery, removes a wedge of skin, fat, muscle, and blood vessels from the abdomen, buttock, or thigh. The flap is transplanted through microsurgical techniques to the chest wall, reattaching the blood vessels that come with it to the blood vessels that supply the breast. The flap techniques take more time and are much more expensive to perform.

The final result of any form of reconstruction surgery, however good, may be somewhat less than a cosmetic triumph. The breast still cannot be restored to its preoperative normal appearance. The woman will look better in a brassiere than in the nude, and the two breasts will most likely be unequal in size. The opposite normal breast can be reduced to match the reconstructed breast, or an inflatable implant can be used in the reconstruction to achieve as much symmetry between the two breasts as possible. Sometimes, several operations may be necessary before the desirable result is achieved, but the less extensive the mastectomy to begin with, the simpler the reconstruction procedure afterward. Extensive postmastectomy irradiation treatment to the chest wall poses a particular difficulty and may make reconstruction almost impossible because of the tissue damage.

If a nipple and areola are to be rebuilt, they will require more surgery, so some women may prefer to do without them. Should reconstruction of the areola be desired, however, a graft can be taken from the other breast. Some doctors are against such areolar sharing because of the possibility of transplanting a present or potential malignancy from the normal breast. Another possible technique is to use a graft from the pigmented skin of the labia minora, which is removed under local anesthesia. A nipple can also be simulated by an implant of scar tissue or cartilage, by nipple sharing from the other breast, or by other surgical methods.

The most appropriate timing of the reconstruction is still a controversial issue, centering primarily on the question of whether the reconstruction may mask and thus delay the discovery of a recurrent cancer. One group of physicians believes that reconstruction should be delayed for 2 years because a local recurrence generally develops within that period. Other surgeons believe in reconstruction at the time of the initial mastectomy. Some prefer to wait a few months to allow the resolution of trauma and scarring and to permit the completion of all postoperative therapy, such as radiation.

Not only when, but also who should have breast reconstruction is also subject to controversy. The easiest candidate to operate on would be a young woman in good health with early cancer, no lymph node involvement, and a simple mastectomy. Women who have had a more extensive modified radical or the classical radical surgery are not excluded but should recognize that the nature of the operation may be more extensive. Breast reconstruction postmastectomy is necessarily subject to the same complications as breast augmentation—the possibility of implant hardness, hematoma, and infection.

If a woman is highly motivated, has made her own decision, and has recognized that there will be improvement but not perfection as a result of the reconstruction, the procedure can be of great value to her. She should be aware, however, of its shortcomings and do it to please herself, not because anyone else wants her to have it done.

Reduction Mammoplasty

Perhaps in the opinion of some men, breasts can never be too large. But ask a woman who has macromastia—breasts that are disproportionately large in relation to her other body dimensions—whether she actually feels twice blessed. Excessive breast size can cause physical discomfort for a woman all her adult life. She may have neck and back pain, deep grooves in her shoulders from her bra straps, chafing, a skin rash and itching under her breasts, and have difficulty in the ordinary movements of walking and running. She would welcome a procedure to reduce mammary tissue and not merely for cosmetic reasons.

The surgical technique of breast reduction is called reduction mammoplasty. Some of the actual breast mass is removed, the skin over the breast is proportionately adjusted, and the nipple and the areola are relocated to a new appropriate position. There is some scarring, and the results are not always perfect and lasting. Most women, however, who have had the operation are very satisfied to get rid of the discomfort and excess weight of their breasts and are able to find and wear clothes that fit for the first time since they were children. In most instances, there is no loss of sensation in the nipples, and women are still able to lactate and nurse a child after surgery, but some doctors recommend that the operation be delayed until childbearing and breast-feeding are no longer desired. Postoperative complications of hematoma and infec-

tion are possible, but the skill and the experience of the surgeon are critical factors in making such complications relatively rare.

Ptosis

Ptosis, or sagging breasts, can occur without macromastia and may sometimes follow pregnancy. The surgical procedure that elevates ptotic breasts is called mastopexy. Sometimes, depending on the patient, it can be done on an outpatient basis under local anesthesia. The surgery is considerably simpler than reduction mammoplasty, although the scarring may be about the same, and there is a lesser incidence of postsurgical complications. When there has been a reduction in breast volume as a result of aging or after pregnancy, a woman may feel it is important to restore the fullness of the breast as well as its elevation. Augmentation with a saline implant can then be combined with mastopexy.

Opinions vary as to whether going braless contributes to sagging breasts. It seems logical that supporting the weight of the breasts against gravity with a brassiere diminishes the stress on the network of connective tissues that supports the fat and glandular elements of the breasts. Larger breasts would be more affected by gravity and are thought to be more subject to "Cooper's droop," the weakening of **Cooper's ligaments**. Women with larger and heavier breasts are usually more comfortable while wearing a bra, anyway.

BREAST CANCER

According to the American Cancer Society, 1 of every 9 American females at birth will someday develop breast cancer. Breast cancer is the most frequent site of female cancer and second only to lung cancer as a killer of women. Every 12 minutes, somewhere in the United States a woman dies of breast cancer. In the late 1960s, more than 65,000 women developed breast cancer and 33,000 died. In 1991, an estimated 175,000 new cases were diagnosed and the death rate at 44,500 was not that different. Now there are nearly 200,000 new cases diagnosed annually and the mortality is 47,000—still not that different. With grim monotony, the incidence of breast cancer continues to increase about 1/2% per year over the past 30–40 years while essentially the same mortality rate persists. Statistically, half the women found to have breast cancer this year will not be alive after 10 years. The various forms of treatment, the dollars poured into research to find a cause, a control, a cure—none of these has thus far been able to extend significantly the lives of women with breast cancer.

With these scary statistics, is there any reason for optimism in the battle against breast cancer? Although it cannot be considered a silver lining, there are some encouraging aspects that have emerged during the campaign. First of all, the increased incidence and the unchanged death rate could mean the survival rate is increasing—a lukewarm victory but heartening nonetheless. Besides, the overall survival rates mean virtually nothing for an individual woman. Not all breast cancer is the same, and there can be many variables, such as the virulence of the cancer or the resistance of the woman. Second, a major contributor to the increased risk is the simple fact that women are living longer and the risk of breast cancer increases with age. The 1 in 9 figure assumes a woman will live to age 85. Third, more localized breast cancer, caught before spread, is being found today than ever before because of increased public awareness and improved technological methods of detection. It is becoming evident that if it is detected early enough and treated promptly, the diagnosis of breast cancer is not an automatic death sentence. Early detection, the discovery of the cancer at a very early stage, before the disease has spread or when the spread is minimal, is the only approach that holds any promise at all of reducing mortality. Women themselves, if they practice monthly self-examination, can come to know their own breasts and develop more sensitive fingers than anyone else. They can detect a small change, an irregularity that could be serious, bet-

ter than their doctors can. Even though only 12% of all women—and no more than that—will ever develop breast cancer, that presents enough of a lifetime risk to make it essential for all women to practice monthly breast self-examination.

If more were known about the causes of breast cancer, more efforts could be directed toward its prevention. There is no way to explain why some women do and other women do not develop the disease. As yet, there has been only the identification of some characteristic risk factors that appear to be associated with an increased frequency of breast cancer. Women who fall into those categories of risk should, in addition to performing monthly self-examination, have more frequent clinical examinations by a physician that include other methods of diagnosis such as routine low-dose mammography, or x-rays, of their breasts.

RISK FACTORS OF BREAST CANCER

The most important risk factor is being a woman. Although breast cancer occurs in men, it is 100 times more frequent in women. The second most important risk factor is age. Breast cancer is rarely found in girls younger than 15, and only 1%–3% of all mammary cancers occur in women younger than age 30. At 45, incidence increases and continues to rise rapidly with age. A woman in her 60s has 20% less risk of developing breast cancer than a woman in her 70s, whose risk is half that of a woman in her 80s.

Having had cancer in one breast increases the risk of developing it in the other breast by 5 to 7 times. As previously indicated, a history of a breast biopsy with a diagnosis of "atypical hyperplasia" may increase the risk 4.4 times beyond that of women who have not been biopsied for benign breast disease. A woman with a family history of breast cancer in a first-degree relative—that is, in a mother or a sister—has a doubled risk of getting breast cancer herself. If she has two affected sisters, her risk before age 40 is increased ninefold compared with women of a similar age; if her sister and her mother both have breast cancer, her risk before age 40 becomes almost 50 times as great as other women her age. Even with affected relatives, however, her own risk substantially decreases as she gets older, and by ages 60–79, her risk is the same as in the general population.

There are other, relatively slight influences on the occurrence of breast cancer that have to do with the reproductive life of a woman. Women whose menarche occurred before age 12 have a slightly increased risk over women who were age 15 or older at menarche, but the relative risk does not increase further with decreasing age at menarche. A late menopause also increases the risk. But if a woman has had an ovariectomy (and thus a surgical menopause) before age 35, the risk is lessened.

Never having had a baby puts a woman at greater risk. Pregnancy is protective, but the evidence currently available suggests that the degree of protection is associated with the age of the woman at the time of the first full-term delivery. The younger she is when she has her first child, the lower her risk for breast cancer. Having five or more children also decreases the risk, but pregnancies interrupted by miscarriage or abortion offer no protection. The risk of breast cancer actually increases with age at first delivery. If a woman has her first baby after 35, her likelihood of developing breast cancer is greater than if she had never had children at all.

For years, it was believed that breast-feeding protected against breast cancer. It seemed logical to correlate the increasing incidence of breast cancer with the greater numbers of women who were not nursing their babies. Although many studies conducted during the 1970s, both in the United States and internationally, had concluded that lactation had little effect either way, later reports revived the theory that prolonged breast-feeding may have a protective effect against the subsequent development of breast cancer (Byers et al., 1985; McTiernan & Thomas, 1986). It was unclear whether the lesser risk was due to a hormonal influence (the delay in reestablishing menstruation after pregnancy) or that lactation had produced changes in the lining of the mammary ducts, the place where more than 80% of breast cancers start.

There has also been the discovery that virus particles very similar to those of mouse mammary tumor virus were present in breast milk in both normal women and women with breast cancer. This led to the hypothesis that there was a viral agent responsible for breast cancer that could be transmitted in human breast milk. There has been no evidence, however, of any association between being breast-fed and the subsequent development of breast cancer. The incidence of breast cancer is the same in women whether or not they were breast-fed as infants, which argues against maternal transmission in milk. But Al-Sumidiae and coworkers (1988) found particles with retrovirus properties in the white blood cells of 98% of a group of women with breast cancer. This suggests that when breast cancer is hereditary, it could be due to a virus transmitted from mother to daughter. If a virus could really be proved to be a cause of breast cancer, there is the potential of immunization against the virus and, thus, against breast cancer.

The relationships among such factors as the length of menstrual activity and childbearing and the development of breast cancer indicate that hormones are involved, but little is definitely known concerning the significance of a woman's own estrogens and ovarian activity relative to her development of breast cancer. While there is little doubt that they are implicated, endogenous estrogens may not actually initiate cancer but may be promoters of cancer. That is, after some other factor—environmental, infectious, or genetic—causes damage to the nucleus of a breast cell, then ovarian hormones, over a period of years, are involved in the processes that lead to the progression of the cancer. Women who have an earlier menarche (a risk factor) and those who have a later natural menopause (another risk factor) are exposed to their own normal estrogens and progesterone for a longer period of their lives than women with a later menarche or an earlier menopause, so long-term exposure to endogenous estrogens may be the important factor. Excess estrogen stimulation in the absence of cyclic progesterone has also been suggested as a risk factor, and several studies have shown an increased risk of breast cancer in women with anovulatory cycles (Cowan, Gordis, Tonascia, & Jones, 1981; Gonzalez, 1983).

Pregnancy is another hormonal event that influences a woman's risk of breast cancer. A first full-term pregnancy that occurs within 5 years after the onset of menarche is protective. One theory to explain the effect suggests that because the hormones of pregnancy cause maturation of the milk ducts of the breast, perhaps when such maturation or differentiation occurs early in life, the milk ducts are not as vulnerable to the long-term cancer-promoting effects of estrogen or any other carcinogen.

During their reproductive lives, women produce three types of estrogen: estradiol, estrone, and estriol. All of these are carcinogenic when administered to laboratory animals. Estradiol is the strongest of the estrogens in biological activity, but it has less carcinogenic potential in animals than estrone. Estriol is the weakest estrogen and has very little or no carcinogenic activity in mice. On this basis, some investigators have credited an increased risk of breast cancer to estradiol and estrone and a protective effect to estriol. During pregnancy, the production of all three estrogens is greatly increased, but estradiol and estrone increase over prepregnancy levels by a hundredfold while estriol increases a thousandfold. This has led to speculation that the higher levels of estriol during pregnancy, acting on the breast, provide the protection against cancer.

As far as exogenous estrogens are concerned, the results of many animal studies have shown that they can induce breast cancer. It would seem reasonable, therefore, to theorize a possible link between the increased use of oral contraceptives, the increased use of estrogen replacement therapy in the menopause, and the increased incidence of breast cancer in the past 40 years. There is conflicting evidence, however, for a cause-and-effect relationship and sometimes conflicting interpretation of the results of the same published data. The Collaborative Group on Hormonal Factors in Breast Cancer used meta-analysis to examine worldwide epidemiological evidence on the relationship between breast cancer and oral contraceptives and analyzed 54 studies that included 53,297 women with breast cancer and 100,239 women without breast cancer (1996). It concluded that while women are taking combined oral contraceptives and in the 10 years after stopping, there is a small increase in the risk of breast cancer, but the resulting tumors were localized and less likely to have spread aggressively beyond the breast. It also concluded that 10 years after stopping use of oral contraceptives, there was no increased significant risk. The methodological limitations in assessing the safety of long-term use of birth control pills are obvious. Not only is it difficult in an epidemiological study to establish the formulation of the pills used (they have changed so much) and know with certainty the duration of use (women forget what they used and how long they used a particular pill), but breast or other cancers may take 20 years to develop and oral contraceptives have been around only 30 years. It may merely be a matter of more time before the issue of pill use and risk of breast cancer is resolved.

There is evidence for an increased risk of breast cancer in postmenopausal women who take estrogen replacement therapy. A study by Steinberg and co-workers (1991) used the sophisticated statistical method of meta-analysis on 16 studies to assess the effect of duration of estrogen replacement therapy on breast cancer risk. They found that 15 years of estrogen use resulted in a 30% increase in the risk of breast cancer. The risk was significantly higher in women with a family history of breast cancer. Colditz, Egan, and Stampfer (1993) reviewed 31 studies and found that a 20%–30% increased risk of breast cancer was associated with current hormone estrogen replacement therapy use for 10 years or longer. Because postmenopausal estrogen is known to cause an increased risk of endometrial cancer, in recent years the addition of progestins to the estrogen has been advocated to avert the possibility. It was speculated that the progestins might have a protective effect against breast cancer as well. But a study of more than 23,000 Swedish women revealed that, while a woman's risk of breast cancer was increased by taking estrogen after menopause, the risk was highest among those women who took estrogen in combination with progestin for extended periods. The researchers concluded that progestins provide no benefit against the risk of breast cancer and may actually do harm (Bergkvist et al., 1989). A large epidemiological study by Colditz et al. published in 1995 concluded that the risk of breast cancer in postmenopausal women who take estrogen is not reduced by the addition of progestins and that the significant increase in the risk of breast cancer should be factored into risk-and-benefit trade-offs of estrogen replacement therapy for older women. A more recent major study published in the Journal of the American Medical Association in early 2000 by Schairer et al. made headline news across the country by affirming, through analysis of data from 46,000 women who participated in the Breast Cancer Detection Demonstration Project—the largest study to date—that combined estrogen-progestin therapies were associated with greater risk for breast cancer than estrogen alone.

Other risk factors besides gender, age, menstrual history, pregnancy, family history, and hormones have been proposed and appear to affect the development of breast cancer. Diets high in saturated fats and obesity in particular, have long been correlated with an increased risk of breast cancer, and there has been ample data to support the theory over the past several decades, especially because a relationship between obesity and breast cancer may have a hormonal basis. After menopause, it is known that estrogens are produced by conversion from androstenedione, a product of the adrenal cortex. This conversion takes place primarily in adipose tissue, and, thus, more estrone is produced in obese women. Moreover, premenopausal obese women also have higher blood levels of estrogen and frequently have irregular menstrual periods and anovulatory cycles. As indicated previously, anovulation may predispose to breast cancer. A further link between diet and estrogen metabolism is suggested by studies that compare vegetarian women with nonvegetarian women. For exam-

ple, Goldin and coworkers (1982) found that vegetarian women had an increased fecal excretion of estrogen and a corresponding decreased level of estrogen in the blood, possibly due to the increased fiber in their diets. The amount of fat and fiber eaten could be a factor explaining the high risk of breast cancer in Western countries where a high fat and animal protein diet is consumed and the much lower risk of breast cancer in Third World countries where women eat vegetarian or semivegetarian low-protein, high-fiber diets. There is also evidence from animal and human studies linking specific vegetables to a beneficial effect. The risk of breast cancer, as well as other cancers, may be lessened when foods rich in selenium, vitamin C, and the cruciferous vegetables (brussels sprouts, cabbage, turnips, broccoli, and cauliflower) are part of the diet. While the lower fat content of a vegetarian diet is believed to be a factor, a further explanation for the protective effect is the presence of carcinogenic inhibitors in the food. The inhibitors are indoles, or plant growth factors, which have been found to prevent tumors in various animals. Michnovicz and Bradlow (1990) provided evidence that the role of indoles in estrogen metabolism may enable them to reduce estrogen-responsive tumors such as breast cancer in humans. The workers extracted an indole from cruciferous vegetables and administered it to a small group of men (to avoid any influence of fluctuating hormone levels and because previous research had indicated that estrogen metabolism is independent of gender). The result was a significant increase in the metabolic conversion of strong estradiol to weak estrogens with little carcinogenic activity.

A number of studies that compared the reported past dietary habits of breast cancer patients with those of matched healthy control women provided data consistent with the hypothesis that increased consumption of fats increases the relative risk of breast cancer. The inherent weakness of such studies is that the current diet may not be the same as the diet during the lengthy period during which the breast cancer cells were becoming malignant, and most women would have difficulty recalling how and what they ate

20–30 years ago. But a review published in the *Journal of the National Cancer Institute* provided very convincing evidence that a diet low in saturated fats and high in fruits and vegetables can reduce the risk of breast cancer (Howe et al., 1990). The paper analyzed the results of the original data from 12 previously conducted studies of diet and breast cancer in populations with very different dietary habits and breast cancer risks. The researchers found a consistent, statistically significant, positive association between breast cancer risk and intake of saturated fats in postmenopausal women and a consistent protective effect for intake of fruits and vegetables. They estimated that dietary modification to reduce fat and increase vegetables and fruits could prevent 24% of breast cancers in postmenopausal women and 16% in premenopausal women.

Body size has also been extensively studied in relation to the risk of breast cancer. In general, increased height is not associated with an increased risk in Western industrialized countries. Concerning relative body weight, obesity does appear to increase the risk of breast cancer, but the effect is seen only in older postmenopausal women (London et al., 1989). Other data imply, however, that a relationship between increased weight and increased risk may have to do with where the excess weight is distributed. Schapira, Kumar, Lyman, and Cox (1990) compared the body measurements of 432 healthy women to 216 women of the same age with breast cancer. The women who were "apple"-shaped, that is, with excess weight around the middle and a waist-to-hip ratio greater than 0.8, were five times more likely to have breast cancer than those with fat hips or thighs, or "pear"-shaped. The waist-to-hip ratio is computed by dividing the waist measurement by the measurement of the hips taken at the widest point between the hips and the buttocks.

Having now discussed a number of investigations indicating that high intake of fat in the diet appears to be associated with an increase in breast cancer risk, a 1999 major epidemiological study published in the Journal of the American Medical Association (Holmes et al.) reported a startling conclusion—that contrary to the prevailing hypotheses, there was *no* evidence that higher total fat intake was associated with an increased risk of breast cancer. The researchers found no increased risk with increased intake of animal fat, polyunsaturated fat, saturated fat, or trans-unsaturated fat. Moreover, there was no decreased risk as a result of eating vegetable fat, and, certainly in contrast to what we have been told, consuming omega-3 fat from fish was associated with an *increased* risk of breast cancer. This is a large, well-designed study and difficult to fault. It began when 121,700 registered nurses, aged 30–55 years, from across the United States (the Nurses' Health Study) answered a mailed questionnaire to identify risk factors and newly diagnosed cases of breast cancer, cardiovascular disease, and other illnesses. The women were then followed up with questionnaires every 2 years. In 1980, a food questionnaire to assess dietary intake was added, which was expanded in 1984, 1986, and 1990. Adjustments were made for all factors that may have confounded the results, such as women who concurrently consumed increased folate, fiber, and vitamin E in foods; who practiced more health-conscious behaviors such as screening mammography; or who underreported fat calorie intake, intentionally or mistakenly. None of these changed the results. This study, however, is not permission to load up on steak and Ben & Jerry's ice cream during the midlife years. The authors suggest that reducing total fat intake is unlikely to prevent breast cancer, and it should receive less emphasis. But reducing animal fats and substituting monounsaturated fats strongly influences the risk of heart disease, which should receive greater emphasis.

Although the data associating excess body weight and consumption of fat to an increased risk of breast cancer have been challenged by the data from the Nurses' Study, it is difficult at this time to accept that study as definitive, given the amount of previous research on diet and breast cancer with opposite conclusions. There is, however, no similar difficulty with the data concerning alcohol intake. All of them show a positive association with an increased risk. In one large study, women who drank two to three drinks per week had a 40% increased risk; those who drank one or more drinks a day experienced a 50% increased risk (Willet et al., 1987). Another examination of 7,188 women found that consumption of any amount of alcohol increased the risk of breast cancer by 50%–100% (Schatzkin et al., 1987). The carcinogenic effect of alcohol on breast cancer must be operating through some biological mechanism, but it is currently unexplained. Caffeine intake, because of its association with benign breast disease and because some kinds of benign breast lumps lead to an increased risk of breast cancer, also has been investigated in a number of studies. There is, however, virtually no evidence to support a relationship between coffee drinking and the risk of breast cancer.

The recently reported nonassociation of dietary intake of fat and fatty acids with the risk of breast cancer becomes particularly puzzling because worldwide geographic differences in breast cancer as well as ethnic and religious differences have been postulated, in the absence of other known reasons, to be due to differences in dietary practices. The amount of fat and fiber eaten could be a factor explaining the high risk of breast cancer in Western countries where a diet high in fat and animal protein is consumed, and the much lower risk of breast cancer in less developed countries where women eat vegetarian or semivegetarian, low-protein, high-fiber diets. Incidence rates are five to six times higher in North America and Europe than in Asia and Africa, and Caucasians have a much higher rate. Eskimo and Yemenite women almost never get breast cancer; the incidence is also very low in women of Asian descent. For example, Japan has a low breast cancer rate and a low average fat intake, and the United States has a high breast cancer rate and an average diet in which 40% of the calories are derived from fat. But if Asians migrate to the West, their incidence rate becomes that of the local population in a few generations.

The mortality from breast cancer is very high in western Europe, particularly in the Netherlands; in the United States it is highest in the northern states. For unknown and puzzling reasons, lower mortality rates occur in the southern or southwestern states, and the lowest rate is in Hawaii. Although the curious cultural and sociological factors that appear to be involved in the incidence of breast cancer must be acting through some biological mechanisms, they have not as yet been identified. What underlies the relationship of breast cancer to diet, or to stress, or to lifestyle? There are no definitive answers, but it is known that breast cancer occurs more frequently in affluent women than in poor women. In one group of Indian women, the Parsis of Bombay, the incidence of breast cancer is three times what it is in the Hindu, Muslim, Christian, and Jewish women in India. Parsi women are wealthier and better educated than the rest of the Indian population.

There is no reason to be overly concerned about risk factors; almost everyone is bound to have one or more of them. Even having all of them does not mean a woman is going to get breast cancer. It means only that her risk is greater than that of other women without the factors. But even with none of the risk factors, a woman still has a greater chance of developing breast cancer if she lives in the United States, and the reasons are unknown. Some American women, however, do have a statistically lower risk of developing breast cancer by the age of 75. These include, in decreasing order of risk, black women, Chinese-American women, Japanese-American women, Hispanic women from New Mexico and Native American women from New Mexico.

When certain groups, such as the Parsis, have a greatly increased incidence, or the Native Americans have a much lower incidence, it would appear that a genetic predisposition or innate resistance to the development of breast cancer may be operating. And when the incidence of breast cancer is higher in women relatives on both sides of a family, it would seem obvious that a genetic basis for the disease exists. Two breast/ovarian cancer genes now have been identified: BRCA-1, located on the long arm of chromosome 17, and BRCA-2, on the long arm of chromosome 13. Everyone has these genes, but only 5%–10% of women and men carry mutations of these genes. Female carriers have a marked predisposition to the development of breast cancer, and male carriers have a small increased risk of developing prostate or colon cancer. The genes are believed to be tumor-suppresser genes. When they function normally, tumor development is inhibited. When BRCA-1 is defective, there is interference with DNA damage repair in other genes, and unchecked cell growth to form a malignant tumor can occur (Gowen et al., 1998; Lancaster, Carney, & Furtreal, 1997). Defective mutations may be distributed throughout both genes, and there is an increased frequency of two distinct mutations of BRCA-1 and one mutation of BRCA-2 in people of Eskanazi Jewish descent. Not all carriers, however, whatever their ethnicity, have the increased risk. Even with a mutation, there is no certainty when and whether a cancer will occur.

With the identification of the possibility of mutations in BRCA-1 and BRCA-2, genetic testing for them when there is a strong familial incidence of breast cancer also became a possibility. But if an individual is determined through testing to carry a mutation, then what? If the woman is young, perhaps in her 20s, she could have repeated mammograms to detect an early curable cancer. The repeated exposure to the radiation of mammography starting at an early age, however, may increase her risk of developing a breast cancer. Other preventive measures such as prophylactic breast or ovary removal are pretty extreme and may not prevent the cancer anyway. Taking a drug like tamoxifen to prevent breast cancer has not been assessed in clinical trials for a long enough time. Also of concern is the potential that a woman may incur insurance discrimination and may have difficulty getting or keeping health insurance, life insurance, or disability insurance. Add the psychological adjustment to knowledge that a woman carries the mutation, and it is obvious that there are pitfalls to genetic testing. If a woman with a strong family history of breast cancer tests negative for the mutation, it could be a true negative, meaning that she really does not carry a defective gene, or a false negative, meaning perhaps that the genetic test was not perfect or that there may be a mutation in a gene other than BRCA-1.

In *The Etiology of Human Breast Cancer,* published in 1974, Papaioannou considered all of the available evidence at the time and set up, in the order of their importance, the possible factors that interact to contribute to the development of breast cancer. He cited genetic predisposition or innate resistance, viruses, hormones, psychogenic stress, dietary fats, environmental carcinogens, and as-yet-unknown factors. He also emphasized the cardinal importance of immunological mechanisms that permit or mediate the action of all the other causative factors. Almost three decades later, there has been no compelling evidence to indicate that the factors or their sequence in this list should be changed.

Some of the research in progress on the causes of breast cancer is highly promising, and eventually some of the questions will be answered. Currently, there are only suggestions and speculations and no definitive information about its etiology. Reducing animal fat consumption in the diet is prudent and sensible, not only as possible prevention of breast and other cancers, but to lessen the risk of the other killer, cardiovascular disease. The only other known method of preventing breast cancer is to bear a child at an early age and then have five more—hardly feasible as a protective measure! Until other means of prevention are known, every woman must recognize that while she may never develop breast cancer, she certainly should place herself in the best possible position for survival if it happens to her. The greatest chance for cure of breast cancer lies in catching it early, and monthly breast self-examination is the best nontechnological way of early detection.

Detection and Diagnosis

Self-Examination.   Breast self-examination, or BSE, is not a difficult technique, and every woman can become as competent, if not more expert, than her physician. There is no need for a woman to doubt her ability to recognize a lump, if it is present. The doctor examines many breasts, but a woman is concerned only with her own two breasts and can become very familiar with what is normal for her. As she continues to practice monthly BSE, she becomes so confident about the topography, the feel, and the appearance of her breasts that she is able to detect the smallest nuance of irregularity. She can easily perceive something that was not there before, the extraordinary from the ordinary.

BSE has been criticized as being unreliable for the detection of breast cancer. Or, more specifically, the woman performing BSE is unreliable. One study reported that 85% of women do not do a good job of examining their breasts (Newcomb et al., 1991). Another source, an editorial in the *Journal of the National Cancer Institute,* speculated that it would be easier and less costly to guarantee quality breast examinations by training a small group of health professionals than by training millions of women in BSE (Morrison, 1991). The underlying premise is that it may be asking too much of the average women to perform self-examination effectively. Do women agree that it is asking too much for them to take the responsibility for the well-being of a part of their bodies, to learn from a pamphlet, book, or doctor a simple, quick effective method that gives them control over their own health? Most things we can do as preventive health measures probably require some expense, giving something up, changing our diet, increasing our exercise, and are generally much more *involved*. But the painless procedure of BSE requires only a little time each month to provide the reassurance that everything is all right—certainly a more positive feeling than an ineffectual fear or anxiety about breast cancer. Even if symptoms appear one month, it rarely means a malignancy. Eight out of 10 lumps are benign. If it is cancer, the chances are excellent that the woman who practices monthly BSE is not going to end up as a mortality statistic. More than likely, the earlier detection means that the cancer is still localized, and the earlier diagnosis and treatment mean cure and survival. What better motivation could a woman have?

When to Perform BSE.

Between menarche and menopause, BSE should become a regular monthly health habit as soon as the menstrual period is over. At that time, levels of ovarian hormones are low, and the breasts are less likely to be painful and nodular. Postmenopausal women should select the first day of the month, the 15th of each month, their birthdates, or any other significant day that will help them to remember to perform self-examination. A premenopausal woman who has had a hysterectomy does not have a menstrual flow to remind her; if she still has an awareness of premenstrual breast tenderness, she should choose the day each month when those symptoms are no longer present.

The incidence of breast cancer is low until age 30, but the American Cancer Society has recently extended its educational efforts concerning BSE to girls of high-school age. They believe it is important to establish a lifetime routine of self-protection early. Many doctors agree, and they instruct their adolescent patients in self-examination when they come for a summer camp checkup or annual physical.

Technique of BSE.

A woman may want to modify the *sequence* of the procedures to be described, depending on her schedule, her privacy, or her inclinations, as long as the three steps—feeling the breast while wet, inspection in front of a mirror, and palpation while lying down—are performed. "Self-examination" can also be performed for a woman by another person as an expression of love and concern. One preferred routine should be chosen and followed regularly, however, to establish total familiarity with the physical characteristics of the breasts. Only in this way can any irregularity be easily identified.

Examination While Wet While taking a shower or a bath, move gently over every part of the wet breasts with a soapy hand. Raise the left arm behind the head and, with the flat fingers of the relaxed right hand, feel the entire left breast, beginning at the outermost top and moving in decreasing concentric circles, finishing at the nipple. Move high into the armpit and all the way over onto the breastbone. Then repeat the procedure for the right breast, using the flat of the left hand and raising the right arm behind the head.

Inspection of Breasts Before getting dressed, sit or stand in front of a mirror with the breasts exposed. There should be a good, strong light, and the mirror should be large enough to allow inspection of the breasts while facing it directly. With arms at the sides, look at the breasts for bulges, asymmetry, or areas of surface flattening. Many women have unequal-sized breasts; they may be surprised at that discovery if this is the first time they are carefully inspecting them. As long as the contours of the breasts are symmetrical, inequality in size is perfectly normal (Figure 7–4).

Continue the inspection, looking for any deviation of a nipple, which could mean that it was being pulled toward an underlying tumor. Check for retraction of the nipple, the areola, or the skin. Examine the breasts for redness, any sore or ulceration of the skin, and for edema of the skin, which can exaggerate the pores so the skin looks like orange peel. Make certain there has been no change from the previous examination.

Next, raise the arms high above the head to expose the sides and undersurfaces of the breasts and repeat the same observations. Cancer can produce retraction of the skin, manifested by anything from a small skin dimple or puckering to shrinkage of the entire breast. Raising the arms moves the muscles under the breast and may cause skin retraction or nipple deviation that may not have been apparent before.

Then, place the palms on the hips and press down to contract the pectoral muscles. Again, changes that are not visible in other positions may become apparent. Bend forward to let the breasts hang free and check for anything unusual.

Lying Down The rest of BSE consists of palpation of the breasts performed while lying down on a bed or a couch. To examine the right breast, a small pillow or a folded bath towel should be placed under the right shoulder. In a woman with anything but very small breasts, this maneuver flattens and spreads out the breast evenly over the chest wall. The right hand is placed behind the neck; this also helps to flatten the breast into a thin layer. Otherwise palpation might be more difficult because of the lateral thickness of the breast.

With the left hand, fingers flat, palpate *gently* in small circular motions around the entire breast as if it were an imaginary clock face. Beginning at the upper outermost top of the right breast for 12 o'clock, move to 1 o'clock, 2, 3, and so forth, all around the outermost part of the breast back to 12 o'clock. A ridge of dense nodular tissue at the lower curve of each breast is the *inframammary fold* and is quite normal. The ridge is frequently tender. Then move the fingers in about an inch toward the nipple and repeat the circling. It may take three or more circles to palpate every part of the breast, *including the nipple*.

The nipple is then gently "milked" between the thumb and forefinger. Most types of discharge that come from both breasts are nothing to worry about. One that looks like skim milk is not cancerous and neither is a bilateral, multicolored, sticky discharge. If a discharge is watery, yellow or pink, or bloody, and occurs only on one side, it is suspicious and should be investigated. A slight scaling on the nipple associated with the menstrual period is not unusual.

The same clock-circling procedure is repeated on the left breast with the right hand, a pillow under the left shoulder and the left hand behind the neck.

What the Breast Is Palpated For. The palpation is done to discover (1) a discrete new lump or mass or any kind, (2) an area of nodularity or thickening that was not present before, (3) any area of tenderness. Essentially, a woman is looking for a change in consistency of the breasts from the previous month's examination.

A good time to start practicing BSE is after a breast examination by the woman's physician, when one is not as likely to be as concerned about the dismaying variations in consistency that one may find. A professional examination is reassuring that all those little irregularities in the breasts are normal. As long as those nodules and thickenings remain the same size and are diffusely scattered through both breasts, there is nothing to worry about. It is the presence of a single dominant mass that was not there before that should arouse suspicion.

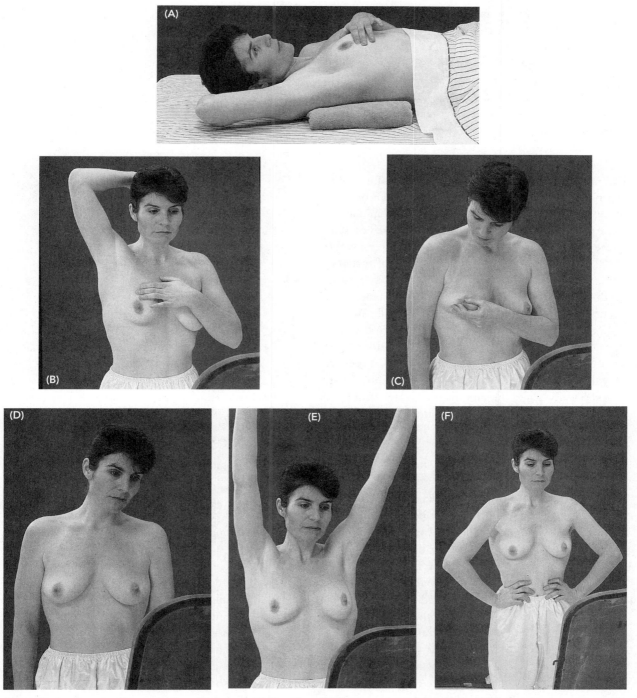

Figure 7–4 Breast self-examination. (A) In bed. (B) Standing. (C) Compression of the nipple. (D) Before a mirror: arms at side. (E) Before a mirror: arms over head. (F) Before a mirror: hands pressed into hips.

If a lump or skin dimple or nipple discharge is discovered during BSE, there is no reason to panic, but there is also no reason to delay in calling for an appointment to see a physician. These findings do not necessarily mean cancer. Actually, most of them turn out *not* to be cancer, but a woman should not put herself through the needless anxiety and sleepless nights worrying about what it *might* be when an immediate visit to her doctor can tell her what it *is.*

Mammography.   The smallest mass or lump that is capable of being felt by palpation during BSE or clinical examination by a doctor is about 1 cm in diameter. At this small size, a cancer may have been present in the breast for many months or even for several years. It is thought that breast cancers are capable of metastasizing to the lymph nodes or to other organs very early in their development. Once this dissemination has occurred, a complete cure becomes virtually impossible, and efforts can be directed only at controlling the disease. But if the cancer can be detected before there are any clinical signs and symptoms and when there is very little probability of spread, if it can be found in an *extremely* early stage, the cure rate is greater than 95% and the death rate can be significantly reduced. Such minimal cancers can be detected by mammography, or x-rays of the breasts (Figure 7–5).

The use of x-rays to identify breast diseases has been known for many years, but the technique has become widely used as a routine examination for breast cancer only since the late 1950s, when it was standardized by radiologist Robert Egan. In mammography, a woman's breasts are alternatively placed on a metal plate and two x-rays of each, from the top and from the side, are taken and developed on photographic film. There are various radiographic abnormalities, such as tiny spots of calcification or areas of increased density and change in breast patterns, that a trained radiologist may recognize as very early cancer. The procedure is not 100% accurate, and much depends on the skill and experience of the interpreter of the films. Generally, the accuracy of mammography is greater in older women, whose breasts are not as

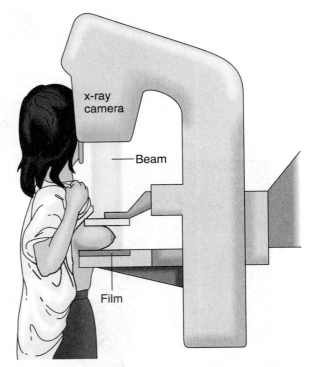

Figure 7–5   X-ray examination of the breast by the film-screen technique of mammography. The woman retracts her right breast as her left breast is positioned for a standard (medial-lateral oblique) view. Note the flattening of her left breast by a plastic plate. The compression produces momentary discomfort but ensures greater detail on the image.

glandular and dense. Xeroradiography and the film-screen technique are refinements of the original mammography. A standard x-ray generator is used as the radiation source for both, but in xeroradiography, the image is recorded xerographically on blue and white paper. In the film-screen system, an x-ray intensifying screen is used in combination with a double-emulsion film. The method allows substantially reduced radiation exposure to all parts of the breast but requires that the breasts are firmly compressed. The tight squeeze during the procedure may produce momentary discomfort. Figure 7–6 is a film-screen mammographic image of the breast of a woman with breast cancer.

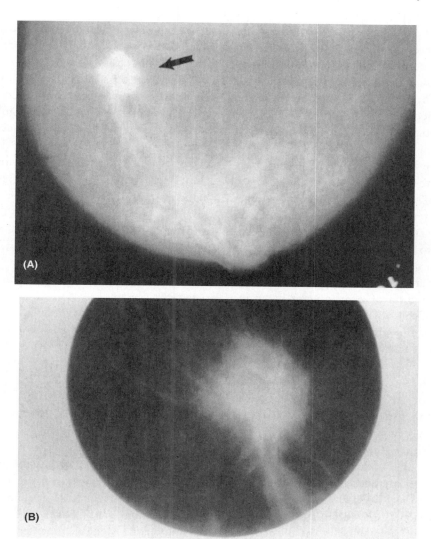

Figure 7–6 (A) A film-screen mammographic image of a breast with a carcinoma (arrow) in the medial aspect. The large vessels are subcutaneous veins. (B) A magnification of the area containing the poorly defined mass. The cancer has a speculated margin and contains several calcifications that are characteristic and verify the diagnosis. (Courtesy of Dr. John Milbrath, Breast Diagnostic Clinic and Treatment Center, S.C., Milwaukee, WI)

Mammography is a major diagnostic tool in the early detection of breast cancer and a valuable adjunct in the treatment of breast cancer. Mammograms can verify a doubtful diagnosis when a mass is discovered by palpation, can determine the exact location of a mass for biopsy or for surgery, and have been shown to play a major role in the reduction of mortality by detecting a substantial proportion of breast cancers, perhaps as many as 45%, that are not as yet apparent by palpation. There are estimates that at the amount of exposure currently being used in mammograms, a woman of age 30 would have to have consecutive annual irradiations until the age of 70 to increase her risk of developing breast cancer by 1%. The American Cancer Society has concluded that the radiation exposure of low-dose mammography is of negligible or virtually no risk. For a woman 50 or over, given the benefits of mammography, any worrying about the carcinogenic potential of a state-of-the-art film-screen mammogram is misplaced concern. Also, 10% of breast cancers occur in women in their 40s and early detection can save their lives.

The use of mammography in women younger than 40 is still somewhat controversial. Younger women live longer. Their hormone-stimulated breasts have more time to be exposed to the cumulative effects of radiation. Moreover, younger women tend to have breasts that are less fatty and of greater density, which makes recognition of early cancers by mammography more difficult.

A screening mammogram is one used to detect breast changes in women who have no sign of breast cancer. A diagnostic mammogram is used to diagnose a breast change such as a lump, pain, nipple discharge, or change in shape or size of the breast. The American Cancer Society's current recommendations for the use of screening mammograms in asymptomatic, apparently healthy women are as follows:

- The basic detection methods for breast cancer are breast self-examination, clinical examination by a health care professional, and mammography.
- Women 20 years of age and older should perform breast self-examination every month and between the ages of 20 and 39 should have a physical examination of the breast by a health professional every 3 years.
- Women 40 years and older should practice breast self-examination, have a clinical examination, and have a mammogram annually.

Women with a family history of breast cancer, especially in a mother or sister, have a higher risk and should discuss more frequent screening with their doctors. Women who have had a previous history of breast cancer and have remaining breast tissue are also at increased risk and should discuss screening schedules with their physician.

There are 52 million American women who fall under the screening guidelines, but only 18 million women regularly follow them. Only one-third of women between 50 and 64 have ever received one mammogram, and utilization of the detection method decreases as the woman gets older. More white women than black women use mammography, and use is higher in women who are more affluent, have more years of formal education, and who are married. Getting the other 34 million women into a mammographic screening program raises issues of cost, access, quality, and convenience.

A high-quality mammogram can be obtained in breast clinics, radiology departments of hospitals, private radiology offices, or mobile vans. All mammography facilities are required to meet certain standards and have certification by the FDA. As of 1999, by federal rules, women who undergo mammograms must receive their results in writing—an easy-to-understand summary within 5 working days if the results of their tests are ambiguous or suggest cancer and within 30 days if the results are normal.

The cost of a mammogram and who pays for it are major problems. The procedure is expensive, averaging $100, and can exceed that figure in some locations. Some state and local health programs, often supported by foundation grants, offer free or very-low-cost mammograms. Medicare, the federal insurance program that covers people over 65, pays for one screening mammogram every year for eligible women, who still have to pay the 20% coinsurance. The majority of American states have passed laws requiring insurers to pay for screening tests, although self-insured employers are exempt from the state laws. This means hundreds of thousands of women, and all of those who do not have health insurance, are not covered for the tests.

Getting the entire medical community to respond to the recommendations also may be a problem. Sometimes physicians themselves become barriers to screening, particularly in women older than 50. Lane and

Messina (1999) surveyed primary care physicians (family doctors and internists) on the staff of 10 community hospitals about their breast cancer screening behavior at three different times: 1988, 1990, and 1995. Although the proportion of doctors who reported that they regularly referred all women aged 50–75 years for mammography significantly increased from 37% to 64% in the 8 years, more than 25% of the respondents to the 1995 survey said they were unaware that breast cancer risk increases with aging and more than 50% did not know that breast cancer detection by mammography is enhanced in older postmenopausal women. There was also a curious reversal of the most frequently performed screening method used by the physicians. In 1988, the doctors more frequently reported performing clinical breast examination on women 50–75 years of age; in 1995, they more frequently reported referring women in this age group for mammography than doing clinical breast examination. All recommendations (NIH, American Cancer Society, American Academy of Family Physicians, American College of Obstetrics and Gynecology) are for both screening methods to be used. The researchers concluded that continuing medical education programs for physicians are needed to improve mammography screening rates. That is certainly unarguable, but if a woman's primary care physician does not perform clinical examination of her breasts and refer her for an annual mammogram after age 50, she must ask for them herself.

Further complicating the issue of providing mammographic screening to all women for whom it is recommended is the fact that mammography, while undeniably valuable, has its limitations. Detecting even a very tiny tumor (less than 1 mm) may not always mean that removing it can result in cure. A fast-growing or very aggressive cancer may already have spread to other parts of the body such as the bone or lung (metastases) and be undetectable (micrometastases). Fortunately, this is not usually the case; the earlier the detection, the more likely the survival. A mammogram fails to reveal a breast cancer 10%–15% of the time, especially in younger women whose denser breasts are harder to evaluate by x-ray. Such false-negative reports can lead a woman (and her doctor) to be falsely reassured, even if she has found a lump by BSE. Unless a breast lump that is discovered disappears on its own within several months, or is found to be a fluid-filled cyst that can be aspirated and does not return, it should be biopsied. A biopsy is a tissue or cell sample removed from the suspicious area for a microscopic examination by a pathologist. An excisional surgical biopsy requires a skin incision and removal of the entire lesion together with a zone of normal tissue around it. A fine-needle aspiration biopsy is performed with a very thin needle to remove tiny bits of tissue and any fluid. Core needle biopsy uses a needle slightly larger in diameter to remove a cylinder of tissue about $\frac{1}{2}$ inch long and $\frac{1}{16}$ inch wide. If the breast lump is large enough to feel, the needle biopsy placement can be by touch; if it is too small to feel, imaging techniques such as ultrasound and stereotactic mammography are used to guide the needle into the right place. The accuracy rates for surgical biopsies and needle biopsies are the same, and each has advantages and disadvantages that should be discussed with the doctor. There are a number of factors to be considered—the size of the breast abnormality, its location, how suspicious of cancer it is, whether there are other lesions present, or whether there may be other medical problems a woman has that may indicate that one type of biopsy may be better for her than another. When the physical examination indicates a breast lump, physicians also need to be more suspicious of negative mammogram reports in young women. A false positive occurs when a mammogram is read as abnormal and no cancer is present, but it has to be followed up with additional procedures such as another diagnostic mammogram, ultrasound, or a biopsy. False positives are more common in younger women. According to the National Cancer Institute, about 97% of women between 40 and 49 who have abnormal mammograms turn out not to have cancer, but 86% of women age 50 and older with abnormal mammograms do not have cancer. They all have to undergo follow-up, of course, which is anxiety provoking and expensive.

Although mammography as a screening test is not perfect and cannot detect breast cancer 100% of the time, it is currently the most sensitive method. Neither the clinical breast examination nor breast self-examination is as good at detecting early breast cancer. A woman should make certain, however, that the mammographic equipment being used on her is technologically state of the art and that the radiologist interpreting her mammograms is board certified. A list of accredited mammography facilities in her area can be obtained from the National Cancer Institute by calling 800-4-CANCER.

Thermography. Thermography is a harmless, inexpensive technique that involves no risk at all to the woman. A thermographic examination involves transferring the infrared heat patterns of the skin of the breast to a visual display that can be photographed, producing a permanent record of the mammary heat pattern. Much like a fingerprint, each woman has her own distinctive thermal print. Because the skin temperature over a cancer is higher than that over normal tissue, it should be possible to use thermography in screening and diagnosis of breast cancer. Unfortunately, a positive thermogram is not specific for cancer. There are a variety of other nonmalignant reasons for an increase in heat, and they may be the cause of false-positive thermograms. Conversely, some cancers may not cause an increased temperature in the skin overlying them, and false-negative results are possible.

Thermography is not as effective as mammography or clinical examination for the detection of breast cancer.

Ultrasound. In the search for a safe, no-risk method of breast cancer detection, ultrasonic examination—the use of sonar to produce echo images of breast tissue—has been tried as a substitute for mammography.

In the breast ultrasound unit, the breasts are scanned with an ultrasound probe. As the reflected high-frequency sound waves bounce off the various fatty and fibrous tissues of the breast, they are converted electronically for display as images. Advantages of ultrasonography over mammography include the ability to visualize a lump in the young, very dense breast and the ability to distinguish between a simple fluid-filled benign cyst and a solid tumorous lump—both are difficult with mammography. The disadvantage of ultrasonography as a screening tool is its inability to find subclinical cancers because the smallest mass detectable by the technique is still too large to be considered a minimal cancer. Some experts have demonstrated masses as small as 2 mm, but in general, ultrasound is not able to find a small and curable cancer. Also, small calcium deposits, an early sign of cancer on a mammogram, are not visible with ultrasound. Future improvements in equipment may make ultrasonograms more useful as a screening method, as researchers in ultrasound claim that the technique could theoretically pick up very tiny lesions. Currently, the greatest contribution of ultrasonography is in the evaluation of a breast lump to differentiate between a cyst and a solid mass (Figure 7–7).

Other Techniques of Early Detection. There are major research efforts to improve the ability of imaging techniques to find cancers smaller than those detectable currently by mammography, to improve the accuracy of breast imaging to distinguish between cancer and benign breast lesions, and to find methods of screening that do not expose a women to x-rays. In nuclear medicine for breasts, a small amount of radioactive substance is injected into an arm vein and the breasts are imaged with a nuclear medicine camera that shows where the radiation has accumulated. The test is not as effective as mammography in distinguishing noncancerous from cancerous areas and is certainly less sensitive, especially when the tumor is small and potentially curable.

Positron emission tomography (PET scanning) is similar in that a radioactive substance is injected and then a special PET scanner is used to form an image. The technique is more successful in the detection of cancer that has spread to other organs because it cannot reliably detect tumors smaller than 1 cm.

In magnetic resonance imaging (MRI) a patient lies within a strong magnetic field that polarizes the

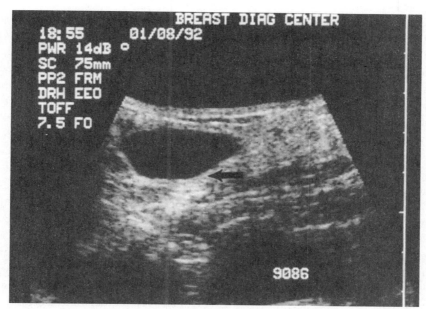

Figure 7–7 Ultrasound image of a cyst. The dark area has well-defined anterior and posterior walls and is totally devoid of internal sound beam echoes, which would appear as white dots. These characteristics, along with the increased whiteness below (arrow) indicate a benign fluid-filled cyst. (Courtesy of Dr. John Milbrath, Breast Diagnostic Clinic and Treatment Center, S.C., Milwaukee, WI)

body cells. When energy in the form of radio waves is introduced, it causes the atomic particles in the tissue to resonate at a different frequency in different tissues and a computer creates a composite picture. Any change from the normal resonance in an organ can then be detected. Breast MRI equipment is specialized and produces higher-quality images than MRI designed for the rest of body scanning. MRI for breast imaging uses an injected contrast material (usually gadolinium DTPA) to improve MRI's capability of visualizing details of breast tissue more clearly. Currently, most hospitals and imaging centers do not own dedicated breast MRI equipment.

Still in a preliminary stage is the use of biochemical markers as detection measures. It has been noted that blood serum levels of certain substances are elevated in breast cancer. Such a biological assay may turn out to be the simplest, most sensitive, least expensive screening test for early breast cancer, but to date no specific biomarker has been found. Right now there is no completely safe, economically feasible, or logistically practical way to

screen all women in the country for breast cancer. Until there is, the only hope of reducing the annual mortality from this disease is through monthly breast self-examination. Early diagnosis means early treatment; early treatment increases the chances of cure.

TREATMENT OF BREAST CANCER

The choice of treatment is influenced by many factors such as size and location of the lesion, tumor stage, lymph node negative or positive status, presence or absence of estrogen and progesterone receptors, and age of the woman and her menopausal status. Because of mammography, the finding of very small cancers is greater than it used to be, and many of them are classified as noninvasive. Cancers that have arisen from the inner lining of the small lobular units or of the ducts but are confined to the walls without penetrating through the membranes of the ducts and the lobules are of two types. **Ductal carcinoma in situ (DCIS)** is a preinvasive malignancy and is likely to progress to cancer if no treatment takes place. With treatment, the outlook for cure is about 98%. **Lobular carcinoma in situ (LCIS),** while it carries a risk of progression to cancer, is generally viewed as not a true malignancy. The chance of developing an invasive cancer after a diagnosis of LCIS is about 25% and the treatment is controversial, ranging from no treatment beyond follow-up with mammography and physical examination to prophylactic mastectomy. About 20% of breast cancers are DCIS or LCIS. The other 80% are invasive cancers. They may be very small and discovered early, but the cells have left the walls of the ducts and lobules and have grown into the breast, where they can gain access to the blood vessels and lymphatics to spread to other parts of the body.

Over the past decades, the management of breast cancer, especially early breast cancer, has markedly changed, but primary treatment remains surgical excision of the tumor.

Surgery

From all historical indications, cancer has been a human affliction probably for as long as we have been human. Breast cancer, being easily accessible, has always been treated by removal. Along with prayer, poultices, and potions, the primary approach in the treatment of breast cancer has been to cut it out, usually damaging or destroying much of the breast in the process. Surgery on the breast, in various forms and techniques, and with heroic endurance on the part of the patient, has been performed in an attempt to cure breast cancer for centuries.

More than 90 years ago, a formalized surgical procedure that has come to be known as the Halsted radical mastectomy was described by Dr. William S. Halsted. He reported that with his operation, he was able to cure 50% of women with breast cancer; very few had ever been cured before his kind of surgery. Halsted's technique was enthusiastically adopted, and it

persisted for years with little challenge. The operation removed the entire breast, a liberal amount of skin, all the subcutaneous fat overlying the breast tissue, the major muscles of the chest wall (pectoralis major and minor), and all the axillary lymph nodes and fat in the armpit. Complications as a result of the surgery included damage to the brachial plexus or network of nerves that supplies the upper arm, forearm, and hand. Another, not infrequent, functional defect was some limitation of shoulder motion; some women had difficulty raising their arms on the affected side to even shoulder height. The anatomical deformity on the chest area could at least be covered by a breast prosthesis and clothing, but a disfiguring and highly visible result of radical mastectomy was often the enlargement or edema of the upper arm that occurred because of the interference with the lymphatic circulation.

The Halsted radical mastectomy became the traditional treatment of choice for breast cancer in this country. It was the preferred method of the great majority of American surgeons, the procedure with which they felt the most secure, and the one that many believed was consistently proven to be the most effective treatment. Even the preoperative procedure became routine. In the one-step procedure, a woman with a suspected breast cancer entered the hospital. There, under general anesthesia, the surgeon performed a biopsy on the tissue. While the woman remained asleep on the operating table, the specimen was rushed to the pathologist in the lab. A frozen section was examined, and if the pathologist said it was malignant, a Halsted radical mastectomy was performed. The woman had been made aware before biopsy that when she awoke, her breast may or may not be there. This routine was the same for everyone—as much for the woman down the block as for a president's wife, Betty Ford.

The Halsted radical remained the standard primary therapy for operable breast cancer for 90 years. Statistically, the number of women who were still living 5 years after surgery with no recurrence of cancer (in medical terms, the disease-free survival rate) was 75% if the cancer was in an early stage and 50% if the cancer was designated more advanced. The 10-year disease-free survival rate was about 70% for women with early cancers and around 40% for women with breast cancers designated as Stage II.

The Halsted radical was designed to remove the cancer mass and the local areas to which it already had or was more likely to spread. The principle on which it was based was consistent with the concept of cancer that prevailed in Halsted's day—that breast cancer is a rather orderly disease that starts at a primary site on the breast, remains there for a certain time, and then spreads through the lymphatic system to the axillary lymph nodes first. The nodes act as barriers for the cancer cells for a while, but when the primary cancer gets large enough, the regional nodes can no longer contain the cancer. The cells metastasize themselves to the bone, liver, brain, and other distant sites.

It now is evident that breast cancer is not just one disease. It probably has a variety of causes, appears in a variety of forms, and varies enormously in its progression and clinical course. The model just cited, while true for some forms of breast cancer, may not be valid for all types. It is now believed that not all cancers progress first to the axillary lymph nodes before spreading. Some cells from certain malignant tumors are capable of bypassing the regional lymph nodes and of metastasizing directly to distant tissues while the original cancer is still very small. No evidence of cancer cells in the lymph nodes at the time of diagnosis of breast cancer may still mean the presence of micrometastases in other tissues. In the 1970s, Dr. Bernard Fisher, at the University of Pittsburgh Medical School, published his theory that many women with breast cancer have disseminated disease by the time the cancer is palpable. Although women are apparently cured by an operation like the Halsted radical mastectomy, it does not necessarily mean that the surgery removed every last cancer cell in the body. It is likely that surgically removing the burden of the growing large tumor may have left sufficiently few cells, which could then be eradicated by the woman's own immunological mechanisms. The newer concepts of tumor biology challenged the continued use of the Halsted radical mastectomy.

Actually, there were other misgivings concerning the routine use of one surgical procedure for all breast cancer patients. Because the Halsted procedure ignored the fact that one of the main routes of lymphatic drainage is through the internal mammary nodes, some surgeons advocated even more extensive surgery, evidently on the premise that getting every last cancer cell in every lymph node produces better results. The "extended radical mastectomy" combined the standard Halsted technique with the additional excision of the internal mammary nodes, and the "super-radical mastectomy" excised the supraclavicular nodes as well. The latter operation required removal of the lateral border of the breastbone and several rib attachments. It proved to do little for the long-term survival of the women on whom it was performed, and it increased morbidity and mortality from the surgery itself.

About the same time, other surgeons began to perform less extensive procedures, either alone or together with postsurgical radiotherapy or chemotherapy. Several alternatives to the orthodox radical operation began to be used. The one that has replaced the Halsted radical in the United States and many other countries is the modified radical mastectomy.

Modified Radical Mastectomy. This procedure is also called conservative radical mastectomy or mastectomy with axillary dissection. The entire breast and the axillary lymph nodes are removed, but the pectoralis major muscles are left in place.

By permitting the pectoralis major muscle to remain, the normal contour of the chest wall and shoulder is maintained, there is less frequent edema and limitation of motion of the arm, and breast reconstruction is easier to perform.

Total, Simple, or Complete Mastectomy. The entire breast, including the nipple and skin over the breast is removed, but the pectoral muscles and the axillary nodes are left in place. Some of the nodes may be dissected, however, and when total mastectomy plus even more axillary node dissection is performed, the procedure becomes a modified radical mastectomy. One of the many controversies in breast cancer treatment is whether the axillary node removal should be performed for therapeutic purposes or merely to determine the stage or extent of the cancer progression. Those believing in the staging, rather than prophylactic value, of axillary node dissection remove only the low axillary and midaxillary nodes. Currently, however, surgery to remove the entire system of 20–30 lymph nodes is still the standard. As a result, about 40% of women who have had axillary node dissection develop lymphedema, a debilitating swelling of the arm. A new procedure called sentinel-node biopsy, developed in 1997, allows identification of the sentinel lymph nodes, the first nodes to which the tumor drains. If the sentinel nodes are negative for metastatic disease, the remaining nodes also are likely to be negative. The technique involves the injection of a blue dye and a radioactive isotope into the breast tissue near the tumor, which are taken up by the lymphatics. Then an incision is made under the arm and the first few sentinel nodes are removed and examined for traces of blue dye or radioactivity. If the sentinel nodes are clear, studies have shown that the rest of the lymph node system is cancer free.

In a subcutaneous mastectomy, as much breast tissue as possible is removed, and the nipple and skin overlying the breast are preserved, so some breast tissue remains under the areola. This procedure makes it easy for an implant to be inserted if reconstruction is desired. Frequently, however, some cosmetic surgery must be performed so that the two breasts will match.

Lumpectomy. In a lumpectomy, the primary tumor, some of the surrounding breast tissue, and usually a small amount of overlying skin are removed. Depending on the varying amounts of breast tissue that are removed with the tumor mass, the operation is also called segmental mastectomy, sector mastectomy, wide extension, partial mastectomy, or quadrantectomy. Most patients undergo some axillary node dissection. This is the most conservative procedure. The operation involves the simple excision of only the breast lump and a narrow margin of normal tissue. If the cancer is not very large, there is no breast deformity. One of the objections to this procedure is that it may leave other microscopic areas of cancer (multicentric foci) in the breast. Radiation therapy is believed to take care of any such potential areas. As generally practiced in the United States, women having this surgery also have some axillary node dissection. Within 1–3 weeks after surgery, supplementary radiation therapy over a 4- to 5-week period is given both to the breasts and to the lymph nodes. A subsequent "booster" dose of radiation, either by external irradiation or by implantation of a radioactive source, is then directed to the quadrant of the breast where the cancer was removed.

Clinical Staging. There is general agreement that no one kind of operation or postoperative therapy routinely should be applied to every woman with breast cancer. The problem is, of course, deciding which operation and which course of treatment should be selected. The classification of the breast cancer and the criteria for treatment are called clinical staging. Every woman with a suspected malignant tumor in her breast should be clinically staged before mastectomy. The whole point of mastectomy is to remove the local disease. If there are already distant metastases, performing even a modified radical mastectomy would be senseless, and other forms of therapy could be used. A few days of assessment before surgery can determine the tumor size, extent, and growth rate; the likelihood of lymph node involvement; and, by x-ray and other scanning techniques, whether or not the cancer has already traveled to the bone or other tissues.

The identification of the anatomical extent of the disease provides a method of assessing the status of the cancer. In this method, T refers to the tumor, N means the regional lymph nodes, and M refers to the distant metastases. Subscripts to these letters indicate the stages of cancer progression in each. Thus, a woman with no breast cancer would be staged at $T_0 N_0 M_0$.

A woman is staged at clinical stage I, II, III, or IV depending on the following factors: size of the tumor

$(T_1–T_4)$; whether the axillary lymph nodes on the same side are palpable but considered negative (N_{1a}) or palpable but considered to have metastatic growth (N_b); whether the lymph nodes or the tumor are fixed to the underlying pectoral fascia, muscles, or chest wall; whether there are any other grave signs, such as edema, ulceration, or pitting of the skin of the breast; and whether there are any distant metastases (M). The overall 10-year survival rate for a woman with Stage I breast cancer is 80%–90%; for a woman with Stage II, it is about 50%. The outlook is not as good for women with Stage III or IV disease, although wide variation owing to individual differences in the woman and in the cancer occur within the clinical stages.

There is no completely accurate way to know whether the cancer has micrometastasized to distant organs, but there are certain methods that can determine the likelihood. A bone scan is performed to see whether the cancer has spread to the bones. Other tests—a computerized tomography (C-T scan) or a magnetic resonance imagery (MRI) scan can be used to detect metastases to the liver, abdominal-pelvic cavity, lungs, or brain. A C-T scan uses focused x-rays to provide thin cross-section slices of the tissues and organs scanned, which are built into an image by computer.

Cancer staging can get very complex, but as an example, clinical Stage I can include a woman who is $T_2 N_{1a} M_0$; that is, her tumor is larger than 2 cm but smaller than 5 cm in its greatest dimension, but the lymph nodes are still considered negative. If the lymph nodes are movable and palpable, are suspected of containing metastases but are still not larger than 2 cm in size or fixed to the underlying connective tissue or any other structures, the woman is considered at Stage II.

Surgical Clinical Trials. No surgeons would currently argue that the Halsted radical is superior to the modified radical mastectomy. There is enough evidence to show that the two procedures are equal in terms of overall survival and disease-free survival. After the conservative breast-prevention methods in the treatment of early breast cancer were introduced, however, they became highly controversial and the focus of great medical debate. A number of controlled, scientific clinical trials were initiated in the 1970s to answer the question of which of the following procedures—the Halsted radical; the modified radical with or without postoperative radiation therapy; the simple mastectomy or the conservative partial mastectomy, both with postoperative irradiation—provided improved survival. Investigators at 34 institutions in the United States and Canada participated in the National Surgical Adjuvant Breast Project (NS-ABP) protocols. In one of the first trials, protocol B-04, women who entered the study with no evidence of cancer in the lymph nodes (that is, clinically negative nodes) were randomly assigned to treatment either with radical mastectomy, total mastectomy followed by radiation of the chest wall and regional lymphatics, or total mastectomy alone. Women with clinically positive (cancerous) nodes were randomized to treatment with either radical mastectomy or total mastectomy and irradiation. Another randomized study compared three groups of women, all of whom had small breast cancers and negative nodes. They received either a modified radical mastectomy, a partial mastectomy plus staging axillary node dissection and no postoperative irradiation, or partial mastectomy plus staging axillary node dissection and postoperative irradiation for 5 weeks. Similar studies were initiated in Milan and other international sites. After many years of follow-up on the women enrolled in these randomized trials, it became evident that the medical controversy comparing surgical procedures should be ended. The results in terms of survival from breast cancer are very similar regardless of what method of surgery is used. Use of the conservative, breast-sparing approach, when combined with radiation therapy, neither improved the survival rate nor decreased it. It would seem logical, then, for a woman with early breast cancer to choose the operation that would be least mutilating and least cosmetically deforming.

The key words, of course, are "early breast cancer." Few doctors would agree that conserving the greater part of the breast is possible for all women with breast cancer, but it has been difficult for many to accept the idea that the less extensive procedures are feasible for even some women with breast cancer. A consensus panel of researchers and medical experts convened by the National Institutes of Health and the National Cancer Institute in 1991 concluded the following:

> *Breast conservation treatment is an appropriate method of primary therapy for the majority of women with Stage I and II breast cancer and is preferable because it provides survival rates equivalent to those of total mastectomy and axillary dissection while preserving the breast.*

Nevertheless, today more lumpectomies are performed in the Northeast and on the West Coast and are still rare in the South and many parts of the Midwest. More and more women, however, particularly in those states that require that women with breast cancer be told of their surgical options, are being given the opportunity to make their own decisions. Some women will choose a modified radical or total mastectomy because they do not want to, or cannot afford to, take the time off for 6 weeks of daily radiation treatments. Access to quality radiation therapy is also a consideration; in some smaller areas, it may not be available or not be of the same technical quality as in a major city. Another factor for some may be the reluctance to retain breast tissue that had a cancer—some women may just feel safer if all of it is removed. The point is, after a biopsy has shown a malignancy, a woman can and should participate in the decision as to why the surgery she will have is the one most appropriate for her. Also, she can take time to think about the options. A delay of several days, or even weeks, except in very rare cases, will not make any difference to the cancer. It has been there for 8 or more years and is not going to get any worse in a couple of days.

Radiation Therapy

Strong doses of x-rays, delivered by a super voltage x-ray machine, damage cells. The irradiation is aimed directly at the abnormally dividing cancer cells and attempts to destroy them without damaging the normal tissue surrounding the tumor (Figure 7–8).

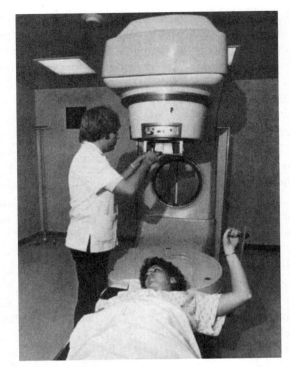

Figure 7–8 Radiation therapy.

Strong radiation is also used to reduce the size of the tumor when it is so large that it is considered inoperable or to palliate (i.e., lessen) the pain in bone or other tissue metastases in advanced cancer.

When it is used as an adjunct to conservative surgery in early breast cancer, radiotherapy is given postoperatively to destroy any cancer cells that may have been left in the breast or the lymph nodes after surgery. Radiation is begun as soon as the wounds have healed, usually after about 2 weeks. Then, over a period of 5–6 weeks, 180–200 rads (or centiGrays) per day are delivered 5 days a week for a total of 4,500–5,000 rads. At the conclusion of the radiation course, there may be a supplemental "boost" of strong radiation given to the area of tumor excision by radioactive pellets implanted for about 36 hours. If chemotherapy is also a part of the treatment, it is integrated with the radiotherapy, sometimes in conjunction with it or sometimes sequentially, depending on the doctor's recommendation.

Chemotherapy

Both surgery and irradiation are local treatments for breast cancer; they are directed at the primary cancer in the breast and at the axillary, internal mammary, and supraclavicular nodes. Neither breast surgery nor radiotherapy is able to affect any tumor cells circulating through the blood or lymph or any groups of cancer cells that have taken up residence in the liver, lung, bone, or brain. Once metastasis has occurred, systemic therapy is necessary to track down and deal with the cancer cells out of reach of the knife and the x-ray beam.

Chemotherapy is the use of cytotoxic drugs to damage or kill malignant cells. The anticancer drugs function at the cellular level to inhibit the growth of, or actually destroy, the susceptible cells. Some of the agents are called antimetabolites, and they interfere with the synthesis of DNA and RNA, the necessary components of cellular function and multiplication. Others are alkylating agents, which cross-link the double helix of DNA and prevent replication; antibiotics, which react with DNA and interfere with its transcription into RNA; and some drugs that prevent cell division by disrupting the orderly processes of mitosis. Table 7–1 lists some of the chemotherapeutic drugs used to treat breast cancer. In addition to those in Table 7–1, newer chemotherapeutic agents for metastatic breast cancer have been developed but have not been subject to as many clinical trials. These include the taxanes—paclitaxel (brand name Taxol) and docetaxel (brand name Taxotere), vinorelbine (brand name Navelbine), and the camptothecins—topotecan (brand name Hycamtin) and irinotecan (brand name Camptosar). These drugs have demonstrated effectiveness and are being investigated. They have adverse or toxic effects similar to those listed in the table for the older drugs.

The compounds that are used in therapy do not selectively seek out the cancer cells for disruption and injury, although sometimes the damage is more extensive to them because they may have altered metabolic processes. Generally, cytotoxic drugs affect all rapidly dividing cells, normal as well as malignant: in the skin, the hair follicles, the mouth, the gastrointestinal tract, and the bone marrow. Reproduction is frequent and rapid in such cells so they are also affected. Side effects, depending on the individual tolerance, can, therefore, include loss of hair, skin changes, sores in the mouth, nausea, and vomiting. Tiredness and lowered resistance to infection may occur as bone-marrow suppression results in fewer red and white blood cells. Some patients are fortunate and have mild or few side effects; others are unable to tolerate a particular drug, which has to be stopped, perhaps to be later resumed.

In the past, chemotherapeutic drugs were used only in advanced breast cancer. They were considered to be the "big guns," to be brought out as a last resort after all else had failed. By then a woman was usually so debilitated that her tolerance to a drug was limited. Over the past three decades, different ideas developed concerning the biology of breast cancer and the use of cytotoxic drugs. Breast cancer is now believed to be a systemic disease; many women may already have small micrometastases in other organs by the time their cancer is diagnosed, especially if the axillary nodes are involved, but even if they are negative. It is also known that small tumors have a greater percentage of actively dividing cells than do large tumors. Since the drugs affect rapidly dividing cells, the cancer with the least mass would be the most susceptible to chemotherapy. It made more sense to use drugs early, as an adjuvant to surgery, rather than as a last ditch effort after recurrence of the cancer. Chemotherapy is now used earlier and in combination form. Several drugs, each independently active but with no overlapping toxic effects, are combined. For the most part, such multiple chemotherapy has supplanted the use of a single drug.

But the questions of *which* women with breast cancer should get chemotherapy after surgery, for how long they should get it, and in what combination, have been subjects of intense medical debate since the late 1980s and right up to the current time. In May of 1988 the National Cancer Institute (NCI), in a clinical alert sent to 11,000 physicians who treated breast cancer patients, recommended that most women whose cancer has not spread to the lymph nodes be offered

TABLE 7–1 Some Chemotherapeutic Drugs Used in Breast Cancer

Generic Name	Trade Name	Mode of Action	Toxic Effects
Antimetabolites Methotrexate	Amethopterin	Blocks folic acid reductase, essential enzyme for nucleic acid synthesis	Nausea, vomiting, bone marrow depression, kidney and liver damage
Fluorouracil (5–fluorouracil, 5-FU)	Adrucil	Blocks thymidylate, synthetase, essential enzyme for nucleic acid synthesis	Nausea and vomiting, bone marrow depression, inflammation of mucous membranes of the mouth and intestine, diarrhea
Alkalating agents Thiotepa (Triethylenethio-phosphoramide)	Thioplex	Exchanges alkyl groups with hydrogens of nucleic acids; modifies nucleic acids; modifies DNA structure, inhibits protein synthesis	Bone marrow depression, anemia, asthma, and phylactic shock
Cyclophosphamide	Cytoxan	Same as above	Bone marrow depression, hair loss, cystitis
Melphalan (L-Phenylalanine mustard, L-PAM, L-Sarcolysin)	Alkeran	Same as above	Bone marrow depression, leukemia, anaphylaxis, anemia, partial hair loss
Vinca alkaloids Vincristine sulfate	Oncovin	Destroys mitotic spindle, stops mitosis	Neuritis, bone marrow depression, nausea and vomiting, hair loss, motion difficulties
Vinblastine	Velban	Destroys mitotic spindle, stops mitosis	Hair loss, bone marrow depression, nausea and vomiting
Antibiotics Doxorubicin	Adriamycin	Modifies DNA functions	Cardiac toxicity, hair loss, oral membrane inflammation, nausea and vomiting

(continues)

TABLE 7–1 *(continued)*

Generic Name	Trade Name	Mode of Action	Toxic Effects
Dactinomycin (Actinomycin D, ACT)	Cosmegen	Modifies DNA function	Hair loss, nausea and vomiting, diarrhea, tongue and oral membrane inflammation, bone marrow depression, liver toxicity, kidney failure
Hormonal agents			
Megestrol Acetate	Megace	Antiestrogen, interferes with growth, may act at cell membrane	Gynecological symptoms, weight gain, abdominal pain
Tamoxifen citrate	Nolvadex	Antiestrogen, growth-factor inhibitor	Gynecological symptoms, hypercalcemia, weight gain, bone marrow depression, thromboembolic disorders
Aminoglutethimide	Cytadren	Antiestrogen, aromatase inhibitor	Adrenocortical insufficiency, hypo-thyroidism
Prednisone	Deltasone	Glucocorticoid, anti-inflammatory	Fluid retention, mood changes, insomnia, peptic ulcers, adrenocortical insufficiency
Miscellaneous			
Mitoxantrone HCl	Novantrone	Tumoricidal effect, inhibition of DNA and RNA synthesis	Congestive heart failure, bone marrow depression, fetal hazard

chemotherapy or hormonal treatment. The recommendation was based upon data from three preliminary studies in the United States that tested the use of combination chemotherapy or hormonal treatment with tamoxifen, an anti-estrogen, and indicated that these treatments reduced the risk of recurrence and increased survival. The difficulty is, when women with breast cancer have negative lymph nodes, 70% of them will never have a recurrence of the cancer. Moreover, there is no way to identify the other 30% in whom the can-

cer will recur, and who are likely to be helped by adjuvant chemotherapy or hormonal treatment. Should all node-negative women get chemotherapy so that the minority might avoid recurrence? An additional quandary developed did not recommend the specific chemotherapeutic drugs to use. The clinical trials tested three different regimens, and they all seemed to provide benefit. In 1990, the Early Breast Cancer Trialists' Collaborative Group published data from 100 randomized trials conducted all over the world. The studies, which involved 40,000 women, evaluated the treatment of early breast cancer with adjuvant tamoxifen, cytotoxic chemotherapy, radiation, and removal of the ovaries and substantiated the earlier NCI recommendation. The overall reduction in death during the first 5 years was 16% for tamoxifen versus no tamoxifen, but was greater for postmenopausal women, and 11% for chemotherapy versus no chemotherapy, but was 25% for women under 50. Radiation therapy in these trials did not appear to provide benefit, and ovariectomy produced results that seemed promising but were based on fewer numbers of women. Although the reduction in mortality may appear modest, even a small decrease in the risk of death, considering the large numbers of women with the diagnosis of breast cancer, can save tens of thousands of lives.

The issue of routine use of adjuvant cytotoxic therapy in early node-negative breast cancer is highly controversial. Proponents believe that women should be given any therapy that has any possibility of curing the disease or prolonging survival. Opponents point out that the chemotherapy drugs are toxic, produce acute side effects, and are carcinogenic in themselves. There is a documented increased incidence of leukemia and other types of cancer following chemotherapy and/or radiation therapy, with evidence that the type of leukemia that occurs is biologically more aggressive and resistant to therapy (Neugut et al., 1990). Because the majority of women with early breast cancer will be cured by the surgical and radiology treatment alone, those who feel it is too soon to assess the risk/benefit ratio say that adjuvant treatment should not be used routinely until it is of proven value. The consensus of a group convened by the National Institutes of Health stated in 1991 that

> the decision to use adjuvant treatment should come after a thorough discussion with the patient about the likely risk of recurrence without adjuvant therapy, the expected reduction in risk with adjuvant therapy, toxic effects of therapy, and the impact of therapy on quality of life.

The group further indicated that although all patients with negative nodes are at some risk for recurrence of the breast cancer, when a woman has a tumor of 1 cm or less, the prognosis is excellent. She may not require adjuvant therapy but should be offered the opportunity to participate in the clinical trials that will ultimately provide the answers. But for the woman with early breast cancer, what to do next remains a problem. According to one whose doctor held the appropriate "thorough discussion" of the options with her, she felt as if she were confronted with the choice of going through "Door Number 1" or "Door Number 2." If she decided against adjuvant therapy and had a recurrence of the cancer, she would be left with "Sorry, you chose the wrong door."

Fortunately, the most thorough analysis of breast cancer patients ever conducted now has provided the strongest evidence to date that all women with breast cancer, even if there is no lymph node involvement, should have adjuvant chemotherapy. A statistical meta-analysis by the Early Breast Cancer Trialists' Group collated the 10-year results of 133 studies involving 75,000 women with breast cancer. It assessed the combined and separate benefits of various treatments in women of different ages and different stages of disease, and published its results in 1992. The research team, led by Richard Peto, director of cancer studies at Oxford University in England, clearly demonstrated that women who had adjuvant therapy had fewer recurrences and lived longer than women who did not receive such treatment. The results in terms of increased 10-year survival were somewhat less in women with Stage I disease but were still significant. The study also suggested some directions for future clinical trials.

At the current time, there are clinical trials (or protocols) all over the world in progress to evaluate the effectiveness of new or different combinations of treatments for early and advanced breast cancer. These include surgical, radiation, chemotherapy, or hormonal approaches. Protocols for studies are divided into phases. A Phase I study determines toxicity and dosages, usually of new drugs or combinations of drugs. It enrolls people with advanced disease who have nothing to lose and everything to gain if the treatment works for them. A Phase II study is initiated if the Phase I has been successful. In breast cancer, Phase II generally looks at therapies administered to women whose cancer has returned but who may not be in a life-threatening state. A Phase III study compares the new treatment to the standard treatment and enrolls patients with all degrees of cancer. Through controlled trials, it is possible to know eventually which patients should get which drugs, when they should get them, for how long, and whether the benefit outweighs the toxicity of the chemotherapy.

Besides waiting years for the outcome of clinical protocols, another way to predict which women should get more aggressive therapy because of possible recurrence has resulted from progress in the field of molecular biology of cancer. In 1971, the National Cancer Act initiated the "War on Cancer." Although it may seem more like a 100-Years War or perhaps another Vietnam in view of cancer mortality statistics, there have been major advances in the understanding of the causes of cancer—the conversion of a single normal cell into a wildly proliferating group of abnormal cells. Two major types of genes have been implicated—the **oncogenes** and the tumor-suppressor genes. The oncogenes are believed to be activated versions of normal cellular growth-promoting genes, or proto-oncogenes. Oncogene activation arises from mutation of a proto-oncogene, and the result is the hyperactivity of growth-promoting genes. Tumor-suppressor genes are believed to function in growth constraint and to retard proliferation of cells. When alterations in these two kinds of genes lead to increased activity of cell growth promoters and decreased activity or inactivation of growth suppressors, the result is uncontrolled growth, or tumor formation. Identification of the number or the state of transformation of these genes in a breast cancer could provide clues to determine whether the cancer will remain confined to a local site, where it can be removed by surgery and irradiation, or whether it is likely to have metastasized and require chemotherapy. In 1987, Dennis Slamon and colleagues discovered an oncogene called HER-2/*neu* in tumors from breast cancer patients that could predict the prognosis, since

an increased number of copies of HER-2/*neu* in the tissue indicated a quicker recurrence and a shorter period of survival. In a 1989 paper, the researchers reported that the gene also was present in ovarian tumors (but not in tumors from the lung, adrenal, and colon) and suggested that the discovery may provide a way of predicting the progress of the disease in patients with ovarian cancer as well. Breast cancer and ovarian cancer already have a number of features in common. Both are influenced by estrogen, and women who develop one cancer are at increased risk for developing the other. The Slamon group's results suggest that the same genetic alterations may contribute to the development of both cancers. Subsequently, research determined that overexpression of the HER-2/neu gene occurs in about 25%–30% of breast cancers and in about 30%–40% of patients with other types of cancers, including stomach, endometrial, salivary gland, pancreatic, and prostate cancer; a type of lung cancer; and colon cancer. The development of a monoclonal antibody called Herceptin (trastuzumab), which works by binding to and blocking the growth factor receptor protein produced by HER-2/neu, thus slowing the growth and causing shrinkage of metastatic breast cancer, is a new and biologic approach to cancer treatment. Monoclonal antibodies are discussed later in this chapter.

Breast cancer that has spread to distant sites has long been considered incurable because the amount of chemotherapy needed to destroy the cancer is also likely to destroy the patient. Conventional chemotherapy produces decreases in white blood count and platelet levels, resulting in immune system suppression and anemia with a slow recovery after a few weeks. High-dose chemotherapy can cause permanent bone marrow damage so that white blood cell and platelet counts return very slowly or are permanently depressed, which can be lethal to the patient. About 15 years ago, some cancer experts and cancer centers across the country began to use high-dose chemotherapy in women with metastatic breast cancer in an attempt to produce prolonged remission (abatement of the cancer) or even a cure (the cancer does not recur for the rest of her life).

To circumvent the problem of bone marrow suppression, a small amount of the marrow is removed from the patient and frozen. Then high doses of chemotherapy are administered. The toxic drugs attempt to kill all the cancer cells but in the process also virtually kill the remaining bone marrow. After completion of chemotherapy, the banked bone marrow is infused back into the patient, but it takes several weeks to a month for the marrow to grow and restore the cells. Until then, without new white blood cells, the patient is highly vulnerable to infection. Without new platelets, the blood is unable to clot, and bleeding problems may result. The technique of removing healthy bone marrow from the patient is called autologous bone marrow transplantation (BMT). When the marrow is donated by an identical twin, the technique is called syngeneic transplantation; it is called allergeneic transplantation when the marrow comes from another person with similar blood and tissue types. BMT has now often been replaced by peripheral blood stem cell transplantation (PBSCT). The stem cells—the source of all blood cells in the marrow—are also found in circulating blood. In PBSCT, the stem cells are removed from the patient's blood and replaced after the high doses of chemotherapy and/or radiation therapy. Both techniques are referred to as stem cell support. High-dose chemotherapy and stem cell support are standard treatment for malignancies other than breast cancer such as the various types of leukemia, lymphoma, and neuroblastoma. The procedure is under study in clinical trials for a number of other malignancies as well. Clearly, this approach pushes the limit of what the body of an individual with cancer can endure. But the end result of advanced, metastatic cancer is death, and while the procedure itself can be lethal, some individuals have been rescued from seemingly terminal disease.

By 1999, an estimated 12,000 women in the United States had undergone high-dose chemotherapy and stem cell support treatment. Initially, many HMOs and health insurers refused to pay for what was considered experimental treatment, but as federal and state governments began to mandate coverage, the procedure came into widespread practice without the usual clinical trials that compared the drastic treatment with conventional chemotherapy. In mid-1999, however, preliminary results from five major studies that looked at the effectiveness of high-dose chemotherapy with bone marrow or stem cell transplants in breast cancer were inconclusive. It appeared, to many breast cancer victims' dismay, that the procedure did not prolong survival overall, although there was benefit to some women. Researchers cautioned that it was too soon to make a final judgment. Three of the trials, which took place in the United States, Scandinavia, and South Africa, enrolled women who had a high risk of recurrence because of more than 10 positive lymph nodes but who had no metastatic involvement. The other two trials, one in the United States and one in France, involved women with metastatic disease and even poorer prognosis. Each of the studies was different in the number of patients enrolled, the characteristics of the patients, and the chemotherapy and doses that were used. Until more research is available, the findings, unfortunately, do not say "here is a treatment that works." Instead, physician proponents of BMT with stem cell support will continue to disagree with physician detractors of the procedure, and women who have to make a decision whether or not to undertake it do not have all the information they need.

Hormonal Therapy

The first kind of systemic therapy employed in breast cancer was endocrine manipulation—attempts to change the hormone environment in the woman. It was recognized late in the 19th century that removal of the ovaries (oophorectomy) would sometimes produce relief of cancer symptoms and prolongation of life in certain premenopausal women. In the years that followed, oophorectomy and irradiation of the ovaries to destroy them became two accepted treatments for advanced breast cancer. Paradoxically, postmenopausal women would sometimes improve when they were given added estrogen, progesterone, and androgen as therapy, although the response rate was variable. In younger women, oophorectomy had been widely used preventively and was often performed immediately after mastectomy.

If a woman benefited from removal of her ovaries, the next procedure, if the cancer continued to progress, was to remove her adrenal glands (adrenalectomy) because these produce estrogen in place of the ovaries. If a relapse occurred, the adrenalectomy was followed by hypophysectomy, the removal of the pituitary gland to get rid of the source of all gonadotropins and adrenocorticotrophic hormones. Should a woman, whose initial surgery had very likely been a radical mastectomy, survive all these additional "ectomies," she would have had to be maintained on a daily replacement of the now missing hormones, some of which are essential to life. Additional morbidity and stress resulting from these successive surgeries could hardly add to the quality of life, but those women who did benefit from endocrine gland removal had relief from pain and prolonged survival, sometimes for as many as 2 years. If there was no improvement, the additional operations only added to their suffering.

Removing one gland after another is hardly the best way of selecting subjects who will benefit from hormonal manipulation, and fortunately there are better methods in use today. Normal breast cells contain receptors for estrogens, progesterone, and androgens. About half of the breast cancers in premenopausal women and perhaps as many as 80% of the breast cancers in postmenopausal women also are hormone dependent; that is, they contain protein estrogen sites in the cytoplasm of the tumor cells that are highly sensitive to estrogen stimulation. If the tumor is analyzed for receptor sites when it is removed and is found to be positive for estrogen receptors (ER), there is a very good chance that the woman will respond to hormonal therapy. There also is a correlation between ER status and prognosis. Women with estrogen receptors in their tumors survive longer and have longer disease-free intervals than women who have ER-negative tumors. This is true regardless of the size of the tumor or the presence or absence of cancer in the axillary nodes, which may mean that ER-positive cancers are slower-growing tumors.

Tamoxifen is a nonsteroid antiestrogen that competes with estrogen binding at the ER sites. It is the only drug known to reduce the risk of recurrence of breast cancer and has been prescribed for more than 25 years. The current treatment for early breast cancer, generally discovered by mammography, is lumpectomy, 6 weeks of radiation, and 5 years of daily treatment with tamoxifen. Whether continuing tamoxifen therapy beyond 5 years is beneficial or harmful is currently an unresolved issue. There is some experimental evidence that after 5 years of taking the drug, resistance to tamoxifen may develop or the drug may actually stimulate tumor growth, but clinical evidence as yet is insufficient. The ongoing ATLAS (Adjuvant Tamoxifen Long Against Short) trial involving 20,000 women randomized to continue or discontinue tamoxifen after 5 years is likely to provide a definitive answer to the question of tamoxifen therapy duration (Swain, 1996). Another unresolved question is the benefit of tamoxifen in women with ER-negative breast cancers.

The use of tamoxifen to prevent breast cancer in healthy women at high risk for the disease is controversial. The National Surgical Adjuvant Breast and Bowel Project, involved for the past 40 years in trials that have influenced breast cancer treatment, initiated the Breast Cancer Prevention Trial in 1992. The trial enrolled 13,388 women who had an increased risk of developing breast cancer and randomly assigned them to tamoxifen or to a placebo. The study was stopped by federal officials a year ahead of schedule with results reported in 1998 because breast cancer was diagnosed nearly 50% less often in women who were assigned to take tamoxifen compared with women who took the placebo. There are other large international multicenter trials in progress testing tamoxifen as prevention of breast cancer, but preliminary results from two of them similar in design have not confirmed the BCPT findings. The National Women's Health Network opposes the use of tamoxifen in healthy women. The Network believes that women with BRCA-1 and BRCA-2 genes, or who have lobular carcinoma in situ, which could progress to cancer, or who have a strong family history of breast cancer in a female relative are candidates for preventive tamoxifen. They believe, however, that the prophylactic taking of tamoxifen to prevent cancer in healthy women who have not been diagnosed with cancer is quite different and may do more harm than good in the long run. The Network's executive director, Cynthia Pearson, testified before an FDA committee on oncology drugs and a U.S. Senate subcommittee expressing reasons for the opposition (1988). Besides affording protection against breast cancer, tamoxifen, taken orally twice a day, has advantages and disadvantages.

While tamoxifen is an antiestrogen in tumors, it mimics the effects of estrogen in other parts of the body. It may decrease osteoporosis and may reduce the risk of heart disease because it decreases the levels of LDL (low-density lipoprotein) cholesterol, the kind that leads to the buildup of artery blockage. There also is evidence, first reported a number of years ago, that tamoxifen reduces the level of certain stimulatory growth factors in the blood (Pollak et al., 1990) and promotes the production of cellular inhibitory growth factors, therefore acting as an inhibitor of tumor growth (Jordon, 1988). There also are numerous reports of the beneficial therapeutic effect of tamoxifen in patients with a wide range of malignancies other than breast cancer (Jordon, 1990). But although tamoxifen has minimal side effects compared with chemotherapy or radiation and does not cause nausea, vomiting, or hair loss, it is not without adverse effects. Many premenopausal women experience menopausal symptoms, which are annoying but not life threatening, such as hot flashes. About 5%–10% get an unusual vaginal discharge. But there are three rare but potentially fatal problems. Tamoxifen has been proven to increase the risk of uterine endometrial cancer; deep vein thrombosis (a blood clot in a major vein); and pulmonary embolism, which can occur when a blood clot travels in the circulation to the lung. In the BCPT, these problems occurred more frequently in women over age 50. Women taking tamoxifen who have not had a hysterectomy need to have annual examinations of uterine endometrial growth by biopsy or transvaginal ultrasound. Other risks that may be more common in women on tamoxifen include visual difficulties, such as an increased incidence of cataracts and macular degeneration.

For most women with breast cancer, the survival benefit of taking the drug outweighs the possible mortality from its adverse effects, however.

Selective Estrogen Receptor Modulators (SERMS). SERMS are "designer" antiestrogens that aim to take advantage of the beneficial effects of tamoxifen (lowering cholesterol, preventing bone loss, killing breast cancer cells) but minimize the adverse effects of tamoxifen (endometrial cancer, deep vein clots, ocular toxicity). Raloxifene, marketed as Evista by Eli Lilly and Company, was originally approved by the FDA for the prevention of osteoporosis in postmenopausal women. The Multiple Outcomes of Raloxifene Evaluation (MORE) was a multicenter, randomized, double-blind trial in which 7,705 women with osteoporosis who took either raloxifene or placebo were followed for 3 years. Women with a history of breast cancer or who were taking estrogen-replacement therapy were excluded from the study. The trial showed that raloxifene, like tamoxifen, had a beneficial effect on bone density and blood lipid levels, increased the risk of deep vein thrombosis, and decreased the risk of invasive breast cancer by 76% in the postmenopausal women with osteoporosis during the 3 years of treatment. Unlike tamoxifen, raloxifene did not increase the risk of endometrial cancer (Cummings et al., 1999). After the results of the MORE study were reported, in 1999 postmenopausal women with an increased risk for breast cancer were being recruited for STAR, the Study of Tamoxifen and Raloxifene. STAR will enroll 22,000 high-risk women at centers all over the country.

Biologic Therapy

Until very recently, there have been few alternatives to what has been called the "slash" (surgery), "burn" (radiation), and "poison" (chemotherapy) treatment of cancer. Major advances in molecular technology, however, have highlighted the promise of biologic therapies such as immune system manipulation, monoclonal antibodies, vaccines, and gene therapy, all formerly considered unsuccessful for the treatment of breast cancer, more promise. And the discovery of the angiogenesis inhibitors provides another avenue to what everyone desires—the prevention and cure of all kinds of cancer.

The immune reaction is the specific response the body has to defend itself against particular foreign invaders such as bacteria, viruses, toxins, or anything that is not recognized as the body's own cells and proteins ("self"). The immune system is made up of the lymphatic tissues and organs located all over the body that communicate with each other by cells carried in the lymphatic and blood circulation. Three types of cells play major roles in immunity: B lymphocytes, T lymphocytes, and macrophages. Other components include the "natural killer" (NK) lymphocytes that are neither B cells nor T cells and that have cytotoxic properties; the lymphokines, a variety of substances produced by T lymphocytes that function as immune response modifiers; plus blood proteins such as complement, which enhances body defenses and antibodies produced by the B lymphocytes in response to an antigen. Figure 7–9 illustrates the components of the immune response. Although much remains to be learned about the immune reaction to cancer, it is believed that when something foreign to the body, like a malignant cell, tries to establish itself, immune system cells detect and destroy the foreign invader. All of the immune mechanisms participate, but the cells responsible for direct destruction are the T killer cells, activated macrophages, and the natural killer (NK) cells. These are the cells responsible for the rejection of organ transplants, and they are also able to recognize malignant cells as "not self" and attack them before the abnormal cells become established as life-threatening tumors. The T-helper cells are hypothesized to improve the immune response to cancer, and the T-suppressors may do the opposite. The theory of immune surveillance suggests that the body is under constant watch by the immune mechanism and that cancer cells are anti-

genic, that is, sufficiently different from the normal to evoke the response of the killer cells. Because abnormal cells probably arise continually in a normal individual as a result of mutations, surveillance is the mechanism of specific defense against them. Recent support for the idea that a healthy immune system is able to destroy early cancers and probably routinely fights tumor cells came from observing transplant patients. Patients who have a kidney or heart transplant and must take drugs to suppress the immune system to prevent rejection have a higher rate of certain cancers, often being stricken many years younger than most people with the same cancers. When the immunosuppressive medication is reduced, their tumors sometimes spontaneously shrink or disappear.

The reason that some tumors escape destruction and continue to grow despite the constant surveillance by the immune system probably is influenced by a number of complex factors, some perhaps mediated by the tumor cells themselves. As more is understood about the immune response to cancer, it may be possible to immunize a person against malignant tumors or to utilize the immune response against cancers that are already actively growing.

There is also evidence that there is a generalized impairment of immune competence in some cancer patients, particularly in advanced malignancy. Because it is reasonable that the better the host defense mechanisms, the better the chances for the host, there have been numerous efforts in the past several decades to treat cancers by immunologic means. Researchers have aimed at enhancing specific anticancer parts of the immune system or augmenting the nonspecific parts, particularly macrophages. Trials are in progress on the effects of various lymphokines such as interleukin-2, interferon, and tumor necrosis factor on cancer regression.

Another way to enhance the tumor-killing capacity of immune cells is by using a tumor-specific antigen vaccine against breast cancer cells. A number of vaccines have been developed and seem to have increased the immune response, but thus far they appear to be more successful when there is only a small amount of tumor present.

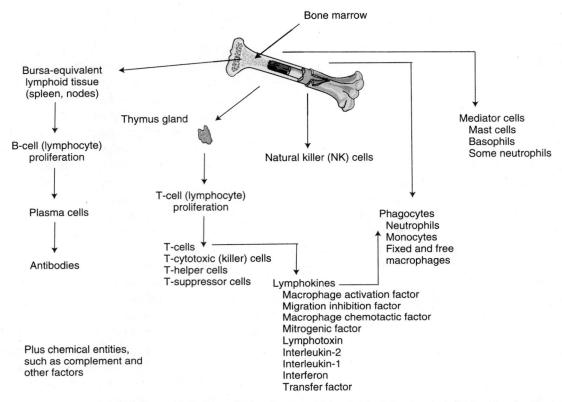

Bone marrow

Bursa-equivalent
lymphoid tissue
(spleen, nodes)

Thymus gland

Mediator cells
Mast cells
Basophils
Some neutrophils

B-cell (lymphocyte)
proliferation

Natural killer (NK) cells

Plasma cells

T-cell (lymphocyte)
proliferation

Antibodies

Phagocytes
Neutrophils
Monocytes
Fixed and free
macrophages

T-cells
T-cytotoxic (killer) cells
T-helper cells
T-suppressor cells

Lymphokines
Macrophage activation factor
Migration inhibition factor
Macrophage chemotactic factor
Mitrogenic factor
Lymphotoxin
Interleukin-2
Interleukin-1
Interferon
Transfer factor

Plus chemical entities,
such as complement and
other factors

Figure 7–9   Components of the immune response. All blood cells originate in the bone marrow. White blood cells, or leukocytes, are involved in the body defense system. Those destined to become lymphocytes mature either in the thymus, and become known as T cells, or in lymphoid tissue like the spleen and lymph nodes, and become the B cells. B cells mature into plasma cells and produce antibodies. Certain T cells further differentiate and acquire special functions. Lymphokines are chemical messages released by sensitized T cells to recruit and activate the macrophages.

Biologic response modifiers (BRMs) are a new category of agents that includes naturally occurring lymphokines such as interferons and interleukin-2 and synthetic compounds such as muramyl tripeptide (MTP-PE). BRMs enhance and stimulate the cancer-killing ability of monocytes, macrophages, and other immune responses. Because it takes 10–20 immune cells to kill one tumor cell, even an enhanced immune response is not effective against large tumor masses. But once 99% of the cancer cells are eradicated, perhaps BRMs can stimulate the immune system to kill the cells left behind after surgery and chemotherapy.

This would be an indication of another promising immunological weapon against metastatic cancer.

Perhaps enhancement of the immune system is possible even without molecular biology techniques. There is growing evidence that emotions such as optimism, techniques such as meditation and visualization, exercise for stress reduction, and the kind of psychological support that helps women to deal with their illness can increase the activity of the immune system. The link between the mental state and the immune system is not proven, but interaction between the immune system and the central nervous system has certainly been shown to exist. Cells of the immune system have been found to have receptors for the neuropeptide transmitters that communicate information from nerve cell to nerve cell in the brain and spinal cord. Physicians such as Bernie Siegal and Carl Simonton, psychologists such as Lawrence LeShan, and laypeople such as Norman Cousins, Marianne Williamson, and Louise Hay have provided additional evidence for the reality of the mind-body connection and the benefit of positive emotions.

Many physicians who tended to scoff at the notion that having the right attitude can help with cancer were virtually stunned by the result of a 10-year study to determine whether psychosocial treatment of women with metastatic breast cancer affects survival. In the study, 50 women were randomly assigned to group therapy and 36 to control. All the women were similar in their disease and continued with the traditional aggressive medical treatments of chemotherapy and radiation, and no one in the therapy group was led to believe that the psychological support would have any effect on the course of their disease. At the 10-year follow-up, three women in the treatment group were still living. From the time of onset of the study, the survival time in the treatment group was approximately 37 months, while the survival time in the control group was only 19 months (Spiegel et al., 1989). This is one of the very few studies to illustrate that psychological factors have a significant effect on mortality.

An exciting advance in immunology that many believe holds the greatest potential for both diagnosis and treatment of breast cancer has been the development of monoclonal antibodies. The technique, known only since 1975, is like an antibody factory—it allows a virtually unlimited number of identical antibodies with a predetermined specificity to be produced in a culture medium. It is based on cell hybridization, the fusion of two different cell lines, usually from different species, to produce a new cell that contains all or part of the genetic information from the parent cells. In the production of monoclonal antibodies, one of the cell lines is from an antibody-producing lymphocyte; the other is from a myeloma, a malignant tumor of the immune system that has the ability to survive indefinitely in cell culture. In 1975, Köhler and Milstein reported that by fusing a cultured mouse myeloma cell with spleen lymphocytes from a mouse that had been immunized against sheep red blood cells (the antigen), a "hybridoma" was produced. This hybrid cell had both the lymphocyte's ability to produce specific antibodies against the sheep red blood cells as well as the immortality characteristic of the myeloma cell. The hybridoma could then be cloned, and the clones could be maintained in culture for indefinite periods, continually producing their pure and identical antibodies to the original antigen—hence the term, monoclonal antibodies. For their achievement, the two researchers were honored in 1984 with both the Nobel Prize in medicine and the Albert Lasker Medical Research award.

The major use of monoclonal antibody technology has been in its application to biological assay techniques—used in a range of products from pregnancy kits to cancer diagnostics—and in the characterization of hormones, viruses, and other biologically active substances. Except for Herceptin, the clinical use of monoclonal antibodies in the treatment of breast cancer has not as yet lived up to expectations, but there are numerous possibilities for their use. Radioactive isotopes or cytotoxins could be attached to monoclonal antibodies to tumor cell antigens, which could then specifically deliver the radioactivity or the toxins to the tumor cells without injuring normal cells. New techniques have greatly improved the chemistry of attaching substances to the antibodies, and there are new ways of manipulating their size, which can affect where they go and how long they last in the body. At the very least, the development of the monoclonal antibody technology has been a significant advance for immunology, genetics, and molecular biology.

Angiogenesis inhibitors, a group of drugs developed by Dr. Judah Folkman and his research team over the past 30 years, seem to hold the greatest promise for control, and just possibly eradication, of cancer. Anti-angiogenesis drugs block the development of new blood vessels in solid tumors, which cannot grow beyond 1–2 mm without inducing the formation of new blood vessels to supply the tumor for its continued growth and nutritional needs. The drugs that are being experimented with stop blood vessel growth by blocking specific molecules involved in new blood vessel formation and literally starving the tumor. Much hope has been raised and the National Cancer Institute has declared the development of angiogenesis inhibitors a top priority. At this writing, the two drugs Folkman has worked with—endostatin and angiostatin—have cured cancer in mice. But Folkman, who never uses the word "cure" for human cancer in talking about his work, has said, "If you have cancer and you are a mouse, we can take good care of you." Researchers long ago learned that what is definitive in mice sometimes turns out to be of little value in humans.

About 20 anti-angiogenesis agents are being tested in clinical human trials. Some are Phase I or II trials, others are in Phase III testing. It could be several years before there are answers concerning their efficacy and safety and whether they really are the hoped-for crack in the enigma of cancer therapy.

The "Best" Strategy of Treatment

What, then, do all these possibilities for treatment mean? Obviously, no single therapeutic approach could possibly be best for all women with breast cancer, and the most beneficial treatment for a particular woman must be selected on an individual basis. A woman who discovers that she has breast cancer is particularly vulnerable to the idea that the doctor knows best, but it is especially important for her at that time, scared and shocked as she may be, to know what the options are. She has to make certain that the status of her condition is appraised before surgery and that she gets a full explanation of the treatment that has been selected for her. She must be assertive enough to let her doctor know that she, too, has some knowledge of breast cancer and its treatments and that she wants to participate in the decisions that are made concerning her.

A woman may be fortunate enough to get herself into the hands of an oncology team, a group in which the surgeon, radiologist, pathologist, and medical oncologist work together. Such teams are usually located in a cancer research center or in a teaching hospital affiliated with a medical school. Most women, regrettably, do not have the opportunity for this kind of treatment and have to rely on a local doctor or a clinic. At least they should insist, difficult as that may be, that their doctors consult with a cancer specialist so that more than one opinion is available. Breast cancer statistics are still too grim for any doctor to feel satisfied about the results of any one treatment. Physicians must be willing to abandon their own prejudices and consider alternatives, particularly in view of the evidence accumulating from the controlled clinical trials that are in progress.

In the midst of all the unknowns concerning the cause and course of breast cancer and the controversy surrounding the most effective treatment, there is one certainty—the earlier the diagnosis, the better the prognosis. When breast cancer is found early, the expectation for cure is greatest.

REFERENCES

Al Sumidiae, A. M., Leinster, S. J., Hart, C. A., et al. (1988). Particles with properties of retrovirus in monocytes from patients with breast cancer. *Lancet, 1*(8375), 5–9.

Bergkvist, L., Adami, H., Persson, I., et al. (1989). The risk of breast cancer after estrogen and estrogen-progestin replacement. *New England Journal of Medicine, 321*(5), 293–297.

Brinton, L. A., & Brown, S. L. (1997). Breast implants and cancer. *Journal of the National Cancer Institute, 89*(18), 1341–1349.

Byers, T., Graham, S. L., Rzepka, T., et al. (1985). Lactation and breast cancer: Evidence for a negative association in premenopausal women. *American Journal of Epidemiology, 121*(5), 664–674.

Colditz, G. A., Egan, K. M., & Stampfer, M. J. (1993). Hormone replacement therapy and risk of breast cancer: Results from epidemiologic studies. *American Journal of Obstetrics and Gynecology, 168*(5), 1473–1480.

Colditz, G. A., Hankinson, S. E., Hunter, D. J., et al. (1995). The use of estrogens and progestins and the risk of breast cancer in postmenopausal women. *New England Journal of Medicine, 332*(24), 1589–1593.

Collaborative Group on Hormonal Factors in Breast Cancer. (1996). Breast cancer and hormonal contraceptives: Collaborative reanalysis of individual data on 53,297 women with breast cancer and 100,239 women without breast cancer from 54 epidemiological studies. *Lancet, 347*(9017), 1713–1727.

Cowan, L. D., Gordis, L., Tonascia, J. A., & Jones, G. S. (1981). Breast cancer incidence in women with a history of progesterone deficiency. *American Journal of Epidemiology, 114,* 209–217.

Cummings, S. R., Eckert, S., Krueger, K. A., et al. (1999). The effect of raloxifene on risk of breast cancer in postmenopausal women: Results from the MORE randomized trial. *Journal of the American Medical Association, 281*(23), 2189–2197.

Deapen, M. D., Pike, M. C., Casagrande, J. T., et al. (1986). The relationship between breast cancer and augmentation mammoplasty: An epidemiologic study. *Plastic and Reconstructive Surgery, 77*(3), 361–368.

Dupont, W. D., & Page, D. L. (1985). Risk factors for breast cancer in women with proliferative breast disease. *New England Journal of Medicine, 312*(3), 146–151.

Early Breast Cancer Trialists' Collaborative Group. (1992). Systemic treatment of early breast cancer by hormonal, cytotoxic, or immune therapy. *Lancet, 339*(8784–8785), 1–15, 71–85.

Gonzalez, E. R. (1983). Chronic anovulation may increase postmenopausal breast cancer risk. *Journal of the American Medical Association, 249,* 445–446.

Goldin, B. R., Adlercreutz, H., Gorbach, S. L., et al. (1982). Estrogen excretion patterns and plasma levels in vegetarian and omnivorous women. *New England Journal of Medicine, 307*(25), 1542–1547.

Gowen, L. C., Avrutskaya, A. V., Latour, A. M., et al. (1998). BRCA1 required for transcription-coupled repair of oxidative DNA damage. *Science, 281*(5379), 1009–1012.

Holmes, M. D., Hunter, D. J., Colditz, G. A., et al. (1999). Association of dietary intake of fat and fatty acids with risk of breast cancer. *Journal of the American Medical Association, 281,* 914–920.

Howe, G. R., Hirhata, T., Hislop, G. T., et al. (1990). Dietary factors and the risk of breast cancer: Combined analysis of 12 case control studies. *Journal of the National Cancer Institute, 82*(7), 561–569.

Jordon, C. V. (1988). Antiestrogen action and breast cancer therapy. In R. J. Santen & E. Juhos (Eds.), *Endocrine-dependent breast cancer: Critical assessment of recent advances.* Toronto, Canada: Hans Huber Publishers.

Jordon, C. V. (1990). Estrogen receptor-mediated direct and indirect antitumor effects of tamoxifen. *Journal of the National Cancer Institute, 82*(21), 1662–1663.

Köhler, G., & Milstein, C. (1975). Continuous cultures of fused cells secreting antibody of predefined specificity. *Nature, 256,* 495–497.

Lancaster, J. M., Carney, M. E., & Furtreal, A. (1997). BRCA1 and 2—A genetic link to familial breast and ovarian cancer. *Medscape Women's Health,* www.medscape.com, *2*(2), 1–8.

Lane, D. S., & Messina, C. R. (1999). Current perspectives on physician barriers to breast cancer screening. *Journal of the American Board of Family Practice, 12*(1), 8–15.

Leis, H. P., Cammarata, A., LaRaja, R., & Cruz, E. (1983, May). Fibrocystic breast disease. *The Female Patient, 8,* 56–77.

London, R. S., Solomon, D. M., & London, E. D. (1978). Mammary dysplasia: Clinical response and urinary excretion of 11-deoxy-17-ketosteroids and pregnanediol following alphatocopherol therapy. *Breast, 4,* 19.

London, R. S., Sundaram, G. S., & Goldstein, P. J. (1982). Medical management of mammary dysplasia. *Obstetrics and Gynecology, 59*(4), 519–523.

London, R. S., Sundaram, G. S., Murphy, L., et al. (1985). The effect of vitamin E on mammary dysplasia: A double-blind study. *Obstetrics and Gynecology, 65*(1), 104–106.

London, S. J., Colditz, G. A., Stampfer, M. J., et al. (1989). Prospective study of relative weight, height, and risk of breast cancer. *Journal of the American Medical Association, 262*(20), 2854–2858.

London, S. J., Connolly, J. L., Schnitt, S. J., et al. (1992). A prospective study of benign breast disease and the risk of breast cancer. *Journal of the American Medical Association, 267*(7), 941–944.

Love, S. (1995). *Dr. Susan Love's breast book* (2nd ed.). Reading, MA: Addison-Wesley Longman.

McTiernan, A., & Thomas, D. B. (1986). Evidence for a protective effect of lactation on risk of breast cancer in young women. *American Journal of Epidemiology, 121*(3), 353–358.

Michnovicz, J. J., & Bradlow H. L. (1990). Induction of estradiol metabolism by dietary indole-3-carbinol in humans. *Journal of the National Cancer Institute, 82*(11), 947–949.

Minton, J. P., Foecking, M. K., Webster, D. J., et al. (1979a). Caffeine, cyclic nucleotides and breast disease. *Surgery, 86,* 105–109.

Minton, J. P., Foecking, M. K., & Webster, D. J. (1979b). Response of fibrocystic disease to caffeine withdrawal and correlation of cyclic nucelotides with breast disease. *American Journal of Obstetrics and Gynecology, 135,* 147–149.

Morrison, A. S. (1990). Is self-examination effective in screening for breast cancer? *Journal of the National Cancer Institute, 83*(4), 226–227.

Neugut, A. I., Robinson, E., Nieves, J., et al. (1990). Poor survival of treatment-related acute nonlymphocytic leukemia. *Journal of the American Medical Association, 264*(8), 1006–1008.

Newcomb, P. A., Weiss, N. S., Storer, B. E., et al. (1991). Breast self-examination in relation to the occurrence of advanced breast cancer. *Journal of the National Cancer Institute, 83*(4), 260–265.

NIH Consensus Conference. (1991). Treatment of early-stage breast cancer. *Journal of the American Medical Association, 265*(3), 391–395.

Papaioannou, A. M. (1974). *The etiology of human breast cancer.* New York: Springer-Verlag.

Pearson, C. (1998, April 22). Testimony before the Subcommittee on Labor, Health and Human Services of the Committee on Appropriations, U.S. Senate. Washington, D.C.

Pearson, C. (1998, September 2). Testimony before the FDA Oncology Drugs Advisory Committee. Washington, D.C.

Pollak, M., Constantino, J., Polychronakos, C., et al. (1990). Effect of tamoxifen on serum insulinlike growth factor I levels in stage I breast cancer patients. *Journal of the National Cancer Institute, 82*(21), 1694–1697.

Schairer, C., Lubin, J., Troisi, R., Sturgeon, S., Brinton, L., & Hoover, R. (2000). Menopausal estrogen and estrogen-progestin replacement therapy and breast cancer risk. *Journal of the American Medical Association, 283,* 485–491.

Schapira, D. V., Kumar, N. B., Lyman, G. H., & Cox, C. (1990). Abdominal obesity and breast cancer. *Annals of Internal Medicine, 112*(10), 798.

Slamon, D. J. (1987). Human breast cancer: Correlation of relapse and survival with amplification of the HER-2neu oncogene. *Science, 235*(4785), 177–182.

Slamon, D. J., Clark, G. M., Wong, W. J., Levin, W. J., Ulrich, A., McGuire, W. L., Godolphin, W., Jones, L. A., et al. (1989). Studies of the Her-2/*neu* proto-oncogene in human breast and ovarian cancer. *Science, 244,* 707–712.

Spiegel, D., Kraemer, H. C., Bloom, J. R., et al. (1989). Effect of psychosocial treatment on survival of patients with metastatic breast cancer. *Lancet, 2,* 888–891.

Steinberg, K. K., Thacker, S. B., Smith, S. J., et al. (1991). A meta-analysis of the effect of estrogen replacement therapy on the risk of breast cancer. *Journal of the American Medical Association, 265*(15), 1985–1990.

Swain, S. (1996). Tamoxifen: The long and short of it. *Journal of the National Cancer Institute, 88,* 1510–1512.

Willet, W. C., Stampfer, M. J., Colditz, G. A., et al. (1987). Moderate alcohol consumption and the risk of breast cancer. *New England Journal of Medicine, 316*(19), 1174–1179.

Zuckerman, D. (1999). No end to breast-implant controversy. *Network News,* National Women's Health Network, *24*(2), 1–2.

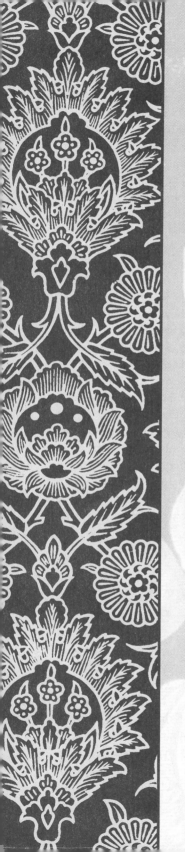

8

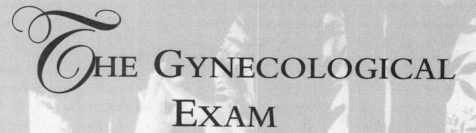

THE GYNECOLOGICAL EXAM

KEY TERMS

Introitus	Pelvic exam
Lithotomy position	Speculum
Pathology	VDRL

$\mathcal{A}$sk any woman how she feels about having a **pelvic exam.** Chances are it will never make the top ten of her favorite things to do. Not that most other preventive or diagnostic procedures are that much fun, either. Who really enjoys having a complete physical, having blood drawn, getting x-rays taken, or going to the dentist? We are pricked, poked, prodded, and subjected to various indignities by health professionals, and we generally accept them with equanimity. But few things make a woman feel as exposed, vulnerable, and downright humiliated as does the gynecological examination. A procedure that requires spread legs in stirrups and a bare bottom hanging over the examining table is at best only tolerable.

Necessity permits the clinician, whether a gynecologist, internist, family physician, or other health care practitioner, as much or greater intimacy with a woman's body than she ordinarily allows herself or her sexual partner. Many women feel more comfortable when the examination is performed by another woman, but a woman gynecologist is no guarantee of greater sensitivity and interpersonal skills. More often than not, the procedure will be performed by a male. The uneasiness or at least mixed feelings that a woman is bound to have as a result of the exam may be compounded by the attitude of the examiner.

Ideally, every OB/GYN would conduct the examination in a sensitive but matter-of-fact manner; listen attentively to what the woman had to say; answer questions unhurriedly; explain what is being done; and, as one adult to another, educate a woman about how to take care of her body. Some are like that, and some are not, and it is not always possible to shop around. Most women have neither the time nor money to try doctor after doctor until they find one with all the right qualities. Many women are geographically limited to the medical care available in their area. There are some things that a woman herself can do, however, if she is not always able to see a doctor who is patient, supportive, communicative, and who respects her dignity as an individual.

Women must remember that the doctor who performs an examination is there to perform a service—the delivery of quality health care. This is the responsibility of the physician, and it is the consumer's right to demand it from the medical profession. But the entire burden for health care is not solely the physician's. Women, too, have a responsibility. They must change their own attitudes about the pelvic examination, rid themselves of their trepidations, and strip it of its mystique and fear. The sexual organs are a part of the body like any other, and there is no need to be embarrassed about their examination. Women must arm themselves with the knowledge to understand what an "internal" is, what it involves, what is taking place during the procedure, and how to recognize a good, thorough, gynecological exam. They must know what kinds of questions to ask, not be afraid to ask them, and they must persist until their questions are answered. Only when women have the information about the medical procedure necessary for their own health maintenance will they be in the position to actively participate in decisions pertaining to their health.

Although some women already know exactly what is taking place during the exam, are medically sophisticated, very knowledgeable, and have no embarrassment concerning the procedure, they still leave the office dissatisfied. They may feel they have been rushed through, brushed off, or that the doctor was authoritarian or judgmental. The physician, male or female, who still treats patients in this way should be challenged. Certainly, it is difficult to sit in a doctor's office or lie on an examining table and criticize the attitude of the physician conducting the examination. But with knowledge, and the power that accompanies knowledge, it is possible for a woman to attempt to change attitudes for the doctor's good as well as her own. A woman can try to educate her doctor, one to one, to the partnership in her health care in which both of them can have responsibility. Confident assertiveness can only improve the relationship between a woman and her doctor. It may never make her feel anything more than just neutral about a pelvic, or any other necessary medical procedure, but at least the examination may become a joint enterprise, one in which she, as well as her pelvis, participates.

How TO KNOW A GOOD GYNECOLOGICAL EXAM

Every human being is a whole person and not a set of organs to be examined and diagnosed. Similarly, the health of the sexual and reproductive organs does not exist in a vacuum. It is part of, and should not be separated from, the total health of the woman. A complete medical history that includes both general medical and gynecological information is an essential part of the first visit to a doctor. If a woman continues to use the same physician, the detailed history does not have to be repeated each time because the information will have been noted on her record. But if on the second visit it appears to her that the doctor has not looked the information over, she should not be reticent about bringing up particular aspects she thinks are relevant. If a woman goes to a clinic, she may not be seeing the same doctor each time, and she should make certain that her record is read.

In the offices of some physicians, the medical history is taken by the receptionist or secretary, or the woman may be asked to fill out a form. A woman who may be reluctant to discuss details of her medical, menstrual, or sexual function with a strange doctor may feel even more uneasy telling her history to a nonprofessional or confessing on paper that, for example, she has had an abortion. It is also possible that information given to someone other than the physician or written down on a form may not reach the doctor before the physical examination. It is better to be asked questions personally by the examining clinician.

It should never be assumed that past or chronic problems are irrelevant to a gynecological difficulty and that they need not be mentioned. A vaginal infection may be associated with diabetes, for example, or with taking antibiotics. If the doctor does not ask about things that the woman may think are important, she should bring them up herself. The following list of questions provides the kind of information that should be obtained from the history. If the questions are not asked, the examination has not been complete, and its quality is questionable.

Family History

Are there any diseases that run in the family: diabetes, heart disease, cancer?

Previous Medical History

Have there been any serious illnesses, either physical or emotional? Any rheumatic fever, any infectious diseases such as TB or VD, any previous gynecological disease? What about operations? For what reason were the surgeries performed and under what kind of anesthesia? Is there any history of allergies in the family? Have there been any urinary difficulties such as frequent bladder infections, stress incontinence (dribbling while coughing, sneezing, or laughing but not at other times), or frequency or urgency not related to stress? Has there ever been blood in the urine?

Gynecological History—Menstrual

What was the age at menarche? Were the initial cycles regular? Is the cycle regular or irregular? How long of an interval between periods? What is the duration and amount of flow? Are external pads or tampons used? Are they "regular" or "super," and how often are they changed? How many are used for the duration of the period? (If the woman has kept a menstrual chart, the pattern of cycles is evident at a glance.) Are there menstrual cramps? When do they occur—before, during, or after the period? Are there any other discomforts besides cramps? Have there always been cramps with menstrual periods, or have the menses only recently become painful? How severe are the cramps, and what is done for them?

Obstetric History

Has there ever been a pregnancy? How many? Any miscarriages and in which month did they occur? Abortions or term deliveries? If a pregnancy was terminated in abortion, what method was used? What kind of labor and delivery was there? Were there any complications? What were the birth weight and sex of each child, and were the babies breast-fed? Are there plans for further pregnancies?

Contraception History

What methods of birth control have been used? What methods, if any, are being used currently?

In taking the medical history, a sensitive physician will not make automatic assumptions of heterosexuality. Doctors who respect women patients as individuals, regardless of their sexual preference, should be aware enough of alternative lifestyles to ask a few courteous questions before attempting to provide birth control information, for example. Neither should lesbian women immediately be equated with sexually active gay men concerning the occurrence of sexually transmitted diseases. Lesbians, at least those who are not bisexual in preference, are at much lower risk for developing venereal diseases than are gay men. The Office on Women's Health in the U.S. Department of Health and Human Services (2000) reports there is no evidence that chlamydia, gonorrhea, and syphilis can be transmitted between women who are sexually active with women.

If the office visit has been for a checkup, breast examination, and a Pap smear, the physical examination should follow the taking of the history. If a woman has come with specific complaints, even more detailed questions that deal with the problem will be asked. The most common gynecological difficulties involve irregularity in uterine bleeding, amenorrhea, pelvic pain, vaginal discharge, the presence of a lump or mass in the abdomen, a protrusion from the vagina, urinary incontinence, hot flashes, infertility, or a problem related to sexual intercourse. A woman should tell the doctor all she can about the onset, severity, and what, if anything, she herself has done thus far about the specific complaint. Her symptoms can direct the physician's approach to her examination. If she suspects what the cause of her problem is, she should say so. She may be guessing incorrectly, but on the other hand, she could be right in her diagnosis.

ℰXTERNAL EXAMINATION

Before going to the doctor, there is no need to take any special cleansing measures at home other than taking a shower or a bath. Advertising to the contrary, a woman's normal secretions are not offensive. A douche should never be used before the examination. If there is a problem with a heavy or odorous vaginal discharge, trying to get rid of it for aesthetic reasons may ruin the diagnosis.

Unless the doctor wants a urine specimen to check for cystitis, the pelvic exam will be more comfortable if the woman urinates before seeing the doctor. Besides, if the bladder is not emptied, its fullness could be mistaken for an abdominal mass, a pregnant uterus, or an ovarian cyst.

If a woman has recently had a checkup, she will not need a complete physical. Some women, however, use their gynecologist as a primary care physician, and then they should not hesitate to ask to have their blood pressure taken; their eyes, ears, nose, and throat examined; and their heart and lungs listened to. If a blood sample is taken, a **VDRL,** the test for syphilis, should be performed on it. A woman should not feel insulted if the test is run on her blood.

The breasts should be examined while the woman is seated and should be palpated while she is lying down. Any questions a woman may have concerning breast self-examination should be asked. If she is uncertain of the method, this is the time to find out how it should be done.

The actual gynecological examination is performed with the woman lying down on the examining table in **lithotomy position;** that is, her feet are up in stirrups, her buttocks are hanging over the end of the table, and a sheet is draped like a tent over the knees and the upper part of her body. This kind of positioning straightens the curvature in the lumbar region of the spine and relaxes the abdominal muscles. It is important for a woman to try not to tense up because it may make the procedure more uncomfortable for her. The usual steps in the procedure are as follows: palpation of the abdomen; breast examination; inspection of the external genitalia; and then, internally, speculum examination of the vagina and cervix, including cell smears for diagnostic analysis, bimanual pelvic examination, and rectal examination.

The doctor will look for any enlargement or tenderness in the abdomen. The vulva and the perineum are examined, and the labia majora and minora are spread apart to see the entrance to the vagina, the hymen, and the urethra. The doctor is looking for any inflammation; scarring; sores; or growths such as warts, cysts, or tumors.

Pushing up the urethral opening against the pubic bone with the tip of the forefinger is called stripping or milking the urethra. In acute urethritis or in gonorrhea, a few drops of pus could be squeezed out from the paraurethral or Skene's glands. The thumb and forefinger are used on either side of the labia majora to palpate for Bartholin's glands, which normally cannot be felt but which may be enlarged and tender if infected.

INTERNAL EXAMINATION

To see the cervix and the inside of the vagina, an instrument called the **speculum** must be used to separate and hold apart the vaginal walls (Figure 8–1). Specula come in various sizes, and the appropriate one to match the size of the **introitus** (vaginal opening) and the length of the vagina is chosen. When the speculum is inside, it may be slightly uncomfortable, but it should not be painful. If it hurts, the woman should say so. Perhaps its position may need to be adjusted.

The bivalve or duck-bill speculum may be made out of steel or plastic. It has two blades, and the posterior, or bottom, one is slightly longer than the anterior blade. It is designed so that it opens after insertion and can be fastened to remain open. The speculum cannot be lubricated with jelly because this would interfere with any analysis of vaginal secretions or cells. Usually, enough natural lubrication is present at the vaginal opening to ease the speculum into place. If not, water can be used.

The sudden entrance of a cold steel unlubricated speculum is a rather startling sensation—one that many women would, just once, wish their male physicians to experience. While one more discomfort added to the entire pelvic exam may not really be that important, it is considerate and more humane to warm the speculum before insertion. Some of the newer examining tables have warming drawers, some doctors keep their specula on a heating pad, and some will warm them by holding them under warm water. Plastic specula do not feel that cold.

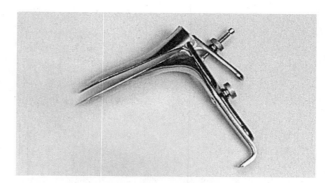

Figure 8–1 Vaginal speculum. Specula are available in different sizes.

The closed speculum is inserted, posterior blade first, into the vagina at about a 45° angle downward. In lithotomy position, the angle of the vagina is down toward the sacrum. When the speculum is in up to the hilt, it is rotated and opened. The entire circumference of the cervix and the vaginal fornices can then be viewed. At this point, a sample of cervical and vaginal cells (Pap smear) or discharge may be taken to test for cervical cancer, vaginal infections, gonorrhea, and chlamydia, or to assess the endocrine status of the woman (Figure 8–2).

The speculum is then slowly withdrawn as the vaginal walls are inspected again to make certain that any redness, cyst, or other damage has not been missed because it was hidden by the blades. The doctor then performs the digital examination, that is, the insertion of the middle and index finger into the vagina. As the examining fingers reach the full length of the vagina, the fornices are explored and palpated for masses or tenderness, and the cervix is palpated for size, shape, and consistency. The woman may be asked to hold her breath and "bear down." This increase in intra-abdominal pressure will reveal any weakness in the muscular supports of the bladder, rectum, or uterus.

The size, shape, position, mobility, and sensitivity of the uterus, ovaries, and fallopian tubes are ascertained by the *bimanual,* or two-handed, examination. The fingers of one hand inside the vagina are placed against the cervix to elevate it while the other hand presses

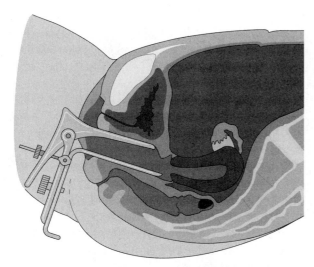

Figure 8–2 Lateral view of the speculum in position.

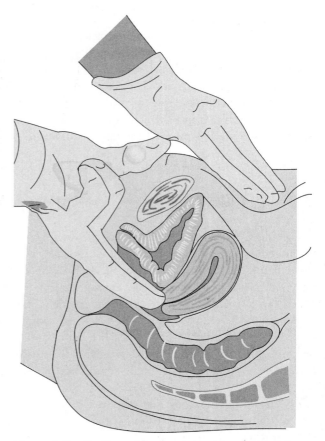

Figure 8–3 Position of the hands in a bimanual pelvic examination.

downward on the lower abdomen. In this way, the body of the uterus can be outlined between the two hands. Then, the physician will try to identify the right and left ovary and tube by placing the vaginally placed fingers in each fornix while palpating abdominally with the other hand. The normal fallopian tube cannot usually be felt as a distinct structure, and the woman may feel a twinge of discomfort as the ovaries are pressed between the external and the internal hands to determine size, shape, and mobility (Figure 8–3).

The pelvic examination should be concluded with the rectal or rectovaginal examination. There are some pelvic structures such as the posterior surface of the uterus, the broad ligaments, the uterosacral ligaments, and the pouch of Douglas that can be felt accurately only through the rectum. At the same time, any abnormal growth that may be present in the rectum could also be located by the examining finger. An internal examination is not complete without a rectal examination (Figure 8–4).

When the physical examination is over, the doctor will tell the woman to get dressed. Some physicians will want to talk to her in the office after she puts her clothes on, but others will discuss the findings and explain any necessary treatment in the examining room. Even if the doctor has provided a running commentary throughout the examination, a woman may still have some unanswered questions. If medication is prescribed, she is entitled to known exactly what the drug is, for what condition it is being taken, and what the potential side effects may be. She should never feel that any question she may have is too "dumb" or trivial to be asked; if something is puzzling her, she should persist until she is satisfied.

It should be noted that in many cities gynecological examinations are performed by nurse-practitioners or nurse-clinicians. Much of what women find distressing about their encounters with a male OB/GYN—the insensitivity, lack of communication, the "busy-doctor"

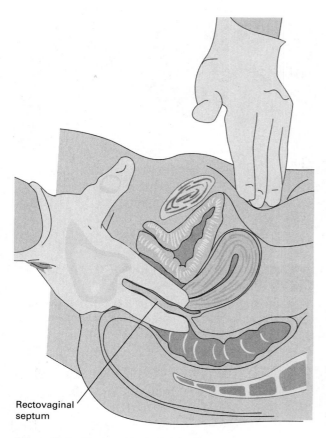

Rectovaginal septum

Figure 8–4   Rectovaginal examination.

attitude—disappear when the examination is conducted by a woman who knows from her own experience what a pelvic is like. Many nurse-practitioners routinely use a mirror and a light during the exam to let the woman see what is going on, and they make a special effort to educate her to understand what she can do to maintain her own gynecological health.

There is no mystery about the gynecological checkup—just a mystique and a vague uneasiness for the woman who cannot see what is happening to her, only feel it while she stares at the ceiling. There is no elaborate instrumentation used—only a speculum, a light, and a cotton swab or a cervical brush for cell specimens. There is no reason to be humiliated by it or feel vulnerable and inferior and uneasy during the procedure—not if one has the knowledge and the confidence to be on

equal footing with the doctor. An MD degree is certainly not necessary to be able to see what the doctor sees inside. Any woman with a tongue depressor, a mirror, and light can look at her own tonsils if she wants to; similarly, any woman with a speculum, a mirror, and light can look at her own cervix, if she wants to.

VAGINAL SELF-EXAMINATION

A plastic, reusable, bivalve speculum usually can be purchased from a medical supply house or from a Planned Parenthood Center if there is one in the area. Depending on where they are purchased, specula cost from $1 to $5, and they come in three sizes—small, medium, and large. About 80% of all women would use the medium size.

To perform self-examination, a woman gets into whatever position she feels is most comfortable for insertion of the speculum. Some may want to squat over a mirror, others may stand with one leg resting on the bathtub or a stool. Many find that a semireclining position on a bed with a back supported by pillows works well. With the aid of a mirror and a high intensity lamp or a strong flashlight, the external genitalia can be examined. After checking the vulva (she will become accustomed rapidly to what is the normal appearance of her genitalia), the woman is ready to examine the vagina and cervix with the use of the speculum.

The tips of the speculum can be lubricated with a little K-Y Jelly or water before insertion. Vaseline should not be used because it can upset the natural balance of organisms in the vagina. While the duck bills are held closed by the fingers of one hand placed between the two sections of the speculum's handle, the labia are separated by the fingers of the other hand. The speculum is then gently inserted sideways at a slight angle into the vagina, aiming downward if the woman is on her back on a bed, or upward if she is standing—similar to the way in which a tampon would be inserted. The speculum should never be forced; if it is uncomfortable or painful, perhaps a smaller size is needed. The valves are inserted as far into the vagina as they will go, and the handle is then rotated up until it is perpendicular to the body. The fingers that are holding the duck bills closed are removed from between the handle sections, and the handles are squeezed together. This opens the valves and spreads the vaginal walls. The finger depression on the shorter handle is then pressed down while pulling up on the longer handle. This locks the speculum into one of three adjustable positions that can be heard clicking into place.

The mirror is then positioned between the legs while the light points into the mirror so that it reflects back a clear view of the vagina. If the cervix is not in view, the speculum may have to be pulled out again slightly and repositioned. Most cervices are not right in the center, and a little gentle searching may be necessary before they appear.

After viewing the cervix and the vagina, the speculum is removed by pulling it straight out without closing it first to avoid pinching the cervix or the vaginal walls. After the speculum is removed, it should be washed with soapy water. There is no need to sterilize it unless it will be used by another woman.

Why Self-Examination? Why Not?

There are reasons for self-examination—there are health and financial benefits for women. There may be some very personal, undefinable reasons for a woman to examine herself. Women who are acquainted with the normal physical appearance of their external genitalia and vaginal and cervical anatomy may be able to detect changes that indicate a developing **pathology** in its early stages. An infection caught early is easier, safer, and cheaper to treat than a full-blown case of itching vaginitis, for example. If a woman has reason to suspect a pregnancy and is familiar with her normal appearance, she may be able to detect its presence through changes in the color and consistency of the cervix and mucus—earlier than is possible through chemical tests. Of course, while regular self-examination can be advantageous for the early recognition of changes, it is *no substitute* for annual or semiannual complete clinical

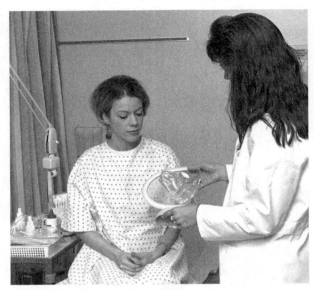

Figure 8–5 Knowledge is power. It can change the traditional doctor–patient relationship into a new and mutually beneficial partnership.

pelvic examinations with a cytological test for cancer. Competent professional backup is a necessary accompaniment to self-care.

Seeing the cervix is not a revelation that can dispel all myths and provide all knowledge. It is an option, another choice that women can make without depending on a physician. It is not the solution, with far-reaching implications, to all the problems women have with the health care system. Women can work toward greater self-determination and responsibility for their own health care with or without a speculum, but for many women it is a way to become more comfortable and knowledgeable about their bodies, to take themselves out of the hands of physicians only and more into their own hands. It is a tool that can be used to take the dominance and mystery out of the doctor's role.

When the physician stands less huge and all knowing, and the woman lies less confused and troubled, the difference in power between them is reduced. Women must find the confidence, however possible, for a more equalized relationship between themselves and their physicians (Figure 8–5).

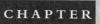

CHAPTER
9

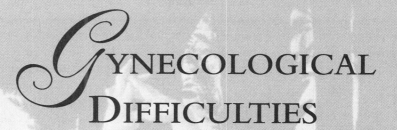

GYNECOLOGICAL DIFFICULTIES

KEY TERMS

Candidiasis

Carcinoma

Chlamydia

Cystitis

Diethylstilbestrol (DES)

Fibroids

Genital warts/
  condylomata

Herpesvirus

Human papillomavirus
  (HPV)

Laparoscopy

Ovarian cyst

Pelvic inflammatory
  disease (PID)

Trichomoniasis

Vaginitis

Truly fortunate, and rare, is the woman who has never suffered an agonizing itch that she cannot scratch in public. And lucky is the woman who has never experienced the burning irritation of a bladder infection; who has never been told she has fibroids, an eroded cervix, or an ovarian cyst; who doesn't know what a menstrual cramp is; and who has never had any of the other "-rrheas." These kinds of

251

gynecological disorders are so common in women and comprise so many of their medical complaints that all women should have a basic understanding of what they are, how to recognize them, and what can be done for them. Some of the more frequent menstrually related problems have been discussed in Chapter 4. This chapter will focus on the vaginal and venereal infections and infestations and on some of the benign and malignant diseases of the reproductive tract.

VAGINITIS AND THE BIG THREE OF INFECTIONS

Vaginitis is the generic term that means inflammation and infection of the vagina. A more correct term is really "vulvovaginitis" because the symptoms are itching and inflammation of the vulva and the vaginal opening and an abnormal vaginal discharge. Pain during sexual intercourse, pain and burning during urination, and local swelling or edema may also occur to varying degrees.

There can be hundreds of causes for vaginitis. In some women it may result from an allergic reaction to soap, laundry detergent, bath oil, feminine deodorant sprays, commercial douche preparations, spermicidal jellies, or even colored toilet paper. Once the allergic contact is known, it can be eliminated and thus the vaginitis will disappear. Sometimes an apparent vaginitis may be caused by a forgotten tampon or perhaps a diaphragm left too long in the vagina. Removal of the object will then remove the vaginitis as well. More often, however, and in more than three-quarters of the women with vaginitis, the cause is infection by one of three organisms—a fungus, *Candida;* a protozoan, *Trichomonas;* or a bacterium, *Gardnerella.*

The normal physiological environment of the vagina is hostile to harmful organisms that cause infection. The lactic acid–producing Döderlein's bacilli, acting on the glycogen stored in the estrogen-influenced vaginal epithelium, are responsible for the lowered pH that protects against invasion. But anything that disturbs the natural healthy balance between the lacto bacilli and the potentially pathogenic micro-organisms—anything that changes the hormonal stimulation, decreases the acidity, or directly damages or kills off the bacilli—can result in the growth and flourishing of infectious organisms and a subsequent vaginitis.

The normal vaginal discharge may vary in amount depending on the stage of the menstrual cycle, but it does not itch, burn, or have an unpleasant odor. Infection and inflammation in the vagina, however, result in an excessive, abnormal discharge called *leukorrhea*. It may be heavy in consistency, white or greenish yellow, sometimes malodorous, and it does produce symptoms by irritating the vulva. The inner walls of the vagina, poorly supplied with nerve endings, are relatively insensitive. In contrast, the vulva and vaginal entrance, richly supplied with nerve endings from the pudendal nerve, respond with pruritus, a distressing and embarrassing itchiness. Leukorrhea and painful outside itching signal a vaginal infection.

Candidiasis

Candidiasis, moniliasis, thrush, fungus infection, and yeast infection are all names for vaginitis caused by the same organism, the genus *Candida,* primarily by the species *Candida albicans.* These yeastlike organisms are commonly found on the skin, in the digestive tract, and may normally inhabit the vaginas of many women (10%–15%), but they remain in a balanced relationship with the other organisms. When certain conditions predispose to the overgrowth of *Candida,* the result may be clinical symptoms of vaginitis. The infection can range in severity from a mild and hardly noticeable irritation to a disseminated, highly dangerous, and potentially fatal disease. Fortunately, systemic candidiasis—affecting the entire body—is very rare.

Causes. Since the introduction of broad-spectrum antibiotics to conquer infection, the incidence of candidiasis has increased dramatically. It is now the most common cause of vaginitis, reportedly outnumbering the other types by a ratio of three to one, or even higher.

Antibiotics, given for some infection elsewhere in the body, suppress the normal bacteria of the vagina that ordinarily keep *Candida* in check. When the harmless and susceptible vaginal bacteria are partially eliminated, the opportunity for the antibiotic-resistant fungus to take over is present. Broad-spectrum antibiotics particularly have been implicated in vaginal candidiasis.

The change in estrogen and progesterone levels during pregnancy also predisposes to the development of *Candida* infections.★ The high hormone levels result in an abundance of glycogen in the vaginal epithelium. The subsequent ample supply of sugars favors a fungal overgrowth. There are data that indicate that for the same hormonal reasons, women on combination oral contraceptives also have a greater incidence of this kind of vaginitis. Of course, the pill may have an effect on the increased frequency of the disease through other than endocrinological mechanisms, since women on the pill are not protected from their partner's possible infections by condoms or contraceptive creams and jellies, which are believed to have an effect in controlling *Candida*.

Diabetes, because it too produces sugar in the urine and a "sweet" environment in the vagina and vulva, has always been suspected of increasing the growth of this yeastlike organism. There have been, however, several large-scale studies that do not support the contention that diabetic women have a greater tendency to *Candida* infection when compared with control populations.

Other reasons for the overgrowth and increase of *Candida* in the vagina include the administration of corticosteroid therapy; malnutrition; a general rundown condition; too-frequent douching, particularly with an alkaline or antiseptic solution; or immunocompromised status, as in individuals with human immunodeficiency virus (HIV) or who are on chemotherapy for cancer.

★Because the infection can be transmitted to the fetus while it is still in the uterus or as it passes through the birth canal, a pregnant woman with candidiasis should not delay treatment. She should immediately see her doctor.

Diagnosis and Treatment. The symptoms of candidiasis are intense itching of the vulva, which is usually worse at night. Because the vulva is frequently red and inflamed, burning, especially after urinating, is also a frequent complaint. The vaginal discharge may be light and watery, but it may also be quite heavy, white, and cottage cheese–like in consistency. Generally it is odorless. Speculum examination may reveal white plaques located on the vaginal walls and variable amounts of the cheesy discharge. Vaginal pH is in the range of 4.3–4.8. The definitive diagnosis is made by a wet smear technique. A cotton swab removes some of the discharge, which is mixed with a few drops of saline solution. One drop of this mixture is placed on a slide, which is then viewed under a microscope to search for the filamentous hyphae and spores characteristic of a fungus (Figure 9–1). Sometimes there is so much cellular debris present that a drop of 10% or 20% potassium hydroxide (KOH) is added to the slide. The KOH dissolves the epithelial cells but leaves the *Candida* undisturbed for easier viewing. *Candida* species appear as oval budding cells plus the filaments or pseudomycelia; other nonpathogenic yeast cells may be present as spores only.

When it has been determined that the vaginitis is the result of a *Candida* infection, it can be treated with intravaginal antifungal preparations such as clotrimazole, miconazole, terconazole, butoconazole, and tioconazole, which are available in prescription and nonprescription forms and are used in regimens that range from 1–7 days. The single dose or 3-day fungicides to be placed into the vagina are said to be as effective as the 7-day course. They may be creams or gels that come with disposable applicators; they may come with one applicator that has to be washed and reused; or they may be in a suppository form, which minimizes the messiness of the oozing creams. These drugs specifically attack *Candida* organisms by disrupting their cell membrane permeability to interfere with mitochondrial enzyme activity in the cell. The preparations are very poorly absorbed from the skin or mucous membranes of the vagina and so do not get into the bloodstream. They apparently have no toxic

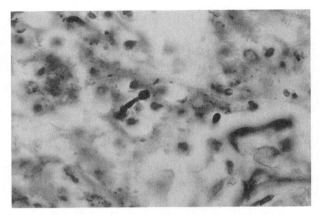

Figure 9–1 Appearance of *Candida albicans* in a smear prepared from vaginal discharge.

effects, and few women are allergic to them. A single-dose pill taken orally is fluconozole (Diflucan), which for many women may work as well as the intravaginal creams. Short-term oral therapy with ketoconazole or itraconazole is also effective. Oral medications are available by prescription only and have the disadvantage of being a systemic treatment, that is, absorbed into the body and transported by the blood to get to the vagina. But sometimes stubborn cases that are resistant to intravaginal therapy may be the result of self-reinfection because women with vaginal candidiasis may also harbor the organisms in their gastrointestinal tracts. Oral preparations, perhaps used in combination with an intravaginal agent, will ensure that no "seeding" of the fungus from the rectum to the vagina takes place.

Another source of reinfection is sexual activity, particularly if the sexual partner is an uncircumcised male. Candidiasis inflammation of the glans under the foreskin is not uncommon, but the infection is rare in circumcised men. It may be helpful for the man to apply an antifungal cream to the glans of the penis before intercourse. *Candida* species have also been found in the semen of males whose partners have frequent vulvovaginal candidiasis. If the fungus does inhabit the reproductive tract of the male, it is generally asymptomatic. This is fortunate because there is no

effective way of treating it in the male. The best protection against "ping-pong" infections is for the man to wear a condom.

Self-Treatment. Getting treatment for an itching, burning yeast infection has traditionally required a visit to the doctor for an examination and a prescription. But during the couple of days it could take to reach the doctor and get the medicine, a woman's quality of life could become pretty miserable. Early in 1991, the ability to get quicker relief and also save the cost of the office visit became possible when two of the most frequently used drugs were made available without prescription. How does a woman know if she should diagnose and treat herself? Itching and inflammation could be the result of an allergic reaction to detergent, soap, colored toilet paper, or a sanitary pad or tampon with deodorant or perfume. The symptoms of candidiasis are distinctive, however, and most women who have already had a yeast infection have no difficulty recognizing the white discharge and intense vaginal itching. Also, if the discharge and itch appear after taking an antibiotic for some other reason, it is virtually a certainty that *Candida* has taken over in the vagina. Severe pain or abdominal pain are *not* symptoms of candidiasis; neither is a bad-smelling, greenish discharge. If symptomatic relief does not occur in a few days on the nonprescription drugs, a health professional should be seen.

The effectiveness of boric acid in treating candidiasis had been known for many years. Van Slyke and colleagues' double-blind controlled study comparing boric acid with nystatin showed that boric acid is even more effective than nystatin. Also, there was little absorption from the vagina, an important consideration because of the known toxicity of ingested boric acid. A daily intravaginal gelatin capsule containing 600–650 mg of boric acid for 14 days is a less expensive alternative to other prescription or over-the-counter agents. Boric acid suppositories could be particularly beneficial when used intermittently to keep symptoms controlled in persistent or recurrent infections. Because in most areas it is necessary to have a physician's prescription to obtain size 0 gelatin capsules to fill with the boric acid powder, the opportunity for self-administration is limited, but women may want to ask their clinicians about the option. No adverse side effects have been reported, but use in pregnancy should probably be avoided.

From an economic standpoint, if a woman's prescription medications are covered by health insurance, even over-the-counter treatments can be unnecessarily costly. She could be better off calling her doctor, who may be willing to phone in a prescription.

When their patients are taking antibiotics for infections, some physicians advise taking acidophilus capsules or eating yogurt to restore the natural intestinal bacterial to the digestive tract. The capsules contain live *Lactobacillus acidophilus* (the same as Döderlein's bacilli) and *Lactobacillus bulgaricus;* yogurt with live culture contains *Lactobacillus bulgaricus.* The tablets and yogurt are said to be useful in avoiding or treating the diarrhea, gas, and other symptoms produced by the antibiotic's destruction of the normal inhabitants of the tract. There is little scientific evidence to support the effectiveness of ingestion of either the tablets or yogurt, but many people claim benefit. Oral antibiotics will also kill off the lactobacilli of the vagina, possibly causing a *Candida* overgrowth with resultant vaginitis. Some women's self-health groups have therefore maintained that the restoring of healthy and friendly bacteria to the vagina early in a fungus infection can actually cut it short before it proceeds into a flaming vaginitis. Two or 3 tablespoons of natural (no fruit!) live-culture yogurt* may be used as a douche, or the yogurt may be directly placed into the vagina with a tampon tube or a vaginal jelly applicator. Most doctors are apt to view this kind of self-treatment as absurd, but there are some who believe the procedure has value. Physiologically, putting the lactobacilli directly into the vagina for candidal vagini-

---

*To determine whether yogurt contains live bacteria, put a couple of tablespoons of the yogurt into a cup of lukewarm milk and leave it overnight in a warm place. If the yogurt contained live culture, the milk will be thickened by morning.

tis makes as much, if not more, sense than eating the bacteria. The method is easy, inexpensive, not harmful, and is worth trying because it may work.

"Trich" Infections

When an itching and burning sensation of the vulva and outer vagina is accompanied by a discharge that is greenish yellow or gray, frothy or bubbly, and possibly malodorous, the microscopic wet smear is likely to reveal the presence of *Trichomonas vaginalis,* a parasitic protozoan that moves by means of four whiplike flagellae (Figure 9–2). The direct wet mount examination is the most common method of detection, but many physicians prefer to use culture methods or an immunoabsorbent assay technique for more accurate diagnosis. There are estimates that 15%–25% of women carry the organism in their vaginas, but many do not experience any symptoms.

Causes. It is known that trichomonas is present more frequently in sexually active women, particularly in those with multiple partners, and the organism is currently considered a venereal disease transmitted through sexual contact. Preadolescent girls occasionally get **trichomoniasis,** however, and because the protozoa are known to survive 30 minutes in tap water and 6 hours in warm saline, it is remotely possible that an infection may be picked up from swimming pools, toilet seats, and wet washcloths. Because an estimated 3%–10% of men also harbor trichomonads, mostly in the urethra or prostate, it is generally recommended that when a woman is infected, both she and her steady sexual partner should be treated simultaneously, whether or not the organism has been shown to be present in the male.

The organisms can remain dormant in the vagina for years, although an asymptomatic woman could develop an active infection at any time. Unlike *Candida albicans,* which happily thrives in the acid environment of the vagina, *Trichomonas vaginalis* finds the normal vaginal pH unfavorable for growth, and circumstances that reduce the vaginal acidity thus

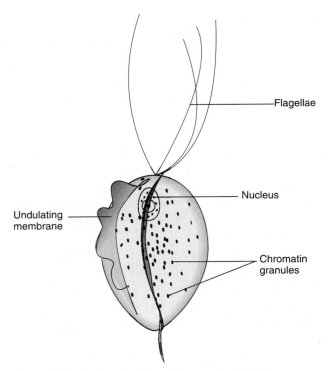

Flagellae

Nucleus

Undulating
membrane

Chromatin
granules

Figure 9–2 *Trichomonas vaginalis.* Seeing motile trichomonads in a drop of vaginal discharge mixed with saline is diagnostic of a "trich" infection.

encourage proliferation of the protozoa. Factors that may result in symptoms of trichomoniasis include pregnancy, trauma to the vaginal walls as a result of childbirth, or even sexual activity. Sometimes a generalized lowered resistance resulting from illness, a crash diet, or even going without enough sleep for a while can induce the growth of trichomonads. Some women experience symptoms after menstruation. In others, growth is triggered by some other factor that produces excessive cervical secretions. Candidiasis or other vaginal infections may activate an infestation with *Trichomonas,* and even an emotional upset will sometimes precipitate or aggravate the symptoms.

Diagnosis and Treatment. The usual treatment for protozoan vaginitis is metronidazole (trade names: Flagyl, by Searle; Metryl, by Lemmon; Protostat, by

Ortho; or Satric, distributed by Savage Laboratories). Metronidazole is one of a group of related chemicals that are effective against anaerobic organisms like *Trichomonas vaginalis* that thrive best only in the absence of oxygen. The current method of treatment with Flagyl is a relatively high dose given over a short period of time. One popular schedule is 500 mg metronidazole (two 250-mg tablets) orally every 12 hours for 5 days for a total of 5 g. One 2-g dosage all at once is usually equally successful and probably better for people who forget or dislike taking medication. The 5-g amount produces a 98% cure rate in nonsexually active women but drops to 50%–85% if treated women are reinfected by sexual partners who harbor the organism. Concomitant treatment is thus recommended. Adverse side effects during treatment occur in 10% of people taking the drug, and these are mostly gastrointestinal—dry mouth, nausea, bitter aftertaste, and sometimes diarrhea and abdominal cramps. Headache, dizziness, and other central nervous system reactions also have been reported. Alcohol should be avoided because drinking during, just before, or after treatment can induce nausea and vomiting.

Metronidazole is an antiprotozoal and antibacterial drug. It is unsurpassed in killing *Trichomonas vaginalis* when taken orally and is effective against other organisms normally occurring in the intestinal or genital tract that can cause infection, given the opportunity and an appropriate set of circumstances. The drug currently is used therapeutically for many kinds of infections and is administered prophylactically before various types of gynecological and other surgeries, including cesarean sections for delivery.

Although there has been no evidence of birth defects as a result of taking metronidazole during pregnancy, it makes sense to avoid the drug in the first 3 months of pregnancy and to take it only if absolutely necessary during the second half of pregnancy.

Metronidazole is, in doctor's language, the "treatment of choice" in the United States. But because women who have a blood or central nervous system disease cannot take oral Flagyl and the drug has very unpleasant side effects for some people, and should not be used in the first 3 months of pregnancy, local topically applied antitrichomonal agents have been used. Several studies have compared such treatments as metronidazole vaginal gel, clotrimazole vaginal suppositories, or other vaginal suppositories containing sulfanilamide or allantoin with oral metronidazole (duBouchet et al., 1997, 1998). Although the vaginal preparations reduced symptoms, none was as effective as oral metronidazole in eradicating the *Trichomonas* infection.

Only 10% of women have the acute classic *Trichomonas* infection—the profuse, frothy, gray malodorous discharge; the severe itching, redness, swelling of the vulva and vaginal opening; the pain on intercourse; the pain on urinating; and the urinary frequency. The other 90% have symptoms that are far less severe, and almost three-quarters of the women harboring trichomonads in their vaginas never have any symptoms at all.

Bacterial Vaginosis

A third common infection of the vagina is bacterial, caused by a gram-negative bacillus formerly called *Hemophilus vaginalis* and now known as *Gardnerella vaginalis*. Formerly, when neither fungi nor protozoa could be identified in the discharge, and a vaginitis was present, the condition was called "nonspecific vaginitis."

Causes.   In 1955, Gardner and Dukes isolated the bacterium from the discharge of women with vaginitis and classified and named it *Hemophilus*. They successfully demonstrated the pathogenicity of the organisms by inoculating them into the vaginas of 15 asymptomatic women and causing vaginitis in 11 of the women.

Diagnosis and Treatment.   The primary symptoms of a *Gardnerella* infection are discharge and a characteristic "stale-fish" odor. Since the bacteria do not ordinarily cause an inflammatory response in the vagina, itching and burning are usually absent.

The discharge is thin, gray white, and homogeneous in consistency. It may be scant, moderate, or profuse enough to soak through several layers of clothing and require the use of pads or tampons. If the secretion

is mixed with a drop of 10% potassium hydroxide on a slide, a characteristic fishy odor caused by the release of two amines is produced. The same odor may be present after intercourse when the vaginal discharge comes in contact with the alkaline semen. The organisms can be diagnosed by saline wet smears because of the presence of characteristic "clue" cells—epithelial cells peppered with myriad small short bacilli. A vaginal pH higher than normal is usual but not diagnostic, and an infection is sometimes confirmed by culture. When it has been determined that the leukorrhea is caused by *Gardnerella,* the reportedly most successful treatment is metronidazole. Alternative antibiotics are oral ampicillin, a semisynthetic antibiotic derived from penicillin, and tetracycline, although local intravaginal therapy (a topical gel form of metronidazole) can also be an option. Sulfonamide creams or suppositories (Sultrin by Ortho and Gantrisin by Roche) or painting the vagina with povidone-iodine are presumably not as successful in curing the infection as any oral therapy unless the local treatment is carried out for at least 14 days. Because *Gardnerella vaginalis* is spread through sexual contact, both partners must be treated, or the woman may become reinfected. If reinfection occurs, it is better to use topical therapy rather than repeated courses of antibiotics, or the original problem could be compounded by an additional *Candida* infection.

When vaginitis is not caused by *Candida, Trichomonas,* or *Gardnerella* as revealed by wet smear, it may be the result of other bacteria, viral infections, cervicitis, or any number of other reasons, allergic or chemical. Unless a specific organism has been verified, there is no point in taking specific medications. Women should also make certain that an accurate diagnosis has been made before permitting treatment. Empirical treatments with various local and systemic medications that attempt to eradicate vaginitis can sometimes make the original condition worse through overtreatment.

Vulvodynia

Vulvodynia is a frustrating condition that is frequently misdiagnosed and treated with conventional therapies for various types of vaginitis or assumed to be psychosomatic. Also known as vulvar vestibulitis or burning vulva syndrome, vulvodynia is characterized by chronic burning or painful itching of the vulva with none of the perceptible physical findings present in the usual forms of vaginitis. Because physicians were unable to find any apparent reasons for the complaint, they initially believed vulvodynia was an unusual psychological problem.

Causes. Although some gynecologists attributed a major role to psychosomatic factors, the work of physician Marilynne McKay and other investigators led to recognition of the condition as a complex disorder with multiple causal factors by the International Society for the Study of Vulvar Disease (ISSVD). McKay (1988, 1989, 1991) studied hundreds of women with the complaint and found there were distinct subsets of disease that were identifiable in her patients. In decreasing order of frequency, these included a number of unrelated conditions such as various skin diseases (dermatoses) of the vulva, cyclic candidiasis, benign skin tumors or papillomas, or essential vulvodynia. "Essential," also termed idiopathic, means inherent with no known cause. Since these subsets may occur simultaneously or sequentially, McKay acknowledged that treatment for one condition may affect the onset of another. In some cases, a subclinical infection with human papillomavirus (HPV) is involved, but vulvodynia also could be related to an as-yet-unidentified virus or to an allergy to something in the environment. It is not believed to be sexually transmitted and occurs just as frequently in nonsexually active women.

Diagnoses and Treatment. The symptoms are, generally, persistent feelings of burning or rawness around the vaginal orifice that can result in anything from mild distress to virtual incapacitation, when even wearing clothing is unbearable. The condition can come and go, or it can linger for a very long time. Examination of the vulvar area with a colposcope (a microscope that allows direct examination of the cells of the vagina and cervix) reveals that the majority of patients have tiny patches of inflamed surface blood vessels (vascular lesions) or marked reddening and tenderness of some of the minor openings of the vestibular glands. Today, vulvodynia is still described as an unexplained vulvar pain syndrome with little to add to what is currently known regarding symptoms, diagnosis, causes, and treatment (Metts, 1999; Bergeron, Binik, Khalife, & Agidas, 1997; Fisher, 1996).

There are no firmly established treatments for vulvodynia. Women with the condition usually consult a number of gynecologists and dermatologists who are unfamiliar with the multifactorial nature of the disease. They have, therefore, been treated unsuccessfully for various kinds of vaginitis, or have been told that their problem is psychological. The anxiety and depression that many women with vulvodynia have is the result and not the cause of the condition, but a number of women have responded to small doses of antidepressant medication. There is evidence that antidepressant medication may relieve pain, possibly by blocking neurotransmitter serotonin uptake by brain neurons. If vulvodynia cannot be attributed to some specific infectious agent such as *Candida* or human papillomavirus, therapies such as cortisone creams, sitz baths with baking soda, or a topical anesthetic cream may provide relief. Symptomatic improvement has also been reported after treatment by the vascular lesion laser, a type of laser surgery also used by plastic surgeons to treat birthmarks and spider veins, and the somewhat drastic procedure of pudendal nerve compression.

How to Prevent Vaginitis

Perhaps, if they are compared to serious diseases of the reproductive tract, common vaginal infections appear insignificant, but women who have suffered with the discomfort and annoyance of a daily vaginal itch never want to have it again. There are several commonsense precautions that all women can take that may help to avoid vaginitis or to prevent its recurrence.

Daily soap and water washing of the vulva and vaginal area is important because all the little moist and dark crevices can provide a good home for organisms and should be kept clean. After defecation, the perineal area should always be wiped from front to back to avoid spreading any bacteria from the anus to the vagina. Of course, the vagina is not sterile, any more than the oral cavity is, but under the same line of reasoning, one should never put anything into the vagina that is too dirty to go into the mouth. If an unwrapped tampon falls on the bathroom floor, for example, it should be thrown away and another should be used.

Very young girls get vaginitis, and so do women who never have sexual intercourse, but since sexual activity plays some role in the transmission of several kinds of vaginitis, the cleanliness of the sexual partner is also important. Once an infection has become established in a woman, she should abstain from sexual intercourse, and her partner should wear a condom or be treated with the same medication to avoid spreading the organism back and forth between them. Condoms are also very helpful for avoiding infections in the first place. There is evidence from laboratory studies that vaginal birth control creams and jellies can be lethal to organisms other than sperm. A woman using spermicidal foam or jelly and a diaphragm may have less trouble with vaginitis.

Obviously, it is important to avoid anything that upsets the natural organisms' balance or the natural pH of the vagina. Antibiotics are useful and necessary drugs but should never be taken without good reason. If they have to be used, eating a lot of live-culture yogurt during treatment may prevent digestive upsets, but whether it will maintain the lactobacilli in the vagina is conjectural. At the first symptom, it could be more effective to use yogurt directly in the vagina.

Too much douching can cause trouble. The normal vaginal discharge varies in amount in different women and from time to time in the same woman with hormonal changes during the menstrual cycle. If a woman wants to douche, she should probably not do it any more often than once every 2 weeks. As for the douche itself, there is some thought that no matter what the solution—vinegar and water, sodium bicarbonate, salt, plain water, or a commercial preparation—the vaginal pH restores itself to normal within 15 minutes. There is probably less chance of disturbing the vaginal chemistry, however, if the solution is kept acidic. The douche bag and apparatus should be kept scrupulously clean; they can harbor mold or bacteria. A woman should never douche while pregnant, and some doctors think that vigorous douching during menstruation may initiate endometriosis by driving the endometrial fragments upward. To douche at all is a personal decision, but if the procedure is used, the douche bag should never be higher than 2 feet above the hips, or the water pressure may be too great.

Mundane as it may sound, one of the greatest preventions for vaginitis is the cotton crotch. Nylon or other synthetic underwear does not "breathe"—the weave is not porous or absorbent enough—and the fabric retains moisture, an ideal environment for the growth of organisms. Pantyhose without a cotton crotch should only be worn with a cotton-lined panty underneath. But wearing cotton-lined underpants will not be as effective if tight jeans, knit pants, or a leotard are worn over them. The point is to cut down on the body heat and resulting dampness that can cause irritation. Loose clothing and the ventilation that cotton underwear provides help to prevent vaginitis. Some studies have shown that *Candida* survives laundering in detergent, so boiling of underpants has been advocated to avoid reinfection by making certain that the yeasts are killed. But since most women are not likely to simmer their lingerie in a saucepan on the stove, one researcher suggested that recurrent yeast infections would be avoided if freshly laundered and damp underpants were routinely microwaved on high for 5 minutes (Masterson, 1988). The underpants must be cotton, of course; nylon would disintegrate.

Women who have difficulties with recurring infections have to be especially careful. They should never sit around in a wet bathing suit, for example. At night in bed even wearing pajamas can cause trouble, and they should wear nightgowns or nothing at all. No perfumed or dyed toilet paper, no "deodorizing" tampons, and no vaginal sprays should ever be used by women who appear to be prone to vaginitis. Bath salts or bath oils should be avoided. All possible sources of irritation should be eliminated.

Despite all the measures taken to prevent it, suppose that a vaginal infection does occur and treatment is necessary. For various reasons, sometimes getting that treatment is delayed. Sitting in a tub of warm water with the hips and buttocks immersed (sitz bath) for 15–20 minutes will help the miserable itching of the swollen and irritated tissues. Between baths, the area should be kept very dry. If a woman has not yet begun using any vaginal tablets or suppositories, wearing a tampon may help because it absorbs the leukorrea inside the vagina and prevents it from spreading onto the sensitive vulvar tissues.

The topical medications used in treating vaginitis have to be inserted high into the vagina. If a vaginal tablet is used, it should be moistened so that insertion is easier; if a cream is used, the applicator should be washed and dried after each use. Because the symptoms usually disappear dramatically after 1 or 2 days of medication and the treatment is sometimes messy and troublesome to use, there is a great temptation to be a therapy dropout. Unless the remedy is continued for the full prescribed time, however, recurrence is likely. It is especially important to carry on treatment right through the menstrual period, but tampons should not then be used because they may soak up all the medication. Even after it has cleared up and no organisms are apparently present in the discharge, a vaginal infection is likely to return after the menstrual period. Application of the jellies or cream that were used on a daily basis to cure the infection should be resumed occasionally or during the first few menstrual periods, even if there are no symptoms or discomfort. Possibly the failure of local treatments to provide long-term cures is due to women not using them for a long enough time in the first place.

NON-HIV SEXUALLY TRANSMITTED DISEASES (STDS)

Perhaps because vaginal infections are not spread exclusively through sexual intercourse, they are not generally seen for what they really are—venereal diseases. For many years, only gonorrhea and syphilis acquired the major social and psychological stigma associated with VD—that they are dirty diseases and that people are promiscuous if they get them. The fear, ignorance, guilt, and anxiety that surrounded gonorrhea and syphilis influenced the ability to effectively treat these diseases and prevent their spread because the public seemed determined to remain unaware that these afflictions are illnesses like any other. Now the foregoing two infections have been joined by "new" sexually transmitted diseases that had never even been considered significant to public health until recently. AIDS, understandably, has eclipsed other diseases as the predominant concern, but the more than 50 diseases and syndromes classified as sexually transmitted diseases are important because these conditions, even excluding AIDS, affect millions of people and account for thousands of deaths annually. All of the STDs, including the lesser-known and rarer ones that few people have ever heard of, have increased over the past decade—a surprising development because public anxiety about AIDS would have suggested a decline in the incidence of STDs.

Most of the non-AIDS STDs are curable with no ill effects if detected and treated early, and although some cannot be cured, they can at least be controlled with proper treatment. The important thing to recognize is that STDs, including AIDS, are mainstream and middle class; they can affect all groups of men and women. Diseases such as genital herpes, chlamydia, anogenital warts, gonorrhea, and syphilis are contagious illnesses, communicated by people, and the only differences between them and other communicable diseases are the parts of the body they affect. They are not spread via air or water, and they are transmitted through very intimate contact. (Syphilis, like AIDS and hepatitis, can also be spread by infected blood and contaminated needles, and not only those shared by intravenous drug users. All such instruments—those used in acupuncture, tattooing, or even ear piercing—must be sterile.) Anyone who is sexually active is at risk for getting a sexually transmitted disease. The only sure method of avoiding infection is celibacy, and even that is uncertain because some vaginal infections become active as a result of factors other than direct transmission. When two virgins meet and remain forever monogamous, the probability of either one getting a STD is virtually nonexistent. There are many in our society like that, but there are also many who are not.

Apart from abstinence, the chances of acquiring a sexually transmitted disease can be reduced substantially by incorporating some changes in the patterns of sexual behavior. People who have active sex lives with several contacts must have a constant awareness of their responsibility for their own good health and for the health of others. There is no need to become paranoid about venereal disease, and it is difficult to regard the person with whom one is involved in a sexual relationship as a potential threat, but it is extremely risky to have sexual contact with a casual acquaintance or someone who cannot be later located. The use of a latex condom with a spermicide containing nonoxynol-9 may be a barrier against transmission of disease but cannot be relied upon to provide infallible protection. Other barrier contraceptives like a diaphragm or cervical cap used with spermicidal jelly protect against pregnancy but provide only partial assurance against STDs. Oral contraceptives are useless against disease transmission. Also, since the symptoms of infection are much more obvious on the exposed genitalia of a man, it is important for a woman to look for them. If any lesion, bump, lump, or sore on the penis or scrotum is seen, she will do herself and her partner a favor by reconsidering sexual contact. If, later, she has any reason to suspect that she has been exposed, and if there are any symptoms, no matter how vague, she must go for diagnosis and treatment. All sex-

ually active women should request tests for syphilis, gonorrhea, and chlamydia with the annual gynecological checkup and should certainly never feel resentful or that their privacy has been invaded if their physicians routinely check for these diseases. If a woman has acquired any STD, she must be willing to have sufficient treatment, come back for follow-up examinations, and identify her contacts so that they can be treated. Gonorrhea and syphilis can be prevented and eradicated and most other STDs can be prevented and controlled if all people behave responsibly, safely, and with concern for others in their sexual relationships.

VIRAL INFECTIONS

Herpes Genitalis

Herpesvirus has an affinity for attacking the skin surfaces and mucous membranes of the body. An infection can be intensely painful, is apt to recur periodically, and as yet there is no cure. At the time of initial onset, compared with almost any other type of vaginal affliction on a misery scale, a herpes infection ranks high. But compared with potentially devastating diseases like gonorrhea, responsible for most female infertility; AIDS; and syphilis, a possible killer, herpes is not even in the running.

Obviously, there is not much good about getting herpes, but neither is it as bad as we have been led to believe. It is incurable but is not a significant health risk for healthy adults, and it is no more life threatening than the common cold, which is also incurable. There are plenty of other incurable diseases, such as arthritis, diabetes, and hypertension, with far more serious consequences for the affected individual than herpes. Herpesvirus is transmitted from person to person by intimate contact that brings mucous membrane surfaces together, but people who have contracted herpes can lead good and active sex lives and never spread the disease as long as they take a few precautions.

Recurrence of herpes becomes less frequent with time, the manifestations become far less severe, and complications of herpes are preventable and manageable.

Causes. Herpes infections are caused by a virus. Viruses are minute infectious agents that are composed of a single molecule core of either deoxyribonucleic acid (DNA) or ribonucleic acid (RNA) and an outer lipid-protein coat or envelope that is largely derived from the components of the host cell's membrane. Viruses can grow only inside living cells. Once a virus has invaded, the virus-DNA or virus-RNA acts as a template to use the host cell's DNA-synthesizing system to make more virus. The foreign virus-DNA units then escape from the cells to infect other cells.

Herpes organisms are DNA viruses with a lipid coat. *Herpesvirus varicellae* are the agents that cause herpes zoster, the painful disease known as shingles; they also result in varicella or chickenpox. *Herpesvirus hominis* is the other group; it causes the herpes simplex virus diseases that can involve the skin, the mucous membranes, the eyes, and in newborn infants cause a disseminated generalized infection that is usually fatal. There are two types of the herpes simplex virus, which were identified in 1962. Type 1, or HSV-1, causes the familiar "fever blisters" or "cold sores" on the lips and face. It can also invade the cornea of the eye. Type 2, HSV-2, is the kind that involves the mucous membranes of the genital tract and is known as herpes genitalis. Today it is believed that approximately 10% of genital herpes infections are caused by HSV-1 and 90% by HSV-2. Research investigation has shown that there are differences in the two strains in terms of recurrence of the disease. Evidently, 60% of type 2 infections recur after an initial episode, but only 14% of infections caused by the type 1 virus recur (Reeves et al., 1981). It also appears that women have fewer recurrences but develop complications of infection more frequently than men. The strain of the virus acquired is irrelevant because both types produce genital herpes with the same clinical symptoms.

As with other foreign invaders, when viruses attack the body cells, specific antibodies are produced by the body to combat them. But unlike some other viruses, which are completely eliminated by the specific antibodies, the herpes viruses persist after an initial or primary infection, remaining latent for long periods of time. The resistance conferred by the antibodies is relative. In some people, the infection may never return; in others, a secondary or recurrent infection can be triggered by any number of factors—a cold, a fever, a gastrointestinal upset, a severe case of sunburn, sexual intercourse, menstruation, or an emotional stress. The antibodies, too, remain in the bloodstream from then on as evidence of a previous herpes infection.

Symptoms. The first episode or primary attack of herpes genitalis is usually the worst and causes a great deal of discomfort. There are some women, however, in whom an initial infection is very mild or completely asymptomatic. A number of adult women, estimates are 15%–20%, have antibodies to type 2 virus in their blood but never remember having had an infection. But, more usually, symptoms begin to appear within 2–20 days following exposure to the infectious virus. First, there may be a tingling or burning sensation, then an intense itching and, as the infection progresses, severe pain. Multiple little blisters appear on the cervix, the vagina, and the vulva or clitoris. They may also be present on the buttock or thigh. In a day or two, they rupture; become secondarily infected; and result in large, shallow, exceedingly painful ulcers covered by a white membrane. There may be systemic symptoms as well—headache; achiness; fever; and tender, swollen inguinal lymph nodes. Painful urination is not uncommon, and there also may be a profuse vaginal discharge. After a week or 10 days, unless the sores have become secondarily infected by bacteria, they will heal spontaneously, leaving no scars. If a secondary bacterial or fungus infection has occurred and remains untreated, the lesions may persist for as long as 6 weeks.

After the sores have healed, the initial active phase of the infection is over, but the virus is still present in the body and enters a latent phase in the nervous system. In oral herpes, the virus lies dormant in a large group of sensory nerve cell bodies (trigeminal ganglion) located near the cheekbone. The genital herpes virus is apt to enter the nerve endings of the lumbosacral nerves and migrate up to the cell bodies that lie next to the lower spinal cord (dorsal root ganglion). When the latent virus is activated, it takes the same nerve pathway back down to skin supplied by the sensory nerve endings. Because the body's defense system is familiar with the virus and has produced antibodies to combat it, the recurrent or second or third infection is of shorter duration and has much milder symptoms. There may be vulvar burning, discharge, and pain, but the severity is considerably less than that of the primary attack. (People who have been exposed previously to HSV but who never had any clinical manifestations will have a first-episode infection that is similar to recurrence—less extensive and less severe.) Many have no warning that a recurrence is going to take place, but some men and women have a premonition or *prodrome* of a tingling, burning, or itching sensation that lasts 6 hours to 2 days before the lesions appear. The virus can be transmitted during the prodrome as well as during the active outbreak. This situation poses a problem for sexual partners of individuals with no prodromal symptoms, but the use of condoms or diaphragms may provide partial protection. More than half of people affected with herpes for the first time will never have a recurrence. Only a very small percentage will have frequent, perhaps once-a-month recurrences. The rest will fall somewhere in between, with rare occasional outbreaks.

Transmission. Contact with an active sore that is "shedding" infectious virus is the primary mode of transmission. The chances of a susceptible person contracting herpes from sexual intercourse with an individual who has active genital lesions is approximately 75%. Kissing a person with cold sores will transmit herpes, and the virus can be passed from the lips to the genitals or vice versa by the hands or by oral sex. Self-inoculation to other sites, particularly to the eyes, is possible, and affected individuals who are in an active stage of the disease should be especially careful to wash the hands before touching or rubbing the eyes. This is particularly essential for contact lens wearers.

Although it is well established that abstention from sexual contact during the prodromal period and until the sores are completely healed is a necessity, whether the virus can be transmitted during asymptomatic periods is controversial. Several studies have demonstrated that small amounts of virus particles can be periodically recovered from the cervices of a small percentage of symptomatic women and the urethrae of an even lesser percentage of asymptomatic men. Brock and colleagues (1990) reported that of 27 women with a history of recurrent HSV infection, 7 of them, or 26%, experienced 11 different episodes of asymptomatic viral shedding from the vulva area, the cervix, or from both areas, which lasted for 1 day. Overall, asymptomatic shedding occurred during only 1% of the days samples were obtained, but the data also suggested that all women with recurrent genital herpes would show asymptomatic viral shedding if they were sampled frequently enough over a longer period of time. The role of such intermittent viral shedding in the transmission of genital herpes is unclear. Spreading the infection from one person to another depends upon the amount of virus shed by the affected individual and the immune susceptibility of the partner. Someone who already has antibodies to oral or genital herpes may not contract the disease after exposure to a small quantity of virus, whereas a nonimmune person could acquire a severe primary infection from a similar exposure. As long as there is a likelihood that people who have herpes may shed the virus in between recurrences, the use of condoms and a diaphragm with jelly (vaginal spermicides may also be virucides) may help prevent transmission to the sexual partner.

It also has been reported that the virus can survive for some hours on inanimate objects (towels, toilet seats, doorknobs) but no one, as yet, has proved that herpes can be acquired from nonhuman contact. Besides, people would have to position themselves on a toilet seat in a highly unusual fashion for a lingering virus to make contact with their genital mucous membranes.

Diagnosis.   It would seem that the presence of blis-
terlike sores on the skin and mucous membranes of
the genitalia would be enough to suggest a herpes
infection, but there are genital lesions or eruptions
from other infections that resemble herpetic lesions,
especially if they are not in the blister stage. The most
reliable method of confirmation is viral culture on living tissue, but a more convenient and cheaper herpes
test, although less accurate than culture, is the Tzanck
smear test. A gentle scraping of fluid from the lesion is
placed on a slide, allowed to air dry, and then stained.
The presence of giant, multinucleated Tzanck cells
that are two to five times as large as white blood cells is
characteristic. A Tzanck smear will not be positive,
however, after the third or fourth day of a recurrent
lesion. A blood test cannot determine whether an
active genital herpes infection is present, but it can
detect antibodies to the virus, which indicate that the
individual has been infected with HSV at some time
and produced antibodies to it. Unlike antibodies to
other viruses, HSV antibodies do not prevent a reacti-
vation of the latent virus. The blood tests also are
unable to tell whether the antibodies are to oral or
genital HSV.

Treatment.   As yet, there is nothing that will cure a
herpes infection. There are, however, ways of preventing secondary infection, lessening the pain, and accel-
erating the healing process.

Keeping the lesions clean and dry is very important in promoting healing and preventing a secondary
infection. The sore or sores can be washed with soap
and water and dried with a blowdryer set on cool. Ice-
cold compresses can provide pain relief during both
the prodromal stage and the outbreak. A local anesthetic, such as lidocaine or 2% xylocaine jelly, and a
painkiller taken systemically will help in an acutely
painful first attack. Any heat to the area only increases
inflammation, and some people cannot even tolerate
warm water; but unless warmth has an adverse effect,
bathing in a warm sitz bath to which a drying agent
such as Epsom salts, Burow's solution, or baking soda
has been added is soothing and relieves discomfort. If

pain is very intense during urination, filling up a tub
of water and voiding into it will prevent the pain and
will also prevent any potential problem with urinary
retention. During an outbreak, loose-fitting clothing
and cotton underwear are recommended to avoid further irritation.

Because drying up the sores and keeping them
clean aids healing and guards against secondary bacterial infection, various salves and ointments one might
think would be helpful are not recommended since
they could actually prolong the outbreak and cause
new lesions to form. These include such self-help
treatments as aloe vera gel, vitamin E oils and creams,
yogurt, or other kinds of herbal or natural remedies.

There are some drugs that are known to act as
antiviral agents; that is, they interfere with the steps
leading toward DNA replication.

Acyclovir, marketed as Zovirax by the Burroughs
Wellcome Company, was approved by the FDA in
1982 in the form of a 5% topical ointment and is now
available in intravenous and oral forms. When applied
to the skin lesions in a first-episode primary herpes
genitalis attack, acyclovir helps shorten the healing
time and reduces pain, itching, and viral shedding.
The oral form of the drug, taken five times a day and
especially when taken within 24 hours of the onset of
symptoms, can shorten the healing time; reduce pain,
itching, and viral shedding; and limit recurrence.
Those who have frequent recurrences can take oral
acyclovir twice a day prophylactically and prevent
most recurrences. Two other drugs—famciclovir
(Famvir) and valacyclovir (Valtrex)—are also FDA
approved for treatment of recurrent episodes of genital
HSV. These drugs are taken less frequently than acyclovir, that is, three times a day for an episode and
once a day to help suppress recurrences. Once suppression is discontinued, however, the recurrences are
likely to take place as frequently as they did prior to
treatment. Currently, suppressive therapy is recommended for individuals with more than six annual
recurrences or who have compromised immune systems. The therapy should be periodically discontinued
to see whether further suppression is necessary. In view

of the large number of cases of herpes in the United States, other virucidal drugs with biochemical activity similar to acyclovir are being pursued avidly by the pharmaceutical industry and are in various stages of clinical evaluation.

Because there is no effective cure for herpes, prevention of the disease by vaccination is an alternative that is getting considerable research attention. Currently, there are several ongoing trials testing the ability of newly developed vaccines to confer immunity and thus protection against herpes. Although the results look promising, these clinical trials will take several more years before there are definite answers on the safety and efficacy of a vaccine, and the concept of protection via vaccination is not without practical problems. Because having the natural infection does not seem to result in immunity to recurrence or autoinoculation to another skin site on the body, at this time the development of a safe vaccine that can actually confer a life-long immunity seems doubtful. Moreover, the cost of mass producing a vaccine is being projected as economically unfeasible, and there are other unanswered questions such as how to administer this expensive vaccine and to whom. There is little doubt, however, given the enormous advances of research in molecular biology that effective vaccination against genital herpes will be possible.

Complications. An active herpes genitalis infection during pregnancy can be very dangerous for the baby. If it occurs during the first 3 months, there is a significantly increased likelihood of miscarriage. If it occurs late in pregnancy, the risk of premature delivery increases. Furthermore, a maternal primary infection can be passed on to the baby by delivery through the infected vagina because there is a high rate of transmission when an infant comes in contact with an active HSV lesion in the birth canal during delivery. There is risk of transmission from asymptomatic shedding, but it is smaller. Fortunately, however, the risk of fetal transmission is much less when the virus is nonactive because maternal herpes antibodies cross the placenta to help protect the fetus even if there is some virus in

the vagina. This is the reason that women with recurrent herpes rarely transmit herpes to their babies during delivery. The American College of Obstetricians and Gynecologists (ACOG) in 1989 provided some recommendations for pregnancy and delivery when there is a risk of herpes in a newborn infant. Any woman who has had herpes genitalis or whose sexual partner is affected is a high-risk mother. She should have weekly cervical and vaginal cultures for HSV starting at a month before delivery. If the cultures are positive for HSV within 2 weeks before delivery, or if she has genital herpes lesions at the time of delivery, a cesarean section should be performed. If vaginal delivery is performed, there should be no fetal monitoring with scalp electrodes to avoid direct inoculation.

The decade-old recommendation of ACOG remains current: vaginal delivery if the woman has HSV but does not have active herpes lesions at the time of delivery. Although the baby is exposed to a risk of infection from possible asymptomatic shedding, the percentage of babies who acquire such an infection is very small, probably because of the maternal antibodies passed through the vagina. Some women request a cesarean section because they want to make certain they are protecting their babies, although a C-section does not offer absolute insurance against infant infection.

The undesirability of a genital herpes infection is obvious, but about 45 million people—one-fourth of the adult population in the United States—are carriers of the virus. With more than 500,000 new cases a year, that means a lot of people have learned to live with it. Also, knowing that some STDs can kill has put a different perspective on herpes, a disease that now could be seen as relatively innocuous. A majority of individuals affected usually are bothered no more than a couple of days a year. Herpes has become an extremely common and, for most people who have it, a mild disease. It is important not to allow its psychological impact to become greater than the physical consequences. Undeniably, however, whether it is mostly dormant or intermittently recurring, a herpes genitalis infection is present for a lifetime. The bottom line is to prevent it.

It is important to remember that the infection is acquired through physical contact with the shed virus, either from a visible sore or just prior to the appearance of an active outbreak. In the case of labial cold sores, this means no kissing or oral–genital contact. In the case of genital herpes, it means no sexual intercourse until the lesions are *completely* healed. The routine use of condoms and spermicidal jellies and foams in between recurrences may reduce the risk of infection because asymptomatic viral shedding, if it occurs, is likely to be in relatively low amounts. These contraceptive methods cannot, however, prevent infection when lesions are present.

If a woman is confronted with a first-episode case of herpes, it is important to remember it is not the end of the world. It may never become reactivated again, and, even if recurrences take place, they reportedly tend to burn themselves out in frequency, usually after about 3 years. Because the virus tends to recur when the body is weakened, doing one's best to maintain good general health could be the best defense.

Hepatitis

The viruses associated with hepatitis or inflammation of the liver are hepatitis A, B, C, D, E, and G. The most prevalent types in America that can cause serious and disabling disease are hepatitis A, B, and C. Hepatitis D (delta) needs the helper function of hepatitis B to replicate and may be acquired as a coinfection of people with chronic hepatitis B. Long-term studies of chronic B carriers with concurrent D infection indicate that more develop liver disease with cirrhosis (progressive damage to liver cells and ultimate failure of their function accompanied by interference with blood flow) when compared with those with hepatitis B infection alone. Hepatitis E is transmitted primarily by fecally contaminated drinking water; almost all cases of acute hepatitis E in the United States have been reported in travelers returning from areas abroad where E is prevalent. Not much is known about hepatitis G except that transmission is bloodborne. It constitutes only 0.3% of acute viral hepatitis, and most

infections are asymptomatic. Hepatitis A is spread via the gastrointestinal tract. It can be acquired by drinking polluted water, eating uncooked shellfish from sewage-contaminated waters, from food handled by a hepatitis carrier with poor hygiene, and from oral/anal sexual contact. Type B is transmissible from saliva, blood serum, semen, menstrual blood, and vaginal secretions. The incidence of hepatitis B has been shown to be higher among promiscuous gay men, prostitutes, and patients attending venereal disease clinics, providing further evidence for its spread through sexual contact. The infectious virus passes through tiny breaks in the skin or across membranes, and the number of asymptomatic chronic carriers is high. Others at high risk include health care professionals, recipients of blood transfusions, and newborn infants of infected women.

Hepatitis C chronically infects almost 4 million Americans. It is serious for some, who develop cirrhosis and liver failure, but not for others who may have some liver damage but do not feel sick and have no long-term effects. Hepatitis C is spread primarily by exposure to blood from a person with the disease. The infected may include anyone who has ever injected street drugs, recipients of blood transfusions or clotting factors prior to 1992, people who have been on long-term kidney dialysis, those whose mother was infected at the time of delivery, health care workers who have had frequent contact with blood, and those who have had sex with an infected person or who have had multiple sex partners. Cases associated with blood transfusions are very rare today, and most new infections are the result of high-risk drug or sexual behaviors. Because many do not realize they have hepatitis C, testing for the disease is recommended for at-risk people. In 1999, the Food and Drug Administration approved a home-testing device that offers the choice to be tested anonymously. The Hepatitis C Check from Home Access Health Inc. does not require a prescription and costs about $70. To use it, an individual pricks a finger with a lancet, puts the blood on special paper, and mails it to Home Access Health's laboratories, and gets results in about 10 days. The home test tells whether a person has ever been infected but not whether an infection is active. Users of the test with positive results should see a physician to determine the status of the infection. There is no vaccine available to prevent hepatitis C, and drug treatment helps about a third of infected patients.

A pregnant woman with an active case of hepatitis B or carrier status can transmit the virus to her fetus across the placenta, but this is relatively uncommon. More frequently, the infection of the baby occurs at birth via contact with body fluids of the mother, and the infected infants then tend to become chronic carriers with a subsequent higher risk of developing liver disease. Hepatitis A evidently is unable to cross the placenta or cause fetal or newborn infection.

Hepatitis A vaccine is very effective in preventing infection. After exposure to hepatitis A, protection or reduction of the impact of the disease can be obtained through a single dose of gamma globulin. Vaccination against hepatitis B has been possible since 1981, when the FDA released a vaccine derived from inactivated virus particles obtained from the plasma of chronic carriers. This vaccine has proved to be both safe and effective, although it still is expensive. This obviously limits the use of the vaccine in underdeveloped countries where hepatitis is a grave public health problem. The incidence of hepatitis B in the United States has declined because of use of the vaccine and currently shows increases only among major risk groups: homosexual men, injection drug users, and sexually active heterosexuals. The Public Health Service advisory committee of the Centers for Disease Control recommends that those adults, health care workers, and all infants receive the vaccine along with their required DPT shots (diphtheria, pertussis, tetanus).

Cytomegalovirus

Cytomegalovirus (CMV) belongs to the herpesvirus family, but unlike infection with HSV-1 or -2 or the varicella/zoster types, it rarely produces any overt clinical symptoms. Most of the population acquires CMV during childhood by respiratory spread, and 40%–80% of the population is infected by puberty. After the age

of 40, between 80% and 100% of adults have antibodies to CMV. This indicates that the virus must be a universal parasite on human populations and, in the vast majority, causes asymptomatic infection. In a few rare instances, the virus results in illness. Occasionally, some people develop a syndrome similar to infectious mononucleosis with the abrupt onset of a high, irregular fever lasting several weeks, tiredness and weakness, and blood cell changes, but the sore throat and enlarged lymph nodes characteristic of infectious mononucleosis are missing. CMV also can become reactivated to result in life-threatening pneumonia or inflammation of the liver in chronically ill patients or people whose immune systems are suppressed. In pregnant women, CMV infection has been incriminated in miscarriage and is able to cross the placenta to infect the fetus, resulting in the birth of an infant with possible mental retardation. Although as many as 95% of all infants infected in this way are asymptomatic at birth, a few may actually be profoundly affected. Several major epidemiological studies have indicated that children in group day care, their parents, and day-care workers have a significantly increased risk of acquiring CMV (Murph, et al., 1991). Because care givers in day care are generally young women of childbearing age, an undetermined potential exists for CMV infection among their own offspring.

The transmission of CMV is by means of contact with body fluids containing the infectious virus material, specifically saliva, urine, tears, and transfused blood. The presence of the virus has been shown to occur in cervical mucus and in semen, making sexual transmission a possibility, although not a certainty.

Genital Warts (Condylomata Acuminata)

Genital warts or **condylomata** (Greek for warts) are caused by the **human papillomavirus (HPV),** a papovavirus similar to those that cause warts any place on the body. In men, genital warts occur most commonly on the glans and urethral opening on the tip of the penis, on the shaft of the penis, and on the scrotum. In women, the most common site is the perineum, but they may also be scattered over the vulva, the vaginal opening, and the skin of the thighs, or they occur within the vagina and on the cervix. For unknown reasons possibly related to hormonal factors, the condylomata have a tendency to become very extensive during pregnancy, and sometimes the growths are so prominent that they may even obstruct the vagina.

Transmission. The means of the transmission of the virus is primarily by sexual intercourse, usually within 8 months of infection, although there have been cases where the warts have appeared in individuals whose only sexual partner does not have them.

Because genital wart infections need not be routinely reported to federal health officials, no one knows the real prevalence of the disease. In 2000, The Centers for Disease Control (CDC) released the first study to provide national data on the HPV's prevalence in the U.S. population. At any one time, the study indicated, an estimated 20 million people in the United States have genital HPV infections that can be transmitted to others, and every year, about 5.5 million people become infected.

HPV and Cancer. The possible association between HPV and cervical cancer is being actively researched. It had long been suspected that cervical cancer is caused by a sexually transmitted agent and a variety of STDs (gonorrhea, syphilis, *Trichomonas,* genital herpes, genital warts) were investigated as possible instigators. Meisels et al. in 1981 had identified atypical, flat, genital warts on the cervix, almost indistinguishable cytologically, histologically, and colposcopically from very early carcinoma of the cervix, and Reid (1982) presented data for the association of condylomata and cervical cancer. Cervical cancer, therefore, was linked to human papillomavirus. Based on epidemiologic evidence in the early 1980s, however, that women with cervical cancer had higher serum levels of antibodies to genital herpes simplex virus than did control women, it was theorized that HSV was the culprit in cervical cancer. After several other epidemiological studies found no relationship between the presence of antibodies to HSV-2 and the development of cervical cancer (Vonka et al., 1984; Adam et al., 1985), doubt was cast on the herpes connection, and interest in the human papillomavirus as a causative agent in cervical cancer was renewed.

There are more than 60 different HPV types, but only 6 have been associated with cervical cancer. Types 6 and 11 are most frequently associated with the typical soft, cauliflowerlike, fleshy genital warts that grow in or around the vagina, anus, or perineum. These virus types generally are not associated with cervical cancer, although they sometimes have been identified in the tissues of vulvar cancer. Cervical cancer is most often associated with HPV types 16 and 18. HPV evidently plays a significant role in the genesis of cervical cancer or other lower tract cancers, but having genital warts or even the identification of HPV DNA in cervical smears is not a predictor of cervical cancer. Although there are suggestions from preliminary studies that the women who harbor HPV-16 may have an increased frequency of progression to cancer compared with women who do not have HPV-16 identified in their Pap smears, no large-scale studies as yet have shown a cause-and-effect relationship. Since there are approximately a million women diagnosed with precancerous cervical changes annually, and only 15,000 actual new cases of cervical cancer diagnosed each year, the vast majority of women who may have HPV found in their cervical samples clearly would have no cervical abnormality. The evidence, therefore, relating HPV to cancer is highly suggestive but not conclusive. It is possible that human papillomavirus, like genital herpes virus, plays a role as a promotor or, perhaps, co-promotor of cervical cancer. It could be that HPV and HSV, together or individually, can function as carcinogens, depending on other factors. One of those factors may be nutrition, in particular, vitamin deficiency. A study of 294 women with cervical dysplasia and 170 controls found that although infection with HPV-16 had the strongest effect on dysplasia risk, inadequate levels of folic acid enhanced the effect of all risk factors, and in particular, that of HSV-16 infection (Butterworth et al. 1992). Another thing is clear. Because cigarette smoking in some way is associated with the development of cervical cancer, women with HPV should definitely not smoke.

Detection. Two screening tests to detect HPV are commercially available. The ViraPap test determines the presence of any of the human papillomaviruses; the ViraType test distinguishes among the strains of HPV. More sensitive is a DNA probe technique such as the *Southern blot,* which requires large amounts of DNA and is very laborious. The most sensitive and sophisticated technique for nucleic acid detection currently available is the *polymerase chain reaction (PCR)* method of DNA amplification.

Treatment. The treatment of genital warts depends on their size and number. If they are not too large or extensive, they can be removed by application of podophyllin, a resin obtained from the mandrake plant that is able to stop mitotic division in cells. The podophyllin, dissolved variously in alcohol, benzoin, or mineral oil in solutions of 15%–25% is painted on the surface of the warts and allowed to remain for 4–6 hours. If it is not washed off thoroughly at that time to remove the residue, the podophyllin can cause severe slow-healing chemical burns. Most people experience considerable pain from treatment; in some it can be persistent and even incapacitating. Two to 4 days after podophyllin application, the warts dry up and slough off, but in some cases, several weekly treatments are necessary. Trichloracetic acid or bichloracetic acid in 90% solution is a treatment for small warts but can be intensely painful. Alternatively, under local anesthesia, the warts can be burned off with electrocautery, frozen off with cryosurgery, or treated with CO_2 laser surgery. Sometimes, many warts coalesce to form a large cauliflowerlike growth, which then has to be removed surgically. Warts often recur after any therapy, most appearing in the first 3 months with a small percentage recurring more than a year later. Two drugs, 5-FU and interferon, have been used for recurrent disease. 5-FU is 5-Fluorouracil, an anticancer drug commonly used in topical form to treat skin cancers. It causes such a high degree of irritation, ulceration, and pain that its use for genital warts has been limited.

*B*ACTERIAL INFECTIONS

Gonorrhea

By law, all cases of gonorrhea must be reported to local health officials, making gonococcal infection the most frequently *reported* communicable disease in the United States today. Two million cases are noted annually, but it is estimated that there may actually be three times that many because of all the infections that private family doctors "forget" to report to the authorities. Only the common cold is more common.

Gonorrhea is a serious and potentially very severe bacterial disease, and it is rapidly becoming more and more resistant to cure. In common with all other STDs, it is an equal opportunity infection—no one is immune to it regardless of race, creed, sex, or sexual preference. Also like other STDs, gonorrhea is not a poor-person disease; anyone at any social or educational level can get it. Of particular significance is the fact that anywhere from 50%–90% of the women who get gonorrhea are totally symptom free. Unlike men who are well aware that they have contracted "a dose of the clap"—they have clear-cut, painful symptoms of urethritis—women may have symptoms that are so vague and nonspecific that they never go to see a doctor with a complaint. There may be no complaint.

Because women are so frequently asymptomatic, they are regarded as the real "problem" in the spread of gonorrhea—an unwitting vast reservoir of infection for unsuspecting males. Of equal, if not greater, concern is the problem of the irresponsible infected man who neglects to inform a woman of her exposure. Because of the widespread prevalence of gonorrhea, a woman must realistically recognize that unless she is celibate or has a mutually monogamous sexual relationship, she is sooner or later likely to be exposed to gonorrhea. A thorough knowledge of all aspects of the disease is essential.

Causes. The organism in gonorrhea is the gram-negative bacterial diplococcus *Neisseria gonorrhoeae*. It grows well only in the moist mucous membranes of the body. Away from the body, the bacteria are very susceptible to drying and lowered temperatures and die within seconds. Although nonvenereal transmission of gonococcal infections has been known to occur in infants through a mother's contaminated hands, it would be extremely difficult to catch the disease from toilet seats, towels, bedclothes, doorknobs, and so forth. One study published in the *New England Journal of Medicine* (Gilbaugh & Fuchs, 1979) demonstrated that when pus from the urethrae of male patients with gonorrhea was *inoculated* onto toilet seats and toilet paper, the organisms could survive in the pus for 2–3 hours. The authors emphasized, however, that this finding alone would not be enough to explain the acquisition of gonorrhea from toilet seats, and some other factor must be involved in transmission. They suggested that "contaminated toilet paper has greater potential as a direct source than do toilet seats." Because it is extremely difficult to imagine circumstances under which individuals would share contaminated toilet paper, nonsexual transmission of gonorrhea, though a possibility, remains unproved.

Gonococcal infection begins with the direct contact of the mucous membranes of an infected person with the mucous membranes of an uninfected person. The surfaces of the gonococci have hairlike projections called pili that enable the invading bacteria to anchor themselves to the mucosal surface and colonize, which they may or may not do successfully. People have varying individual resistance to the disease. It is estimated that in one penile-vaginal sexual contact with an infected partner, a man has a 20%–50% chance of contracting gonorrhea, and a woman has more than a 50% chance. Of course, repeated sexual activity with an infected person virtually ensures that the disease will be acquired. Rectal intercourse may result in inoculation of the bacteria into the anus and rectum, and oral-genital contact can result in gonorrheal pharyngitis or tonsillitis. Mouth-to-mouth kissing alone cannot transfer gonorrhea bacteria.

After an infecting exposure, almost all men (an estimated 10% are asymptomatic) know that they have caught something. After only 1 day or as much as 2 weeks later, there will be a thick, pus-laden discharge from the urethra at the tip of the penis, and urination will be very painful. The urine is cloudy with pus and sometimes even a little bloody. Many men also have enlarged and tender lymph nodes in the groin. These signs are hard to miss or ignore. The severe discomfort, coupled with the campaigns that have made VD a household word, are motivation enough to send men off to the clinic, the private doctor, or the student health service for diagnosis and treatment.

Symptoms. In women, the characteristic symptoms, if there are any at all, are vaginal discharge and painful and perhaps frequent urination. The discharge is distinctively green or yellow in color with an unpleasant odor, but there is so little of it that it may be unnoticed. Besides, these kinds of symptoms are so common to women throughout their nonsexual and sexual lives that they are very likely to completely ignore them.

If the disease remains local, that is, confined to the lower genital tract, the bacteria may involve the urethra, vagina, and the cervix. If Skene's glands are invaded, pushing up on the urethra will result in a pus-filled discharge from their ducts. Bartholin's glands may also become infected and their ducts obstructed. In a small percentage of women, one gland may become abscessed and produce tenderness that makes walking or sitting extremely painful. (Not all Bartholin's gland abscesses, however, are caused by gonorrhea.) The organisms can lodge in the glands of the cervix and cause the production of a profuse and irritating gonorrheal discharge. Gonorrhea bacteria also can remain in the cervix, silently and latently, and later proliferate and become the source of an upper reproductive tract infection. The cervix can look normal with no unusual discharge, but a culture of material from the endocervical canal will provide evidence of the presence of the organisms. The anus and rectum may also be sites of involvement. The condition, called gonococcal proctitis, develops in 40%–60% of women with gonorrhea and is usually the result of the bacteria traveling from the infectious vaginal discharge to the anus. Few women notice any symptoms, although there may be a little itching in the perineal area or a little mucus drainage from the anus.

Sometimes, a local gonorrhea infection is self-limiting. There is no further spread—the disease either undergoes a spontaneous regression, or a woman can become an asymptomatic carrier. Actually, the first recognition that a gonorrhea infection is present may occur after several months when, in about 50% of untreated women, the bacteria spread to the upper genital tract and cause major complications. Undiagnosed and untreated, or inadequately treated, the disease ascends upward through the endocervical canal to the endometrial cavity of the uterus, further on to the fallopian tubes, and out into the peritoneal cavity. Although the cervix usually acts as a barrier to the spread of disease organisms, the cervix is dilated at menstruation, and the gonococci rise into the uterus where they rapidly propagate on the dead cells, glandular secretions, and blood from the sloughing endometrium. The inflammation of the fallopian tubes, or *salpingitis,* can be acute, with pain in one or both sides of the lower abdomen, a temperature of 102° or higher, and nausea and vomiting. Usually, fever and nausea mean that the organisms and their inflammatory products have spilled out of the fimbriated ends of the tubes into the body cavity. When the peritoneum and the ovaries become involved, the condition is known as *acute gonorrheal salpingo-oophoritis,* less accurately called **pelvic inflammatory disease (PID).** A significant further complication of gonorrheal PID is tubal and/or ovarian abscess. A ruptured tubo-ovarian abscess necessitates surgery with removal of the uterus and both ovaries and tubes. Fitz-Hugh-Curtis syndrome is another major complication in which the gonococci migrate to the liver. The severe pain is similar to, and has to be distinguished from, the pain of acute hepatitis, pneumonia, perforated ulcer, kidney stones, and gallstones.

Subacute salpingitis produces much milder symptoms so similar to those caused by other gynecological problems that it is difficult to diagnose. Even if cured by treatment, the damage done by acute or subacute salpingitis remains permanently. The scarring of the fallopian tubes that results is a major reason for infertility and is a possible contributing factor in ectopic pregnancy. PID can become chronic, flaring up at intervals with recurrences of acute inflammation.

More rarely, and only in about 1% of untreated gonorrhea cases, the gonococci enter the bloodstream, a condition called disseminated infection. Occurring predominantly in women, a disseminated gonococcal infection produces a characteristic skin rash, chills, fever, and arthritic joint pains in the wrist, ankles, knees, and feet. If disseminated infection is unrecognized and untreated, or if treatment is delayed, the joints become permanently damaged. Occasionally the gonorrhea bacteria can also invade the heart (endocarditis), the brain (meningitis), and the liver (toxic hepatitis).

If a pregnant woman has gonorrhea when she delivers her baby, the infection is transmitted to the infant's eyes as it travels through the cervix and vagina. The eye infection, called *gonococcal ophthalmia neonatorum,* can cause blindness. It is prevented by dropping a silver nitrate or penicillin solution into all newborns' eyes immediately after delivery. As better protection against neonatal eye infections, pregnant women should be screened for possible gonorrhea early in pregnancy and also several times during the last months.

Diagnosis and Treatment of Gonorrhea. The presence of a gonorrhea infection can be diagnosed by a microscopic examination of a stained smear of secretions from the patient. This bacterial stain test is more accurate for men but not very sensitive for women—only one in two women with gonorrhea have a positive test. The inaccuracy of this method has resulted in its replacement by a bacteriological culture test. Specimens obtained from the major anatomical sites the bacteria invade—the urethra, cervix, rectum, and pharynx—are streaked across a special nutrient jelly. A widely used new test, as accurate as the culture, involves the detection of bacterial DNA in a cervical swab.

Neisseria gonorrhoeae are not easy to culture; they need special media that contain antibiotics to inhibit the growth of other organisms and incubation in an atmosphere with increased carbon dioxide. In a positive culture, colonies of gonorrhea bacteria appear on the incubated medium within 24–48 hours.

There was a time when the gonococcus was very sensitive to penicillin, and 200,000 units of that drug would destroy the bacteria. Now, after widespread use of penicillin and its availability in many parts of the world without prescription, it takes 4.8 million units, and the gonococci are becoming more resistant all the time. In the late 1970s, reports began to appear of gonococcal strains that were not susceptible to penicillin no matter how large a dose was administered. Evidently, some of the *Neisseria gonorrhoeae* strains had acquired the ability to produce an enzyme, beta-lactamase, or penicillinase, that inactivated penicillin and made it valueless in treatment. The penicillinase-producing *Neisseria gonorrhoeae* (PPNG) strains that penicillin is powerless to eliminate could originally be cured by spectinomycin. Subsequently, the penicillin-resistant strain spread and developed a resistance to spectinomycin as well. The double-trouble organisms, resistant to both penicillin and spectinomycin, were treated with yet other antibiotics: ceftriaxone, cefixime, ciprofloxacin, or ofloxacin. Currently, the relative or absolute resistance of some strains of gonococci to antibiotics has become a major problem throughout the United States. In some parts of the country, a virtual epidemic of gonorrhea caused by resistant strains affects all age, ethnic, and economic groups, in part driven by "dope dating"—people having sex in exchange for drugs, usually cocaine. A national surveillance system to monitor trends in antimicrobial resistant *Neisseria gonorrhoeae* found that penicillin-resistant gonorrhea increased 131% in a year. As a result of the surveillance data, the CDC revised the national policy for treating gonorrhea infections. Penicillin, ampicillin, amoxicillin, and tetracycline are no longer recommended as therapy.

The current first-line treatment for uncomplicated gonorrhea is a single dose of ceftriaxone, 250 mg intramuscularly, combined with doxycycline, 100 mg orally twice daily for 7 days. At the present time, such sequential therapy can cure antimicrobial-resistant gonorrhea and also eradicate *Chlamydia trachomatis,* present in 20%–50% of persons with gonorrhea. But the probable next chapter in the antibiotic resistance story is obvious.

Equally worrisome about the resistant gonococci is their possible ability to spread their talent for resistance to other bacteria. The genetic information for producing the penicillin- or tetracycline-deactivating enzymes is transmitted by gonococcal plasmids, small circular extrachromosomal DNA molecules found in the bacteria's cytoplasm. Plasmids may be transferred between microorganisms by bacterial conjugation, a process somewhat analogous to sexual reproduction. Such plasmid interchanges can take place between different bacterial species, although the more distant the relationship, the less efficient the transfer. But the possibility of PPNG organisms incorporating their trait into the bacteria that cause meningitis, for example, is another nightmare for public health officials.

As with other STDs, a vaccine against the organisms that cause infection would be a significant breakthrough. Several kinds of gonorrhea vaccines are being tested in the laboratory and clinically.

Syphilis

The prevalence of infectious syphilis is nowhere that of gonorrhea but has recently shown an alarming trend by increasing to its highest level in the past 40 years. By 1950, most states had passed laws requiring syphilis cases to be reported to health officials, and the disease was thought to have been brought under control through education and the tracing of sexual contacts of reported cases. Syphilis now has made a dangerous comeback nationwide, with the number of cases doubling since 1986. The current explosive rise in primary and secondary syphilis has occurred primarily in urban minority groups. While some of the increase may be influenced by the interaction of drug abuse and sexual behavior ("sex for crack") in some segments of the population, the whole story behind the inner-city rise in all STDs also includes poverty, despair, prejudice, and inadequate health care and education, which can result in crime, substance abuse, and prostitution. Although the number of cases of syphilis annually (an estimated 100,000) is nowhere near the 2 million cases of gonorrhea, the long-term significance of syphilis is much greater. It can be a killer. Untreated, syphilis can affect the central nervous system to produce blindness, deafness, insanity, and ultimately, death.

Part of the difficulty with the treatment of syphilis may result from its lower incidence. Not expecting to see it, private physicians may misdiagnose the condition or miss it completely. In women, the infection can be clinically unapparent in the primary and secondary stages, only becoming obvious in the tertiary stage. Even then, the visible lesions that are present are similar to those found in perhaps 20 other diseases, and the confirmation of syphilis must be made by expensive and time-consuming tests. Blood tests for syphilis are mandatory in most states for people obtaining a marriage license, giving blood, or joining the army, and they are performed on all pregnant women. A woman not in any of those categories can easily remain undiagnosed and untreated.

Causes.   The microorganism that causes syphilis is a spirochete, *Treponema pallidum.* Its length is about the diameter of the largest white blood cell, but it is so thin it is almost undetectable by light microscopy and must be viewed with a darkfield microscope. It is an extremely delicate organism, very sensitive to drying and temperature, so transmission via inanimate objects is virtually impossible. An open lesion is highly infectious, and there have been instances in which doctors, dentists, or nurses in their professional work have contracted the disease through a break in the skin. The usual transfer of the spirochete, however, results from vaginal, anal, or oral-genital sexual intercourse.

The *Treponema* organisms invade any moist mucosal surface, although they can also enter through a minute break in intact skin, and they reach the bloodstream. Within 24 hours, they spread throughout the body. After an incubation period averaging about 3 weeks (it may be as short as 9 days or as long as 90 days), during which the infected individual has no symptoms, a primary lesion called a chancre appears at the site of contact. The chancre is a hard, painless ulcer that in women appears on the vulva, vagina, or cervix. Treated or not, the primary lesion will spontaneously heal, leaving no evidence, but the blood is still infectious. If the chancre is on the vagina or cervix and a woman has had no other reason to see a gynecologist, the disease will remain undetected and untreated.

The secondary stage appears 2–6 months after the initial exposure, sometimes occurring at the same time the primary chancre is subsiding. The only symptoms of the second phase may be flulike—headache, slight fever, loss of appetite, perhaps a general achiness. In addition, there may be a generalized nonitching skin rash on the body. In the genital areas, the syphilitic rash may form *condylomata lata,* growths that are similar to genital warts. These lesions are swarming with spirochetes and are highly contagious. It is during the secondary stage in a pregnant woman that *Treponema pallidum* is able to cross the placenta and infect the developing fetus. There are innumerable other diseases that syphilis mimics in the secondary stage—anything from "mono" to allergies have many of the same symptoms. Less common manifestations are hair loss and the presence of grayish-white lesions in the mucous membrane of the mouth and throat. If there are eruptions on the oral membrane, kissing could be contagious, especially if the person being kissed by the infected individual has broken skin in or around the mouth.

Left alone, untreated, the symptoms of the secondary stage also will go away, although they may recur during the following 2 years. The disease has now progressed into the latent stage, and after a few years have passed, it is no longer infectious. In two-thirds of the people with untreated syphilis, that is the end of it; they are no longer contagious to their contacts, they have no further symptoms, and they may live out the rest of their lives without ever knowing that they had syphilis. A blood test will always be positive, however, and in an untreated pregnant woman with latent syphilis, the spirochetes in maternal blood can pass to the unborn child. Syphilis during pregnancy contributes to spontaneous abortion (miscarriage) and stillbirths. If the pregnancy goes to completion, most full-term deliveries result in a baby with congenital syphilis, having marked and severe deformities. Unfortunately, the incidence of congenital syphilis is far greater than it used to be. Blood tests for syphilis are a routine part of prenatal examination, and if the infection is discovered early enough, treatment produces protection for the infant. Even if the fetus is already infected, control of the disease is possible, and further damage is prevented.

In the remaining one-third of the untreated latent syphilitics, the disease progresses to the tertiary or late syphilis stage. The complications of late syphilis can affect any part of the body. They may be benign, producing only a skin lesion, called a *gumma,* with no further disability, or there may be a massive body reaction to the long-term presence of the spirochetes that involves the brain and spinal cord (neurosyphilis), the heart and lungs, and many other systems of the body. For 10% of individuals affected with tertiary syphilis, it is fatal. There is no way of knowing which cases of latent syphilis will get tertiary syphilis or how severe and extensive the complications will be.

Diagnosis and Treatment.   Syphilis can be diagnosed by examining the fluid from a lesion for spirochetes under a darkfield microscope. All of the blood or serological tests are based on antigen—antibody reactions that occur between *Treponema* and the host. The VDRL (Venereal Disease Research Laboratory) test is widely used because of its low cost and simplicity, but it has its limitations. Evidently, any number of conditions—chickenpox, various collagen diseases such as arthritis or systemic lupus erythematosus, measles, pneumonia, even drug abuse or pregnancy—may falsely give a positive VDRL. It can also give a false-negative result since it is positive in only about 70% of patients with primary syphilis. A negative

VDRL, therefore, cannot rule out active disease. Another widely used method, sensitive enough to detect all stages of syphilis and specific enough to result in very few false positives, is the FTA-ABS (Fluorescent Treponemal Antibody-Absorption) test. The TPI, or Treponema Pallidum Immobilization, is also a highly specific test that is currently used only for confirmation in problem cases because of its expense and difficulty. Tests used in screening large populations are the TPHA (Treponema Pallidum Hemagglutinin Assay) and the RPR (Rapid Plasma Reagin). Any positives or doubtfuls showing up with these rapid and simple tests can be evaluated further with more sensitive procedures.

The treatment of syphilis in any stage is easy: penicillin, in amounts appropriate to maintain a continuous low blood level for a number of days. *Treponema pallidum* has fortunately not developed a resistance to penicillin and can be eliminated by it. An alternative drug for individuals with a penicillin allergy is tetracycline, but this antibiotic, if given during the first 3 months of pregnancy, may result in birth defects and causes fetal teeth and skeletal problems if given in later stages of pregnancy. The recommended drug for a pregnant woman sensitive to penicillin is erythromycin. Treatment for syphilis must always have follow-up examinations and repeated blood tests for at least a year to make certain that a cure has taken place.

A recent research breakthrough that is likely to make it possible for the development of a vaccine against syphilis as well as provide better diagnosis and treatment is the sequencing of the DNA (genome) of *Treponema pallidum.* Knowing the genetic blueprint of the bacterium eventually should enable scientists to prevent the disease, identify it quickly, and cure it with targeted antibiotics (Fraser et al., 1998).

Although gonorrhea and syphilis are two very different diseases, it is obvious that they have many things in common. Both, except in very rare instances, are transmitted through sexual contact. Both present a danger to the unborn child when a pregnant woman is infected. Having either one of the diseases once does not confer any kind of immunity from future infection; it is possible to contract either gonorrhea or syphilis immediately after cure. It is even possible to contract them both and have them exist simultaneously. Both diseases are found to a great extent in younger people. The majority of reported cases of gonorrhea and syphilis in the United States are found among individuals between the ages of 15 and 29. Finally, the social and behavioral factors in the incidence and spread of both diseases may be equal to, if not more important than, the medical aspects.

*C*HLAMYDIAL INFECTIONS

A ubiquitous little bacterialike organism, *Chlamydia trachomatis,* probably has edged out herpes genitalis for the dubious title of agent that causes the most prevalent venereal disease in the United States. It is now responsible for more cases of pelvic inflammatory disease and its resultant infertility or ectopic pregnancy than gonorrhea. As with herpes, it is not required that cases of chlamydia infection be reported to local health officials.

Chlamydia infection is an inclusive term that describes three major groups of diseases caused by 15 recognized serotypes or strains of *Chlamydia trachomatis.* Serotypes A, B, Ba, and C are responsible for a chronic eye inflammation called trachoma. Trachoma has long been endemic, or continually prevalent, mainly in Africa, the Middle East, and Southeast Asia where it affects hundreds of millions of people. It is highly contagious in early stages and, untreated, results in scarring of the eyelids to blindness.

Serotypes L-1, L-2, and L-3 cause lymphogranuloma venereum (LGV), a sexually transmitted condition that causes genital or rectal sores; possible inguinal lymph node involvement; and, in the later stages, massive swelling (elephantiasis) of the penis or vulva as a result of inflammation of the genital lymphatic vessels. LGV is relatively rare in the United States and is more common in tropical and semitropical climates, although one manifestation of the disease, anal procti-

tis, has become a greater problem for homosexual men. The remaining serotypes D, E, F, G, H, I, J, and K are the sexually transmitted strains that cause genitourinary infections in men and women associated with a variety of complications and acute eye infections or chlamydial pneumonia in newborn infants who have acquired these diseases in passing through the infected mother's genital tract.

Nongonococcal urethritis (NGU), as the name implies, is urethritis that is not caused by *Neiserria gonorrhoea.* NGU is estimated by the CDC as being twice as prevalent as gonorrhea, and about half of the cases of NGU are caused by chlamydia infection. Males show more symptoms of NGU than females. In men, the infection differs from the urethritis produced by gonorrhea in that the discharge is watery rather than thick and mucoid and is more profuse. The pain on urination, however, is less severe; men are likely to complain more of smarting or stinging and not of burning. The mildness of the symptoms frequently leads them to delay treatment, and complications such as epididymitis can occur. Moreover, lack of treatment provides more opportunity for the infections to be transmitted to their sex partners. Women are often asymptomatic carriers, unaware that they harbor the infection. They are, hence, diagnosed and treated less often than men. Unattended and untreated, however, the disease can lead to serious complications, which include pelvic inflammatory disease; acute salpingitis that can result in subsequent infertility; acute inflammation of the tissues surrounding the liver; or, in pregnant women, the possibility of transmitting the infection to the baby during delivery.

An infant delivered vaginally through the cervix of a woman with chlamydial cervicitis has a 50%–70% risk of acquiring the infection. More than 100,000 newborns are infected annually. About 15%–25% of these exposed children develop an acute eye infection called inclusion conjunctivitis within the first 2 weeks of life, and 20% develop pneumonia within 2–3 months. Conjunctivitis and pneumonia are the two well-established sequelae of neonatal infection, but there is some evidence that chlamydia is involved in middle ear infections, nasal passage obstruction, inflammation of the bronchioles, and even in sudden infant death syndrome as a result of an inability to breathe.

Diagnosis and Treatment. Because the majority of women who harbor chlamydia are asymptomatic and thus untreated, the disease is a potential risk to their health and any children they may have. It would seem reasonable to screen pregnant women for chlamydial infections so that they may be treated to eradicate the disease. This would protect the infant and reduce the risk of maternal complications. Until recently, the barrier to maternal screening has been the lack of an easy, inexpensive diagnostic test for chlamydia infection. A simple stained smear test, used to confirm many kinds of infections, is only 40% accurate in identifying chlamydia, and formerly the only certain method of verification was by special tissue culture techniques that are both expensive and time consuming. Gene detection technology has resulted in the development of other more expensive tests, but they have the advantage of being able to screen for chlamydial disease using only urine samples in asymptomatic men and women. These newer tests are equally if not more sensitive than the cell culture tests. Because they do not require a pelvic exam and cervical swab, researchers believe the gene technology tests are worth the extra cost in large-scale screening. Another research breakthrough in 1998 that should help in diagnosis and treatment is the sequencing of the *Chlamydia trachomatis* genome. The availability of inexpensive screening tests would have a significant impact on maternal and infant infection and on the treatment of the millions of nonpregnant women as well as men with the disease. Teenagers have a higher infection rate than any other age group with one out of four in some populations harboring chlamydia. The typical high-risk patient is under 20 years of age, is sexually active with more than one partner, has had a history of STD, and does not regularly use condoms. If all doctors recognized the prevalence of the often asymptomatic infection and screened for it, some of its tragic reproductive effects might be avoided.

Chlamydia infection is curable with the right antibiotics: these include tetracycline, doxycycline, or erythromycin stearate if the woman is allergic to tetracycline or is pregnant. According to the CDC, any exposure to chlamydia (as in sex partners of NGU cases) requires antibiotic treatment even if testing for the organism is not available. As previously indicated, all gonorrhea cases currently are treated with ceftrioxone and antichlamydial therapy. The disease is so widespread in the United States that 40%–60% of gonorrhea patients have coexisting chlamydia infections.

INFESTATIONS THAT ITCH— "CRABS" AND SCABIES

The general term for infestation of the skin and hair by lice is called pediculosis. Closely related to the head louse and the body louse, the insect that attaches itself to pubic hairs to cause the condition commonly known as "crabs" is *Phthirus pubis*. When viewed under the microscope, the louse, between 1–4 mm in length, looks very much like a tiny crab (Figure 9–3). The blood-sucking lice attach themselves to the skin at the base of pubic hairs and feed off the tiny capillaries in the skin. They are hard to see unless a hand magnifier is used. Lice do not move very much, and they look like little brown freckles on the vulva. The female lays her eggs or "nits" at the base of the pubic hair. In 7–9 days, the nits hatch and attach themselves to the skin.

Pubic lice are transmitted by sexual contact. Occasionally, infestation can occur from toilet seats, towels, or infected clothing or bedding, but the louse dies if it is separated from its human host for more than 24 hours. Most people with this infestation have intolerable itching, but others do not have any symptoms at all. Difficult as it may be to understand, some individuals have crab lice that they can pass on to others and evidently may never be aware of it. The treatment is easy—a prescription drug called lindane, or gamma benzene hexachloride (brand name Kwell) that comes in a cream, lotion, or shampoo. Used as

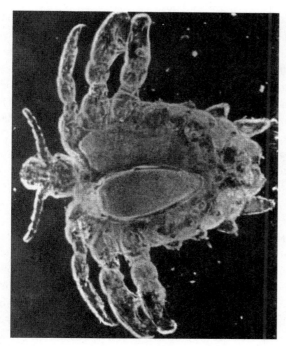

Figure 9–3 An adult female pubic louse. (Courtesy of Reed & Carnick Pharmaceuticals, Piscataway, NJ.)

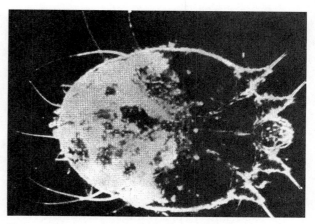

Figure 9–4 *Sarcoptes scabiei,* the mite that causes scabies or the "itch." (Courtesy of Reed & Carnick Pharmaceuticals, Piscataway, NJ.)

directed, Kwell gets rid of the organisms and brings rapid relief from the itching. It should never be used more frequently than the package insert recommends. Like other chlorinated hydrocarbon insecticides, Kwell is potentially toxic to the central nervous system if it gets into the bloodstream at sufficiently high-dose levels. Because it can be absorbed through the skin, exceeding the recommended usage by larger or more frequent doses can be hazardous, especially to children.

After treatment, all underwear, towels, washcloths, and bed linen should be freshly laundered before using, but an outer clothing that has not been worn for 24 hours can be worn again. The lice are not able to survive for any longer than that away from the body.

Infestation with head lice *(Pediculus humanus capitis)* is most common in children but can affect adults as well. Like many other infections, head lice have developed resistance and no longer respond easily to the standard over-the-counter insecticidal shampoos that used to eliminate them. Using lindane shampoo, an

old remedy, on children is risky because overuse can cause neurological damage, so newer prescription treatments for resistant head lice include ivermectus, an oral drug approved for treating intestinal parasites, or trimethoprim sulfanethoxazole (Bactrim), an oral antibiotic that kills bacteria in the lice that are necessary for their survival (Burkhart, Burkhart, & Burkhart, 1998; Morsy et al., 1996).

Scabies, usually called "the itch," is caused by a mite (Figure 9–4). The female burrows into the epidermis of the skin and lays her eggs along the tunnel. After an incubation period of 4 weeks or more, the signs of infestation—a fine, wavy dark track with a small intensely itchy bump at the end—become evident. Scabies is transmitted by intimate sexual or close body contact with an infected person. It is also treated with Kwell or with benzyl benzoate preparations.

URINARY TRACT INFECTIONS

The term urinary tract infection (UTI) is a catchall phrase used to describe conditions responsible for the symptoms of dysuria, or burning pain on urination, and urgency, the feeling of having to pass urine immediately and often, even right after having voided. Other symptoms of **cystitis,** or bladder infection, include dull, aching pain above the pubic bone and passing urine that is either pink, blood-streaked, or frankly bloody enough to redden the toilet bowl. The initial dysuria/frequency symptoms of cystitis can be alleviated or sometimes even cured by drinking a lot of water, but once the infection really takes hold or there is any blood in the urine, it is not going to get better or go away by itself. It means the lining of the bladder is severely inflamed, and a doctor should be seen as soon as possible. Urethritis and cystitis are lower UTIs; they produce misery but are easily treated and cause no complications. Untreated bladder infections, however, can progress to a kidney infection, an upper UTI that is potentially a far more serious disease. Symptoms of a renal infection are chills followed by fever higher than 101°F, pain and tenderness in the flanks, and nausea and vomiting.

Sometimes painful urination is caused by infection unrelated to the urinary tract. Vaginitis that results from *Trichomonas, Candida,* or *Gardnerella* infections can cause burning on urination as the urine (especially the last few drops) passes over the tender, inflamed vulva. This kind of pain on urinating is described by women as feeling "external" and is usually unaccompanied by urgency or blood in the urine. It has not been established whether the three organisms that cause vaginitis cause urinary symptoms because they actually infect the urethra or whether the dysuria is the result of the labia-irritating discharge; but clearing up the vaginitis or the chronic cervicitis will often completely relieve the urinary symptoms.

In women without vaginitis, symptoms of cystitis result from two other groups of organisms. The sexually transmitted pathogens—chlamydial, gonorrheal, or herpes—can cause "internal" dysuria and frequency but rarely cause blood in the urine. A urine sample will show either no pus cells in the urine or what is referred to as sterile pyuria, that is, pus cells in the absence of demonstrable bacterial organisms. This latter finding is often due to chlamydial or gonococcal infection that must be treated by the appropriate antibiotic.

Causes. The most common cause of nonsexually transmitted UTI in women is the result of their own bowel organisms, primarily *Escherichia coli,* but also *Staphylococcus saprophyticus* and *Klebsiella* species. These bacteria, found in the colon but also on the perineum and in the vagina, can ascend the short (2-inch), straight urethra in women and migrate up into the bladder, there to reproduce to millions of bacteria within 24 hours. This is likely to happen at least once during the lifetime of almost all women; in some unlucky ones, it returns again and again and again. Why some women experience recurrent bladder infections while others have one or none is unknown, but there are several theories. It is speculated that those with frequent infections are more susceptible because they (1) are unable to produce local antibodies or lack the antibacterial defense mechanisms to fight their own colon bacteria once they get into the urethra or bladder; (2) lack the specific competing organisms that would inhibit the growth of colon bacteria; (3) possess colon bacteria strains that have an enhanced ability, perhaps through specialized attachment organelles, perhaps by unique virulence properties, that enable them to infect the urinary tract; or (4) have unique factors about their own cells lining the urinary tract that allow them to be more hospitable to the attachment of colon bacteria.

A sudden increase in the frequency of sexual activity results in bladder infections (honeymoon cystitis) for some women. The rectal bacteria have inadvertently been thrust up into the urethra during foreplay or intercourse. Urinating them away immediately after coitus can help rid the urethra of the unwanted invaders before they have the opportunity to spread and multiply. It may be, however, that a poorly fit diaphragm used for birth control can be an obstruction to the necessary washing out of the bacteria. A contraceptive diaphragm that is fit too large may press against the bladder neck and constrict the flow of urine by changing the urethrovesical angle. A general rule in diaphragm fitting is that if it can be felt by the woman, she has been fit with too big a size.

Even in women who are not diaphragm users, recurrent UTIs can often be traced to some factor and thus prevented. It is very important to try to empty the bladder completely when voiding; a small amount of urine left at the bottom of the bladder pools to form a culture medium for avid bacterial growth. Drinking a lot of water daily is another significant method of prevention. It flushes the urine as well as any bacteria out of the bladder. Drinking cranberry juice, which contains hippuric acid in order to acidify the urine and make it less hospitable to bacteria, has also been advocated. Initially, there was little scientific basis for the theory, and it was assumed that the volume of the fluid consumed was probably more important than its content. A study in Israel, however, reported that antiadhesive agents in cranberry juice and blueberry juice inhibited the *Escherichia coli* "adhesins"—the tiny protrusions on the bacterial surface that enable the organisms to cling to the cells of the urinary bladder and thrive, despite natural cleansing mechanisms and normal nutrient deprivation. The researchers identified one of the agents in the juices as fructose, a simple sugar constituent present in all juice. The other inhibiting compound, a high molecular-weight polymer as yet unidentified, was found only in cranberry and blueberry juice and not in the grapefruit, guava, mango, orange, and pineapple juices tested (Ofek et al., 1991). A number of subsequent studies by other investigators, among them Fleet (1994) and Avorn (1994), have substantiated the beneficial role of drinking cranberry juice (even "cranberry juice cocktail" with only 27%–30% cranberry juice) in the prevention of recurrent UTIs. Taking vitamin C (ascorbic acid) also acidifies the urine, but it is best to keep the amount below 1,000 mg daily. There is some evidence that long-term megadose amounts greater than 1 g in some individuals may increase oxalic acid levels in the kidneys and promote kidney stone formation.

Other possible factors that have been implicated in recurrent bouts of cystitis include allergy to spermicidal jelly or cream, too-tight jeans, wearing synthetics instead of cotton in the crotch area, bath salts, or colored toilet paper. For women with a truly "touchy" urethra, symptoms of dysuria/frequency can result from exercise, the vibrations of long auto rides, or the pressure from the narrow seat of a 10-speed bicycle.

Diagnosis and Treatment. For a confirmed, culture-proven urinary tract infection, the conventional treatment is antibiotic treatment. Women with chlamydial infection should be treated with tetracycline. It is least expensive in generic form but must be taken on an empty stomach and is apt to cause gastrointestinal symptoms. Doxycycline is synthetic tetracycline, much more expensive but more easily tolerated. It is also frequently prescribed for nonchlamydial UTIs. Other antibiotics used to treat the common *Escherichia coli* bacterial form of bladder infection are amoxicillin, ampicillin, and cephalexin, the latter more frequently used during pregnancy. Nitrofurantoin (Macrodantin) should be taken with food or antacids to avoid gastrointestinal difficulties. Sulfamethoxazole (Gantanol) and sulfisoxazole (Gantrisin) are old standbys. The trouble with the standard forms of treatment is that having to take one to two pills four times a day, sometimes for 7–10 days, especially if they cause stomach upset, leads many women to forget about them once the initial symptoms disappear. Relapse or reinfection are then very likely to occur. After 1980, a number of reports in the medical literature described the success of single-dose, 1-day or 3-day treatment, as long as the UTI was confined to the lower urinary tract. Depending on the antibiotic used, cure rates of 90%–100% have been reported. The choices include amoxicillin in a single 3-g dose, sulfisoxazole in 2-g dose, or double-strength trimethoprim/sulfamethoxazole (Bactrim or Septra), usually taken as three tablets. A woman should discuss the less expensive, more easily tolerated option of single-dose treatment with her clinician.

Multiple recurrences of UTI, or a chronic infection that appears to be intractable to the usual antibiotic therapy, may have to be investigated for the possibility of a structural abnormality of the urinary tract or for kidney involvement. Cystoscopy (an x-ray of the bladder after it is filled with opaque fluid) and an intravenous pyelogram (IVP), in which contrast medium is injected into a vein to be eventually excreted and show up on kidney x-rays, are diagnostic methods to identify congenital obstructions, stones, or other anatomical abnormalities. When the urinary system has been determined to be structurally normal and the cystitis frequently recurs, the exact therapy is controversial. Some clinicians treat each recurrence with antibiotic as though it were a new episode. Others will prescribe a long-term antibiotic in a low dose prophylactically. A 5-year period of low-dose prophylaxis in 51 women prone to UTI was shown to be effective and well tolerated (Stamm et al., 1991). The patients studied, however, were older women, less sexually active, and they infrequently used diaphragms. In young women, taking an antibiotic after sexual intercourse has been found to be an effective prevention against recurrent urinary tract infections. In the study, 16 university students with a history of at least two culture-documented UTIs in the previous year took a tablet of trimethoprim-sulfamethoxazole (Bactrim) after sexual intercourse. Eleven other women similar with respect to age, diaphragm use, frequency of intercourse, number of sexual partners, and the same history of recurrent cystitis, took a postcoital placebo. After 6 months, 9 of the 11 placebo-taking group developed a UTI while only 2 of the 16 who took Bactrim after sex had an infection (Stapleton, Latham, Johnson, & Stamm, 1990). Pfau (1991) found postcoital administration of cinoxacin or cephalexin to be equally effective. Repeated dilations of the urethra, a painful procedure advocated and practiced by some urologists, in an attempt to stretch the urethra so that the bladder can more easily empty completely, is viewed by other urologists as a futile and unnecessarily traumatizing treatment for recurrent cystitis.

BENIGN AND MALIGNANT CONDITIONS OF THE CERVIX

The cervix is the lower constricted part of the uterus. Half of the cervix projects into the vagina and is called the *portio vaginalis* or the vaginal cervix. It is covered with pale pink stratified squamous epithelium that is continuous with the rest of the epithelial lining of the vagina. The external os is the opening into the cervix

from the vagina. It leads into the endocervical canal, which opens into the uterine cavity at the level of the internal os. The endocervical canal, about 3 cm long, is lined by a different kind of epithelium. Here the cells, arranged in single rows, are tall, columnar shaped, and ciliated. There are about 100 infoldings of the endocervical epithelium that are called cervical glands. The cervical glands contain many mucus-secreting cells.

The junction of the red columnar epithelium of the endocervical canal with the pale pink stratified squamous epithelium of the vaginal cervix is called the squamocolumnar junction. The color change between the two different epithelia is obvious; it has been described as being the same as that between the skin around the mouth and the red of the lips. In the majority of women, the union of the squamous epithelium and the columnar epithelium is not sharp and well defined. Rather, there is a zone of cells in which there is a gradual transition between the two types of linings, a transitional or transformation zone in which the cells can differentiate either into squamous or columnar cells. Most cervical cancers arise in this transformation zone.

The most common benign conditions of the cervix are cervical erosions, cervicitis, and cervical polyps (Figure 9–5). Some of these conditions are so common that many authorities believe that the "normal" cervix—the perfectly healthy cervix—is only the ideal and is rarely seen. Most of the descriptive terms for the cervical appearance were originated when the cervix could be examined only with the naked eye. With the introduction of the colposcope, an instrument that allows direct stereoscopic visualization of the cervix with magnifications of 6–40 times, it became evident that much of what were formerly considered "conditions" were actually normal and physiological (Figure 9–6).

Erosions and Cervicitis

Cervical erosions are a misnomer because nothing is actually eroded or missing, and there is no loss of epithelium. In colposcopic terminology, an erosion is called an

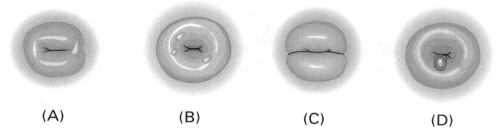

Figure 9–5   Benign conditions of the cervix. (A) An eversion, misnamed an erosion. (B) Nabothian cysts. (C) Laceration with eversion after pregnancy. (D) A cervical polyp.

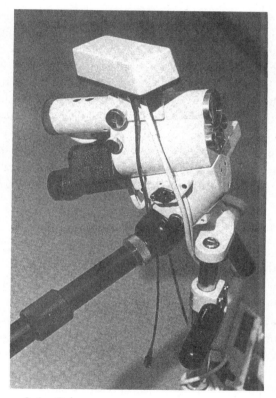

Figure 9–6   Colposcope.

cervix. The patches, which have a soft and velvety appearance, contain the same glands as the regular lining of the endocervical canal, and they produce the same clear mucus. Why the endocervical mucosa moves from its ordinary location is not really understood, but it is assumed that the movements are influenced by a woman's hormonal status and, possibly, by local environmental factors in the vagina. In adult women, it has been postulated that cervical erosion may be associated with a previous inflammation of the cervix, with oral contraceptives, with the hormonal influence of pregnancy, or with the trauma of childbirth.

Erosions commonly cause no symptoms, although in some women more than the usual amount of a clear nonirritating vaginal discharge may be produced. A normal sequel to a cervical erosion is the inward growth of the flat squamous epithelium to replace the endocervical epithelium in its normal limits. When this occurs, it is called *squamous metaplasia*. If this ingrowth of squamous epithelium obstructs the openings of some of the endocervical glands, the cervical mucus continues to accumulate but has no way of exiting. It accumulates as little round bumps or nabothian cysts, named after an 18th-century anatomist, Martin Naboth.

When speculum examination reveals a red patch and nabothian cysts on the cervix, and there are no symptoms, opinions vary as to what to do about such an "erosion." Some doctors regard all cervices that are not covered by squamous epithelium with suspicion, believing that any change in the normal growth pattern of cells in the transformation zone can be a forerunner

ectropion; that is, the endocervical lining is found outside of its normal boundaries. In a so-called erosion, patches of the red columnar epithelium of the endocervical canal have shifted position and have extended out beyond the original squamocolumnar junction to replace the paler squamous epithelium of the vaginal of cervical cancer. They use electrocautery (burning) or cryosurgery (freezing) to destroy the area of displaced tissue. The epithelium regenerates and heals over, restoring the cervix to a more normal appearance. Since sensory nerve endings on the surface of the cervix are very sparse, extremes in temperature produce little or no discomfort. Electrocautery and cryosurgery can be performed in the doctor's office without anesthesia.

There is evidence that the destruction of cellular overgrowth does prevent the progression to cervical cancer, but, of course, not all cervices become cancerous. If a woman has no discomfort or distressing symptoms as a result of the condition, it may not be necessary to treat it at all. Even minor surgical procedures on the cervix carry some risk of complication and may be viewed as both medically and economically unwarranted. But the criteria of symptomatic or asymptomatic may not be enough to guarantee that erosions or ectropions should be treated or left alone. First, there must be a differentiation between a perfectly normal benign overgrowth of endocervical mucosa and a malignant process, and there is no way that the naked eye can do that. A Papanicolaou test (Pap smear) must be made. If the Pap smear is negative, no symptoms can be taken as an indication for no therapy.

Cervicitis

Chronic cervicitis is a catchall term that implies the presence of chronic inflammation or infection. It is used to describe everything from symptomless erosions, which are not caused by infection, to an obviously inflamed everted cervix, which bleeds on contact and produces quantities of a thick yellow-white purulent discharge containing organisms not ordinarily found in the vagina. Women with the latter kind of chronic cervicitis may also complain of backache, feelings of urgency and frequency of urination, and spotting or bleeding after intercourse. Symptomatic cervicitis is indistinguishable from cervical malignancy, and colposcopy or cytological smears and tissue biopsy must be performed. Once cervical cancer

has been ruled out, the usual treatment for chronic cervicitis is electrocautery or cryosurgery.

Acute cervicitis is an acute infection, accompanied by vaginitis, and can be caused by any of the conditions already described—gonorrhea, syphilis, candidiasis, trichomoniasis—as well as almost any pathogenic bacterial agent and a number of viruses. The treatment of acute cervicitis is the appropriate therapy for the specific organism that has caused it.

Cervical Polyps

Cervical polyps are small extensions of the uterine endometrium or the endocervical canal that look like a little tail coming out of the external os. They may be single or multiple and are most common after age 40. If the extruded part is manipulated, even slightly, the polyp will bleed easily. Polyps very rarely become cancerous, but they also have little tendency to spontaneously disappear. Small polyps can be removed by a simple twist at their base and then cauterization of the base to prevent bleeding. Larger polyps may require a more extensive surgical procedure.

Cervical Incompetence

Cervical incompetence is a term used to describe a situation in which the internal os is too wide and is actually not competent to contain a fetus for the full 9 months. The result is spontaneous abortion in the second trimester (3 months) of pregnancy. Typically, when miscarriage is caused by an incompetent cervix, the cervix painlessly dilates, there are no labor contractions, there is very little bleeding, and the fetal membranes (bag of waters) rupture with a gush shortly before delivery. If a woman has an obstetrical history of repeated miscarriage after the first 3 months, it is likely that she has an incompetent cervix. If she is not pregnant, this diagnosis can be tested by determining whether it is possible to insert a dilator 6–8 mm in diameter through the external os into the endocervical canal without discomfort—a procedure that ordinarily would be very painful and require an anesthetic. A hysterogram, or x-ray of the uterus after an opaque dye has been injected through the cervix, may show widening at the level of the internal os. Ultrasonography has also been used to confirm the diagnosis.

An incompetent cervix can be caused by a congenital anatomical defect, but many cases are caused by trauma. Dilation of the cervix to alleviate menstrual cramps, a procedure that has proved to be useless but may still be practiced, often causes damage resulting in later cervical incompetence. Sometimes a previous delivery caused cervical lacerations that were not recognized at the time and hence not adequately repaired, or perhaps a woman has undergone an overly enthusiastic dilation of the cervix when she had a therapeutic or diagnostic D and C (dilatation and curettage).

If a woman wants to become pregnant after the diagnosis of incompetent cervix, a surgical treatment, known as the Shirodkar procedure or the Macdonald modification, is performed. A strip of suture material or nylon ribbon is stitched around the cervix in a purse-string fashion in order to keep it tight. The operation, said to have about a 75% success rate, does not guarantee that the pregnancy will be maintained. A woman who has had the procedure should be aware that any signs of impending miscarriage, such as contractions or bleeding, mean that she must *immediately* get to the hospital. There can be serious consequences during labor if the circular suture is not released. If the pregnancy has proceeded to term, either the purse string is cut for vaginal delivery or a cesarean section is performed.

The Pap Test for Cervical Cancer

In 1928, George Papanicolaou, an American scientist, first described the use of the vaginal smear for the diagnosis of early genital cancer. His special staining technique for cervical and vaginal cells forms the basis of the Pap smear, a test that should be performed at regular intervals on every woman. Because of this test, there has been a steady decrease in the number of deaths from cervical cancer; it is now one-third the rate of 40 years ago.

To perform the test, cells from the squamocolumnar junction and the endocervical canal are aspirated with a glass pipette, or scraped off with a cotton-tipped applicator, wooden spatula, or plastic brush and smeared onto a glass slide. The smear is immediately "fixed" to prevent deterioration of the cells by spraying with a commercial fixative or by dropping the slide into 95% ethyl alcohol solution. The cells are later stained and examined microscopically for malignant changes by a cytologist or a cytotechnologist, experts in cell analyses. The technique of the physician in collecting the sample and preparing the smear is as important as the interpretation of the cytology laboratory in obtaining accurate results.

The following is the classification used for reporting the results of the smears:

Satisfactory/within normal limits

Atypical squamous cells of undetermined significance (ASCUS, recommended for follow-up specifying type of further investigation)

Low-grade squamous intraepithelial lesion (LGSIL) encompassing (1) changes associated with HPV, (2) mild (slight) dysplasia/cervical intraepithelial dysplasia Grade I (CIN I)

High-grade squamous intraepithelial lesion (HGSIL), encompassing (1) moderate dysplasia/CIN II, (2) severe dysplasia/CIN III, or (3) carcinoma in situ/CIN III

Squamous cell carcinoma

Cervical Cancer

The report of an abnormal Pap test would understandably frighten any woman, but it does not necessarily mean that she has cervical cancer. It indicates only that some of the cells shed from the epithelium of the cervix or endocervical canal are atypical and that there should be further investigation. If she has been having annual tests, a positive smear more than likely means that a possible premalignant condition has been uncovered. It can be treated and cured, making certain that further development to cancer cannot take place.

The Pap test is the best kind of preventive medicine; if all women were screened, deaths from invasive cancer of the cervix could be completely prevented. For many reasons, based on social, political, and economic issues that make adequate health maintenance unavailable to large segments of the population, relatively few American women are being routinely screened by Pap tests. The incidence of cervical cancer is higher in low-income groups, and there is a higher rate among smokers, and women of color than among whites. The disease is rare among nuns, virgins, and lesbians, and it is accepted that there is a direct relationship between sexual activity and cancer of the cervix, with a growing body of evidence pointing to human papillomavirus as the link.

Cytological screening could eliminate further mortality from cervical cancer since the disease in its invasive or life-threatening form does not just suddenly appear out of nowhere. There is every indication that true cancer of the cervix, a malignancy that has spread, may take 10 or more years to develop. The cancer first exists as a mild abnormality of atypical cells, which progresses through a series of intermediate stages, each more atypical than the last. Some of these early stages have the ability to regress to normal or, in a number of instances, may remain stable without further progression for an indefinite period. Even if untreated, an area of abnormality does not inevitably go ahead and become cancerous. The Pap test, however, picks up the early changes from the normal when they are preclinical and preinvasive, and the possible evolution to cancer can be stopped.

How frequently should Pap smears be taken? For many years all women were told to have an annual Pap smear, but the most recent recommendation of the American Cancer Society is that all women who are or have been sexually active or who have reached the age of 18 years should have an annual Pap test and pelvic examination. After a woman has had three or more consecutive satisfactory normal annual examinations, the Pap test can be performed less frequently at the discretion of her physician. This recommendation has been adopted by the National Cancer Institute, the American Medical Association, and the American College of Obstetricians and Gynecologists. The latter group also recommends annual Pap smears for women who are at high risk for cervical cancer. A high-risk woman would be one who is a cigarette smoker (there is a strong relationship between smoking and cervical cancer), has had more than two sexual partners, or who began having sex before age 20. This is consistent with the epidemiological evidence associating cervical cancer with a sexually transmitted virus. Low risk is defined as women who are celibate or in a mutually monogamous relationship, are nonsmokers, or have had a total hysterectomy for benign disease. Many health professionals still believe in an annual Pap test for all women, since the majority of women are likely to have begun sexual activity before age 20 and have had two sex partners. An individual woman's decision on the frequency of her Pap smears should take into account her own risk status for cervical cancer. Of course, many women in a low-risk group will continue to have an annual relatively inexpensive Pap smear anyway in conjunction with their yearly breast and pelvic examination.

Most cancer of the cervix begins in the transformation zone of the squamocolumnar junction, where the cells have the ability to differentiate into squamous or columnar cells. More than 90% of cervical cancer is squamous cell carcinoma on the outside of the cervix; the rest are adenocarcinomas or malignancies of the glandular columnar cells of the endocervical canal. The natural progression of a squamous cell carcinoma is believed to be as follows:

Normal squamous epithelium $\longrightarrow$

cervical intraepithelial neoplasia (CIN)

dysplasia $\longrightarrow$ carcinoma in situ
Grade 1 $\longrightarrow$ (mild) Grade 2 (moderate) $\longrightarrow$
Grade 3 (severe)
$\downarrow$
microinvasive cancer
$\downarrow$
invasive cancer

Cervical intraepithelial neoplasia (CIN) is the first abnormality in the normal squamous epithelium of the vaginal cervix that may possibly evolve into invasive cancer. It means that there are atypical cells starting in the lowermost layer of the epithelium and extending to the upper layers of the epithelium and that the cellular arrangement is no longer orderly. The nuclei are enlarged and stain darkly, and some cells are multinucleated. According to the numbers of atypical cells, CIN is characterized as very mild or mild (CIN-I or Grade 1) dysplasia, moderate (CIN-II or Grade 2) dysplasia, and severe (CIN-III or Grade 3) dysplasia and carcinoma in situ, depending upon how much of the epithelium is involved in the proliferation of the abnormal cells. Cases of dysplasia may regress and return to normal epithelium, but the likelihood of regression is decreased as the amount of atypical cells increases; that is, severe dysplasia has a greater malignant potential than mild to moderate dysplasia.

Carcinoma in situ (CIS), literally cancer-in-place, is the next stage in progression. While the malignant nuclear and cytoplasmic changes do not differ that much qualitatively from those in dysplasia, in carcinoma in situ, the entire thickness of the epithelial cell layer is involved. This stage is still a superficial condition, considered pre- or noninvasive because the abnormality has not broken through the epithelium into the connective tissue or stroma lying underneath. It has been widely accepted, although there is little direct evidence, that if cases of carcinoma in situ are left untreated, many of them will progress to invasive cancer within 10 years. Carcinoma in situ has, therefore, long been considered the "intraepithelial neoplasm." Once diagnosed, carcinoma in situ has generally been treated by hysterectomy with removal of the cervix, unless the woman still wants to have children, when a temporary lesser procedure called *conization* is used. In contrast, a diagnosis of dysplasia may be treated with cautery, conization, laser beam therapy, or sometimes ignored. Many clinicians, cytologists, and histopathologists have argued that overdiagnosis and overtreatment are as bad as underdiagnosis and undertreatment—that the standard practice of surgical removal of the uterus when atypical cell changes involve five or six cell layers of the epithelium, but leaving the uterus intact when the atypical occurs in only two or three cell layers should be reexamined. More current thinking supports the concept that dysplasia and carcinoma in situ are part of a disease continuum, beginning with a mild abnormality and ending with invasive carcinoma and extending over a whole spectrum of changes. All degrees of dysplasia and carcinoma in situ are currently referred to as cervical intraepithelial neoplasia (CIN), with the implication that once CIN is diagnosed, there is the capability for progression to invasion if it is untreated. Each case, however, should be considered individually, and the most suitable treatment based on the severity of the abnormality determined by several diagnostic methods, the age of the woman, and whether or not she wants any or more children.

An abnormal Pap test, then, may mean any phase in the transition from normal cervical epithelium to a true cancer that has spread beyond the cervix. Further investigation by tissue biopsy is necessary.

Because it is not unusual for no visible difference to exist between a normal cervix and one with CIN, colposcopy or the Schiller test is utilized to aid in defining the suspicious area that should be biopsied after a positive Pap smear report. The Schiller test is based on the fact that normal cervical epithelium cells contain glycogen and will stain dark brown when painted with a 3% potassium iodide solution. Abnormal cells do not store glycogen and will, therefore, remain unstained. A pinching forceps is used to take a punch biopsy of the abnormal area—a "bite" of tissue that is then prepared for microscopic examination. If the histological or tissue examination indicates only a mild dysplasia, the area is treated by cautery or cryosurgery and there is frequent follow-up by Pap smears. When the site for biopsy has been directed by colposcopy, it is possible that the entire cervical lesion has been removed, and there is now no further treatment necessary.

If the pathologist's diagnosis is that the biopsy has revealed severe dysplasia, most doctors will then perform a conization, or cone biopsy. In this procedure, carried out in a hospital with the woman under general anesthesia, a cone-shaped piece of tissue is removed from the cervix with a scalpel.

The operation is apt to be a bloody one and is associated with a number of postoperative complications, unless the cone is shallow, which may not provide the pathologist with enough tissue to rule out invasive cancer. When the cone is deep and extends up into the endocervical canal, damage to the internal os and the canal itself is not uncommon. The subsequent scarring can threaten a woman's ability to conceive and deliver a child. The most common method of investigating an abnormal Pap smear, however, is by conization (Figure 9–7).

Physicians who are trained in the use of the colposcope, which magnifies up to 20 times, or colpomicroscope, which magnifies up to 180 times, believe that conization is too extreme to be used for diagnosis purposes. They claim that in 90% of the cases in which there are visible cervical lesions, the entire extent of the abnormality can be seen with the colposcope, and invasive cancer can be ruled out. The lesion can then be removed in the doctor's office by electrocautery, cryosurgery, or laser beam painlessly without the use of anesthesia. Like a cone biopsy, these lesser approaches can also prevent the development of invasive disease but without endangering a woman's fertility.

When carcinoma in situ has been diagnosed, there are the usual differences of opinion concerning the most appropriate way of treating it. Women should be aware that a body of evidence and a belief among many clinicians exists that hysterectomy is rarely indicated for carcinoma in situ. Several studies have found the results of conization to be as effective as hysterectomy in preventing invasive cancer from developing in the cervix or elsewhere. There are proponents of even more conservative outpatient procedures—electrocautery, cryosurgery, and laser therapy. Carbon dioxide laser surgery is a newer method of treating CIN that has many advocates. Laser is an acronym for *light amplification by stimulated emission of radiation*. CO_2 laser refers to the production of energy in the form of

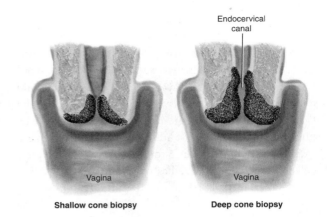

Figure 9–7 Cone biopsy. The shaded area represents the extent of the cone. The procedure requires a general anesthetic and carries a 10% postoperative complication rate. Hemorrhage is a common problem after deep conizations.

an infrared light beam that literally vaporizes cells by turning their intracellular water to steam. Since the laser instrument is used in conjunction with an operating microscope, the beam of heat, highly accurate and controllable, is said to provide a preciseness of tissue excision greater than that of a surgical scalpel. Laser surgery is considerably more expensive than cautery or cryosurgery. Another method is the loop electrosurgical excision procedure (LEEP), which utilizes a low-voltage high-frequency radio wave run through a thin wire loop. After the lesion is identified by colposcopy, LEEP allows the abnormal tissue to be excised as a button-shaped specimen rather than to be vaporized by a laser beam. The intact tissue can also serve as the biopsy specimen that can be sent to the laboratory for examination for invasive cancer.

If a woman gets a diagnosis of preinvasive carcinoma and a hysterectomy has been advised, there is plenty of time in which to get a second, or even a third, opinion. It takes an estimated 10 years for an untreated lesion, diagnosed as cervical carcinoma in situ, to progress to clinical invasion. There is some evidence that implies that only 10% of carcinoma in situ actually develop into invasive cancer. Other authorities are equally adamant in their belief that as many as

60%–70% of in situ cancers become invasive. Many clinicians are convinced that the recurrence rate for subsequent disease is lower when the uterus is removed.

Invasive Cancer of the Cervix

True cancer of the cervix that has gone further than the epithelium is staged as follows:

Stage 1   Strictly limited to the cervix (Stage Ia is for cases of microscopic invasion)

Stage 2   Spread to beyond the cervix, the upper two-thirds of the vagina, but not to the lateral pelvic walls

Stage 3   Has extended to either lateral pelvic wall and the lower third of the vagina

Stage 4   Involves the urinary bladder and/or the rectum or has metastasized beyond the true pelvis

Invasive cancer has been most commonly treated by radiation therapy, either externally by a supervoltage x-ray or cobalt source and/or internally by way of a radium implant inserted into the cervical canal. In some cases, a radical hysterectomy, removing the uterus, upper part of the vagina, all the adjacent tissues, and the lymph nodes, is performed. Pelvic exenteration, an even more extensive operation, which removes the bladder and the rectum, is used in late stages of the disease or when irradiation has failed.

Early in 1999, the National Cancer Institute released a clinical statement for physicians announcing that the results of five randomized Phase III trials indicated that concurrent chemotherapy along with radiation conferred an overall survival advantage in women with advanced cervical cancer. The benefit of such chemoradiation was so apparent that the NCI not only allowed an early release of the results but also closed off the radiation-only part of an ongoing study in which women had been enrolled. As mentioned previously, however, the results of therapy for cervical intraepithelial neoplasia are virtually 100% effective.

The best treatment for invasive cancer of the cervix is prevention—by regular Pap smears.

DES MOTHERS AND CHILDREN

Diethylstilbestrol (DES) is a nonsteroid synthetic estrogen that has estrogenic properties, is effective when taken orally, and is less expensive than the real thing. First synthesized in 1936, the drug was released for clinical use in the United States in 1941 and gained immediate popularity. It was used as replacement therapy in the postmenopause in the management of dysfunctional uterine bleeding, and frequently to "dry up" the breasts of women who did not want to nurse after delivery. In the late 1940s and for the following 2 decades, DES was widely prescribed for the treatment and prevention of habitual and threatened miscarriage and to prevent late complications of pregnancy that might be hazardous to the mother and fetus. Its use in pregnant women is a prime example of an increasingly frequent medical phenomenon—the therapeutic time bomb. A drug or a particular form of therapy, for example, x-rays, is generally used in accordance with accepted medical practice and believed to be safe and free of adverse effects. Many years later, the administration of the drug or therapy is discovered to have been a mistake—and often a tragic one.

DES and Cancer

In the late 1960s, eight cases of vaginal clear cell adenocarcinoma, a very rare type of cancer, were found in Boston among adolescent girls. Vaginal cancer is infrequent, making up less than 2% of all genital cancers. When it does occur, it is usually in women over 50, and most often of the squamous cell variety. Because of the unusual circumstances, further investigation took place. It was determined that the mothers of seven of these girls with vaginal cancer had received DES to prevent miscarriage during the first weeks of pregnancy, and the dose had been steadily increased during the remainder of the pregnancy.

Arthur L. Herbst, the physician at the Harvard Medical School who discovered the relationship between prenatal exposure to DES and clear cell adenocarcinoma (CCA), set up a national clearinghouse, the Registry for Research on Hormonal Transplacental Carcinogenesis (also called the Herbst Registry)★ to study CCA and other types of genital cancers. By 1997, approximately 695 cases of CCA with about 15% mortality had been reported to the Registry. Sixty percent of those cases were associated with prenatal exposure to DES. Most often the cancers developed in young women aged 15–27 years, but the upper age limit for the development of CCA is currently unknown and the average age of diagnosis appears to be rising. In the past decade, several DES daughters in their 40s have developed CCA, indicating that there is no specific age after which the risk is over. Analysis of the Registry cases suggests that CCA is more likely to develop if the daughter was prenatally exposed to DES prior to the 12th week of pregnancy, she was born in the fall of the year, and the mother had a history of at least one previous miscarriage (Herbst et al., 1986). On the basis of the data collected to date, it would appear that the risk of CCA developing in an exposed woman is low; it is currently estimated at 1 in 1,000. If CCA is caught early (Stage I), survival rates have been reported as 92% at 5 years and 88% at 10 years by the Registry. Women with Stage II vaginal clear cell adenocarcinomas have a survival rate of 83% and 62%, respectively, (Senekjian et al., 1987; Senekjian, Frey, Stone, & Herbst, 1988). The con-

sumer group DES Action USA, however, reported cases of recurrence and subsequent deaths from cancer some 8–20 years after the initial diagnosis of CCA. These are anecdotal incidents and as yet there is no published data on the unusually late recurrences.

DES and Adenosis

Fortunately, the most common abnormality related to DES exposure is not cancer but a benign condition of the vaginal epithelium called *adenosis*. In vaginal adenosis, the junction of the columnar glandular epithelium of the endocervical canal with the squamous epithelium of the cervix—the so-called transformation zone—occurs not just around the external os where it belongs but extends over the whole vaginal portion of the cervix and sometimes involves almost the entire vagina. The incidence of vaginal adenosis as well as such other vaginal or cervical irregularities as abnormal transverse cervical or vaginal ridges (variously described as cockscomb cervix, cervical hood, pseudopolyp cervix) is about 35% according to Herbst, but more than 90% according to Stafl and Mattingly (1974). These investigators, after studying 280 DES daughters, were concerned about the abnormal colposcopic findings in the cervices and vaginas of more than 90% of the women. Pointing out that the incidence of squamous cell carcinoma of the vagina and cervix is known to be greatly increased in the presence of such atypical colposcopic lesions, they maintained that the major clinical danger from prenatal exposure to DES was not the development of clear cell adenocarcinoma, which infrequently occurs, but rather the subsequent progression of the abnormalities to squamous cell cervical and vaginal cancer when the exposed girls reached middle age. The researchers predicted an increase in the occurrence of cervical cancer in DES daughters, placing their risk at 10–20 times greater than that for prenatally DES-unexposed women. Studies in the early 1980s of whether cervical cancer was more prevalent in DES daughters were not definitive, probably because not enough time had elapsed and insufficient data had been collected. Later

---

★Current address is Department of Obstetrics and Gynecology, University of Chicago, 5841 S. Maryland Avenue, MC 2050, Chicago, IL 60637. Phone 773-702-6671. For related resource information, women can call the National Cancer Institute, 800-4-CANCER for DES publications; DES Action USA, 800-DES-9288, a nonprofit national consumer organization representing exposed mothers and children and dedicated to informing the public about DES; or the DES Cancer Network, 800-DESNET4, a nonprofit support organization made up of women who have had CCA.

it became evident that Stafl and Mattingly were right in their predictions of increased risk. Robboy and coworkers in 1984 studied nearly 4,000 DES-exposed women. In comparing the exposed women with unexposed matched control women, the researchers found that the incidence of CIN and CIS was increased 2–4 times in the DES-exposed group. Virtually no cases of precancerous conditions occurred in DES-exposed virgins, however, reaffirming that STDs also play a role in the development of the disease. The authors suggested that perhaps exposure causes changes in the vaginal and cervical epithelium that may result in greater susceptibility to the risk factors of early coitus and multiple partners. Although a later investigation by Ben-Baruch in Israel (1991) found that abnormal cervical cytology and colposcopic findings were consistently higher in a small sample of Israeli women who are otherwise at low risk for development of cervical neoplasia, a subsequent study of cancer incidence other than CCA in a large cohort of DES-exposed daughters compared with unexposed women found that, at least to the date of the study, there was no increased risk of cancer in other sites. Because the exposed daughters were, on average, only 38 years at the time of the study, the authors cautioned that continued follow-up is necessary, particularly during the menopausal years (Hatch et al., 1998).

DES and Other Complications

Another concern raised by several researchers was the possibility of a relationship between prenatal exposure to DES and subsequent ovarian cancer (Schmidt & Fowler, 1982; Walker et al., 1988). Whether these findings are significant will also be substantiated with time. What is clear, however, is that the more DES-exposed progeny were studied, the more problems became apparent. The following physiological and structural abnormalities have been demonstrated in DES daughters: uterine abnormalities; distortions of the fallopian tubes; menstrual irregularities; infertility; a greater incidence of pelvic adhesions and benign ovarian cysts; abnormal healing response to cautery, cryosurgery, or

other minor outpatient procedures; hirsutism or increased facial hair; higher male hormone levels; and a generalized dysfunction of the hypthalamic-pituitary-ovarian axis (Schmidt & Fowler, 1982; Fowler et al., 1981; Peress, Tsai, Mathur, & Williamson, 1982; Senekjian, Potkul, Frey, & Herbst, 1988).

The risks and the abnormalities as a result of DES exposure are not limited only to the female offspring. DES-exposed sons have been found to have lower ejaculate volume, more abnormal sperm, and a lower sperm count. Also reported are a significantly higher incidence of cysts in the epididymis, small penis (microphallus), undescended testes (cryptorchidism), underdeveloped testes (testicular hypoplasia), other urogenital abnormalities, and a possible greater incidence of testicular cancer (Bibbo et al., 1977; Gill, Schumacher, & Bibbo, 1976; Beral & Colwell, 1981; Moss et al., 1986; Gershman & Stolley, 1988). Beral and her colleagues further found that a greater proportion of hormone-exposed men were either not married or not living with a woman, suggesting that interference with normal sexual function is a not uncommon aftermath to DES exposure in males.

The DES mothers, the women who were given the drug to protect their pregnancies from miscarriage, have also been reported to suffer adverse effects. In 1978, Marluce Bibbo and her coworkers found that women who had been exposed to a maximum of 12 g of DES had a slight excess of breast cancer, 4.6%, compared with a control group of women who had not taken DES during pregnancy, in whom the occurrence of breast cancer was 3.1%. This was not considered to be statistically significant, although there were more deaths from breast cancer among the exposed group, due in part to the early onset of the disease. There was also a slightly increased incidence of other endocrine-related cancers (ovary, endometrium, cervix, colon) in the exposed mothers, with an excess number of deaths occurring in the same order of magnitude as for breast cancer. Beral and Colwell's follow-up study of DES mothers (1980) found 4 cases of breast cancer in 80 exposed women and none in 76 nonexposed women. Brian and coworkers, however, found no association between DES exposure and breast cancer in their study (1980). Results of a 1984 study (Greenberg et al.) clearly pointed to an increased risk of breast cancer later in life when a woman is exposed to DES during pregnancy. The risk became greater in women over 60 years of age but was not as great as that associated with a family history of breast cancer. Currently, there is no conclusive evidence that DES-exposed mothers experience an increased risk of breast cancer. The guidelines for mammographic screening and breast examination in exposed mothers are the same as for unexposed women.

The further discovery that the health risk spans three generations, that not only the women who took the drug and their sons and daughters, but possibly their grandchildren may be affected, is perhaps a not unexpected and tragic continuation of the DES story. The many anatomical abnormalities and distortions of the upper and lower reproductive tract in DES daughters are necessarily associated with altered function. Women whose mothers took DES during pregnancy 30 years ago may have greater difficulty in delivering a healthy, viable baby of their own. A number of studies have shown that DES daughters have a higher proportion of spontaneous abortions, incompetent cervix, ectopic pregnancy, premature delivery, and greater infant mortality (Veridiano, Delke, Rogers, & Tancer, 1981; Herbst et al., 1981; Ben-Baruch, Menczer, Mashiach, & Seer, 1981; Stillman, 1982; Senekjian et al., 1988; Herbst, Senekjian, & Frey, 1989).

The greatest use of DES during pregnancy was in the 1950s when an estimated 4%–7% of all pregnant women in the United States received it. A popular dose schedule was to administer 2.5 mg daily during or before the 6th week of pregnancy, increase to 5 mg by the 7th week, and to increase by 5 mg every other week until the 15th week when 25 mg was given. Every month thereafter, the dosage was increased by 25 mg until a maximum dose of 150 mg per day was given by the 35th week of pregnancy. As early as 1953 and during the 1960s, there were published reports doubting the therapeutic value of DES during pregnancy. A decline in its use resulted, but it was still pre-scribed by many doctors, and in some areas of the country, the peak prescribing occurred during the middle 1960s. It was not banned by the FDA for use during pregnancy until November 1971. By then an estimated total of 5 million American women had taken DES. No one born before 1941 could possibly have been exposed to DES, but it is obvious that there are hundreds of thousands of DES offspring.

It is evident that both the sons and the daughters of women who took DES, as well as the women themselves, should be alerted to the need for periodic and frequent examinations to detect possible abnormalities at as early a stage as possible. The problem is, who are all the DES offspring and the several million mothers? Many woman who took DES do not remember taking it or were not aware or informed that it was given to them. Obviously, therefore, not every woman or man is in a position to know or to find out whether she or he has a history of exposure to DES in utero. Most of the knowledge concerning the DES hazards was originally provided through the activity of Dr. Sidney Wolfe, director of the Washington-based Health Research Group, and by cancer epidemiologist Kay Weiss. A number of widely read books by Gena Corea, Barbara and Gideon Seaman, Cynthia Orenberg, and others covered the complete DES story in detail. The entire population at risk, however, could not be reached by books and magazine articles dealing with women's health. Wolfe called for governmental action to require follow-up studies by medical centers that supplied DES to pregnant women and to request that all private physicians search their files for DES-exposed women and notify them. The NCI, by way of a Task Force Summary Report issued in 1978, recommended that all women who received DES in pregnancy, as well as their exposed offspring, be informed of their risk by a public information campaign and that individuals be notified by their private physicians. No federal funds were provided for implementation of these recommendations, however, and until recently there have been no large-scale efforts by government agencies, by the doctors who prescribed the drug, or by the pharmaceutical companies who profited by its sales to inform individuals that they may be at increased risk for genital abnormalities and the development of cancer. In 1997, however, Congress passed legislation authorizing DES research until the year 2003 and establishing a National DES Education Program under the authority of the Secretary of the Department of Health and Human Services. Now major research concerns—what is the actual impact on DES sons, whether DES-exposed women should take estrogen replacement therapy, is there a genetic effect on the third generation—can be addressed. Because the DES Education and Research Amendments bill was attached to the women's health bill covering breast and cervical cancer research, the funding for implementation is available.

The DES issue has become an ongoing medicolegal morass. After a number of successful class action and individual suits against the pharmaceutical firms that manufactured the drug for injuries arising from administration of DES, thousands of lawsuits were filed by DES daughters. The New York courts have allowed women to sue individual drug companies such as Eli Lilly and Company, the largest DES manufacturer, under the legal principle of "joint-enterprise liability" of all DES producers, regardless of the actual manufacturer. The most recent suits are attempting to continue the legal battle against the manufacturers of DES by representing the third generation, children who were not directly exposed to the drug themselves but whose grandmothers took the drug while pregnant. In one case in Maryland, the parents of a 13-year-old girl who died of CCA filed suit against Lilly, charging that the girl's father was exposed. Another suit in New York is on behalf of a 9-year-old with severe cerebral palsy whose injuries as a result of a premature birth were related, the parents claim, to DES her grandmother took 30 years ago.

Clearly, continued DES research is needed. As more DES mothers become postmenopausal, and the sons and daughters move into middle age, it is important to determine the long-term effects of DES exposure, which are still unknown, to recognize potential new problems that may appear, and to find out whether a third generation effect on the offspring of DES-exposed parents exists.

The health of millions of young men and women is at risk through no fault of their own but because their mothers were given DES. Routine physical examinations can detect and reduce the consequences of their exposure, but evidently the full responsibility and the major expense that accompany the avoidance of these medically induced abnormalities are to be borne by the DES sons and daughters and their mothers. Any woman who knows or suspects that she was given DES or a chemically related substance while pregnant with her son or daughter must have frequent physical examinations herself. Unless their mothers have assured them that there was no pill taking during pregnancy for a possible miscarriage or late complication of pregnancy, men and women born after 1941 can logically presume that they may have been prenatally exposed to diethylstilbestrol. For males, the preliminary data suggest that functional abnormalities that could interfere with fertility may be a problem, but future investigations are necessary. DES exposure before birth in young women is likely to be revealed by vaginal adenosis and cervical abnormalities. Gynecological examinations have to be more extensive than usual when there is a presumed or definite history of prenatal DES exposure. The Schiller test or a colposcopic examination has to be made. It is also necessary that a Pap smear from all quadrants of the vagina be taken separately from a smear of the cervix.

The biological effect of DES in creating an increased risk of cancer in both mothers and their daughters is not known. One clue may be the evidence from mouse studies that DES evidently suppresses the activity of the Wnt-7a gene that is important in the normal development of the male and female mouse reproductive tracts (Miller, Degenhardt, & Sassoon, 1998). Additional investigations to determine how DES works are important even though it has not been taken by women for more than 30 years because of other estrogenlike compounds that exist in the environment or are prescribed for women. It may be that DES, in similar fashion to other estrogens, lays the groundwork for the possibility of future malignant changes. Perhaps DES reacts with other factors to result in the development of cancer at a later time or acts to speed up the onset of cancer. It may be possible that later exposure to more exogenous estrogen could be a critical and triggering factor. For this reason, the identification of DES-exposed women and men is doubly important. They need to have this information, not only so that they can obtain what could be lifesaving examinations on a regular basis, but so that they can avoid any additional ingestion of estrogen. Because of the hormones added to the food supply, this might be difficult.

When steroid hormones are added to farm animal and poultry feed, they accelerate growth. Without these growth hormones, it takes 30 more days and 500 more pounds of feed to produce a 1,000-lb steer. Obviously, meat producers can get livestock to market earlier and save feed by using hormones, and they maintain that without them, the cost of production would be raised by 70%–100%. The hormone given to cattle as a feed additive or as a pellet implant for many years was DES. After the evidence linking DES to cancer, and because the Delany clause of the Food, Drug and Cosmetic Act prohibits the use of any food additive known to be carcinogenic, the use of DES was banned by the FDA in the early 1970s and finally implemented in 1979, although cattle on hundreds of feedlots in many states were still being illegally treated with DES as late as 1983. Currently, there are six steroid growth hormones approved by the FDA for use in cattle: testosterone, estradiol, progesterone, trenbolone acetate, melengestrol acetate, and zeranol. Government regulations allow hormone-containing capsules to be implanted in the ear, far from the edible parts of the animal. If the implants are done correctly, they are safe, says the FDA, and any residues of hormones remaining in the beef can be safely ingested. To what extent all meat producers use the proper procedures is unknown. Also unknown are the possible effects of ingestion of even minimal amounts of steroids when there has been initial exposure as in DES offspring. It could be that, from a nutritional point of view, the high saturated fat content of meat is more of a health hazard than the tiny amount of hormones, but Europeans apparently have major concerns about the way cattle are raised in the United States. In 1989, the 12-nation European Union banned all imports of U.S. beef, citing the health risk posed by treatment with hormones. As of this writing, the European Union has refused to lift the ban.

Tumors of the Uterus

The most common gynecological tumors are benign masses of muscle and connective tissue in the uterus called **fibroids** or *leiomyomas*. Their true incidence is unknown, but there are estimates that they occur in anywhere from 20%–50% of women after the age of 35. They are very rare before menarche and after menopause, and estrogen is evidently important in their development. Estrogen definitely appears to stimulate their growth. Genetic factors, too, may play a role in their incidence. Fibroids are found somewhat more frequently in Jewish women, and it is well recognized that for no known physiological reason, they occur much more commonly, appear earlier, and grow more rapidly in black women.

Fibroids

Fibroids may be single or multiple; they may be microscopic in size, or they may grow to be enormous. The largest one ever reported in the medical literature was in 1888—it weighed 144 lb! Although tumors of 40–50 lb are still occasionally seen, earlier and better diagnosis has made excessively huge ones quite uncommon in the United States. Most of them average about 4–5 cm in diameter. They are round, smooth, quite firm in consistency, and when they are cut open, display pinkish white whorls and lines of muscle bundles.

The name, fibroids, implies that the tumors originate in fibrous connective tissue. Although they do contain varying amounts of fibrous elements, they are actually composed of smooth muscle cells and are more appropriately called myomas or leiomyomas (from *leios,* smooth, and *myos,* muscle). Depending on their location in the uterus, fibroids are classified as intramural, submucous, and subserous. Intramural are the most common and are found in the center of the uterine muscular wall. If they are small, they are frequently asymptomatic. Submucous fibroids grow between the endometrial lining and the uterine muscle. They may project into the uterine cavity and distort and stretch the endometrium. The subsequent increase in the surface of the endometrial lining may result in excessive menstrual bleeding. Submucosal fibroids may also be a cause of habitual miscarriage because they can interfere with the anchoring site of the placenta. Subserous tumors develop between the uterine wall and the external peritoneal covering or serosa. Because they have so much space in which to grow, these fibroids may attain sizes many times greater than that of the uterus itself. They also have a tendency to become pedunculated, that is, attached by a stalk or pedicle to the uterus. Occasionally, subserosal pedunculated fibroids can even become totally separated from the uterus and move away from it, becoming known as parasitic or wandering fibroids.

The most frequent reason for hysterectomy is a diagnosis of fibroids. Just because fibroids are discovered on bimanual pelvic examination, however, does not mean that they necessarily have to be treated. The vast majority of small fibroids are symptomless, grow very slowly, and have to be watched only from time to time. If they are not showing any evidence of rapid growth and are not causing any trouble, they are best left alone. Large fibroids may encroach on the bladder or rectum and cause pressure symptoms, such as urinary frequency, constipation, or sensations of abdominal fullness. Fibroids have also been shown to increase uterine contractility, suggesting a reason for the menstrual pain and irregularity that some women have. But if a woman is close to menopause and the symptoms are those she can live with, the discomfort will disappear with the climacteric as the tumor or tumors stop growing and diminish in size (unless, of course, she is on estrogen replacement therapy). The risk of fibroids becoming malignant is very small—less than 0.3%—but the operative mortality risk of hysterectomy in the average American hospital is 1%.

In younger women, the presence of fibroids, even if they produce no symptoms, may be associated with infertility problems if they obstruct the opening of the fallopian tubes. If pregnancy does occur, small fibroids generally do not affect the course of the pregnancy. Conversely, neither does pregnancy affect the fibroids. If the fibroids are large, however, they may interfere with implantation and cause spontaneous abortion, or block the birth canal to prevent vaginal delivery. Myomectomy, the removal of only the fibroids and not the entire uterus, is performed when a woman is younger than her late 30s and wants to bear a child. The operation is technically more difficult than hysterectomy, and the fibroids may recur at a later date. The probability of pregnancy following myomectomy has been estimated as between 40%–50%, and it is generally necessary to deliver a baby by a cesarean section to avoid rupture of the uterus at the site of the incision for myomectomy. When fibroids are present in younger women, they should be aware that oral contraceptives may cause more rapid growth of the tumors.

When a woman is over 40, has a fibroid larger than a grapefruit with an excessively rapid growth rate, has severe pain, pressure, or bleeding, and nonsurgical treatment for the symptoms has been unsuccessful, hysterectomy, performed abdominally or vaginally, is the most specific form of treatment. Anyone who has virtually hemorrhaged her way through painful monthly periods that last for 9 days or longer or that occur more frequently than every 21 days and have made her anemic, is not going to be surprised to find out that a hysterectomy is indicated. She will be relieved to discover that the cause is benign and not malignant and recognizes that there is little chance that the procedure is being performed unnecessarily. If, on the other hand, a woman is advised that she needs a hysterectomy for asymptomatic or very mild symptoms of fibroids, a second opinion is mandatory.

Total hysterectomy, which removes the cervix as well as the uterus has today almost completely replaced the subtotal or supra-cervical operation. The majority of doctors advocate oophorectomy if the woman is 40 or older at the time of hysterectomy. The assumption is that the ovaries will stop functioning in a few years anyway and there is a 1% risk of ovarian cancer in women over the age of 40. Ovarian cancer undeniably is difficult to diagnose and even more difficult to cure. On the other hand, prophylactic removal of the ovaries creates a surgical menopause, and hormone replacement therapy may be required. It has been noted that surgical castration occurring 10 years or more before expected menopause contributes to the increased incidence of coronary heart disease, atherosclerosis, and osteoporosis. There has also been the suggestion that the ovaries may continue to function for many years after menopause. So even if removal is recommended by her physician, a woman still has to weigh the advantages and disadvantages to her, and make her own decision. Other organs of the body, for example, the prostate gland, pose an even greater risk for the development of cancer but are not routinely removed. Whether male physicians would be as definitive about taking them out if the word "testes" were substituted for "ovaries" is conjectural.

Cancer of the Uterus

More than 90% of uterine cancer is **carcinoma** of the endometrial lining. It is primarily a disease of older women, occurring postmenopausally at an average age of 55. Only a small percentage of cases occur in women under the age of 40 and there has been the suggestion that risk factors for the disease are related directly or indirectly to long-term or excessive estrogen stimulation. The number of new cases of endometrial cancer annually had been increasing since the 1950s, peaked in 1975, and declined through the 1980s, perhaps not coincidentally with the decrease in the prescribing of estrogen replacement therapy for postmenopausal women. The overall mortality rate as a result of endometrial cancer is about 3,000 per year,

1.9 deaths per 100,000 women. Actually, the death rate is distributed as 1.8 per 100,000 white women and 3.0 per 100,000 black women, which probably indicates more about health care access and treatment than about the behavior of the cancer in African-Americans. Authorities are still cautious about making a case for estrogen as the cause of endometrial cancer, but many investigators believe it to be an associated factor. It is recognized that when estrogenic stimulation of the endometrium is prolonged and unopposed by progesterone, the risk of the disease increases. Women who, for various reasons, do not ovulate (no progesterone is produced) or who have estrogen-producing ovarian tumors have a greater incidence of uterine cancer. Also with an underlying hormonal basis, so do white women of high socioeconomic status who are more than 30% overweight, have not had any children, have had a late menopause, diabetes mellitus, high blood pressure, or prolonged estrogen-replacement therapy.

The major initial symptom is abnormal and painless vaginal bleeding. Any episode of bright red bleeding, either scant or moderate in amount, that occurs after menopause should immediately send a woman to her doctor. Just before menopause, irregularity is so common that it is sometimes difficult to distinguish normal from abnormal bleeding. At any age, however, a bloody discharge, intermittent spotting, or steady bleeding that takes place between menstrual periods should be investigated. Abnormal uterine bleeding is very rarely the result of uterine malignancy in a young woman. In the postmenopause, however, it should be regarded with suspicion. Depending on which authority is quoted, bleeding that occurs 6 months after menstruation has stopped indicates that a cancer is present someplace in the genital tract 20%–50% of the time. But because the symptom is such an early sign of the disease and an endometrial cancer tends to be such a slow-growing tumor, the chances of cure are very good if medical advice is sought quickly.

Diagnosis of the cause of abnormal bleeding is made by biopsy of the lining of the uterus. The sample can be taken in the doctor's office with only a local anesthesia to the cervix. In microcurettage, a small strip of endometrium is scraped away with a sharp spoon-shaped instrument called a curette. Larger curettes are used for more generous samples. In suction biopsy, the curette tip is incorporated into a hollow tube inserted into the uterine cavity. When light suction is applied, the tissue sample is drawn out through the tube. Samples can also be taken by "jet-washing," brushing, or scraping cells from the endometrial surface, but these methods are seen as less effective. A Pap smear is also considered unreliable in ruling out endometrial cancer.

A positive diagnosis through endometrial biopsy is conclusive evidence of cancer, but a negative finding does not necessarily exclude it. The carcinoma may have been missed in an area that was not sampled. The most definitive diagnosis is made by the conventional D and C that includes a thorough systematic curettage.

Early endometrial cancer is treated by total hysterectomy plus removal of the fallopian tubes and the ovaries. More extensive carcinoma is generally considered an indication for preoperative radium treatment followed by surgery. When metastases to the vagina, pelvis, and lungs occur, chemotherapy in the form of massive doses of progestins has produced remissions. As in all cancers, increasing the rate of cures depends on early diagnoses. Vaginal bleeding in the post-menopause is a definite warning that could mean malignancy. It should not be ignored by a woman or her doctor.

OVARIAN TUMORS

The ovary is physiologically, normally, and naturally a "cyst-y" kind of organ. Every month between menarche and menopause, follicles develop and become little sacs filled with fluid—actually cysts. One of them, outdistancing all the others, grows to the size of 1.5–2 cm in diameter, bulges on the surface of the ovary, and bursts. The egg is released in a gush of follicular fluid, the large follicle is replaced by a corpus luteum, and all of the other follicular cysts disappear.

Quite commonly and probably due to some alteration in the usual hypothalamic-pituitary-ovarian hormonal axis, a follicle does not ovulate but continues to grow, accumulate fluid, and produce estrogen. More rarely, the corpus luteum may not regress normally but continues to grow and produce progesterone. The hormones secreted by such a functional *follicular cyst* or *corpus luteum cyst* may produce dysfunctional bleeding—delayed onset of menstruation, prolonged menstruation, or perhaps a period every 2 weeks for a month or two. There may be some abdominal pain as a result of pressure from the cyst on the ovarian connective tissue capsule. These retention cysts will spontaneously disappear by fluid absorption or rupture within a month or two and do not have to be treated, by surgery or any other method, unless there is some complication.

Functional follicular and corpus luteum cysts occur frequently, and women are probably seldom aware of their existence. There is no reason to be upset if an enlarged ovary or ovarian cyst is detected on pelvic examination; it can be watched for several months with repeated ultrasonography. A true neoplastic or tumorous growth in the ovary will persist and progressively enlarge, but follicular and corpus luteum cysts will eventually vanish. Occasionally, a retention cyst will rupture through a small blood vessel on the surface of the ovary, producing intraperitoneal bleeding. If the bleeding is scant and spontaneously stops, there may be few symptoms. If the bleeding is extensive, the source can be diagnosed by laparoscopy (the examination of the pelvic cavity by an instrument inserted through a small incision in the abdominal wall). Surgery may then be necessary to control the bleeding and repair the ovary.

Unfortunately, as several authorities have recognized, too many doctors fail to appreciate the fact that the ovaries are normally cystic, and treat persistent follicular and corpus luteum cysts—physiological in origin—by surgical removal. In Max Bloom's words, the large number of ovaries that have been "needlessly incised, resected, bisected, tinkered, punctured, wedged, suspended, and even ablated for no good reason at all . . ." bear silent testimony to that fact.

The unnecessary removal of wedges of ovarian tissue as treatment for polycystic ovary syndrome is an example. This condition, an endocrinological disorder also known as a type of Stein-Leventhal disease, is manifested by a failure of ovulation, large numbers of follicular cysts, enlarged ovaries with thick capsules, excessive androgen production, and amenorrhea. Previously, the therapy for this disease was the removal of up to 50% of the ovarian tissue to decrease the production of androgens and presumably permit ovulation. Today it is believed that there is little indication for doing this type of operation. Any endocrine abnormalities can be corrected with hormonal treatment.

In actuality, cystic ovaries are not ovarian cysts; that is, functional cysts in the ovary are not considered to be *neoplastic,* or new growths. True ovarian neoplasms, both benign and malignant, occur much less often but are far more significant. Growth that is new, a tumor, can increase to a very large size and must always be removed to exclude the possibility of cancer.

Neoplastic tumors of the ovary are classified according to their cellular origin, that is, whether the growth started in the surface epithelium of the ovary, in the germ cells themselves, in the connective tissue stroma, or other miscellaneous cells. There are more than 60 kinds of ovarian tumors, but only the most common will be described.

Benign *serous cystadenomas* form about 20%–25% of all ovarian neoplasms occurring at any age but most often between the ages of 40 and 50. Most of the time a cyst will be found on only one ovary, but they also occur bilaterally in 20%–30% of the cases. A cyst may be very small and hardly palpable, but it may also be large enough to fill up the entire abdomen. Serous cystadenomas contain a clear, watery, protein-rich fluid, yellow in color or chocolate brown as a result of bleeding into the cyst. The type called *papillary serous cystadenomas* have the greatest likelihood for malignant change, and about half of that kind actually are, or potentially will be, cancerous.

Mucinous cystadenomas are filled with a thick, gelatinous, viscous fluid. They can attain an enormous size but become secondarily malignant much less fre-

quently than the serous variety. They are usually unilateral.

Dermoid cysts, or benign cystic teratomas, make up about 20% of benign ovarian tumors. They can occur at any age but are most frequently found between the ages of 18 and 35. Dermoids are a strange kind of growth that contain multiple tissues, which are derivatives of all the three embryonic germ layers. Inside a dermoid are skin, sebaceous and sweat glands, and long strands of hair that bear no relationship to the hair color of the woman with the cyst. Cartilage, bone, and several well-developed teeth are not unusual, and even intestines and thyroid gland have been found. The tumors vary in size but average 6–8 cm in diameter. They very rarely become malignant.

Dermoid cysts have been known since antiquity, and speculations concerning their origin have been many and disputed. One theory holds that a dermoid cyst develops by parthenogenesis, the reproduction of an ovum that has not been fertilized by a sperm. Another postulates that a dermoid is actually a woman's underdeveloped twin. Neither idea is universally accepted.

Dermoid cysts have a tendency to be found in both ovaries. For this reason, at the time of surgical removal of the cyst, the other ovary, even if it appears completely normal, has to be carefully inspected for a very small dermoid.

Malignant Neoplasms of the Ovary

Ovarian cancers are considered the worst of gynecological malignancies, primarily because they sometimes develop slowly and remain silent and symptomless until it is too late. There is no practical and certain way of detecting early cancer of the ovary—Pap smears are virtually useless for this—and it is usually found by chance. The highest incidence occurs in women between 55 and 65. While an ovarian mass could be observed for several months in a younger woman, in the postmenopause any enlargement of the ovaries is suspicious. One larger than 5 cm in diameter is an indication for immediate investigation. Frequently, there are no obvious symptoms until advanced stages. As the tumor enlarges, it may press on surrounding organs and result in constipation, urinary frequency, or vague feelings of abdominal pressure or gastrointestinal discomfort.

Several screening techniques for early detection of ovarian cancer have been developed, but as yet none has proved sensitive, specific enough, or inexpensive enough to be of great value in screening large populations of women. CA-125, for example, is an antigen found in blood serum that becomes elevated in ovarian cancer. It is also increased in other gynecological and nongynecological cancers as well as in a number of benign conditions, including endometriosis and early pregnancy. But a large pilot study in Great Britain by Ian Jacobs and coworkers (1999) found that when an elevated CA-125 is combined with vaginal ultrasound to measure for increased ovarian volume and followed up with continued surveillance, this kind of screening can save lives by detecting cancer early when it is symptomless and confined to the ovaries.

A major hurdle to massive ovarian cancer screening is that, deadly as the disease may be if it has spread beyond the ovaries, only 1 in 2,000 postmenopausal women in Western countries contract it annually, although 15,000 women die of ovarian cancer in the United States each year. For some women, however, frequent screening is more important. Five to 10% of breast and ovarian cancers are associated with two inherited susceptibility genes, BRCA-1 and BRCA-2. The lifetime risk of breast and/or ovarian cancer for a woman who carries a mutated BRCA-1 or BRCA-2 gene is increased, and women should consider getting genetic testing if three or more closely related family members have had either type of cancer. Positive test results are a good reason for more frequent mammograms and ovarian cancer screening.

M. Steven Piver (1989), who started the Family Ovarian Cancer Registry in 1981 at the Roswell Park Cancer Institute in Buffalo, New York, maintains that women with a family history, that is, two or more first-degree relatives who had ovarian cancer, should begin periodic ultrasonography and CA-125 assays in their early 30s. Gilda Radner, the comedian who died in 1988 at the age of 42, was unaware of her family history. She had two, and possibly three, blood relatives who had died of ovarian cancer. In her book, *It's Always Something,* she described how she was sick for 9 months with bloating and abdominal cramps, going from doctor to doctor, before she was finally diagnosed with cancer that had already spread.

Malignancy of the ovary, when found, is always treated by aggressive and radical surgery. Depending on the clinical stage of the disease when detected, surgical treatment may be supplemented by radiation and chemotherapy. Some doctors do exploratory abdominal surgery or "second-look" operations on selected patients to determine the progress of the treatments, particularly after long-term chemotherapy.

Every year, cancer of the ovary kills more women than all the other gynecological malignancies combined. But with early diagnosis and treatment, 85%–95% currently survive 5 years or longer. Once the cancer is advanced, the survival rate falls to 23%. Even in later stages, advances in the use of combination chemotherapy have made a diagnosis of cancer of the ovaries—although no reason for super-optimism—at least not as gloomy as before.

Like breast cancer, ovarian cancer occurs more frequently in highly industrialized countries. Epidemiologists have looked at a number of factors that might be involved as etiological agents—talc, asbestos, coffee ingestion, amount of dietary fat consumed—but the results of studies are still inconclusive. Fathalla (1971) first suggested that "incessant ovulation," without respite from pregnancy or breast-feeding, was traumatic for the ovarian surface and could predispose to ovarian cancer. Additional support for that theory is provided by research that found that more pregnancies, early age at first pregnancy, oral contraceptives, a late menarche, and an early menopause all appear to have a protective effect against the development of ovarian cancer. British epidemiologist Valerie Beral noted that ovarian cancer is infrequent in populations that do not practice birth control. She pointed out that the death rate from this malignancy is lower in Catholic women, who until recently had an average family size greater than that of Protestant or Jewish women.

REFERENCES

Adam, E., Kaufman, R. H., Adler-Storthz, K., et al. (1985). A prospective study of association of herpes simplex virus and human papillomavirus with cervical neoplasia in women exposed to diethylstilbesterol in utero. *International Journal of Cancer, 35,* 19–27.

Avorn, J., Monane, M., Gurwitz, J. H., et al. (1994). Reduction of bacteriuria and pyuria after ingestion of cranberry juice. *Journal of the American Medical Association, 271*(10), 751–754.

Ben-Baruch, G., Menczer, J., Mashiach, S., & Seer, D. M. (1981). Uterine anomalies in diethylstilbestrol-exposed women with fertility disorders. *Acta Obstetrica et Gynecologica Scandinavica, 60*(14), 395–397.

Ben-Baruch, G., Rothenberg, O., Modan, M., & Menczer, J. (1991). Abnormal cervical cytologic, colposcopic and histologic findings in exposed DES young Israeli Jewish women. *Clinical and Experimental Obstetrics and Gynecology, 18*(2), 71–74.

Beral, V., & Colwell, L. (1980). Randomized trial of high doses of stilbestrol and ethisterone in pregnancy: Long-term follow-up of mothers. *British Medical Journal, 281*(6248), 1098–1101.

Beral, V., & Colwell, L. (1981). Randomized trial of high doses of stilbestrol and ethisterone in pregnancy: Long-term follow-up of the children. *Journal of Epidemiology and Community Health, 35*(3), 155–160.

Beral, V., Fraser, P., & Chilvers, D. (1978). Does pregnancy protect against ovarian cancer? *Lancet, 8073,* 1083–1986.

Bergeron, S., Binik, Y. M., Khalife, S., & Agidas, D. (1997). Vulvar vestibulitis syndrome: A critical review. *Clinical Journal of Pain, 13*(1), 27–42.

Bibbo, M., Gill, W. B., Freidoon, et al. (1977). Follow-up study of male and female offspring of DES-exposed mothers. *Obstetrics and Gynecology, 49*(1), 1–8.

Brian, D. D., Tilley, B. C., Labar, D. R., et al. (1980). Breast cancer in DES-exposed mothers: Absence of association. *Mayo Clinic Proceedings, 55*(2), 89–93.

Brock, B. V., Selke, S., Benedetti, J., et al. (1990). Frequency of asymptomatic shedding of herpes simplex virus in women with genital herpes. *Journal of the American Medical Association, 263*(3), 418–420.

Burkhart, C. G., Burkhart, C. N., & Burkhart, K. M. (1998). An assessment of topical and oral prescription and over-the-counter treatments for head lice. *Journal of the American Academy of Dermatology, 38*(6 Pt. 1), 979–982.

Butterworth, C. E., Hatch, K. D., Macaluso, M., et al. (1992). Folate deficiency and cervical dysplasia. *Journal of the American Medical Association, 267*(4), 528–533.

DuBouchet, L., McGregor, J. A., Ismail, M., & McCormack, W. M. (1998). A pilot study of metronidazole vaginal gel versus oral metronidazole for the treatment of *Trichomonas vaginalis* vaginitis. *Sexually Transmitted Diseases, 25*(3), 176–179.

DuBouchet, L., Spence, M. R., Rein, M. F., et al. (1997). Multicenter comparison of clotrimazole vaginal tablets, oral metronidazole, and vaginal suppositories containing sulfanilamide, aminacrine hydrochloride, and allantoin in the treatment of symptomatic trichomoniasis. *Sexually Transmitted Diseases, 24*(3), 156–160.

Fathalla, M. F. (1971). "Incessant ovulation" and ovarian cancer. *Lancet, 2,* 163–168.

Fisher, G. O. (1996). The commonest causes of symptomatic vulvar disease: A dermatologist's perspective. *Australasian Journal of Dermatology, 37*(1), 12–18.

Fleet, J. C. (1994). New support for a folk remedy: Cranberry juice reduces bacteriuria and pyuria in elderly women. *Nutrition Reviews, 52*(5), 168–170.

Fowler, W. C., Schmidt, G., Edelman, D. A., et al. (1981). Risks of cervical intraepithelial neoplasia among DES-exposed women. *Obstetrics and Gynecology, 58*(6), 720–724.

Fraser, C. M. et al. (1998). Complete genome sequence of *Treponema pallidum,* the syphilis spirochete. *Science, 281,* 375–387.

Gardner, H. L., & Dukes, C. D. (1955). *Hemophilus vaginalis* vaginitis. *American Journal of Obstetrics and Gynecology, 69*(5), 962–975.

Gershman, S. T., & Stolley, P. D. (1988). A case-control study of testicular cancer using Connecticut tumour registry data. *International Journal of Epidemiology, 17*(4), 738–742.

Gilbaugh, J., & Fuchs, P. (1979). The gonococcus and the toilet seat. *New England Journal of Medicine, 301*(2), 91–93.

Gill, W. B., Schumacher, G., & Bibbo, M. (1976). Structural and functional abnormalities in the sex organs of male offspring of mothers treated with diethylstilbestrol (DES). *Journal of Reproductive Medicine, 16*(4), 147–153.

Greenberg, E. R., Barnes, A. B., Resseguie, L., et al. (1984). Breast cancer in mothers given diethylstilbestrol in pregnancy. *New England Journal of Medicine, 311*(22), 1393–1398.

Hatch, E. E., Palmer, J. R., Titus-Ernstoff, L., et al. (1998). Cancer risk in women exposed to diethylstilbestrol in utero. *Journal of the American Medical Association, 280*(7), 630–634.

Herbst, A. L. et al. (1981). Reproductive and gynecologic surgical experience in diethylstilbestrol-exposed daughters. *American Journal of Obstetrics and Gynecology, 141*(8), 1019–1028.

Herbst, A. L., Anderson, S., Hubby, M. M., et al. (1986). Risk factors for the development of diethylstilbestrol associated clear cell adenocarcinoma. *American Journal of Obstetrics and Gynecology, 154,* 814–820.

Herbst, A. L., Senekjian, E. K., & Frey, K. W. (1989). Abortion and pregnancy loss among diethylstilbestrol-exposed women. *Seminars in Reproductive Endocrinology, 7,* 124–129.

Jacobs., I. J., Skates, S. J., MacDonald, N., et al. (1999). Screening for ovarian cancer: A pilot randomised controlled trial. *Lancet, 353*(9160), 1207–1211.

Masterson, B. J. (1988, June 24). Microwaving underwear helps kill yeast infections, doctor says. *Milwaukee Sentinal.*

McKay, M. (1988). Subsets of vulvodynia. *Journal of Reproductive Medicine, 33,* 695–698.

McKay, M. (1989). Vulvodynia. A multifactorial clinical problem. *Archives of Dermatology, 125*(2), 256–262.

McKay, M., Frankman, O., Horowitz, B. J., et al. (1991). Vulvar vestibulitis and vestibular papillomatosis. Report of the ISSVD committee on vulvodynia. *Journal of Reproductive Medicine, 36*(6), 413–415.

Meisels, A., Roy, M., Fortier, M., et al. (1981). Human papillomavirus virus infection of the cervix: The atypical condyloma. *Acta Cytologica, 25*(1), 7–16.

Metts, J. F. (1999). Vulvodynia and vulvar vestibulitis: Challenges in diagnosis and management. *American Family Physician, 59*(6), 1547–1556, 1561–1562.

Miller, C., Degenhardt, K., & Sassoon, D. A. (1998). Fetal exposure to DES results in deregulation of Wnt7A during uterine morphogenesis. *Nature Genetics, 20*(3), 228–230.

Morsy, T. A., Ramadan, N. I., Mahmoud, M. S., et al. (1996). On the efficacy of Cotrimoxazole as an oral treatment for pediculosis capitis infestation. *Journal of the Egyptian Society of Parasitologists, 26*(1), 73–77.

Moss, A. R., Osmond, D., Bacchetti, P., et al. (1986). Hormonal risk factors in testicular cancer. A case-control study. *American Journal of Epidemiology, 124*(1), 39–52.

Murph, J. R., Baron, J. C., Brown, C. K., et al. (1991). The occupational risk of cytomegalovirus infection among day-care providers. *Journal of the American Medical Association, 265*(5), 603–608.

Ofek, I., Goldhar, J., Zafrir, D., et al. (1991). *Anti-escherichia coli* activity of cranberry and blueberry juices [Letter]. *New England Journal of Medicine, 324*(22), 1599.

Peress, M. R., Tsai, C. C., Mathur, R. S., & Williamson, H. O. (1982). Hirsutism and menstrual patterns in women exposed to diethylstilbestrol in utero. *American Journal of Obstetrics and Gynecology, 144*(2), 135–140.

Pfau, A. (1991). Sex and recurrent UTI in young women. *Medical Aspects of Human Sexuality, 6,* 34–39.

Reeves, W. C., Corey, L., Adams, H. G., et al. (1981). Risk of recurrence after first episodes of genital herpes: Relation to HSV type and antibody response. *New England Journal of Medicine, 305,* 315–319.

Reid, R., Stanhope, R., Herschman, B. R., et al. (1982). Genital warts and cervical cancer. *Cancer, 50,* 377–383.

Robboy, S. J., Noller, K. L., O'Brien, P., et al. (1984). Increased incidence of cervical and vaginal dysplasias in 3,980 diethylstilbestrol-exposed young women. *Journal of the American Medical Association, 252*(21), 2979–2983.

Schmidt, G., & Fowler, W. D. (1982a). Gynecologic operative experience in women exposed to DES in utero. *Southern Medical Journal, 75*(3), 260–263.

Schmidt, G., & Fowler, W. D. (1982b). Ovarian cystadenofibromas in three women with antenatal exposure to diethylstilbestrol. *Gynecologic Oncology, 14*(2), 175–184.

Senekjian, E. K., Frey, K. W., Anderson, D., et al. (1987). Local therapy in stage I clear cell carcinoma of the vagina. *Cancer, 60,* 1319–1324.

Senekjian, E. K., Frey, K. W., Stone, C., & Herbst, A. L. (1988). An evaluation of stage II vaginal clear cell adenocarcinoma according to substages. *Gynecologic Oncology, 31*(1), 56–64.

Senekjian, E. K., Potkul, R. K., Frey, K. W., & Herbst, A. L. (1988). Infertility among daughters either exposed or not exposed to diethylstilbestrol. *American Journal of Obstetrics and Gynecology, 158*(3 Pt. 1), 493–498.

Stafl, A., & Mattingly, R. F. (1974). Vaginal adenosis: A precancerous lesion? *American Journal of Obstetrics and Gynecology, 120*(5), 666–673.

Stamm, W. (1991). Long-term prophylaxis effective against recurrent urinary tract infections. *Reviews of Infectious Diseases, 13,* 77–84.

Stapleton, A., Latham, R. H., Johnson, C., & Stamm, W. E. (1990). Postcoital antimicrobial prophylaxis for recurrent urinary tract infection. *Journal of the American Medical Association, 264*(6), 703–706.

Stillman, R. J. (1982). In utero exposure to diethylstilbestrol: Adverse effects on the reproductive tract and reproductive performance in male and female offspring. *American Journal of Obstetrics and Gynecology, 142*(7), 905–1021.

Van Slyke, K. K., Michel, V. P., & Rein, M. (1981). Treatment of vulvovaginal candidiasis with boric acid powder. *American Journal of Obstetrics and Gynecology, 142*(2), 145–148.

Veridiano, N. P., Delke, I., Rogers, J., & Tancer, M. L. (1981). Reproductive performance of DES-exposed female progency. *Obstetrics and Gynecology, 58*(1), 58–61.

Vonka, V., Kanka, J. Hirsch, I., et al. (1984). A prospective study of the relationship between cervical neoplasia and herpes simplex type-2 virus. *International Journal of Cancer,* 33:61–70.

Walker, A. H., Ross, R. K., Haile, R. W., et al. (1988). Hormonal factors and risk of ovarian germ cell cancer in young women. *British Journal of Cancer, 57*(4), 418–422.

$\mathcal{H}$IV/AIDS IN WOMEN

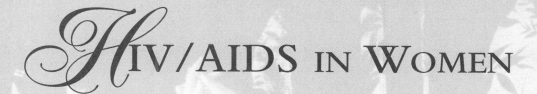

KEY TERMS

Acquired immuno-
deficiency syndrome
(AIDS)
AZT
CD4 receptor
Highly active antiretroviral
therapy (HAART)
Human immunodeficiency
virus (HIV)

Kaposi's sarcoma
Pneumocystis carinii
pneumonia
Retroviruses
Seroconversion
T-helper lymphocytes

$\mathcal{O}$n June 5, 1981, the Centers for Disease Control (CDC) published a brief report on an outbreak of a mysterious illness among five gay men in Los Angeles. The disease was *Pneumocystis carinii pneumonia,* a type of pneumonia previously seen only in cancer patients with profoundly suppressed immune systems. This short article, found on the second page of the federal agency's *Morbidity and Mortality Weekly Report,* marked the beginning of the **acquired** immunodeficiency syndrome (AIDS) epidemic. The disease at that time was of unknown cause, unknown transmission, and unknown potential for fatality. It had been spreading, however, extensively and silently long before it was recognized. Within months there were hundreds of cases; within a few years, there were thousands, and almost half of the patients had died. It took 8 years for 100,000 cases to be reported. It took only 26 months more for the AIDS count to reach the next 100,000. By January of 1992, 206,392 people with AIDS had been diagnosed and 133,232 (65%) had died of the disease. AIDS had become the second leading cause of death among men aged 25–44 years, one of the five leading causes of death among women aged 15–44 years nationwide, and the leading cause of death for women aged 25–34 in New York City.

By the end of the century, AIDS had become the world's most deadly infectious disease, having moved ahead of tuberculosis to fourth place among all causes of mortality and causing about 2.28 million deaths worldwide, according to the World Health Organization. About 33 million people in the world were estimated to be infected with the disease, and in Africa AIDS was the leading cause of death, accounting for 19% of fatalities. In the United States, women constituted the fastest-rising group at risk for contracting AIDS. Although at the beginning of the epidemic homosexual or bisexual men and people with a history of injecting drugs accounted for the largest number of AIDS cases, there had been a steady increase in heterosexuals affected, especially in racial and ethnic minorities of both sexes and their sexual partners. Cases of AIDS were occurring more frequently among women than among men, and 75% of the victims were black and Hispanic women. Cases in children as a result of mother-to-infant transmission at the time of birth had steadily increased and in some locations became a major cause of death among infants and young children. Only the number of AIDS cases associated with blood transfusions had stabilized. In epidemiology, fatality rate, in all social, legal, ethical, and political aspects, AIDS had become a public health crisis and

had generated more concern than any other infectious disease in modern medical history. Currently, there is no cure for the disease.

CAUSE OF INFECTION

The agent that causes AIDS is **human immunodeficiency virus (HIV)**. HIV belongs to a viral class called **retroviruses** (from the Latin word for reverse), which store their genetic information in the form of RNA rather than DNA. Retroviruses are composed of a core of RNA surrounded by a protein coat further surrounded by a protein envelope, and they produce a unique enzyme called reverse transcriptase. This enzyme allows a reverse of the usual flow of genetic information in the synthesis of new protein, that is, DNA→RNA→protein. Reverse transcriptase enables the virus-RNA to synthesize virus-DNA within the infected cell using the RNA as a template—backward, so to speak. The newly formed virus-DNA moves to the nucleus to become incorporated into the host cell's DNA. The integrated viral and host DNA then is used by the host cell's normal protein-synthesizing machinery to make more virus-RNA.

The structure of HIV in cross section is shown diagrammatically in Figure 10–1. The external envelope is studded by 72 spikes formed by two major viral-envelope proteins, gp120 and gp41 (gp is the abbreviation for glycoprotein). The viral core of HIV contains two copies of single-stranded RNA that carry the virus's genetic information and the enzyme reverse transcriptase. Coat proteins (p24, p17, p9, and p7) make up the rest of the core.

The target cells in the body attacked by HIV are those that have a cell surface receptor molecule called CD4. The **CD4 receptor** binds with high affinity specifically with the gp120 envelope protein of the virus. After binding, the bound virus particle fuses with the host cell's membrane so it can enter the cell, and, once inside, the virus sheds its outer protein coat. The exposed viral RNA core is released into the inte-

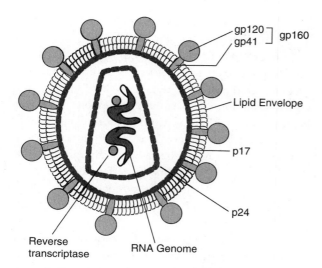

Figure 10–1 Schematic diagram of the human immuno-deficiency virus. Viral proteins (gp120 and gp41) make up the spikes on the outer envelope. The CD4 receptor on host cells binds with the gp120 envelope protein. Coat proteins surround the diploid RNA, which is associated with reverse transcriptase.

rior, ready to make viral DNA with the aid of reverse transcriptase. The DNA made by the virus is then integrated into the DNA of the target cell.

CD4 receptor protein is present on certain white blood cells or leukocytes, namely, a lymphocyte population known as **T-helper lymphocytes.** T-helper cells help other lymphocytes combat foreign antigens. CD4 receptors are also found on monocytes and macrophages, blood cells that attack and engulf cells infected by viruses and bacteria. HIV may also infect some other types of cells, including supporting cells in the nervous system, cells lining the digestive tract, and certain bone marrow cells. Infection of these target cells may be why mental deterioration, intractable diarrhea, and various blood abnormalities are associated with full-blown AIDS.

Although most retroviruses do not kill the cells they infect, when HIV infects T-helper cells, it rapidly results in their death. The killing off of the T-helper cells in an infected individual gradually depletes their numbers and profoundly compromises the ability of the immune system to fight off infection. This causes the person to become vulnerable to the life-threatening diseases characterized by AIDS. But when HIV enters CD4-positive cells other than T-helper lymphocytes, it does not kill them. Some of the infected monocytes and macrophages continue to produce and release more HIV particles, but the majority establish a persistent state of infection; that is, they retain the viral-DNA in the host chromosomes in a latent state, ready to be reactivated and produce particles of virus at a later date. Thus, monocytes and macrophages serve as an important reservoir for the virus and could explain why many years may elapse from the time of an initial HIV infection and the development of full-blown AIDS.

*E*FFECTS OF HIV INFECTION

AIDS is the most advanced stage in a continuum of effects of HIV infection. After initial infection the individual undergoes **seroconversion;** that is, he or she produces antibodies to HIV, which indicate its presence. Generally, there are few initial signs of illness. Some infected people may have symptoms of fever and malaise and swollen glands similar to those in mononucleosis, but many remain asymptomatic for variable periods—an average of 9–11 years. During the asymptomatic period, a person may be totally unaware of the infection but can spread the virus to others because the body fluids contain HIV and are infective. With the passage of time, many HIV-infected persons exhibit clinical symptoms, usually of a nonspecific nature, such as swollen lymph nodes (lymphadenopathy), unexplained weight loss, bumps or a rash on the skin, chronic fatigue, fever, night sweats, diarrhea, cough, and shortness of breath.

The last stage of the progressive HIV infection is AIDS. With the continued depletion of the T-helper lymphocytes and immune system failure, "opportunistic" infections—those caused by organisms that ordinarily would be unable to produce disease in healthy individuals—can take hold in the immunosuppressed with life-threatening effects. Key opportunistic diseases associated with profound immunosuppression are *Pneumocystis carinii* pneumonia; herpes simplex; toxoplasmosis; cytomegalovirus; candidiasis; tuberculosis; and, in women, such gender-specific diseases as pelvic inflammatory disease and vaginal candidiasis. Because the immune system also defends the body against cancer, AIDS patients may develop malignancies such as **Kaposi's sarcoma** and non-Hodgkin's lymphoma, and abnormal Pap smears indicating cervical disease in women. They can also suffer from a "wasting syndrome" of weight loss, persistent and relentless diarrhea, fever, and an AIDS-related dementia that impairs mental function. Before the development of **highly active antiretroviral therapy (HAART)** and the remarkable benefits resulting from its use, there were estimates that more than 70% of people infected with HIV would develop AIDS within 8 or more years after infection.

DIAGNOSIS: THE HIV ANTIBODY TEST

The most commonly used test that detects the presence of circulating antibodies to HIV virus proteins in blood serum is the inexpensive and efficient enzyme-linked immunosorbent assay (ELISA). Current ELISA tests are said to have an accuracy of more than 99.9%; that is, the frequency of false positives (non-HIV-infected individuals would test antibody positive) is less than 1 in 1,000. Antibodies to HIV are produced shortly after infection, depending on the host and the viral characteristics, but may be at low levels and undetectable. The earlier assays detected antibody 6–12 weeks after infection; the newer forms of tests are able to detect antibody at about 3–4 weeks after infection. A screening test such as ELISA that produces a positive result generally is repeated, and if the serum sample is positive again, the results are confirmed by the western blot or another very specific test.

Other screening tests are the "rapid test," which can be performed in less than 30 minutes and is as accurate as the ELISA test, and the "simple test," which takes longer than 30 minutes but easily can be performed without instrumentation. Confirmatory tests include the western blot, the indirect fluorescent antibody assay, or the radioimmunoprecipitation assay. When these are properly performed and interpreted, they eliminate false-positive results. They take more effort and are more expensive than the screening tests.

As technology has evolved, alternatives to blood sample testing, such as saliva tests and urine tests, have been approved by the FDA. And as of May 1997, the FDA approved the use of home collection of blood via a finger stick. The sample is mailed to a laboratory and subjected to ELISA tests. Results and counseling are by telephone.

Individuals exposed to HIV are considered to be uninfected if they are negative for antibodies 6 months after exposure and remain negative for another 6 months.

The HIV-antibody tests became widely available in the mid-1980s and were controversial from the beginning. Although the traditional public health approaches to the control of sexually transmitted disease include screening, reporting of infected individuals to confidential registries of public health departments, and partner notification and treatment, it was argued successfully that HIV infection was different and should constitute an exception to the usual methods of reporting and identification. Although clinical AIDS is a reportable condition, HIV infection is not. Many were concerned that the identification of HIV-infected individuals could lead not only to ostracism because of the attached stigma of homosexuality but also to loss of employment, medical insurance, or housing. Testing for HIV has been for the most part voluntary and could not be performed without an individual's permission. The notification of partners has also been voluntary, and sex partners have not been systematically traced. As the epidemic grew to more alarming proportions, and particularly as the disease moved out of the gay male community and became of greater concern to many Americans, some public health officials and physicians believed that control of the epidemic should have priority over confidentiality. Strong measures were advocated, such as widespread mandatory screening and the removal of infected individuals from schools, jobs, or neighborhoods. After the first documented cases in which HIV from an infected dentist was transmitted in some unknown fashion to five of his patients, and despite no evidence of any transmission in several thousand patients of some 20 other infected health care workers who had also performed invasive procedures, some of the anxious public demanded mandatory testing of all health care workers so they could be prevented from practicing if they were infected. In turn, many health workers called for mandatory testing of patients for HIV, pointing out that they are at greater risk of infection from patients from accidental sticks by contaminated needles, for example, than patients are of being infected by providers. The general consensus in the Centers for Disease Control, American Medical Association, and American Dental Association is that with the appropriate techniques, which include strict adherence to the usual and standard precautions against infection, training in proper infection control measures, and monitoring of appropriate techniques for disinfection and sterilization of instruments, the risk of health care provider-to-patient transmission is very low and for most procedures is zero. Moreover, most analyses of the costs versus benefits of a national program of mandatory testing have concluded that it would not be worth the expense. In view of the many false negatives and false positives that would occur, mandatory testing of huge groups would be an inefficient and ineffective use of resources that could be better utilized for research, treatment, and prevention of infection.

TRANSMISSION OF HIV

The virus is transmitted by intimate sexual contact, by needle sharing for intravenous drug use, from mother to fetus during pregnancy, or by transfusion of blood or blood products. In an infected individual, HIV is present in certain cells and certain of the body fluids and secretions that contain those cells. HIV-infected cells are found in high concentrations in semen, cervical and vaginal fluids, blood, and cerebrospinal fluid. Other fluids, such as tears, saliva, sweat, urine, and feces, have a low concentration of HIV-infected cells and are of little or no importance in transmission between individuals. Outside the body, HIV is fragile and dies when exposed to air. It is, therefore, not airborne or waterborne and cannot be transmitted through sneezes and coughs of an infected person; by sharing food, dishes, cooking utensils, napkins, or towels; by using the same toilet seat or telephone; or by handshakes and hugs—all the behaviors generally referred to as "casual contact."

Sexual Transmission

Transmission via intimate sexual contact increases with the number of acts of intercourse with an infected person or with the number of sexual partners, probably because of the greater likelihood of sex with an infected person. But reducing the number of partners does not eliminate the risk; HIV can be acquired from a single exposure. It is unknown why some people will contract the virus after a single act of intercourse while others have intercourse without using condoms with an infected partner for years and remain uninfected. Transmission is enhanced by concurrent infection with other sexually transmitted diseases, particularly those that cause open sores or ulcers. STDs also increase the number of white blood cells in the genital tract and provide additional opportunity for viral infection of CD4-positive cells. Uncircumcised men are more likely to contract infection than circumcised men, perhaps because they tend to have more genital ulcers than their circumcised counterparts. Women who have sex with infected men are about 10–14 times more likely to catch HIV than are men who have intercourse with infected women because the virus is more concentrated in semen than in vaginal fluid. The risk of transmission from women to men is increased, however, by intercourse during menstruation.

Sexual practices also influence transmission. Any sexual activity that allows HIV-contaminated body fluid (semen, vaginal fluid, or menstrual blood) to come into direct contact with a target site (the vagina, anus, mouth, or an open cut or sore on the skin) is a high-risk activity. The best protection against transmission, therefore, is (1) to choose abstention from sex or (2) to be in a mutually faithful relationship between two uninfected partners. For those who want to continue sexual activity and find that the second alternative is not an option, there are sexual practices that reduce the risk of transmitting HIV from one individual to another and have been called "safer sex."

Safer sex practices include nonpenetrative activities such as dry kissing, caressing, masturbation of the male as long as the ejaculation of semen is away from the body or only on healthy unbroken skin, and oral sex on a man using a latex (not natural membrane) condom to contain the semen. Some women have used a latex barrier such as a dental dam for receiving oral sex. Unlike condoms, however, the 6-by-6-inch dental dams have not been specifically tested for transmission of HIV or other STDs and are, necessarily, more awkward to use and keep in place. There is little information concerning the risk of HIV transmission among lesbian women, but there have been cases reported in the literature, so women who have sex with other women should be careful and practice safer sex. Use of a latex barrier (dental dam) when a woman is in contact with the vaginal secretions of another woman, for example, may help reduce the risk of transmission. The dental dam should be cleaned with a dilution of bleach and water

after use. An alternative for women receiving oral sex, whether lesbian or heterosexual, is to place plastic wrap over the genital area.

Less risky sex practices include use of a latex condom for vaginal or anal sex. Anal sex with a condom is riskier than vaginal sex for a woman because a condom has a greater risk of tearing during anal sex. Open-mouth or wet kissing has a very low potential for transmission but transmission is theoretically possible because of the HIV-infected cells in saliva and the presence of macrophages in the mucosal lining of the pharynx. It is, therefore, one category down from safer sex.

Risky sex practices include oral sex on a woman, oral sex on a man without a condom, or semen ejaculation on irritated or broken skin.

Dangerous sex practices include vaginal or anal sex without any condom. The association of drugs or alcohol with sexual activity is dangerous because substance abuse can lead people to forget the differences between safer and risky or dangerous sexual behavior.

Transmission Through Injections

HIV-infected needles and syringes can transmit the virus when they are shared by drug users, when health workers in a medical setting have accidentally stuck themselves when drawing blood or starting an IV solution, or when needles and syringes are reused without adequate sterilization. Drug abuse is a major mode of transmission, but because there is a low probability of transmission from contaminated needles and syringes in a medical setting, health workers are advised to be careful, to wear gloves (or double gloves) for all clinical procedures, and to use standard sterile techniques.

Transmission Through Blood Transfusions

To reduce the risk to the public of contracting AIDS through a blood transfusion, procedures at blood banks have been established to discourage blood donation from individuals who may be infected, and all donated blood is screened. Before 1984, the year the screening test for HIV antibodies was begun on blood supplies, it was estimated that the previous year, more than 7,000 people had become infected by contaminated blood or blood products. Currently, the risk of HIV transmission in the blood in the United States is estimated at 1 in 440,000–660,000 donations in blood screened negative for HIV antibody (Lackritz, 1998). Despite the low risk, blood collection agencies and policy makers continue to search for more sensitive HIV screening tests. Even though the risk is very low, screening cannot detect all possible contamination, so it makes good sense to make use of autologous blood transfusions (use of one's own blood banked until needed after surgery) whenever possible.

TREATMENT OF HIV/AIDS

Medical research efforts focus on searching for a vaccine to prevent infection, finding antiviral compounds to interfere with or block infection, bolstering an immune system weakened by the loss of T-helper lymphocytes, and finding better ways to treat opportunistic diseases and cancers.

There are three major classes of antiretroviral treatment of HIV that form the foundation of highly active antiretroviral therapy (HAART) and have led to remarkable progress in the suppression of HIV replication and the enthusiastic recognition that HIV is now a manageable disease. The first antiretroviral drug approved by the FDA was zidovudine (AZT, also called ZDV or Retrovir). **AZT** is a reverse transcriptase inhibitor. It inhibits an enzyme crucial to an early stage of HIV replication. The two types of reverse transcriptase inhibitors are nucleoside analogs and nonnucleoside analogs. The third class of HAART is the protease inhibitors, which target protease, an enzyme that functions near the end of HIV replication and slows or stops the production of proteins required by the virus.

Combination therapy with these drugs generally involves two nucleoside analogs and a protease inhibitor. The regimens have major side effects, and many patients have great difficulty in adhering to them because of the side effects and having to take numerous drugs on a very strict schedule. If a patient under treatment skips doses or does not take them on schedule, the consequences can be serious. Currently, there are about 14 antiretroviral drugs available and more are in development, so treatment of HIV has become very medically complex for the physician and the patient. There is the strong possibility of developing drug resistance, which can limit long-term effectiveness. Also, the long-term safety of the drugs is unknown. HAART therapy lowers the viral load in the blood, that is, the amount of HIV in the blood, and increases the number of CD4 lymphocyte cells. For many patients who undergo the standard multiple-drug treatment, there are no detectable levels of HIV in their bloodstream, sometimes for years. Although it is known that the virus hides out in certain cells of the body not easily attacked by drugs, it was hoped that continued use of antiretroviral therapy could eventually kill all traces of infection. Two recent studies, however, have shown that, despite sustained suppression of plasma levels of the virus by antiretroviral drugs, infectious virus is not totally eradicated, persists in CD4 lymphocytes, and could become reactivated despite intensive treatment. The researchers suggest that different antiretrovirals, higher doses, and a longer time may achieve the long-term goal of total eradication of the HIV virus (Furtadol et al., 1999; Zhang et al., 1999).

Deciding whether to start treatment is not difficult for those with symptoms of advanced disease, but for an asymptomatic patient who has tested HIV positive, the decision is far less clear-cut. Not only is there a potential risk of limiting future treatment options by using available drugs during early disease, but how long the available drug regimens work or their long-term toxicity is unknown. The general recommendations currently for asymptomatic patients is treatment when the CD4 cells are less than 500 and the viral load (the amount of HIV in the blood plasma) is 10,000 as measured by the bDNA test or 20,000 as measured by the RT-PCR method.

A very effective prevention of HIV would be a vaccine to produce a defense and block infection in an immunized individual. Vaccine development has been a top research priority since the mid-1980s but presents a major challenge because the virus infects T-helper cells and macrophages—some of the very cells of the immune system that play a critical role in the immune defense. That HIV is a retrovirus increases the problem. The virus inserts its own genes into the genes of the cells it infects, thereby creating a permanent infection and enabling it to not be "seen" by the cells of the immune system. Thus, it can successfully evade the body defenses. Moreover, the virus has an unusual tendency to mutate and form variants, particularly of the gene that codes for one of its envelope proteins. Despite the difficulties, however, researchers are confident that HIV is not invulnerable. Many experimental vaccines have been developed and are being studied.

HIV/AIDS IN WOMEN

The natural history of HIV in women has not been studied the way it has been in men. Little is known about the consequences of infection in women; most of the information has been extrapolated from the studies of gay men. What currently is known is principally derived from studies of infected pregnant women where the greatest focus has been on perinatal effects. Women with AIDS get many of the same opportunistic infections described for men, but Kaposi's sarcoma is rarely seen in women patients. They are more likely to exhibit a range of gynecological disorders that point to immunosuppression—chronic recurring vaginal candidiasis; more frequent and severe recurrences of herpes, perhaps atypical in location and appearance; or pelvic inflammatory disease (PID), which appears to manifest itself differently when HIV infection is pres-

ent. A study of HIV-infected women with PID indicated a significant trend toward more abscesses and the necessity for more surgical intervention (Des Jarlais et al., 1990). HIV infection may also produce unique genital ulcers. Minkoff and DeHovitz (1991) reported that they have cared for several women whose genital ulcers were not associated with herpes, chancroid, or other STDs and that responded only to administration of AZT. These authors also noted that infections with STDs such as herpes and syphilis appear to be more aggressive in HIV-infected individuals. They urge that the dosage of antibiotic treatment for women coinfected by HIV and syphilis reflect this knowledge.

Compared with men, women are often diagnosed at a more advanced stage of the disease, do not receive equivalent treatment, and have died sooner, frequently because they were unaware they were infected. Because men—stereotypically gay, white men—represented the epidemic early on, they were the subject of the most study. It took a long time to recognize that the clinical manifestations of HIV/AIDS are different for men and for women. In many areas of the country, a person must have a diagnosis of AIDS based on the CDC definition of the disease, which includes a variety of clinical conditions based on studies in men. When these are coupled with a positive HIV antibody test, it allows the formal diagnosis of AIDS. It was not until 1993 that an expanded case definition was implemented that added many of the opportunistic infections that affect women. This meant that the more restrictive definition, prior to its broadening to include women, denied or delayed the claims of poor women and children for the federal financial aid and services provided to people with HIV/AIDs in their area, unless their community was willing to provide help to people without the CDC diagnosis of AIDS.

There is research to indicate that women's viral loads may be equivalent to men's viral loads when checked but that women may be at a more advanced disease stage than the men and should be started on HAART sooner than they are under the guidelines that are largely based on the experience of men (Fang et al., 1997). This is only one of the special problems encountered by infected women. Women are still regarded as a low-risk population even though they constitute the fastest-growing group of people with the disease in the country. Because women generally have been excluded from research drug trials based on the possibility of their pregnancy, little is known concerning the differences in efficacy and toxicity of antiretroviral drugs between women and men.

Impact of HIV Infection During Pregnancy

Statistics indicate that in the absence of maternal antiretroviral therapy, there is about a 30% chance that a baby born to an HIV-infected mother will be infected. For the majority of infants who are not infected, maternal HIV has not been associated with fetal malformations, premature birth, or complications of pregnancy. HIV may be transmitted from the mother during fetal development, during delivery, and postpartum by breast-feeding. Factors believed to influence transmission are the HIV viral load in the blood, the length of time the mother is infected, the amount of immunosuppression, her general health at the time of pregnancy, older maternal age, cigarette smoking during pregnancy, and the presence of malnutrition or other infections. The discovery that zidovudine (AZT) given to the woman during pregnancy and to the infant after birth resulted in a 70% decrease in the risk of HIV transmission has resulted in AZT being offered to all HIV-infected pregnant women after 14 weeks of gestation and to their infants for 6 weeks. Because the risks of antiretroviral therapy during the first trimester of pregnancy are unknown, the Public Health Service Guidelines recommend that HIV-infected women who have not yet initiated HAART should consider delaying therapy until after the 10th to 12th week of gestation. If a woman is already receiving combination antiretroviral therapy when pregnancy is detected, she should consider temporarily suspending it during the first trimester and restarting therapy after 14 weeks. If

AZT had not been included in the patient's antiretroviral regimen, it should be added or substituted for one of the other nucleoside analogs that had been part of her therapy (Centers for Disease Control and Prevention, 1998).

Women and Self-Responsibility

There are also social issues associated with women and HIV/AIDS infection. More than 70% of the women diagnosed with AIDS are women of color, specifically black and Hispanic women, who are disproportionately affected relative to the number of black and Hispanic females in the population. Minority women are likely to be poorly educated, have low incomes, and have limited access to the health care system, making them double victims.

Moreover, infected women are viewed as a vast reservoir of infection to others, especially their future children and sex partners. The limited reproductive choices for women in the United States are further restricted for HIV-infected women. Either their access to abortion services is restricted or they get biased urging of abortion and sterilization.

There is an urgent need for all women to be informed about HIV transmission and infection; to share the knowledge they have with other women; and to work to influence legislators, public health officials, and the entire health care establishment toward policies to stop the HIV epidemic. Research toward treatment and cure is tremendously important, but the major key to prevention of transmission of the virus is education.

That many people have misconceptions about the spread of the disease is apparent when they are surveyed. In a study of 8,450 women aged 15–44, the National Center for Health Statistics discovered the following erroneous ideas: nearly 20% of women interviewed thought that AIDS can be caught by *donating* blood, 22% thought it could be transmitted by an insect bite, 10% said it could not be transmitted by sharing hypodermic needles, 6% said it could be transmitted by casual contact, and an amazing 29% believed that a woman could not get AIDS from a person who tested positive for antibodies but had not developed full-blown AIDS (McNally & Mosher, 1991). Even health care workers, who should know better, are confused about how AIDS is spread. In another survey of 606 health professionals in six states that included physicians, nurses, and medical students, one-quarter of the *doctors* believed that being spat upon could transmit the virus; one-third thought it could be transmitted during cardiopulmonary resuscitation; and a little more than 10% said HIV could be spread by donating blood, sharing cigarettes, or by mosquito bites.

Sometimes the AIDS message evidently fails to reach people despite the availability of programs aimed at educating them. University students have been warned about AIDS for years in classes, campus newspapers, and by college health officials. But given the high incidence of STDs like chlamydia and papillomavirus infection on college campuses, it appears that most students still think of condoms as a form of birth control rather than disease prevention and have not modified their sex practices to reflect the dangers of AIDS. Thus far, AIDS has been a relatively slim risk for students on college campuses. But although the rate is far lower than that of populations known to be at high risk, there is an obvious potential for the further spread on the university campus. Evidently, the realization that the AIDS epidemic can and is affecting everybody, however, and not just members of high-risk groups, is often ignored. Quoted in the *New York Times,* a junior at a major university admitted she does not insist that the man use a condom. "I have an attitude—it may be wrong—that any guy I would sleep with would not have AIDS," she said. Another article relates the story of the 20-year-old student at a prestigious college who had had only two sexual partners in her life. One was her high school sweetheart, the other was a man she met on a ski vacation. When she found out he had used drugs, she refused to see him again. But during her annual gynecological examination, although she felt strong and healthy, she found out she had been infected by him with HIV. Clearly, as long as women think that for some reason they are invulnerable and do not need to protect themselves because they are young, healthy, and heterosexual, the disease will continue to spread. The best way for women to protect themselves against transmission of HIV is by having the male partner use a condom. When a male partner refuses to wear a condom, Planned Parenthood says that an assertive stance of "protected sex or no sex" should work. If it does not, women are advised not to take the risk with that partner.

REFERENCES

Centers for Disease Control. (1991). The HIV/AIDS epidemic: The first 10 years. *Morbidity and Mortality Weekly Report, 40*(22), 357–360.

Centers for Disease Control and Prevention. (1998). U.S. Public Health Service Task Force recommendations for the use of antiretroviral drugs in pregnant women for maternal health and reducing perinatal HIV-1 transmission in the United States. *Morbidity and Mortality Weekly Report, 47* (No. RR-2).

Des Jarlais, D., Abdul-Quadar, A., Minkoff, H. L., et al. (1990).

Crack use and multiple AIDS risk behaviors. *Journal of Acquired Immune Deficiency Syndromes, 3,* 1135–1138.

Fang, G., Siegal, F. P., Weiser, B., et al. (1997). Measurement of human immunodeficiency (HIV) type 1 RNA load distinguishes progressive infection from nonprogressive HIV-1 infection in men and women. *Clinical Infectious Diseases, 25*(2), 332–333.

Furtado, M. R., Callaway, D. S., Phair, J. P., et al. (1999). Persistence of HIV-1 transcription in peripheral-blood mononuclear cells in patients receiving potent antiretroviral therapy. *New England Journal of Medicine, 340*(21), 1672–1674.

Lackritz, E. M. (1998). Prevention of HIV transmission by blood transfusion in the developing world: Achievements and continuing challenges. *AIDS, 12,* Suppl A, S81-6.

McNally, J. H., & Mosher, W. D. (1991). *AIDS-related knowledge and behavior among women 15–44 years of age: United States, 1988.* Bethesda, MD: National Center for Health Statistics.

Minkoff, H. L., & DeHovitz, J. A. (1991). Care of women infected with the human immunodeficiency virus. *Journal of the American Medical Association, 266*(16), 2253–2258.

Zhang, L., Ramratnam, B., Tenner-Racz, K. et al. (1999). Quantifying residual HIV-1 replication in patients receiving combination antiretroviral therapy. *New England Journal of Medicine, 340*(21), 1605–1613.

11

PREGNANCY, LABOR, AND DELIVERY

KEY TERMS

Abortion

Apgar score

Braxton Hicks
    contractions

Cesarean section

Contraction stress test
    (CST)

Eclampsia

Epidural anesthesia

Episiotomy

Fetal alcohol syndrome
    (FAS)

Human chorionic
    gonadotropin (HCG)

Lamaze method

Parturition

Placenta

Placenta previa

Preeclampsia

Uterus

*H*aving a baby now is a very different experience from childbirth in previous generations. Any woman over the age of 60 will probably remember having had a mask slapped on her face, her hands being tied down, and waking up with a baby. Then she probably spent a week in the hospital recovering. Today, a lot has changed, even the vocabulary. People go to prepared childbirth classes. They talk about "birthing," "imprinting," "bonding," "Lamaze"—words that had no meaning for their mothers and grandmothers. Today, women want to be in control of the process. There are also many women who are having their babies at an older age than their mothers. They recognize that giving birth could happen only once or twice in their lifetimes and they want to be there, awake and participating. They view pregnancy and delivery as a normal physiological process and reject the "sickness" view of the past.

The major changes in childbirth came about because many women were no longer content to approach childbirth passively, letting the doctor take over. They wanted to make decisions about the manner of delivery, the procedure, the drugs, the instruments. Today, if the birth is in a hospital, it probably will not take place in the old labor and delivery room with its surgical look. It will happen in a "birthing room" with a homelike atmosphere and where the presence of the father or other partner is welcomed. Delivery also could be outside of the hospital in a childbirth center or even at home, surrounded by friends and family, and attended by an obstetrician who does home deliveries, or by a midwife.

These are progressive and positive innovations. They represent a return of control to the mother and began to emerge with the rise of the women's movement and the struggle for control in other areas of a woman's life. The demands for birthing alternatives changed the attitudes of hospital administrators and physicians and stimulated research evaluating the benefits of different methods of childbirth.

Today's emphasis is on the pleasures and the joys, rather than the trials and tribulations, of pregnancy and delivery. The options in birth, however, are mostly available to the middle- and upper-class women who have planned pregnancy and have chosen to bear a child. A pregnant woman who already has more children than she wants, who is worried about how she is going to manage, who has neither the knowledge nor the money to get the best kind of prenatal nutrition or care, whose medical treatment is given in overcrowded county or city facilities, is not likely to place much value on a beautiful birthing experience. Neither is a pregnant teenager, who is physically immature, subsisting on an improper or perhaps even bizarre diet, and probably more concerned with hiding the pregnancy for as long as possible. Only when a pregnancy is planned and wanted, and the parent or parents have the money and time for options, can all the experiences and sensations of childbirth be truly understood and appreciated. The goal of increased alternatives in maternity care is of great value and should not be underestimated, but it must be accompanied by a continued effort toward better health care for *all* women, and it must also include the right to choose whether to be pregnant at all.

Our discussion of childbirth, then, makes the assumption that the woman made a decision to have a baby and that she is ready to deal with all the joys, discomforts, highs, lows, and ambivalences of pregnancy. It is probably most relevant for the woman who has been fortunate enough to demand a certain standard of health care.

GETTING PREGNANT

All things considered, the act of conception is essentially inconceivable. To say merely that it occurs when the sperm unites with the egg is deceptively simple. Getting them both together at the right time involves an intricate interplay of hormonal preparation and an overwhelming number of natural barriers. That it happens at all seems amazing; that the world should be overpopulated as a result seems extraordinary.

For a pregnancy to occur, a healthy ovum has to be liberated from the ovary; pass into a normal, open fallopian tube; and start being transported downward. The ovum must be mature but cannot get too ripe. If fertilization does not occur within less than a day after ovulation, the egg begins to deteriorate and die. If coitus does occur around the time of ovulation, between 250 and 400 million sperm in the ejaculate are deposited in the vaginal canal—for them, a very hostile environment. Not only can the acidity of the vagina be fatal, but sperm are subject to attack and ingestion by wandering leucocytes. It is essential for survival that they get out of the vagina and into the uterus in a hurry. So, with a limited amount of stored energy, they must swim upstream to a destination 7 in. away—7,000 times their own length. (In humans this distance is the equivalent of 8 miles, or half the English Channel!) Many of the sperm start off in the wrong direction and get lost in the crevices of the vagina. Many more of them never make it up through the endocervical canal of the cervix. Even in the middle of the menstrual cycle when the cervical mucus is more watery, penetrating the cervix is still no small task. Presumably, with the aid of additional hormones—oxytocin is present in the female and prostaglandins are found in semen—and the muscular contractions of the uterus and the fallopian tubes, some of the sperm finally make it to the ampulla of the oviduct.

Animal studies have shown that after the sperm are ejaculated, they remain motionless in the isthmus of the fallopian tube until an ovulated egg appears in the ampulla of the tube. The sperm then resume their motility and reach the ovum within minutes. A study in Israel found that the ovum signals the sperm to get moving again by releasing an as-yet-unidentified chemical factor into the follicular fluid. The authors suggest that if this kind of chemical communication between the egg and the sperm is a necessary interaction for successful fertilization to take place, the absence of the substance could be an explanation for infertility of unknown origin (Ralt et al., 1991).

The sperm that actually get to the ovum, and only about 0.0001% do, find further formidable barriers. The egg is surrounded by a clear protein layer, the *zona pellucida,* and then outside of that, a densely arranged layer of cells, the *corona radiata.* The actual mechanisms of sperm penetration in the human are not completely known. It is generally believed that the sperm must undergo "capacitation," or the removal of surface-coating materials from their heads. Only then are they able to undergo the acrosomal reaction, that is, to secrete digestive enzymes and create a pathway

through the corona radiata and the zona pellucida. Only one sperm actually penetrates the egg cytoplasm to fertilize it. Any others are blocked at the zona. Once the sperm gets to the plasma membrane, the egg resumes meiosis and forms a nucleus with half the number of chromosomes and a second polar body. The climax of all this effort is the union of the nuclei of the sperm and the egg. The two nuclei approach each other, make contact, lose their respective nuclear membranes, and combine their maternal and paternal chromosomes. The zygote, the beginning of a new individual, has been formed.

This event has been observed on human ova cultured in blood serum or follicular fluid and has even been filmed, using microcinematography. When scenes showing human fertilization are incorporated into television specials or other educational films, the approach of the sperm to the egg is generally accompanied by a rising crescendo of music. Then, at the very moment of conception, the drums roll and the cymbals crash—most appropriate for a happening this momentous. In real-life fallopian tubes, with no camera and no music, there is absolutely no awareness on the part of a woman that a potential pregnancy has been initiated. Whether she has been trying to get pregnant for more than a year, or whether pregnancy is the last thing in the world that she wants, there is no physiological signal for any woman that says, this is it, now you are pregnant, and barring other circumstances, you will deliver a baby in 38 weeks! Several weeks will elapse before even one of the presumptive signs of pregnancy—missing the first menstrual period—will take place.

Influencing the Sex of the Child

Getting pregnant as soon as possible is generally the first priority when a couple decides to have a baby. Producing a daughter rather than a son, or vice versa, may not be of any particular concern unless the family already consists of two or more children of the same sex or sex-linked genetic disorders are an issue. It was explained previously (Chapter 5) that sex determination occurs at the time of fertilization and depends on whether the egg is fertilized by a Y-bearing sperm or an X-bearing sperm. An XX zygote will be a female, an XY will become a male. The chances of having a daughter or a son are 50:50. Statistically speaking, on any particular day throughout the world, about half of the babies conceived will be girls and half will be boys. Because it is possible to make certain that only X-sperm or only Y-sperm reach the egg first, it is then possible to select for a particular sex. Why might this be important? Sorting the sperm to get those with X chromosomes rather than Y chromosomes and then artificially inseminating the woman with the X-bearing sperm would result in a greater likelihood of producing a healthy daughter instead of a son. This would decrease the risk of transmitting a sex-linked genetic disease such as hemophilia, X-linked hydrocephalus, or Duchenne's muscular dystrophy. A sperm-sorting method called the Beltsville Sperm Sexing Technology for livestock reproduction and developed by the U.S. Department of Agriculture is used at the Genetics and IVF Institute in Virginia in human pregnancy. The technique is based on the difference in the amount of DNA in X-bearing sperm and Y-bearing sperm. The sperm are treated with a fluorescent marker dye that attaches to the sperm proportionate to the amount of DNA present. The sperm are then passed through a flow cytometer cell sorter, where a laser beam generates ultraviolet light and illuminates the dye. The X-bearing sperm glow brighter because of the greater amount of DNA and are sorted accordingly.

Although the sperm sorting/artificial insemination technique was used first in 1995 by the Genetics and IVF Institute researchers to prevent an X-linked disorder—a medical indication—patients treated at the institute subsequently wanted to "balance out their families"—clearly a lifestyle decision. The Virginia clinic has allowed choosing a child's gender for nonmedical reasons, a decision not endorsed by other researchers.

If having an offspring of a particular gender is terribly important to a couple, there are some other methods of sex selection that have been applied to humans that involve the techniques of sperm separation and artificial insemination used in livestock. But separating X- and Y-bearing sperm by sedimentation, centrifugation, or electrophoresis (running an electrical charge through the sperm in solution) has, thus far, been more successful in bull sperm than in human semen. One of the more publicized methods was patented by Ronald Ericsson, a California biotechnician who founded a company called Gametrics, Ltd. in Montana with many centers worldwide. Ericsson's procedure starts with diluted human ejaculate layered onto a column of human serum albumin. The Y-bearing sperm, faster swimmers than the heavier X-bearing sperm, evidently move more quickly into the boundary between the semen solution and the albumin. After concentrating the sperm through two more albumin layers, the resultant sperm disc, now presumably containing 85% of the Y-bearing type, is resuspended in solution and inseminated into the woman's vagina near the cervix. The technique allegedly enhances the chances of conceiving a male to 75% (Beernink & Ericsson, 1982). The laboratory fees for Ericsson's sex-selection method are expensive even without including physician's costs for the insemination. Thus, only the relatively affluent who live near a Gametrics center and are willing to have sperm manipulation and artificial insemination can increase their chances of having a son by 25%.

According to the American Society of Fertility registry, there are numerous practitioners offering sex selection in the United States. With some modifications, techniques similar to Ericsson's are used to separate X-bearing from Y-bearing sperm, either to increase the chances of a baby of a particular sex or to avoid the transmission of X-linked genetic diseases. One such program in Minnesota costs close to $1,400 for sperm examination, separation, insemination, and subsequent tests.

Currently, the only completely reliable method of ensuring an offspring of the desired sex is through selective abortion after amniocentesis—a procedure with physical risk and of questionable ethics when used for preselection. Most couples are primarily interested in having a healthy baby and are willing to take their 50:50 chances on its sex.

After Fertilization

When the egg is fertilized by a sperm, any symptoms of pregnancy are still weeks in the future, but for the fertilized egg, or zygote, a great deal of immediate activity takes place. The zygote somehow seals itself off so that no other sperm may penetrate it. The first cleavage take place about 20 hours after fertilization, then the second and then the third, all the while the conceptus is slowly being transported into the uterine cavity as a result of the tubal muscular movements. After there are four cleavages, the 16 cells appear as a solid ball or *morula,* meaning "little mulberry." The morula reaches the uterine cavity 72–80 hours after fertilization. Once there, cell division continues rapidly. Within the morula, an off-center fluid-filled space appears, transforming it into a hollow ball of cells, the *blastocyst.* On one aspect of the inner surface of the blastocyst is a mound of cells destined to become the embryo—the *inner cell mass.* The outer wall of the tiny ball becomes the *trophoblast,* containing the cells that will be responsible for the invasion of the uterine lining. By 6 days after ovulation, the pole of the blastocyst that contains the inner cell mass has attached itself to the endometrium of the uterus. Up until now, the developing conceptus has been nourished by the secretions of the tube and the uterus, but its further growth requires more food and oxygen. The blastocyst gains access to the maternal blood supply by burrowing into the uterine lining and becoming completely implanted in it. The trophoblast secretes enzymes that dissolve the cells of the endometrial blood vessels, glands, and connective tissue, and eventually the blastocyst comes to lie in a pool of maternal blood. Now the trophoblast cells proliferate to form branching sprouts, the primitive villi, which increase the surface area of the blastocyst and make it easier for the developing embryo to tap the maternal arteries for nourishment. The thick prepared endometrium is called the *decidua,* meaning "to shed." The portion of the endometrium under the blastocyst

is the *decidua basalis;* this will become the maternal portion of the placenta. Figure 11–1 is a diagrammatic summary of the developmental events during the first week after fertilization.

Concurrent with the development of the trophoblast and implantation there is further differentiation of the inner cell mass. Some of the cells will become the embryo itself, and others will give rise to the membranes that surround and protect it. Three embryonic layers of cells—the ectoderm, the endoderm, and the mesoderm—are formed (Figure 11–2A). The outer ectoderm will give rise to such structures as the entire nervous system and the special senses, the skin, and some of the endocrine glands. From the inner endoderm rises the digestive and respiratory systems and parts of the reproductive system. The middle layer, or mesoderm, differentiates into the future skeletal, urinary, circulatory, and reproductive systems. A cavity, the amniotic sac, develops from a cleft in the ectoderm. By about the 13th day, a second cavity—the yolk sac or primitive gut—appears in the endoderm (Figure 11–2B). As the amniotic cavity enlarges, it becomes filled with a clear and watery fluid and will expand until its roof, the *amnion,* reaches the wall of the blastocyst. As the embryo develops, it is protected and cushioned by amniotic fluid within the amniotic sac. The second fetal membrane, or *chorion,* consists of the trophoblast cells and a mesoderm lining (Figure 11–2C). The trophoblast primitive villi, now with a mesoderm core, proliferate and branch to become the chorionic villi. Blood vessels develop in the mesoderm of the chorionic villi. They become attached to the body stalk connected to the embryo, formed when the two edges of the amniotic sac came together. The body stalk is the future umbilical cord (Figure 11–2D).

Originally the chorionic villi are present over the whole surface of the blastocyst, but as the blastocyst enlarges, the surface that projects into the uterine cavity loses its villi and becomes smooth. This part of the chorion is known as the *chorion laeve* (smooth chorion). At the opposite side of the blastocyst, the chorionic villi branch and enlarge. This area becomes

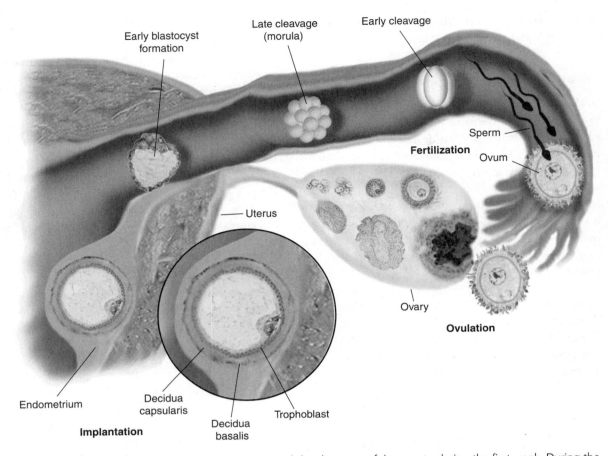

Figure 11–1 Summary of the ovarian cycle, fertilization, and development of the zygote during the first week. During the second and third days after fertilization, the fertilized egg grows from two cells into the 16-cell morula stage. The next stage, the blastocyst, remains free in the uterine cavity during days four and five. By the sixth day, the blastocyst begins to attach itself to the endometrium of the uterus.

known as the *chorion frondosum* (bushy chorion). The connecting stalk of the embryo is attached to the wall of the blastocyst at the *chorion frondosum,* which will become the fetal part of the special structure for fetal–maternal exchange, the **placenta.** A very complicated network develops in which the fetal villi are surrounded by and bathed in the maternal blood sinuses of the *decidua basalis.* Later, the fetal blood vessels, two umbilical arteries and one umbilical vein, are carried in the umbilical cord, which attaches to the

fetal side of the placenta. These blood vessels continue on into the villi. Figure 11–3 is a diagrammatic section showing fetal and maternal tissues in the placenta.

At no time during the pregnancy is there any direct connection between the blood of the fetus and the blood of the mother, so that there can never be any mixing of blood. There are always layers of fetal tissues that separate the maternal and the fetal blood. This is the so-called placental barrier. Materials can be interchanged only through diffusion. The food and

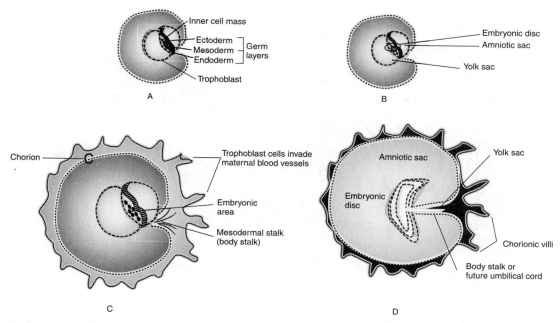

Figure 11–2 Further development of the embryo and formation of the fetal membranes. (A) Formation of the germ layers. (B) Two small cavities, the amniotic sac and the yolk sac, appear. (C) Projections of trophoblast cells (primitive villi) invade blood vessels in the endometrium, and a circulation between the uterine vessels and the embryo begins to be established. The second fetal membrane or chorion forms. (D) The amniotic sac expands until it reaches the wall of the blastocyst. The two edges of the sac come together to enfold the yolk sac and form the body stalk. The blood vessels from the embryo extend along the stalk to become continuous with the vessels in the chorionic villi, ultimately giving rise to the umbilical arteries and the umbilical vein.

oxygen delivered by the maternal uterine arteries diffuse across the placental barrier into the bloodstream of the fetus to provide its life-support system. The waste products from the fetus travel in the opposite direction and are carried away by the mother's uterine veins. When the baby is born, it is still connected to the placenta by the umbilical cord. The mature placenta, approximately 7 in. in diameter and 1 in. thick, is dark red and weighs about a pound. It is delivered from the uterus after the baby, and the umbilical cord must be cut and tied off.

The placenta functions as a transfer vehicle for oxygen and nutritional substances passing from the maternal blood to the fetal circulation, and for carbon dioxide and waste materials from the fetus in the

opposite direction. As the maternal blood enters the placenta, there is a fall in blood pressure that slows its passage and facilitates the respiratory, nutritional, and excretory transfer. The placenta is not only a transfer organ but a factory as well. It is capable of synthesizing enzymes and proteins, and it manufactures fats and carbohydrates that serve as a source of stored energy. The placenta is also a unique kind of endocrine gland; it has a feature possessed by no other endocrine organ—the ability to form both protein and steroid hormones. The hypothalamic-pituitary-ovarian hormones of the mother have set the stage for ovulation, conception, and implantation, but very early in pregnancy, the placenta begins to synthesize hormones. Placental **human chorionic gonadotropin (HCG)**

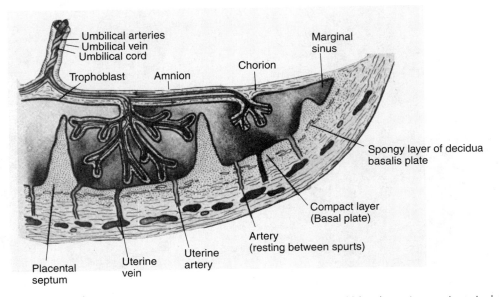

Figure 11–3 Diagram of the maternal-fetal blood flow through the placenta. Maternal blood carrying nutrients is delivered in spurts through the ends of the eroded uterine arteries into the intervillus spaces to bathe the chorionic villi. Nutrients and wastes are exchanged between the chorionic villi from the fetus and the pools of maternal blood.

is secreted very early by the cells of the trophoblast. In biological effects, HCG is similar to luteinizing hormone. Its function is to preserve the corpus luteum and its progesterone production so that the endometrial lining of the uterus, and hence pregnancy, is maintained. The production of HCG begins soon after implantation, rises to a peak production between the 8th and 12th weeks of pregnancy, and then falls to a much lower level for the remainder of gestation. Its presence in blood or urine is used as the basis for pregnancy tests. *Human placental lactogen,* similar in function and chemical structure to both pituitary growth hormone and prolactin, is also known as human *somatomammotropin.* But there is some evidence that the placenta also produces adrenocorticotropin, growth hormone, and possibly thyrotropin as well. After about the 8th week, the placenta is a major source of progesterone, which it produces in large quantities to maintain the pregnancy. The placenta forms estrogen from androgen precursors, many of which are provided by the fetal endocrine glands.

The Period of Gestation

The first few days of human development after fertilization are spent in the fallopian tube, with the zygote busily cleaving itself into the eight-cell stage. In the next 2–3 days, the morula and then the blastocyst are free in the uterine cavity, but by the end of the first week, the blastocyst is superficially imbedded in the endometrial lining of the uterus. It will not be completely implanted until 2½ weeks have elapsed.

The third week of development coincides with the first indication for the woman that she may be pregnant—the missed period. It is not unusual, however, for vaginal bleeding as a result of hemorrhage from the implantation site to occur. Such bleeding, when it is misconstrued as menstruation, commonly results in a faulty calculation of the delivery date. Between the third and fourth week of pregnancy, the first organ system in the embryo becomes functional. The primitive heart tube is linked to the blood vessels in the connecting stalk and chorion, and there is now a cardiovascular system in the embryo, which can draw on the maternal blood supply in the uterus. With the formation and differentiation of a heart and blood circulation, the rest of the full development can take place. In the next few weeks, all the organ systems of the embryo rapidly become established. By the end of the eighth week of pregnancy, the beginnings of all the major internal and external structures are present. Up until this time, the general body form was that of any mammalian embryo, but now it has taken on unquestionably human characteristics. With the change to a recognizable human, the developing zygote is no longer called an embryo. From the ninth week until birth, it is known as a fetus.

The entire gestational period is commonly divided into three parts or trimesters, each consisting of three calendar months. The first trimester is a critical period of development because of the great sensitivity of the fetus to teratogens, agents that can induce malformations. By the end of the first trimester, all of the major organ systems are developed. The rest of the fetal period is concerned with the further growth and differentiation of the organs.

The rate of body growth is astonishing. At the end of the first week of life, the embryo is smaller than the period at the end of this sentence. At the end of the first trimester, the fetus weighs a little over 1 oz and its length from the top of its head to the end of its spine is the length of one's middle finger. In 9 months of fetal life, the ovum will average a daily increase of 1½ mm in length and will increase its weight 6 billion times. If it kept growing like that after birth, a 10-year-old child would be 20 ft tall and weigh several trillion times as much as the earth!

By the end of the second trimester, 24 weeks after fertilization, the crown-rump length of the fetus is equal to the span of one's hand. It weighs about 1½ lb with very little subcutaneous fat stored under its skin. Consequently, the fetus looks wrinkled and wizened with more of the characteristics associated with old age than with infancy. Although all of its organs are well developed, the respiratory system of a fetus born prematurely at this time is generally too immature to permit it to survive.

Beginning late in the seventh month the fetus accumulates rapidly increasing amounts of fat. As term approaches, it begins to take on the rosy plumpness of a newborn infant. Mortality rates are still high for fetuses born between 26 and 29 weeks, but some do survive independently. The last 3 weeks of fetal life, 35–38 weeks after fertilization, put on the finishing touches. Growth slows as birth approaches. On the average, fetuses reach a crown-rump length of 360 mm (14 in.), total length 20–22 in., and weigh about 7½ lb. Male fetuses grow somewhat more rapidly than female fetuses, and baby boys tend to weigh about 3 oz more than baby girls at birth. All newborns' eyes are the same color, blue-gray, and it is impossible to predict their later hue.

Multiple Pregnancy

Only one offspring at a time is the usual condition in humans and other large mammals. The most common type of human twinning occurs when two eggs are simultaneously ovulated from separate follicles and are fertilized by different sperms to implant in two separate but closely opposed areas in the uterus. These are fraternal or *dizygotic* twins. They may be the same or of opposite sexes, and they resemble each other as much as any other siblings. *Monozygotic* twins originate from one fertilized egg. This kind of twinning usually starts at the end of the first week with the division of the inner cell mass into two embryos. Such twins are the same sex, genetically identical, and obviously are identical in physical appearance unless there has been some environmental factor during fetal life to cause a difference between them.

Twins occur about once every 87 births in the United States, and most of them are the fraternal type. The tendency toward dizygotic twinning is genetically influenced, being greater in blacks and less in Japanese, for example. The likelihood of twins increases with the age of the mother, and once a woman has given birth to twins, a multiple birth is about five times more likely to occur the next time. There are various opinions concerning the inheritability of monozygotic or identical twins, but it is agreed that age of the mother is not a factor. "Siamese" or joined monozygotic twins occur as a result of incomplete duplication about 1 in every 400 identical twin pregnancies.

Multiple births other than twins can be of the identical type, the fraternal type, or combinations of the two. Triplets are said to occur once in 7,000 births (87^2) and quadruplets once in 660,000 births (87^3). In recent years, the use of drugs to induce ovulation has resulted in a greater frequency of quadruplets, quintuplets, sextuplets, and even octuplets.

DIAGNOSIS OF PREGNANCY

In the old movies, pregnancy was always diagnosed by telephone. The phone would ring, the prospective mother would pick it up, listen, and then announce to whomever was around, "The rabbit died!" A whole generation of young moviegoers grew up thinking that dead rabbits were somehow integral to being pregnant.

The rabbit did not just die, of course. It had to be killed so that its ovaries could be examined for ruptured follicles. Urine from a presumably pregnant woman was injected into the ear vein of a mature virgin female rabbit. The chorionic gonadotropin in the urine, if the woman was indeed pregnant, induced ovulation in the rabbit within 16–48 hours after injection. This constituted the Friedman test, one of the biologic methods for determining pregnancy. The test animals for the Aschheim-Zondek test were immature mice, and other biological tests were developed using immature rats, female toads, or male frogs. They were all based on the same principle—that chorionic gonadotropin present in the blood and urine of pregnant women will cause an effect in the reproductive tracts of test animals.

Although these biological tests were reliable, they required destroying test animals, took several days for determination, and gave the best results only after about 2 weeks past the missed period. After 1960, immunological tests to detect the presence of chorionic gonadotropin became available and have largely replaced the animal tests.

Immunological pregnancy tests are either slide tests or tube tests. In the slide tests, the woman's urine is mixed with the blood serum that contains antibodies to human chorionic gonadotropin (HCG). Latex particles coated with pure HCG are then added to the mixture. If the woman is pregnant, no clumping or agglutination of the latex particles takes place and the test is considered positive. If she is not pregnant, the agglutination of the particles can be observed, and the test is then negative. The basis for the test is that if there is HCG in the woman's urine, it neutralizes or inhibits the serum antibodies. The antibodies are then unavailable to react with the purified HCG that had been coated onto the latex particles; hence, there is no agglutination. Some slide tests are simplified to a quick one-step procedure. The latex particles, coated with anti-HCG serum, are mixed with the urine. If there is HCG in the urine, the particles agglutinate (positive test); if HCG is absent, there is no agglutination (negative test).

The tube tests are based on the same kind of agglutination inhibition, but the purified HCG is coated on sheep red blood cells. When anti-HCG serum, the coated blood cells, and pregnancy urine containing HCG are mixed in a tube, the HCG in the urine will neutralize the antiserum. The unagglutinated red blood cells sink to the bottom of the tube and form a ring of cells in a doughnut pattern, positive for pregnancy. The absence of the ring indicates a negative test, that is, no HCG in the urine.

There are a number of slide and tube immunoassay tests supplied to clinics, laboratories, and doctors in the form of pregnancy kits. No test is ideal, and all will occasionally produce false results. False-positive results, incorrectly diagnosing pregnancy in women who are not pregnant, are relatively infrequent but can occur when certain drugs, particularly tranquilizers, are taken. Protein or blood in the urine, common in bladder infections, also can result in false positives. False-negative results, which indicate nonpregnancy in women who are actually pregnant, are more common, particularly in early pregnancy. Some of the tube and slide tests have greater sensitivity for detecting low levels of HCG, but all of the routine immunoassays that are performed in a physician's office or at home are basically qualitative tests.

Immunoassay tests are much more sensitive than the slide and tube tests, are capable of detecting very low levels of HCG in the blood serum instead of the urine even before the first missed period, and are usually quantitative tests. The earliest way of detecting HCG is by means of the immunoassay for the beta subunit of HCG, the portion of the molecule responsible for its biological properties. The beta subunit is produced by the trophoblast cells of the embryo 7–9 days after ovulation, and the test can be performed in about 2 hours by a laboratory that has the appropriate equipment. Because the beta-HCG test is able to pick up such very small amounts of the hormone in the blood, it is especially useful in the diagnosis of ectopic pregnancy, which is associated with very low levels of HCG. Currently, the most popular pregnancy tests used in clinics and doctor's offices are the enzyme-linked immunosorbent assays (ELISA). The technique utilizes two monoclonal anti-HCG antibodies for two separate binding sites on the HCG molecule: one for the alpha subunit and the other for the beta subunit. An enzyme bonded to the second anti-HCG monoclonal antibody will induce a visible color reaction if HCG is present in the urine or blood serum sample. The test requires only minutes to perform and is sensitive to 25 milli-international units of HCG per milliliter of sample.

Although home pregnancy tests had been sold over the counter in Canada and Europe for many years, it was not until early 1978 that the first home pregnancy kit was licensed for sale at about $10 in the United States. Today, a woman has several products from which to choose. Not all of the kits are equally effective, but the ELISA tests have made it possible to get the sensitivity of the best home pregnancy tests (not necessarily the most expensive—read the label) to the range at which a woman can get a positive result within 1 day of a delayed period or even before.

Pregnancy tests are tools to establish the diagnosis of pregnancy when the physical signs are still inconclusive. By confirming a pregnancy, they can reassure a woman who is very anxious to have a baby. They can allay anxiety by confirming nonpregnancy in a woman who is not. If a termination of the pregnancy is desired, a pregnancy test is useful because early abortions are safer. If a woman wants to be pregnant, she can start a program of prenatal care and avoid needlessly exposing the fetus to drugs, smoking, or alcohol. Pregnancy tests, however, are rarely necessary for a wanted pregnancy. Within 2 weeks after a missed period, there are usually enough subjective symptoms so that a woman can be reasonably certain she is pregnant. At that time, a pelvic examination by an experienced practitioner can establish the diagnosis of pregnancy with accuracy.

Signs and Symptoms of Pregnancy

Traditionally, the portents of pregnancy have been grouped into those that are presumptive and experienced by the woman herself; those that are probable, and observed by the clinical examiner; and finally the positive, beyond-the-shadow-of-a-doubt signs. The latter are not evident until the 16th to 18th week of gestation.

The most obvious presumptive symptom is the absence of menstruation. Of course, just being late or even skipping a period is not a reliable sign of pregnancy, but when the cessation of menstruation is accompanied by morning nausea, fatigue, breast tenderness, and frequency of urination, pregnancy is very likely. Every woman is different, and these early complaints may not be present. But when several of them are associated with a missed period there is a 2:1 chance of pregnancy.

A woman accustomed to vaginal self-examination would notice color changes from the usual pink to a dusky blue in the walls of the vagina and the cervix. This is caused by increased blood supply and venous congestion and is called Chadwick's sign. Such a color change can be present, however, in heart disease or with a pelvic tumor.

A rather reliable indication of pregnancy is an elevation of the basal body temperature (BBT). A woman who keeps a record of her BBT would know she is pregnant if a level of 98.8°F–99.8°F remained for 3 weeks after ovulation.

Probable signs of pregnancy are those that appear on physical examination. Changes in the size, shape, and consistency of the uterus can be observed. Soon after implantation of the fertilized ovum, a soft bulge at the implantation site appears on one side of the uterus. Skilled hands can detect this softening of the uterus on one side while the other side remains firm (Piskacek's sign). Goodell's sign, a softening of the cervix, also appears early. Hegar's sign refers to the softening of the neck or isthmus of the uterus, the narrow part between the body and the cervix. First detectable at about 6 weeks, Hegar's sign disappears later when the entire cervix and the uterus have become soft and spongy in consistency.

The positive signs of pregnancy refer to proof that there is, beyond any doubt, a fetus growing in the uterus. Around 16–18 weeks, a woman will begin to feel a sort of fluttering feeling (often mistaken for gas in a first pregnancy) that is known as quickening, or "feeling life." For the doctor or nurse-midwife, hearing the fetal heart sounds, a fetal electrocardiogram, or an ultrasound outline of the fetus within the fetal sac, identifiable by the fifth or sixth week, are all signs that make the diagnosis of pregnancy a certainty. By 14 weeks, a procedure called internal ballottement can be performed gently during a vaginal examination. With the finger up against the cervix, the cervix is gently tapped. The fetus within the amniotic sac bounces up against the top of the uterus, and, as it sinks back down, the rebound is felt against the finger. By 24 weeks, external ballottement—a push on one side of the abdomen with one hand in order to feel the fetus bounce to the other side and hit the other hand—can be performed.

Waiting to get these kinds of confirmation of pregnancy may seem to be unnecessary, but there are circumstances when demonstrating the presence of a fetus is the only way of distinguishing pregnancy from another condition, such as an ovarian cyst or multiple fibroids. Every now and then, a case is reported in which a woman, usually very obese, actually delivers a baby as her first indication of pregnancy.

Calculation of the Due Date

Should a woman be fortunate enough to know the date of conception, she can, based on statistical averages, expect to deliver a baby 266 days, or 38 weeks, later. Because the precise time of fertilization is ordinarily not known, the usual rule of thumb is to date the pregnancy from the onset of the first day of the last menstrual period that occurred—a total of 280 days, or 40 weeks, or 10 lunar months, or 9 calendar months. The estimated delivery date is obtained by taking the first day of the last menstruation, subtracting 3 months from that date, and then adding 1 week. If, for example, the first day of the last menstrual period was February 21, the termination of the pregnancy will be on or about November 28. This calculation assumes that ovulation, and hence fertilization, occurred 14 days after the onset of the menstrual period. This is only true in a 28-day cycle. Ovulation is known to occur 14 days *prior* to a menstrual period, but if a woman is pregnant, that is the menstrual period she will not have. The point is, the due date is only a time frame; delivery can normally occur 2–3 weeks before or after it.

MATERNAL CHANGES DURING PREGNANCY

Pregnancy is a physiologically normal condition and not an illness. This does not mean that a woman will feel terrific and tranquil for the entire 9 months. Who does, pregnant or not, for the better part of a year? Treating pregnant women as though they were ill and women thinking of themselves as such is one extreme. The other is denying that pregnancy can be anything but a healthy, happy, productive, problem-free period.

Sometimes all the emphasis on the "naturalness" of pregnancy can produce unrealistic expectations about how a healthy and emotionally stable woman "should" feel and behave. But consider that there are profound and multiple physiological adjustments of all body systems that begin at the moment of conception, even before a woman is aware that anything has taken place. These changes continue throughout pregnancy, and some of them may not be reversed until 6 weeks after delivery of the baby. Such alterations are bound to be the basis for some symptoms. How a woman reacts and copes with them has a lot to do with her personality, life situation, relationship with her partner and the rest of her family, and her feelings about having a baby. It would seem logical that there may be more ambivalence, regret, or conflict when the pregnancy was unplanned. But even a planned and wanted baby is no guarantee that the period of waiting for it will be gratifying and free from minor problems and complaints.

Everyone is different and unique. A great many women can sail through pregnancy experiencing no difficulties and enjoying every minute of it. No nausea, no backaches, no swelling mars their expectancy. They bloom, they glow; they apparently have no trouble with their skin or hair, and they don't get hemorrhoids, stretch marks, or varicose veins. Other women may have some or all of these symptoms, and they will obviously not get as much pleasure out of being pregnant. But whatever the ups and downs of pregnancy, and they do exist, a woman can have the underlying knowledge that she is participating in something exceptional—the process of creating another human being. The physical aspects of pregnancy are frequently unpredictable and sometimes uncomfortable, but an understanding of what is taking place and why, and an appreciation that other women have similar experiences, can provide a woman with the knowledge to work with her body and not against it.

Changes in the Reproductive System

Uterus. The **uterus,** which in a nonpregnant woman weighs 2 oz, has a capacity of 2 ml, and measures 3 by 2 by 1 in., undergoes a spectacular increase in size. At full term it weighs 2 lb, is about five to six times larger, and has increased its capacity by 2,000 times to accommodate the developing fetus. This enormous enlargement of the pregnant uterus is accomplished by growth of the individual smooth muscle cells, or fibers, which become wider and longer. The blood vessels elongate, enlarge, dilate, and sprout new branches to support and nourish the growing muscle tissue, and the increase in uterine weight is accompanied by a large increase in uterine blood flow. Uterine contractility is evidently enhanced. Spontaneous, irregular, and painless contractions, called **Braxton Hicks contractions,** begin in the first trimester. They continue throughout pregnancy, becoming especially noticeable during the last month when they function in thinning out or effacing the cervix before delivery.

The uterus is still in the pelvic cavity for the first 3 months, after which it progressively ascends into the abdomen. As the uterus grows, it presses on the urinary bladder and causes the increased frequency of urination noticed in early pregnancy. By 20 weeks, the fundus, or top of the uterus, is at the level of the umbilicus. Thereafter, the growth of the fetus can be determined by measuring the distance from the pubic symphysis to the top of the uterine fundus. The expanding uterus begins to "show" around the fourth to fifth month, although the waistline seems to thicken earlier in subsequent pregnancies. Figure 11–4 shows the change in abdominal shape in a woman who is 7 months pregnant.

Cervix. Softening of the cervix by the sixth week (Goodell's sign) has been mentioned. Along with the softening, which is the result of vasocongestion, the endocervical glands increase in size and number and produce more cervical mucus. Under the influence of progesterone, a thick mucous plug is formed, which blocks the cervical os and protects the developing conceptus from bacterial invasion. The increase in cervical secretions results in leukorrhea, or increased vaginal secretion. The secretion is markedly acidic, which also helps in preventing bacterial infection.

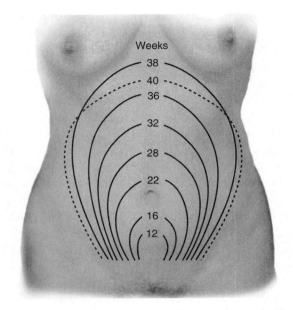

Figure 11–4 Pregnancy during the seventh month. The top of the uterine fundus is about three finger breadths above the umbilicus. By the ninth month, it will rise to about 1½ in. below the breastbone.

The cervix is composed almost completely of connective tissue with very little smooth muscle. The cervix at term can be compared to a combination of rubber bands and salt water taffy. Under a slow steady pull, the cervix stretches but has very little rebound and can, therefore, progressively dilate.

Ovaries and Tubes. The increased blood supply to the ovaries and tubes causes them to become somewhat enlarged and elongated, and they tend to hang down alongside the uterus. The ovary that contains the corpus luteum, which reaches a maximum development during the third month of pregnancy, is even more pronounced in its enlargement. After the placenta takes over the major production of progesterone, the corpus luteum of pregnancy regresses. The anterior pituitary gland is inhibited by the large amounts of circulating steroid hormones, and no follicles mature or ovulate during pregnancy.

Vagina. Ordinarily a highly distensible organ, the vagina prepares for even greater distensibility during delivery by a thickening of the vaginal lining, a reduction in the density of the connective tissue, and an increased growth of the muscle tissue. The increased blood supply results in the color change previously mentioned.

Breasts. Many women experience a tenderness and enlargement of the breasts during the progestational phase of each menstrual cycle. This sensitivity remains and becomes intensified in early pregnancy. Tingling and soreness are common in the first 2 months; thereafter, the breasts become enlarged and even more tender and nodular. A woman accustomed to sleeping on her stomach may not be able to because her breasts hurt. Wearing a bra all the time, even at night, to support the breasts will help. The nipples enlarge and become more erectile and deeply pigmented. As seen in Figure 11–5, the primary areolae become wider and deepen in color and Montgomery's glands are more prominent. Under the influence of steroids from the corpus luteum and the placenta, from placental lactogen, prolactin, and chorionic gonadotropin, the ducts, lobules, and alveolae of the gland tissue proliferate tremendously. By the 10th week of gestation, colostrum can be expressed from the nipples, but actual milk synthesis is inhibited by the high sex steroid hormone levels. If a woman is planning to nurse her baby, certain preparations can be made during the last 2 months of pregnancy. The colostrum should be massaged out of the breasts twice daily, and a wet washcloth should be used on the nipples and areolae to remove any crusting. Inverted nipples may have to be pulled out each day to encourage protraction. Some women's breasts become dry and chapped, and a petroleum jelly-based cream can be massaged into the skin.

Changes in the Digestive System

Morning Sickness. One of the most annoying symptoms of early pregnancy, experienced by

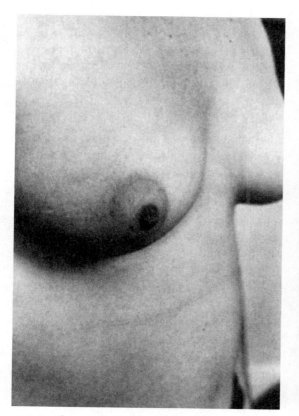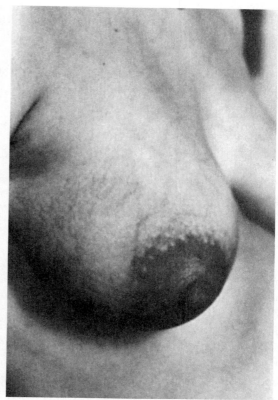

Figure 11–5 Comparison of the breasts of a nonpregnant woman (left) with the breast of a woman who is 7 months pregnant (right). Note the size, the deeply pigmented areola, signs of increased vascularity, and prominent Montgomery's gland elevations in the breast during pregnancy. The second areola, a further pigmented mottling effect surrounding the primary areola, is evident.

50%–80% of pregnant women, is the nausea and vomiting familiarly known as "morning sickness." While it occurs most often in the morning, the nauseated feeling can be present in the afternoon or evening, and some women have it all day. The nausea is not a dizzy nausea, the kind one gets with the flu, but is of sudden onset and seems to be associated with hunger pains, although it can be precipitated by odors from cooking, paint, cigarettes, and so forth. For many women, nausea can be eliminated by avoiding an empty-stomach situation. If the nausea is the mild prebreakfast type, munching a few crackers or dry toast in bed before arising may be the answer. For a particular woman, a period of trial and error may be necessary to find something that alleviates her nausea. With hot tea, fruit juices, candy drops, several small meals instead of three large ones, nonfat foods, and high protein foods, many women can solve this problem. Evidently, it is the frequency of eating rather than the quantity that is important.

The physiological basis for morning sickness is essentially unknown. There are various theories that attempt to link the nausea and vomiting with the high levels of human chorionic gonadotropin, high levels of circulating estrogens, reduced stomach acidity, and the lowered tone and motility of the digestive tract.

The principal nutrient utilized by the fetus is glucose, and it derives its supply from the mother's blood. As a result of the placental transfer of glucose, the pregnant woman's fasting blood sugar level is about 10% lower than normal. This, and other changes in maternal carbohydrate metabolism, may play a role in morning sickness, since drinking a sweet beverage on arising often can prevent nausea and vomiting.

There are some women who try soda crackers, juice, hard candy, ice water—all the measures that apparently work for other people—without success and still experience multiple daily episodes of vomiting. Relatively rarely, the nausea and vomiting of pregnancy can develop into *hyperemesis gravidarum,* which as the name implies, is a severe and persistent vomiting that produces dehydration and disturbances in acid-base balance and requires hospitalization for intravenous feeding and other measures to relieve it. There is an analytic school of thought that associates hyperemesis with an unwanted pregnancy. "There is no doubt," stated one OB/GYN text, "that most instances of excessive persistent vomiting (hyperemesis gravidarum) are due to deep-rooted psychological factors which result from a subconscious rejection of the pregnancy" (Page, Villee, & Villee, 1976). Another text on obstetrical practice, edited by Aladjem and presumably used to teach medical students, unequivocally states that hyperemesis is psychogenic vomiting and that a woman is unconsciously trying to "vomit up the baby" because she either rejects it or is frightened of having a baby with a serious birth defect. In Dunnihoo's text, emotional and psychological factors are said to instigate or aggravate hyperemesis. Women who have it are characterized as "being of moderate intelligence with histrionic personalities. . . . with strong maternal attachments and have demonstrated immature behavior."

Certainly, the involvement of the emotions with physical complaints is well recognized, and there may be cases in which excessive nausea and vomiting has a psychosomatic basis. Despite psychiatric conviction, however, there can be little actual evidence to prove or disprove this explanation because unconscious motivation is obviously difficult to validate. A woman whose morning sickness has become serious and persistent enough to put her in the hospital probably would have considerable anxiety as a result, and it would not be surprising if she very *consciously* rejected the whole idea of being pregnant at that point. In addition, labeling a woman with a preconceived psychological evaluation could easily lead physicians to ignore a consideration of other conditions, such as food poisoning or intestinal obstruction, that could cause hyperemesis.

The safety of any drug taken during pregnancy, including those to relieve nausea and vomiting, is questionable. Drugs should be avoided if at all possible, but women whose morning (or all day) sickness drastically interferes with their daily lives, is unresponsive to the usual nondrug remedies, generally makes them miserable for months on end, and can develop into hyperemesis with its accompanying metabolic disturbances would have to weigh the benefits of taking an antiemetic drug against its potential risks. From the time of its introduction in 1956, an estimated 33 million women worldwide took such a proprietary antinauseant called Bendectin in the United States and Canada, Debendox in Great Britain, Lenotan in Germany, and Merbental in South America. When its manufacturer, Merrell Dow Pharmaceuticals, ceased production in June 1983 and took it off the market, about 25% of the pregnant women in this country were taking Bendectin. Composed of an antihistamine (10 mg of doxylamine succinate) and a vitamin (10 mg of pyridoxine hydrochloride), Bendectin was the only medication for nausea and vomiting of early pregnancy that had specifically been approved by the FDA.

Because it was the most commonly taken prescription drug during early pregnancy, it also was the most thoroughly studied for the risk of birth defects. Its widespread use, however, contributed to the inconsistency of the results. The incidence of birth defects in the general population—the risk that everyone faces—is 3%. Since one-quarter of all pregnant women in the United States (an estimated 400,000 annually) took Bendectin in the first trimester of pregnancy, there were babies born with congenital abnormalities who also were exposed to a drug, but this does not prove that Bendectin caused the defect. A cause-and-effect relationship between Bendectin and congenital malformations has never been clearly or consistently demonstrated, but there have been a number of studies that associated its use with birth defects that included digestive tract abnormalities, sternum concavities (funnel chest), heart defects, and cleft palates or lips.

A panel of experts convened by the FDA in 1980 examined the data from animal studies and 13 epidemiological studies and concluded that the incidence of malformations in the offspring of women who took Bendectin was no greater than the incidence in women who had not been exposed to Bendectin.

In 1982, the FDA, prompted by public concern and publicity about animal data that again raised questions about the safety of the drug, decided to reexamine all the Bendectin studies. An investigation had suggested an association between exposure to Bendectin in the first trimester of pregnancy and diaphragmatic hernias, a potentially fatal defect in which the abdominal organs herniate up into the lung cavity through a hole in the diaphragm, and a rat study in West Germany demonstrated a similar relationship. A monkey study in which the pregnant animals were treated with Bendectin at 10–20 times the human dose by weight linked the drug to a heart defect. Subsequent epidemiological studies, however, provided no evidence for a relationship between Bendectin use and such adverse effects as skeletal abnormalities, limb deformities, cleft lip or palate, or cardiac defects (Michaelis, Michaelis, Gluck, & Koller, 1983; Aselton & Jick, 1983; Golding, Vivian, & Baldwin, 1983). Only one retrospective investigation, by Yale researchers Eskanazi and Bracken in 1982, found that Bendectin appeared to be strongly associated with the occurrence of pyloric stenosis, a stricture or narrowing of the opening between the stomach and the small intestine. Even those findings were refuted in late 1983 by researchers at Boston University, who reported that in their study of 325 infants with pyloric stenosis and 3,153 babies with other defects, Bendectin did not increase the likelihood of pyloric stenosis or any other congenital malformation (Mitchell et al., 1983).

But despite a lack of a statistical evidence that Bendectin causes birth defects, an anguished woman who has been exposed to Bendectin and delivers a child with a congenital abnormality is going to be convinced that Bendectin caused the birth defect, and juries may feel the same way. By early 1983, there were 300 lawsuits pending against Merrell Dow Pharmaceuticals, and the company's insurance rate was $1 million a month. After a jury recommended an award of $750,000 to the parents of a child with limb deformities, Merrell Dow voluntarily discontinued production of Bendectin, based on its economic decision that it could not afford to pay the insurance and the costs arising from the suits. In 1985, 1,000 lawsuits against Merrell Dow were consolidated in one federal court trial. After months of deliberation, the jury decided that Bendectin did not cause the clubbed feet, missing limbs, and other birth defects in the children of women who took the drug to alleviate nausea. The plaintiffs initiated an appeal process, which took another 4 years, but in 1989, a federal court of appeals panel absolved Bendectin from any role in causing birth defects. Despite the vindication of the drug, Merrell Dow stated that it would never reintroduce Bendectin. Said a spokesperson, "We just find that marketing products for use during pregnancy is just an invitation to litigation" (Ross, 1989).

Bendectin was the only antinausea drug approved by the FDA for use during pregnancy. Now that it is unavailable, there are likely to be pregnant women who really require such aid. They even may be reluctant to have a second pregnancy after experiencing the first one without the help of an antinauseant. Mild or moderate morning sickness is bearable, but for many women, months of severe nausea and vomiting is not. Although the ingredients in Bendectin are readily available, physicians, like the Merrell Dow pharmaceutical company, are unlikely to risk litigation by prescribing them. One OB/GYN text, however, points out that vitamin B_6 has some effectiveness alone and could be tried first. Doxylamine (as Unisom, a sleep aid) also can be obtained over the counter, so a combination similar to that of Bendectin can be made

(Niebyl, 1990). Whether to take doxylamine and pyridoxine hydrochloride for morning sickness could, therefore, be an individual woman's choice. Of course, no drug should be taken during pregnancy unless absolutely necessary. The fact that the majority of epidemiological studies have found no association between Bendectin and birth defects could still be viewed as inconclusive because no one of them is able to prove beyond a doubt that Bendectin can or cannot cause birth defects. It is significant, however, that since 1983 when the drug was taken off the market, there has been no decline in the birth defects that had been attributed to its use. They still occur at the same rate.

There is much less information known about other antivomiting aids. Highly potent antiemetic drugs such as phenothiazines have not routinely been used for morning sickness but have been reserved for the treatment of hyperemesis, for which they produce a rapid and gratifying response. But safety of phenothiazines during pregnancy has not been as well established as it has for Bendectin, and their potential for producing severe side effects in the mother (liver damage, blood difficulties) makes them even more controversial than Bendectin. Should phenothiazines be necessary, however, a pregnant woman can be reassured by the lack of consistent evidence for their teratogenicity, that is, ability to cause abnormalities.

Other Gastrointestinal Tract Difficulties. Digestive tract complaints may include excessive salivation, which occasionally occurs and then spontaneously disappears by the middle of the second trimester. Heartburn is somewhat more universal, especially during the last 3 months. It is caused by regurgitation of the stomach contents into the upper esophagus and may be associated with the general relaxed muscle tone of the entire gastrointestinal tract during pregnancy, a hormonal effect. The cardiac sphincter at the junction of the esophagus and the stomach, which normally constricts to prevent reflux of the acid gastric juices into the esophagus, is more relaxed. When this relative atony of the sphincter is coupled with the increased pressure from the growing uterus pressing on the stomach, heartburn results. It is not due to hyperacidity in the stomach, but antacids such as calcium carbonate, magnesium trisilicate, or aluminum hydroxide preparations relieve the symptom. Baking soda or other antacids commonly used for heartburn, should not be taken because of their high sodium content. Other solutions for heartburn are avoiding spicy or greasy foods, small frequent meals, and sleeping on several pillows so that the head is elevated.

The decreased muscle tone in the large intestine results in decreased motility and increased water absorption and leads to another common complaint: constipation and flatulence, or gas. Adequate roughage in the diet and exercise will usually minimize the problem.

A hormonal effect on the gums in the mouth may cause gingivitis—swollen, spongy gums that bleed easily. The condition may be improved by taking vitamin C; the difficulty will spontaneously disappear after delivery. There is no truth to the old wives' tale that pregnancy results in more tooth decay. The calcium in the teeth is fixed and is not withdrawn. Dental repair can be done at any stage, but because of exposure to the anesthetic, pregnancy is not the best time to have one's wisdom teeth extracted. Oral surgery should be postponed, if possible.

Changes in the Circulatory System

Cardiovascular alterations occur early in pregnancy. These changes are necessary to meet the demands of the enlarging uterus and the placenta for more blood and more oxygen. A pregnant woman is, after all, oxygenating the blood of the fetus as well as her own. The heart works harder and pumps more blood. By the end of the first trimester, cardiac output has increased by 25%–50%, and there is an accompanying increase in the blood volume. By the end of the pregnancy, blood volume will increase 40%–90%, depending on the size of the mother, the size of the fetus, and on which investigator is reporting the data. The number of red blood cells also increases, but there is a greater rise in the plasma volume as a result of hormonal factors and sodium and water retention. The hemoglobin concentration falls, the heart rate increases and rises to a maximum of 15 beats above the nonpregnant state. Arterial blood pressure drops, reaches its low point at about 22 weeks of gestation, and thereafter slowly rises to prepregnant levels until term. The ability of the blood to clot increases significantly (hypercoagulability), but there is no increase in the incidence of thrombosis, or formation of blood clots, during pregnancy.

Varicose veins in the legs and the vulva are common during pregnancy. There may be a genetic predisposition to weakened venous walls and supporting tissues; women whose mothers or other family members have varicosities are more likely to have them. The developing uterus presses on the veins returning blood from the legs and impedes the flow of venous blood. This slowing of circulation, coupled with the engorgement of the pelvic veins, causes the blood to back up in the veins of the legs and exert increasing pressure on their walls. If the venous walls are not strong enough to withstand this increased pressure, they stretch and thin out to become the large, tortuous varicose veins. They may not produce any symptoms, but some women have varying amounts of discomfort ranging from mild burning and itching to aching pain. Relief can be obtained by avoiding standing for long periods, elevating the legs whenever possible, and wearing support hose. In severe cases, putting on elastic stockings or bandages in the morning when the veins are collapsed and empty will help.

Hemorrhoids are varicosities of the rectal veins and can be very annoying during pregnancy. Constipation aggravates hemorrhoids, and straining during defecation may cause bleeding. There are various hemorrhoidal ointments that may provide relief.

Some women get occasional mild nosebleeds during pregnancy that may be related to the increased blood volume and resultant capillary pressure. These can usually be controlled by remaining upright, bending the head forward, and pinching the nostrils together.

Early in pregnancy, there is an increase in the minute respiratory volume—the total amount of air moved into the lungs each minute. The number of breaths per minute does not increase, but the amount of air breathed in with each breath does. Later in gestation there are anatomical changes as well. Even though the uterus in the abdominal cavity pushes up on the diaphragm and elevates it, the entire thoracic cavity compensates by an increase in its dimensions so that more air can be inspired. Shortness of breath, or dyspnea, develops in slightly more than half of pregnant women in the last month. Since the breathing capacity is not limited, the mechanism is unknown. It may be related to pressure on the diaphragm and lungs. Dyspnea usually subsides when "lightening," the settling of the fetal head into the true pelvis, occurs. Lightening is experienced several weeks before labor begins with a first baby, but usually takes place during labor in a woman who has already borne a child.

Changes in the Excretory System

Urinary frequency occurs at the beginning of pregnancy and also near the end. Early in pregnancy, the enlarging uterus causes traction on the muscles of the bladder neck and results in the sensation of having to urinate often. As the uterus rises out of the pelvis, the frequency of urination subsides, but it returns in late pregnancy because of lack of room for the bladder to fill. There is little a woman can do about this symptom.

Probably as a result of hormonal influences, the ureters leading from the kidneys to the bladder become dilated by the 10th week of pregnancy. The right side is generally more affected than the left side. In some women, this enlargement may predispose to kidney infections.

Total body water and electrolytes are normally increased in pregnant women. Ankle swelling is very common and of little significance. A generalized body edema with swollen fingers and puffy eyelids occurs in about 25% of pregnant women. When it is accompanied by a rapid weight gain (1½ lb in a week), an increase in blood pressure, and protein appearing in the urine, it may signal the beginnings of difficulties. In the absence of these signs, however, generalized swelling is of no consequence. There should be no attempts to reduce the edema with diuretics. Whether sodium restriction is helpful or harmful is uncertain. It is generally believed that the most prudent course is to neither increase nor decrease sodium intake, but to salt foods as usual and to rely on kidney mechanisms to maintain a normal salt balance.

Musculoskeletal Changes

By the 10th to 12th week of pregnancy, and under hormonal influence, the ligaments that hold the sacroiliac joints and the pubic symphysis in place begin to soften and stretch, and the articulations between the joints widen and become more movable. The hormones involved are estrogen and progesterone and relaxin, a peptide produced by the corpus luteum of pregnancy and placenta. Relaxin was originally identified in the blood serum of pregnant rabbits, rodents, and pigs.

The relaxation of the joints is progressive and becomes maximal by the beginning of the third trimester. The purpose of the changes is to increase the size of the pelvic cavity and to make delivery easier. But the instability and looseness of the joints may cause discomfort in the pubic and lumbar regions. In an attempt to keep the joints "locked" during locomotion, a pregnant woman will assume the characteristic duck-waddling walk of late pregnancy.

The postural changes of pregnancy—an increased swayback and an upper spine extension to compensate for the enlarging abdomen—coupled with the loosening of the sacroiliac joints may result in lower back pain. The backaches can be relieved by heat, rest, a bed board under the mattress, and by exercises that strengthen abdominal and back muscles.

Many women experience leg cramps during the last few months of pregnancy. A painful spasm of the gastrocnemius (calf) muscle is most likely to occur when lying in bed in a supine position. Immediate relief of the cramp can be obtained by flexing the foot upward so that the toes point toward the face while simultaneously pushing down on the knee to straighten the leg. There are claims that high dietary phosphorus or insufficient calcium provokes leg cramps, but attempts to prevent them by adding calcium preparations or restricting dietary phosphorus are not always successful.

Some women notice occasional sensations in their hands, ranging from tingling or pins and needles (paresthesia) to actual pain that comes and goes. The symptoms are similar to those in carpal tunnel syndrome, pain and paresthesia of the hand and forearm as a result of compression of the hand's median nerve. Incidence of carpal tunnel-like symptoms in pregnancy has been reported in up to 50% of women. Although some have related the condition to relaxin, fluid retention in pregnant women is more likely responsible for the symptoms.

Skin Changes

Many pregnant women are justifiably concerned about stretch marks, skin problems, and falling hair. Unfortunately, little is known about how to avoid them, and maintaining a healthy program of eating well and getting enough rest may be the best preventives.

Striae gravidarum, or stretch marks, are irregular reddish streaks that appear on the abdomen, breasts and buttocks in about half of pregnant women after the fifth month (Figure 11–6). After delivery, the red discoloration disappears but the striae persist indefi-

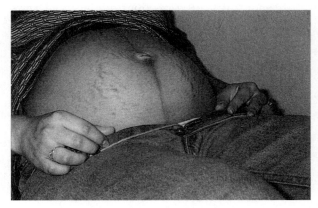

Figure 11–6 Stretch marks (striae gravidarum) on the stomach of a woman who is pregnant.

nitely as whitish lines. The striae are the result of changes in the collagen and elastic fibers in the lower layers of the skin and have little or nothing to do with weight gain. They may be related to normal hyperactivity of the adrenal gland. Controlling weight within limits is sensible, but dieting to avoid stretch marks is useless and harmful to the fetus.

Complexion changes are not unusual. Clear skin sometimes develops acne, and problem skin sometimes clears up. The increased pigmentation that occurs on the breasts and genitalia may develop in other areas as well. Dark-haired women may notice a brownish-black line (linea nigra) appearing down the middle of the abdomen. Some women develop irregular patches of freckles on the forehead and cheeks to form the mask of pregnancy, or chloasma. (The same pigmentation may occur in women taking oral contraceptives.) Chloasma gradually disappears after delivery.

Another skin manifestation, believed to be secondary to the high estrogen concentrations, is the appearance of vascular "spiders," bright red circular areas of branching and dilated capillaries. These occur on the face, neck, thorax, and arms and are especially obvious in white women but disappear after childbirth.

The blood flow to the extremities is increased. Women who have always had cold hands and feet will find them characteristically warm and even clammy during pregnancy.

Some women notice an acceleration in fingernail and hair growth during pregnancy. The hair follicles on the scalp and on the rest of the body normally undergo a growing and a resting phase. The resting phase is followed by a loss of hairs, which are then replaced by new ones. During pregnancy, fewer hair follicles go into the resting phase, and after delivery, there is a catching-up period with subsequent loss of hair until the follicles get back into their normal cycle. A similar hair loss sometimes occurs in women on oral contraceptives.

Staying Calm and Coping

The preceding list of physiological and anatomical alterations with their accompanying symptoms may sound discouraging, especially if one has never been pregnant. Almost all changes, however, disappear within a short time after birth, and a woman returns to her prepregnant state. Almost all the complaints are minor, rarely incapacitating, and more annoying than anything else. They have to be viewed with common sense and an attitude of acceptance. There are bound to be good days and bad days, and it would be unrealistic to expect only positive feelings for a period of 9-plus months. The point to remember is that pregnancy is not a test. No one passes or fails it. Neither is it a contest to see who can have the best or the worst one. Having the most "normal" pregnancy ever, and working right up until the moment of delivery is fine for some women, but it is just as normal not to, and it need not be a goal. The real goals are good health for the mother and the baby, and the foundations for health, as they are at any time in life, are good nutrition, exercise, and enough rest. A woman should listen to what her body tells her; it will indicate how to respond and what is right for her. If she feels like continuing her usual activities during pregnancy, then she should do so. But when she feels like resting, then she should rest. No woman has to prove anything to anyone with her pregnancy.

COMPLICATIONS OF PREGNANCY

Preeclampsia-Eclampsia

Healthy, middle-class women, over age 17 and under age 34, with no serious physical illnesses, who are well nourished and have the opportunity to obtain good prenatal care, are considered low-risk pregnancy prospects. They approach term in good health and can expect to have a completely normal delivery. For them, the 15 or so prenatal visits to the obstetrician's office appear superfluous, and even boring. They may sit around in the waiting room for several hours only to give up their morning urine specimen to the technologist, get weighed, then have their blood pressure taken, and finally have a brief abdominal examination by the physician. It may seem to them that they are getting very little health care, and less caring. With subsequent pregnancies, these women have such a lackluster feeling about seeing the doctor that there is a tendency to delay prenatal care until the fifth month or even later.

These monthly, then bimonthly, and later, weekly visits are more important than are generally realized, however. It takes just a few minutes for the examiner to establish that all is progressing normally and well. For example, the evaluation of these three things—blood pressure, urine, and weight gain—is necessary to detect the onset of a real and major difficulty: a group of disorders formerly called toxemia of pregnancy and now known as pregnancy-induced hypertension (PIH).

PIH occurs in about 6%–8% of pregnant women and is a leading cause of maternal and fetal illness and death. The term pregnancy-induced hypertension is a general one used to designate a number of conditions characterized by high blood pressure. The disorder known as **preeclampsia,** is a combination of symptoms that includes hypertension, edema, and proteinuria (protein in the urine) and is categorized as mild or severe. A progression of preeclampsia into a more severe state with convulsions and coma is called eclampsia. Unless controlled, **eclampsia** may be fatal.

Despite a century of investigation, the cause of PIH or preeclampsia is basically unknown, but currently there are several mechanisms that have been suggested. One is that PIH is due to widespread vasospasm, or constriction of the smooth muscle lining the blood vessels. In a woman with PIH, the constriction is mainly the result of an enhanced sensitivity to normal body substances (pressors) that raise blood pressure by causing vasoconstriction of the small blood vessels, or arterioles. The constriction narrows the diameter of the blood vessels, which increases their resistance to the flow of blood, which increases blood pressure. Another suggested reason for the development of PIH is an imbalance in the production of certain prostaglandins

(thromboxane A_2 and prostacyclin) that also results in the vasoconstriction of arterioles, impairment of the blood clotting mechanism, and a reduction of uterine blood flow. The reduced blood supply to the uterus and placenta may cause the release of protein substances that can affect blood pressure, kidney function, and capillary permeability. A familial, or genetic, factor has been suggested as a possible cause, and so has the breakdown of maternal immunologic tolerance to the fetus. Generally speaking, the characterization of eclampsia as a "disease of theories" by a German physician in 1916 still holds true today.

A case-control study examined 139 women with preeclampsia to determine whether there were any risk factors that would make it possible to predict who develops it. The researchers found that never having borne a child (nulliparity) or having a previous history of eclampsia greatly increased a woman's risk, as did having a greater body mass prior to pregnancy compared with the control women. Also, there was a greater incidence of both preeclampsia and eclampsia in black women compared with white women, whether or not the black women had preexisting high blood pressure. Working during pregnancy increased the risk for preeclampsia regardless of the kind of job—factory work, clerical, or professional/managerial (Eskanazi, Fenster, & Sidney, 1991).

The first in the triad of symptoms associated with preeclampsia is a rapid weight gain of at least 2 lb in 1 week. Since the weekly gain normally should be less than a pound during the last 6 months of pregnancy, a greater gain indicates salt and water retention and causes a generalized swelling. This is the basis of the concern about an edema not limited to the ankles. The edema of preeclampsia is the deeply pitting type; an indentation or pit remains for a period of time if a finger is poked into the swollen tissue. The second symptom is a rise in systolic blood pressure to 30 mm Hg above the normal readings and a diastolic pressure of at least 15 mm Hg above normal. The third event is the appearance of protein excreted in the urine on 2 successive days. A woman who is not having her weight, blood pressure, and urine routinely checked may not notice the symptoms. As the preeclampsia becomes more severe, symptoms of headache, dizziness, and blurred vision occur. Pain under the sternum, an indication of liver enlargement, is a serious sign. When it is accompanied by vomiting and scanty urination, it means that convulsions are going to occur.

The prognosis for a mild eclampsia is good if it is detected early enough. Because the only definitive cure is the delivery of the baby, treatment involves reducing the symptoms, preventing progression to the more severe stages, and trying to maintain the pregnancy until the fetus is able to live independently. For a mild form, if the blood pressure is not too high, bed rest at home and a high protein diet with vitamin supplements may result in improvement. More severe preeclampsia requires hospitalization and sedation. As soon as it is practical, labor is induced with drugs or a cesarean section is performed.

Because very little is known about the cause of preeclampsia, there is little known about how it can be prevented. A number of published reports have suggested that low-dose aspirin may be effective in reducing PIH. Imperiale and Petrulis (1991) used the statistical technique of meta-analysis to evaluate six published clinical trials. They found that aspirin in low doses (60 mg to 100 mg or one-quarter or one-half of a 5-grain tablet per day) taken during the second and third trimesters of pregnancy reduced the risk of PIH, was protective against severely low birth weights in infants, reduced the risk of cesarean section by 66%, and appeared to have no adverse effects on mother or child. The authors concluded that low-dose aspirin appears to be an effective and safe preventive for PIH and its consequences, but until further clinical trials definitely establish the benefits and risks of routine use of low-dose aspirin, therapy should be reserved for the high-risk woman. There also is evidence that good maternal nutrition, with a high protein diet and appropriate vitamin and mineral supplements when necessary, may reduce the frequency of PIH. Careful watching for early symptoms can reduce the progression of preeclampsia to the more severe and life-threatening form.

Spontaneous Abortion

Abortion means the termination of pregnancy before the fetus is able to live independently. Usually, a fetus is not deemed legally viable unless it has reached 500 g and 20 gestational weeks, although few infants survive delivery before 24 weeks. Abortion may be spontaneous, that is, an involuntary expulsion from the uterus, or it may be induced intentionally by trained personnel in an appropriate facility. The familiar term for spontaneous abortion is miscarriage.

Of all recognized pregnancies, one out of six—an astounding number—terminates by spontaneous abortion. For all we know, there may be as many or even more that occur before the diagnosis of pregnancy and are considered to be only delayed menstrual periods. Taking into account the number of fertilized eggs that for some reason fail to implant, it is estimated that 50% of all pregnancies are aborted naturally.

Early spontaneous abortions are usually the results of defects in the fetus and may not actually be the tragedies they appear to be at the time. Although they may be disappointing, spontaneous abortions should be viewed as desirable in most instances. Studies on aborted fetuses have shown that 20%–60% of them have abnormal chromosomes. Late abortions, which occur in the middle trimester (only 2%), are more likely to be caused by an incompetent cervix, uterine abnormalities, PIH, or preexisting chronic maternal disease.

Having a miscarriage during the first 3 months of pregnancy does not necessarily mean that a woman will have another one, although some authorities believe that her chances may increase. Habitual abortion, a term used when a woman has miscarried three or more consecutive times, is rare and occurs in only 1 out of 300 women. Even after three spontaneous abortions, the risk of another is only 25%.

When abortion is recurrent, it is an indication for genetic counseling and chromosome karyotyping of both parents because one may have a chromosomal abnormality. Sometimes it is not possible to determine a specific cause. Nutritional deficiencies, genital tract abnormalities, endocrine disturbances, and exposure to environmental agents have all been recognized as factors in spontaneous abortions. Evidence is accumulating that links chemicals and other hazards encountered by women working in hospitals and as industrial workers with the growing incidence of spontaneous abortions, stillbirths, and birth defects. Once detected, correction and elimination of a known condition in habitual aborters can often produce an uninterrupted pregnancy with a successful outcome.

The first sign of the possibility of abortion is vaginal bleeding, with or without cramping. Not all uterine bleeding, of course, indicates an abortion. Slight bleeding may be associated with implantation, or it may be originating from the cervix, the vagina, or the vulva. If the bleeding is occurring from the uterus without any dilatation of the cervical opening and, usually, without pain, it is termed a *threatened abortion*. The treatment is to wait and see what happens. Sometimes the symptoms subside within several days and the pregnancy continues. Continued bleeding accompanied by uterine cramps and dilatation of the cervix means that progression to *inevitable abortion* has occurred. As the term implies, the abortion is going to take place, and any attempt to maintain the pregnancy is useless.

In most instances of abortion, the death of the fetus has taken place several weeks before the first symptoms. The stimulus of the growing conceptus is no longer there to cause the placental production of hormones that maintain the integrity of the endometrium and the placenta. Regression and placental separation follow. Obviously, if the bleeding in a threatened abortion is the result of fetal death, there is no way of preventing it. Going to bed or taking hormones is not going to change the ultimate course. If the early bleeding is not the result of a dead embryo and the pregnancy continues, the threatened abortion has little effect on later fetal development. It does not increase the probability that the baby will be stillborn or be born with a serious congenital defect.

The administration of progestational agents formerly was prescribed by some physicians as prevention or treatment for threatened abortion. Unless labora-tory tests have confirmed that the miscarriage is due to insufficient progesterone production by the corpus luteum—a rare condition—hormone administration has no value and only delays expulsion of the fetus.

In a *complete abortion*, the placenta and the embryo are totally evacuated, and the bleeding and cramping stops. More often, the abortion is *incomplete*. Some placental tissue remains in the uterus and has to be removed by curettage. Occasionally, long after fetal death, the fetal and placental tissue are retained in the uterus, and there are no signs of abortion. This is called *missed abortion*. The signs and symptoms of pregnancy gradually disappear, and curettage is usually necessary. Eventually the uterine contents will spontaneously be expelled, but it could take several months. By then, the amniotic fluid has been reabsorbed and the fetus is apt to be mummified or calcified.

If a fetus is meant to stay within the uterus for 9½ months, it will. Tennis, horseback riding, or any other kind of physical activity will not result in its being expelled. The physical trauma of a fall or a blow, or even, in many instances, the crushing injuries to the pelvis in automobile accidents, have not resulted in interrupted pregnancy. Although it is generally believed that severe emotional shock may bring on an abortion, verification is difficult. As expected, the "rejection-of-motherhood-as-a-result-of-deep-seated-emotional-factors" theory has also been suggested by some psychiatrists as a cause of abortion, particularly in habitual aborters, but substantiation is obviously difficult. Presumably, blood flow to the placenta could be affected by autonomic factors as a result of emotional stimulation, and physiologically, the possibility for a psychological basis for pregnancy termination exists.

Placental Bleeding

Vaginal bleeding in the first 28 weeks of pregnancy may signify the onset of spontaneous abortion, but 15% of women who have bleeding retain the pregnancy with no adverse consequences. Ultrasound has become a valuable method for diagnosing the reason for bleeding in early pregnancy. Vaginal bleeding in the last trimester may be due to two other complications of late pregnancy—*placenta previa* or *abruptio placentae.*

Placenta previa, which occurs in 1 out of 200 pregnancies, is the result of implantation of the fertilized ovum in the lower part of the uterus instead of its more usual site higher up in the fundus. The placenta is then formed very close to, partially covering, or completely covering, the internal os of the cervix (Figure 11–7). Late in pregnancy or at the time of delivery, a part of the lower edge of the placenta may separate from its attachment to cause characteristically painless bleeding that is bright red in color.

If placenta previa is diagnosed at the time of labor, the baby is delivered by cesarean section. If the bleeding has occurred as early as 32 weeks, the pregnancy is allowed to continue with hospitalization, bed rest, and careful watching and waiting. As soon as there is no risk to the life of the fetus, a cesarean is performed.

When the placenta is normally located in the upper segment of the uterus but separates before the birth of the baby, the condition is known as abruptio placentae. Such premature separation occurs in only 1% of pregnant women and may be associated with hypertensive or chronic kidney disorders. The rate of abruptio placentae dramatically increases when a pregnant woman uses cocaine. It has been speculated that the hypertension produced by cocaine use is responsible for the increased incidence of abruptio placentae. Even if the woman abstains from the drug during the second and third trimesters, cocaine use apparently causes early damage to the placental and uterine vessels and places the pregnancy at continued risk (Chasnoff et al., 1989).

WEIGHT GAIN AND NUTRITION

For years it had been believed that excessive weight gain during pregnancy was associated with several complications, particularly preeclampsia, and was further related to mechanical difficulties in labor and birth. Pregnant women were advised by their doctors to restrict caloric intake, sometimes drastically, to avoid excessive weight gain. The problem with this recommendation was that the definition of what constituted excessive varied considerably among different physicians. At one point it was generally agreed that weight increases should be limited to 20 lb over the course of pregnancy, but many women were more severely restricted to as little as 16 lb by their well-meaning but overzealous doctors. Some may even have been given diet pills (amphetamine appetite suppressants) to achieve that goal. It was also considered appropriate for overweight women to reduce while pregnant. Gains of nothing at all or just a few pounds were presumed safe for the fetus and for the mother if she was obese prior to pregnancy. Many women may remember how they dreaded that monthly visit to the office, reluctant to step on the scale and ashamed to face the physician because a "good" patient was one who strictly adhered to the proposed weight control.

The idea that excessive weight gain predisposed to preeclampsia-eclampsia arose from rather specious evidence. During World War I, it was reported that there had been a startling reduction in the incidence of toxemia of pregnancy in central Europe. Because the

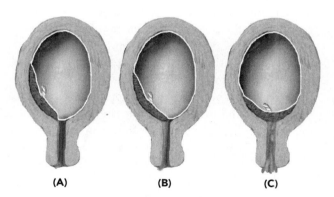

Figure 11–7 Types of placenta previa. (A) Marginal, in which the margin of the placenta extends to the edge of the cervical opening. (B) Partial or lateral, in which the placenta covers only a part of the cervical opening. (C) Complete, in which the placenta extends across the entire cervical opening.

(A) **(B)** **(C)**

incidence of toxemia reverted to its former frequency as soon as the war was over, the change, without any further study, was attributed to the food blockade that had existed during the war. A theory that dietary restriction was protection against eclampsia developed, persisted, and was taught to several generations of physicians. There have been studies since that have attempted to prove a cause-and-effect relationship between diet and obstetric complications, but confirmation is lacking. Some investigations have noted an apparent relationship between the incidence of PIH and prepregnancy obesity or overall maternal weight gain, but there have also been studies showing just the opposite. Underweight women seem to have an increased frequency of eclampsia, and there has been the suggestion that dietary deficiency and malnutrition pose greater risks for the development of toxemia of pregnancy. A report of the National Research Council's Committee on Maternal Nutrition concluded that there was no evidence that caloric restriction to limit weight gain in pregnancy had any effect on the incidence of preeclampsia-eclampsia.

There is a great deal of evidence, however, that indicates that there is a relationship between weight gain during pregnancy and the birth weight of the infant. Babies who are smaller and lighter than normal, who are born at term weighing 2,500 g (5½ lb) or less, have an increased susceptibility to illness and an increased rate of mortality compared with heavier babies. A woman whose weight gain is limited and inadequate during pregnancy has a substantially increased risk of delivering a baby of low birth weight.

Of course, not all low-birth-weight infants are the result of maternal malnourishment only. Some babies are premature, but they are the right size for their fetal age. But when a baby is born at term and weighs disproportionately less than what is considered to be a healthy weight, it is said to be a small for gestational age (SGA) infant. In SGA babies, some factor or combination of factors has retarded their intrauterine growth. Fetal growth retardation can be caused by the biological immaturity of the mother if she is younger than 17. It can be associated, not necessarily in order

of importance, with pregnancy in women who have twins or triplets, who have had many prior pregnancies, who are short and small women themselves, or who may have been underweight and in a poor nutritional state before pregnancy. Additional known factors that influence fetal growth adversely are smoking, chronic maternal disease, certain infections, or some maternal vascular problem that interferes with the blood supply to the placenta. In study after study, however, one cause stands out as a major determinant of fetal weight, and that is maternal weight gain. Pitkin believes that maternal weight gain is second in importance only to the length of pregnancy in responsibility for the birth weight of the infant.

Until recently, it was generally believed that the developing fetus could get everything it needed at the expense of the mother, as long as she received plenty of vitamins. This concept has been challenged by investigational studies. The fetus is no longer seen as a complete parasite, miraculously able to draw on all the maternal tissues and remain unaffected even though the mother is malnourished. Animal studies have shown that maternal malnutrition decreases the ability of the placenta to transfer nutrients from the blood of the mother to the blood of the fetus. Prenatal malnutrition has also been shown to cause a reduction in cell size and number of cells in fetal tissues, with disproportionate effects occurring in the brain (Barker, 1997; Schieve, Cogswell, & Scanlon, 1998; Grantham, McGregor & Fernald, 1997). Furthermore, in nonhuman animals, food deprivation during pregnancy always reduces the fetal weight proportionately more than it does the maternal weight, and there are data that suggest that the situation is similar in humans.

Two major episodes of human malnutrition that occurred during World War II were studied extensively and provided corroborating evidence that there is a strong positive correlation between maternal nutrition and infant birth weight. The siege of Leningrad in 1942 and the Nazi-induced famine in western Holland in the winter of 1944–1945 resulted in severe nutritional restriction, and hundreds of people died of starvation each month. The babies that were born during those periods of calorie deprivation were of significantly lower birth weight than those born before and after the famines. The infants also suffered excessive morbidity and mortality after birth.

The Leningrad and Dutch experiences of the effects of maternal undernutrition on the developing fetus were the result of profound deprivation. It is evident, however, that less-than-adequate maternal nutrition, which is far short of actual starvation, also has an effect on the babies produced. For many years it has been known that birth weights were lower in developing countries and that more smaller and lighter infants were delivered to poor women than to rich women in this country. Several nutritional intervention studies that took place in Formosa, Guatemala, and New York City provided additional evidence that calorie supplementation for the mother during pregnancy increases the birth weight and decreases the infant mortality rate. Experimental animal studies have pointed to an association between maternal malnutrition and brain development and function. Some human studies have suggested that malnutrition in early infancy, particularly when combined with low birth weight, can affect mental development. The full implications of maternal nutrition and malnutrition are not known, but it is obviously essential that the undesirability of imposing restrictions on weight gain during pregnancy be recognized.

The current view is that there is probably no one ideal value for the weight gain in pregnancy that would be appropriate for all women. A woman's age, prepregnancy nutritional status, and activity level during pregnancy are modifying factors, but it is generally agreed that she should gain at least 24 lb to support the changes in her body and in the developing fetus. With that increase, the fetus and placenta account for about 11 lb. The remaining 13 lb are distributed as about 8 lb in increased maternal blood volume and extracellular fluid, about 3 lb for additional uterine and breast tissue, and approximately 2 lb of extra fat tissue. Underweight women should gain more—about 30 lb. Increases in the range of 22–30 lb are seen as normal and commensurate with the fewest obstetrical complications and the most favorable outcome of the pregnancy. Less gain

than that contributes to the likelihood of delivering a low-birth-weight infant. A gain of more than that, perhaps 40–50 lb, will result in excessive fat deposition, be more difficult to lose after delivery, and contribute to future obesity. The total accumulation, however, is less significant than the *rate* of gain. By the end of the first 3 months of pregnancy, when the fetus still weighs only 1 oz, the total gain should have been only 2–4 lb. After that, during the next 6 months, the gain should be ½–1 lb weekly. Thus, the weight is gained gradually, and only when there is a sudden and large increase should there be any reason for concern.

According to Roy Pitkin, who has written extensively on maternal nutrition, a weight gain of 1 kg (2.2 lb) per month in the second and third trimesters is inadequate. Four pounds per month is optimal, but 6–7 lb or more each month is excessive and will lead to postpartum obesity. Women who are overweight should not try to lose weight during pregnancy but should gain at the appropriate rate. Pregnancy is no time to diet, and even obese women must put on the 24–30 lb all pregnant women should gain. A woman who is reducing is likely to eliminate some of the essential nutrients from her diet. Moreover dieting results in an increased fat metabolism, which elevates the level of ketone bodies in the blood. Not only is ketosis undesirable for a pregnant woman, it is potentially extremely dangerous for the fetus.

Thinking Nutritionally

The fact that a woman is encouraged to gain up to 30 lb during pregnancy cannot be construed as permission to indulge in all the high-calorie, empty-calorie goodies she may have always denied herself. The quality of the food chosen—its nutrient properties—is extremely important so that the weight gained is not merely excess fat. Building an entire new person inside one's body while simultaneously increasing one's own uterine and breast tissue and blood volume is not possible on junk food. It requires the basic nutrients, proteins, fats, carbohydrates, vitamins, minerals, and water in the correct amounts. The problem with eating potato chips, ice cream, or pastries is not that they are completely without nutrition, but that they are loaded with fat and sugar. They do have some nutrient value, but they can be so filling that there may be less appetite for the really necessary foods.

There is no necessity to eat everything in sight even if it is nutritious. A woman is not really eating for two—she is actually eating for about one (herself) and one-seventh. The calorie requirements, averaged out over the entire 9 months, are not as much as one thinks. The total energy needs, 80,000 calories, are about 300 extra calories per day, an amount equal to 15% over the prepregnant state. Those additional calories can be obtained from a peanut butter sandwich on whole wheat bread with a glass of milk, which would be excellent. A doughnut and coffee with cream and sugar provide the same calories, but little nutrition.

A woman who selects her diet carefully will assure herself of the essential nutrients. The physiological adjustments of the body to pregnancy and the optimal growth of the fetus do require, however, that special attention be paid to getting additional amounts of some nutrients.

Milk.   Milk is very important for an expectant mother. It is a source of calcium, phosphorus, protein, and vitamins as well as some valuable minerals. The entire daily requirement for calcium during pregnancy is contained in 1 quart of milk. Three 8-oz glasses of whole or skim milk are recommended daily during the first trimester, increasing to four glasses during the next 6 months. This would be an inordinate amount to drink for a woman with a small appetite and would be virtually impossible for someone who actively dislikes milk. Fortunately, milk can be flavored, or it can be disguised in cream soups, custards, or puddings. When ⅓ cup of nonfat dry milk is added to a glass of milk, the result is "double milk"—the equivalent of two 8-oz glasses. Buttermilk can also be substituted for regular milk. A 1½-oz chunk of hard cheese, 1½ cups of creamed cottage cheese, or a carton of yogurt is the equivalent in nutrients (except for vitamin D) of a glass of milk. So is 1½ cups of ice cream or ice milk, but the extra fat and sugar are hardly bonuses.

Proteins.   Protein needs double during pregnancy. Nonpregnant women need 0.8 g of protein for every 2.2 lb (kilogram) of body weight. This increases to 1.3 g per kilogram during pregnancy. In most American diets, the amount of protein consumed daily, primarily obtained from meat, is already way above the requirement. Under most circumstances, women do not need to deliberately increase their protein intake since the recommended dietary allowance already includes a buffer against protein deficiency. Neither does the source of the protein have to be an expensive steak or filet of whitefish. Eggs, canned tuna, or several slices of luncheon meat (but watch the fat content), or good old peanut butter on whole wheat can be used for the requirement. One-half cup of cottage cheese contains 20 g of complete protein. Nuts, beans, lentils, or peas combined with grain or a small amount of animal protein become complete. A vegetarian who eats milk and eggs would have no problems in getting ample amounts of protein when pregnant, but a non-lacto-ovo-vegetarian may have to select her foods more carefully to ensure that they are appropriately combined.

Iron.   Iron is necessary for life. Approximately 70% of the body iron is incorporated into the "heme" part of the hemoglobin molecule, the oxygen carrier present in the red blood cells. Smaller amounts of iron, about 5%–10%, are necessary for the synthesis of muscle protein, or myoglobin, and also form parts of certain cellular respiratory enzymes, essential in the extraction of energy from oxygen and food. The rest of the iron in the body, 20%–30%, is bound to proteins for iron transport or is stored in the liver, spleen, and bone marrow. In adults, the levels of iron necessary for the body's needs are controlled by very efficient mechanisms that balance the daily intestinal absorption of iron in the diet with the daily loss of iron in body excretions and sloughed-off dead cells. Men absorb about 1 mg of dietary iron daily to replace the iron lost from the skin and from the intestinal tract. Women, who during their reproductive years lose an additional 15–60 mg each month by menstruation, need more and absorb more to compensate for the additional loss.

People who eat nutritious diets consume iron-rich foods. A woman who eats meats, fish and poultry, green vegetables, and enriched flour or breakfast cereals has no problems with iron deficiency. Certain foods such as prune juice, dried apricots, molasses, or dried beans and peas are very high in iron. During pregnancy, however, there are additional requirements for iron. The blood volume increases, and more iron is needed to provide hemoglobin for the increased number of maternal red blood cells for the placenta and for potential blood loss during childbirth. The iron is also needed for the fetal hemoglobin, the fetal myoglobin, and the fetal cellular enzymes. The fetus draws more heavily on the maternal iron in the last months of pregnancy. Because both breast and cow's milk are iron deficient, and a newborn is able to absorb very little iron anyway, the fetus must accumulate enough storage iron to last for the first 3 months or so after birth.

The fetus will take what it needs from the iron stores of the mother whatever her state of iron sufficiency, and if there is not enough, it is the pregnant woman who will become anemic, not her offspring. It is generally presumed that women's dietary intake is likely to be inadequate to meet the needs, and iron supplements in the form of 30–60 mg of ferrous iron salts are almost universally prescribed for pregnant women in the last half of pregnancy. Such routine supplementation is done to eliminate possible iron-deficiency anemia as a pregnancy complication.

The need for across-the-board administration of iron salts to all pregnant women is debatable, however. Women need a total of 500–750 mg additional iron during pregnancy. Pregnant women absorb dietary iron from the intestine at twice the usual rate and an adult woman can store as much as 1,000 mg of iron, depending on her size and prepregnancy diet. Unless she has been living on a marginal diet, has had multiple past pregnancies within a short period of time, or has had excessive menstrual or other blood loss, her own reservoirs and her dietary intake will be sufficient for her needs and that of the fetus. The amount of supplemental iron in the daily dose would probably not be harmful, but some of the possible side effects of taking iron pills—nausea, heartburn, constipation, burping—are already experienced by many pregnant women. If iron is unnecessary, why supplement their gastrointestinal symptoms? It would seem obvious that iron salts should be administered only if a simple blood test has determined that a pregnant woman is actually iron deficient.

Folic Acid. Folic acid, also known as folacin and folate, is a water-soluble B vitamin that is involved in the formation of DNA and in the maturation of red and white blood cells. Because cell division increases so greatly during pregnancy, folate requirements are increased as well and are set at twice the recommended dietary allowance for the nonpregnant woman.

There is compelling evidence that daily oral folic acid supplements taken before conception and during early pregnancy reduce the risk of neural tube defects (NTDs), conditions in which the embryonic neural tube, from which the brain and spinal cord develop, fails to close, leaving an open groove or seam. If the opening occurs at the head region of the tube, the brain fails to grow and remains primitive or never develops at all—a defect called anencephaly. Spina bifida is another NTD, an inclusive term for a number of conditions associated with failure of the neural arches of the vertebrae to meet each other and enclose the spinal cord, which may protrude through the unclosed arch and result in permanent damage to the cord and spinal nerves. NTDs occur in about 1 in every 1,000 births, but women who have had an infant or fetus with a NTD have a 2%–3% increased risk for recurrence.

A study by the British Medical Research Council, which began in 1983 but was halted in 1991 so that all women could receive the benefits of supplementation, reported that daily intake of 4 mg of folic acid starting before conception and continuing through the first trimester of pregnancy reduced the recurrence of NTDs by 71%. The idea that folic acid may prevent NTDs is not a new one. Other researchers have shown that women who had infants with NTDs had diets low in folic acid and lower blood levels of folic acid. On the basis of the British study and other similar findings, the Centers for Disease Control (CDC), in their Morbidity and Mortality Weekly Report, issued a recommendation for folic acid supplementation. Women who previously have had an infant or fetus with an NTD and plan to become pregnant again should take a 4-mg daily dose of folic acid starting from at least 4 weeks before conception and continuing through the first 3 months of pregnancy.

Protection against having a fetus or infant with an NTD for women who have not had a previous pregnancy resulting in neural tube defect may be obtained from far lower levels of folic acid than 4 mg. A 1989 study by Milunsky and coworkers found that women who take multivitamins in general, and folic acid in particular, during the first 6 weeks of pregnancy have a significantly reduced prevalence of NTDs in their babies. In the study population of more than 22,000 women, those who took multivitamins containing at least 100 mcg of folic acid in weeks 1 through 6 of pregnancy had a 50%–70% decreased risk of delivering an infant with NTD.

Obviously, a major difficulty in trying to protect against NTDs by taking vitamins containing folic acid or making certain that the diet contains enough folic acid for the first 6 weeks of pregnancy is that many women may not know they are pregnant until that amount of time has elapsed. Mulinare, Cordereo, Erickson, and Berry reported in 1988 that the use of multivitamins for 3 months before and 3 months after conception was protective against the occurrence of neural tube defects. It makes sense for all women who could become pregnant or who are trying to get pregnant to consume at least 400 mcg of folic acid per day from food (the recommended daily allowance for pregnant women) or take a multivitamin supplement containing that amount. After pregnancy is confirmed, a multivitamin that contains 800 mcg of folic acid could be taken, but high-dose vitamin supplements that may contain excessive amounts of vitamin A or vitamin D should be avoided.

It is possible, but somewhat more difficult, to obtain the required daily amount of folic acid from the diet. A number of foods are rich in the vitamin: liver, dark green leafy vegetables, broccoli, asparagus, legumes, and in particular, oranges and orange juice. Three oz of chicken livers contain more than 600 mcg, and 1 cup of cooked lentils has nearly 400 mcg. Kidney, pinto, and lima beans are good sources, and so are all cruciferous vegetables. Folate is relatively unstable, however, and exposure of some foods to air and light results in the loss of much of the vitamin. For this reason, if fresh fruits or vegetables are not readily available on a daily basis, a vitamin supplement would be a good idea.

Other Nutrients. Besides additional protein, calcium, iron, and folate, a pregnant woman needs the daily amounts of the rest of the vitamins and other important nutrients she should have ordinarily. The recommended daily allowances for other vitamins and minerals are not significantly increased over those in the prepregnant state. Sodium, for example, should neither be increased nor decreased. One can continue salting one's food in the usual way with no attempts at restriction. Common sense indicates that larger amounts than ordinary of salted foods should not be ingested.

In certain instances, an overabundance of a vitamin can be as harmful as an insufficiency. There is some evidence suggesting that there is an association between maternal hypervitaminosis for vitamin D and the development of severe fetal abnormalities. For this reason, a woman is advised not to increase vitamin D over prepregnancy levels.

Obstetricians are likely to prescribe multiple vitamin and mineral supplements during pregnancy in a shotgun approach. They recognize that such routine supplementation may not be helpful, but they presume it is not harmful and believe that it provides a margin of safety since women probably will disregard a recommended diet. This generally low opinion of the ability of women to understand or follow a food plan is almost universal and is held by some women themselves, who claim that they like to eat food and not servings of nutrients. Many women have learned to question their own capacity for maintaining a nutritional diet, perhaps as a result of the paucity of specific dietary advice that doctors give them. The nutritional counseling provided may be "eat a balanced diet" or "watch your weight" accompanied by a pamphlet. They are not told what to do. Few physicians utilize the services of a professional nutritionist in their obstetrical practice. It is not unusual for women who can afford a busy private obstetrician to get less nutrition advice than women with fewer socioeconomic advantages who are seen at federally funded clinics.

Women can certainly be presumed intelligent enough to make themselves nutritionally aware. A food plan during pregnancy or at any other time in life requires individualization and extra time. A woman's lifestyle, family situation, food preferences, and a number of other ethnic, economic, psychological, and physical factors influence her eating patterns. Some of the dietary leaflets may sound patronizing or be written in a picture-book style, but the information is helpful and can easily be applied to one's own dietary plan.

Table 11–1 is a guide to the daily essentials. Whether they are consumed in three meals, five meals, or many meals and snacks is not important, as long as all the nutrients are included. If, after the basics are eaten, there is still room for junk food, that is the time to eat it.

There is no need to curb calories, within commonsense limits, as long as the essentials are consumed.

If the total weight gained has not exceeded 24–30 lb, a woman can count on losing 18–20 of them within a week after delivery. The rest of the pounds are likely to be completely gone by 3 months after delivery, especially if a woman is breastfeeding. If she is not lactating, she can speed up the weight loss by restricting calories (not nutrients). Under no circumstances should a woman embark on a fad diet, particularly the low-carbohydrate type. The best and only long-term solution to a weight problem, after a woman has learned to eat "right," is to continue in the right way but with smaller portions.

PRENATAL CHILD ABUSE— EFFECTS OF DRUGS ON THE FETUS

Every year in the United States, about a quarter of a million children are born with a birth defect. Some have an obvious structural malformation; their limbs are crippled, they have a cleft palate, or a heart,

Table 11–1 Daily Guide to Essential Foods		
	Servings Each Day	
To Be Consumed	**Pregnant**	**Breastfeeding**
Milk and milk products	4	4–5
Protein source (meat, fish, poultry, eggs, cheese, and at least one vegetable protein)	4	4–5
Leafy green vegetable	1–2	1–2
Source of vitamin C	1	1
Other fruits and vegetables	1	1
Whole grain breads and cereals	3	3–4
Water and other liquids (milk may be included in total)	6	6

gastrointestinal, or kidney defect. Others may be mentally retarded, be born blind or deaf, or have a metabolic disorder. Some may have problems that do not show up for years. Not too long ago, birth defects were attributed to a peculiarity of behavior of the mother, who could mark her child. Before that, deformities were blamed on witchcraft. Today, we are enlightened enough to know that structural and functional malformations are the result of genetic, viral, or chemical influences or, in many instances, are the result of interactions between genetic and environmental influences. Gene mutations or chromosomal aberrations are said to be the cause of about 25% of birth defects. Certain virus infections, drugs, and exposure to radiation are known to give rise to another small percentage. But at our current state of knowledge, the reason for 60%–70% of human abnormalities is essentially unknown and is presumed to arise from the interplay of several factors.

The recognition that environment influences prenatal development is astonishingly recent. The role of rubella, or German measles, infection in a pregnant woman causing fetal deformities was not established until 1941. And, incredibly enough, it was not until the thalidomide tragedy of the early 1960s that it became generally recognized that drugs taken by pregnant women may produce abnormalities in the developing children.

It had always been assumed that a placental barrier existed—that all the tissues through which materials must pass in maternal exchange constituted an effective obstacle that prevented an adverse effect on the fetus. What was safe for the mother to take was therefore considered safe for the fetus. When the new tranquilizer, thalidomide, became available in many countries, it was believed to be so safe that it was sold without prescriptions. Besides, it had been extensively tested in pregnant rats and had produced no effects in the offspring. People took thalidomide for a variety of maladies, and pregnant women used it for morning sickness, anxiety, headache, and whatever else was bothering them. It is generally agreed that had it not been for the distinctive abnormalities caused by thalidomide—it particularly affected the long bones in the arms and the legs—the drug might not have been recognized as a *teratogen,* an agent that caused a high proportion of exposed embryos to develop malformations. When a virtual epidemic of deformed children appeared in 1961, the search narrowed to thalidomide as the causative agent. By the time the drug was withdrawn from the market, an estimated 12,000 children throughout the world had been born with birth defects, many with phocomelia, abnormally short or absent arms and legs.

After that disaster it became mandatory for all drugs to be tested not only for their toxicity to humans, but for their teratogenicity on fetal development. In the past 30 years, a new discipline, fetal pharmacology, or the effects of drugs on the fetus, has generated a great deal of research. Symposia have been held, reviews have been written, central registers for birth defects have been established—much effort has been devoted to identifying those compounds that are able to cross the placenta. What is becoming increasingly recognized is the extent of the inadequacy of current knowledge. Relatively few chemical agents are positively known to be teratogenic, many are suspected, and probably all have the potential. Some drugs may be safe in animals (thalidomide is a case in point), but some drugs, considered harmless and not specifically associated with malformations in the fetus, have been known to induce deformities in several animal species.

The timing and the dosage of a chemical agent, that is, when it was taken during fetal development and how much, are very important to the possible occurrence of a congenital malformation. For the first 2 weeks after fertilization, the embryo is believed to be resistant to environmental influences. If it is affected, presumably it undergoes such severe damage that implantation does not occur, and death and early abortion result. Animal studies, however, have shown that a number of chemical agents can actually penetrate the oviduct fluid to reach the fertilized egg. Fabro and Sieber were able to recover such substances as caffeine, nicotine, DDT, and phenobarbital in a rabbit blastocyst before implantation when those chemicals had been injected into pregnant rabbits (1969). Whether the ability of such substances to penetrate into the preimplantation embryo is of teratogenic significance is unknown, but the possibility exists.

The most critical period for disturbance of development of the embryo is from approximately day 15 to day 56, the time when all of the organs are forming. Each of the organs has its own particularly sensitive period, and interference by a teratogen at that time can result in malformations. Because the development time of many organ systems overlaps, the outcome could be a whole group of abnormalities (Figure 11–8). The effect of rubella, for example, is known to be most harmful if the disease occurs within the 4 or 5 weeks after fertilization when the brain, heart, eyes, and ears are undergoing rapid development. Although the risk to the child is greatest during the first trimester, susceptibility to environmental influences can continue. Brain development, for example, takes place throughout gestation and even extends into the postnatal period.

It has been determined that compounds that are positively or negatively charged, that are not soluble in lipids, are of high molecular weight, or are bound to large protein macro-molecules, are not able to cross the placenta as rapidly as those drugs that are not ionized (charged), highly lipid soluble, or of low molecular weight. The majority of drugs, however, are likely to be transmitted across to the fetus despite the physical properties if a high enough level persists in the maternal bloodstream for an adequate amount of time. For all practical purposes, the placenta does not constitute much of a barrier.

The problem is further compounded by the diversity of ways in which a drug can affect the fetus. Even if agents are not able to cross the placenta, they are still potentially harmful. Some drugs pass across the membranes of the placenta and directly enter the bloodstream of the fetus to exert a toxic effect; others may be transformed by the liver of the mother into a toxic metabolite. Very little is known about the ability of the placenta itself to metabolize, detoxify, or in other ways affect the dose of the drug received by the fetus. There

is the possibility that the placenta could convert an innocuous chemical into an active teratogen, mutagen, or carcinogen.

Two drugs, neither of which is particularly teratogenic, may interact to produce an adverse effect. It may be that a drug could be potentiated by genetic or other predisposing factors and is then able to cause a malformation. This might explain the puzzling fact that not all women who are exposed to a particular chemical agent or infection will deliver a child with defects. A woman's overall health before pregnancy, her nutritional status during pregnancy, perhaps her own unique genetic susceptibility, the amount of alcohol she drinks, or the number of cigarettes she smokes—all these can be factors.

A drug may indirectly produce abnormalities by interfering with the activity of another substance. The antitumor drug, aminopterin, is a folic acid antagonist that is known to induce abortion. Although it usually resulted in the deaths of the embryos when it was administered in early pregnancy, some of the fetuses that survived to term were grossly deformed. Methotrexate, another chemotherapeutic drug and an aminopterin derivative, has also been implicated as a teratogen.

The appearance of reproductive abnormalities in the sons and daughters of women given DES during pregnancy is a prime example of how unforeseen and even carcinogenic effects can be produced 15–20 years after exposure.

A strong teratogen—one that produces a specific abnormality in virtually all fetuses exposed at any time in the first trimester to any dose—should be relatively easy to spot in the population because the sudden increase in the incidence of that unique defect would stimulate an intensive search for the cause. Unfortunately, most human teratogens rarely act that way. That a substance produces adverse effects in offspring when the mother takes it during pregnancy is difficult to verify, given the overall 2.7%–3% incidence of birth defects in the population. As described previously for Bendectin, published reports that associate a drug with congenital abnormalities do not constitute a cause-and-effect relationship.

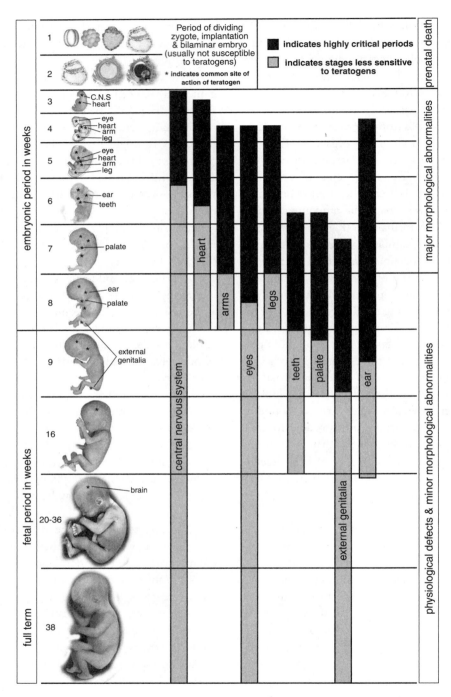

Figure 11–8 Schematic illustration of the sensitive periods in human development. The embryo is not believed to be susceptible to teratogens during the first 2 weeks of development. The dark part of the bar indicates highly critical periods; the light portion indicates stages less sensitive to teratogens.

The association may be the result of the way the information was collected or analyzed. The sample size may have been very small, or the results may be of borderline statistical significance.

Information that appears in the medical literature may be in the form of a case report, in which an individual case of malformation and a history of drug exposure appeared so interesting or unusual that the physician decided to write it up and submit it to a journal. Although the drug may become suspect as a result of case reports, more information and further studies are needed to verify its potential teratogenicity. Epidemiological studies of the exposed populations compared with control populations can then be made to confirm or disprove the suspicion and to provide an evaluation of the risk of taking the drug. An estimate of risk can be obtained by a retrospective *case-control study,* in which the exposure to a drug is determined in a group of women who delivered babies with a birth defect compared with a control group of women who are comparable in all respects except that they delivered normal babies. The extent of exposure may be determined by interviews with the women, by examination of their medical records, or both.

In a prospective *cohort study,* the frequency of occurrence of a birth defect in the offspring of a group of women who were exposed to a drug in question is compared with that in a group of control women who did not take the drug. Prospective studies are viewed as more reliable, since the ultimate proof of teratogenicity of a drug could come only from observations of the consequences of exposure to an agent in a well-controlled experiment. But because it is unthinkable to set up a study in which half of the women receive a suspected drug and half of them do not to see whether an adverse effect on their babies occurs, another way of assessing the teratogenicity of substances is to accumulate data from animal experimentation in the laboratory. Animal studies, however, also present problems. The differences in the metabolism and development of different species, the way in which drugs are absorbed and excreted in rodents and primates, and the basic difficulty in extrapolation of animal data to human populations make estimations of human risk of a drug from its animal teratogenicity prone to under- or overestimation. Teratogenicity has been *established* for only a very few infectious or chemical agents, but some of the drugs that have been associated with the production of congenital malformations are listed in Table 11–2. There is no way of knowing how many drugs may be low-risk teratogens, that is, cause some adverse effects in some fetuses but no actual malformations. It is obviously important to determine which drugs result in major defects and which do not. Then if drug therapy during pregnancy is required, the least hazardous medication can be chosen. It is probable that any chemical agent, taken at a sensitive time of development and in a high enough dose, can affect an embryo or a fetus. At our current state of knowledge, it is reasonable to assume that *drugs* are teratogenic, but some are more so than others. It would be prudent for a woman to avoid drugs unless she is certain that she is not pregnant.

This creates a dilemma for a pregnant woman who has heart disease, high blood pressure, toxemia of pregnancy, epilepsy, bacterial infections, or any other disorder for which drug therapy is indicated. Obviously, the risk of untreated maternal illness may be greater for the woman and for the fetus than the possible harmful effect of a drug. If a complete evaluation of the condition and all of its ramifications has been satisfactorily explained to the parents, if it has been determined that the drug is essential and that the least hazardous drug has been chosen, and if the beneficial effects of the therapy are greater than the potential harmful effects, then the decision to take the drug can be made by a woman and her doctor.

Over-the-Counter Drugs

The drugs ingested during pregnancy are hardly limited to those prescribed by a physician. A woman who claims to have taken no drugs while pregnant has forgotten the times she sprayed the African violets, had her hair dyed, drank diet cola, painted the baby's room, or put aspartame in her coffee. People seem to forget that aspirins are drugs; that cigarettes and alcohol are drugs;

Table 11–2 Known Human Teratogens

Medications

Thalidomide	Limb reduction defects, ear anomalies
Diethylstilbestrol	Vaginal adenosis/adenocarcinoma, cervical erosion and ridges
Warfarin	Nasal hypoplasia, stippled epiphyses, CNS defects
Hydantoin	Dysmorphic facial features, hypoplastic nails, growth and developmental retardation
Trimethadione	Developmental retardation, dysmorphic facial features
Aminopterin and methotrexate	Pregnancy loss, hydrocephalus, low birth weight, dysmorphic facial features
Streptomycin	Hearing loss
Tetracycline	Stained teeth, enamel hypoplasia
Valproic acid	Neural tube defects, dysmorphic facial features
Isotretinoin	Pregnancy loss, hydrocephalus, other CNS defects, small or absent thymus, microtia/anotia, conotruncal heart defects
Antithyroid drugs	Hypothyroidism, goiter
Androgens and high doses of norpro-gesterones	Masculinization of external female genitalia
Penicillamine	Cutis laxa
ACE inhibitors	Renal dysgenesis, oligohydramnios sequence, skull ossification defects
Carbamazepine	Neural tube defects
Cocaine	Pregnancy loss, placental abruption, growth retardation, microcephaly
Lithium	Ebstein anomaly

Chemicals

Methylmercury	Cerebral atrophy, spasticity, mental retardation
Lead	Pregnancy loss, CNS damage
Polychlorobiphenyls (PCBs—ingested)	Low birth weight, skin discoloration

Maternal Disorders

Insulin-dependent diabetes mellitus	Congenital heart defects, caudal deficiency, neural tube defects, limb defects, holoprosencephaly, pregnancy loss
Hypo/hyperthyroidism	Goiter, growth and developmental retardation

(continues)

Table 11–2 *(continued)*

Maternal Disorders	
Phenylketonuria	Pregnancy loss, microcephaly, mental retardation, facial dysmorphism, congenital heart defects
Hypertension	Intrauterine growth retardation
Autoimmune disorders	Congenital heart block, pregnancy loss
Reproductive Toxins	
Cigarette smoking	Pregnancy loss, low birth weight
Hyperthermia	Neural tube defects
Chronic alcoholism	Growth and developmental retardation, microcephaly, craniofacial dysmorphism
Therapeutic radiation	Growth and developmental retardation, microcephaly

Source: Teratogen Update (1995) vol. 12. Published in *The Genetic Drift Online*. Retrieved from the World Wide Web; http://www.mostgene.org. Published by Mountain States Genetic Network.

that vitamins, cough drops, nose drops, antacids, laxatives, and antihistamines are drugs; and that coffee and tea are drugs when 10–15 cups are consumed daily.

Little is known about the potential hazards of over-the-counter drugs. Lynn Woodward and her colleagues (1982) interviewed 304 women who had recently delivered normal babies and found that they had consumed 93 different drug products, excluding alcohol, tobacco, and vitamins. The nonprescription drugs most frequently taken were, in order of decreasing consumption, Tylenol, Rolaids, aspirin, Maalox, Robitussin, Sudafed (an oral-nasal decongestant), Alka-Seltzer, and Massengill Disposable Douche. Although some of the 93 preparations or their ingredients have been amply investigated for adverse or toxic effects during pregnancy, Woodward found no documentation on the potential teratogenicity or safety of fully two-thirds of the drugs or drug ingredients that the women consumed.

Aspartame (NutraSweet). There has been no evidence thus far that the ingestion of aspartame-sweetened diet drinks during pregnancy is any risk to the fetus. Aspartame is metabolized by the body into phenylalanine, a necessary amino acid nutrient, and presents no problem to most people.

Nearly 300 American babies each year, however, are born with phenylketonuria, or PKU. They have inherited a genetic defect from both their parents that results in the accumulation of toxic high levels of phenylalanine in their blood and subjects their developing brains to irrevocable damage and mental retardation if they are not treated. Fortunately, a simple screening test, mandatory in all 50 states, can identify PKU babies so they can be placed on a special phenylalanine-free diet and retardation can be prevented. Lifelong restriction is recommended, but many adults give the diet up after childhood. Pregnant women with PKU who have discontinued their phenylalanine-free diets are at significantly higher risk to have a PKU infant and should, of course, never have aspartame. But about 1 in 60 people is a heterozygote for the recessive PKU gene, is perfectly normal, and is usually unaware of the carrier status. It is highly unlikely, but remotely possible, that *excessive* aspartame intake in a PKU carrier mother (or in any pregnant woman) might approach a blood level of phenylalanine that could be damaging to the fetal developing central nervous system. Until more information on the safety of aspartame during pregnancy is available, it would be prudent for women to avoid large quantities of it.

Tobacco.

Cigarette smoking in a pregnant woman is unquestionably related to low birth weight in the infant she delivers, and more than 50 studies have confirmed this finding. The relationship is dose dependent; that is, the amount of growth retardation is directly correlated to the number of cigarettes smoked. The reduced birth weight with maternal smoking has been shown to be independent of all the other factors that may influence the size of the offspring, such as size of the mother, her race, socioeconomic status, birth order, or sex of the child. Although it is possible that heavy smokers have lower maternal weight gain, which could concurrently retard fetal growth, the cause of the decrease in fetal weight (an average of 6 oz) is probably related to the presence of excess carbon monoxide in the mother's blood. Repeated studies have shown that the level of fetal carboxyhemoglobin, the amount of hemoglobin combined with carbon monoxide, is up to 10 times higher in infants born of smoking mothers than in infants born of nonsmoking mothers. Hemoglobin that is tied up by carbon monoxide is not available to carry oxygen. Animal research has indicated that high levels of carbon monoxide can limit the oxygen supply to the fetus and affect the development of the brain cells. It has also been shown that sidestream smoke, that produced off the end of the cigarette, contains four times as much carbon monoxide as does mainstream smoke, that which is inhaled by the smoker. This means that pregnant women smokers who also spend long periods of time in a smoke-filled room or automobile could have alarming amounts of carbon monoxide buildup in their bloodstreams.

King and Fabro's review (1982) of the further effects of cigarette smoking on pregnancy and pregnancy outcome documents an association of smoking and an increased frequency of spontaneous abortions and a greater incidence of pregnancy complications such as bleeding. The long-term growth and development of the offspring born to smoking mothers is also affected. There is even evidence that significant differences in height as well as reading and math abilities exist in children whose mothers smoked 10 or more cigarettes daily during pregnancy, and a number of studies have linked maternal smoking with a greater incidence of sudden infant death syndrome. A study in Israel that examined the smoking habits of more than 16,000 mothers found that infants delivered by pregnant women aged 35 years and older who smoked had an increased rate of major malformations such as cleft palate, heart defects, and central nervous system anomalies and a significantly higher risk for minor malformations (Seidman, Ever-Hadani, & Gale, 1990). There also is evidence that prenatal exposure to the mother's cigarette smoking increases the risk of cancer in the offspring. Epidemiologist Esther John and her colleagues (1991) studied 223 children with cancer and 196 controls and reported an association between maternal smoking and leukemia and lymphoma in children. The risk of cancer was greater for male children, confirming previous evidence that prenatal exposure to cigarette smoking affects male and female fetuses differently. These workers also noted an increase in the risk of leukemia, lymphoma, and brain cancer in children whose fathers smoked but whose mothers did not. Although the effect may be due to the passive exposure of the mother to the father's smoking, the research suggests the possibility of a mutation effect on the father's sperm.

Caffeine.

Animal studies, in which high doses of caffeine (equivalent to 12–24 cups of coffee daily) were fed to rats, produced skeletal abnormalities in the rat pups. On this basis, suspicion has been leveled at overindulgence in coffee or tea drinking during pregnancy, but it is evidently unwarranted. Two epidemiological studies, one by Rosenberg, Mitchell, Shapiro, and Slone (1982) and the other by Linn and colleagues (1982), found no association between caffeine consumption and birth defects. Linn's group studied more than 12,000 pregnancies and discovered that women who reported that they drank more than 4 cups of coffee or tea daily had babies with a malformation rate of 2.0 per 1,000 live births, and women who drank no coffee or tea at all during pregnancy delivered infants with a birth defect rate of 2.5 per 1,000. On the basis of current evidence, it would appear that a pregnant women need not give up her morning cup of coffee or tea that contains between 100 and 200 mg of caffeine, but it would be prudent to keep the caffeine consumption in a reasonable range. A chocolate bar contains about 25 mg and a cup of cocoa or hot chocolate about half that much. Twelve ounces of noncaffeine-free sodas, however, contain between 30 and 60 mg of caffeine.

Maternal Alcohol Consumption, or One for My Baby.

Certainly, no mother in her right mind would give a glass of wine, beer, or hard liquor to her newborn infant. But alcohol, unlike some other drugs, passes with ease across the placenta. An embryo or fetus, therefore, is exposed to the same blood alcohol concentration as the mother, and when the mother drinks, so does her unborn child. The teratogenic effects of alcoholism or heavy maternal drinking have been recognized since 1973, when **fetal alcohol syndrome (FAS)** was first described. FAS is a pattern of defects that may be completely or partially expressed and includes low birth weight and fetal growth retardation, especially microcephaly; facial abnormalities, such as small eye slits, short pug nose, underdeveloped jaws, and nonparallel low-set ears; a number of cardiac, urogenital, cutaneous, and musculoskeletal defects; and later developmental delay and mental retardation.

FAS currently is the major cause of mental retardation in the United States, surpassing Down syndrome or any other genetic defect. As yet, full-blown FAS has been diagnosed only in the offspring of chronic alcoholic mothers, for whom the risk may be as high as 30%, but there is no simple dose-response relationship that can be used to predict its occurrence. FAS should be viewed as the most severe outcome in a range of disabilities caused by maternal alcohol consumption during pregnancy. Nor is FAS just a childhood disorder. Ann Streissguth and colleagues (1991) were the first to do a long-term follow-up on a group of infants born with FAS. As the study group of 61 FAS children progressed into adolescence and adulthood, their facial abnormalities tended to be not as distinctive, but their central nervous system abnormalities persisted. The patients functioned at second- to fourth-grade levels; had an average IQ of 68; and exhibited, in the words of the researchers, "maladaptive behaviors."

There also is ample evidence that a woman need not be an alcoholic to run a greater than normal risk of having a deformed or retarded child. Studies comparing heavy drinkers (five or six drinks on some occasions with an average of two drinks daily) with moderate drinkers found that heavy drinkers had babies with twice as many congenital, growth, and functional abnormalities as did the moderate drinkers. But one analysis of the effects of only moderate drinking during pregnancy found decrements in the children's IQ and learning problems at age 7½ years (Streissguth, Barr, & Sampson, 1990). Even light drinking, defined as having a drink once a week, has been linked to an increased risk of miscarriage and low birth weight.

What is unknown currently is whether there is a minimal amount of alcohol safe to drink during pregnancy. An occasional glass of wine could be harmless, but it makes more sense to assume that any alcohol use can be harmful to the fetus. Most women know that they should quit drinking during pregnancy, but when nonpregnant women of reproductive age drink, there can be what researcher Marcia Russell calls the "window of vulnerability"—the time lag between conception and the recognition of the pregnancy that may put substantial numbers of children at risk (1991).

Children with FAS, "crack babies," infants born addicted to heroin, are the tragic consequences of maternal substance abuse and they represent a new generation of sufferers. To many experts, the only ways to lessen the devastating impact of drug abuse in women and their babies are better and more available drug treatment services and educational programs.

Women should be aware that ingestion of "social" drugs during pregnancy may not be the only source of risk to the fetus. Researchers who investigated women's drug taking during pregnancy discovered that 65%–95% of women self-medicate with over-the-counter preparations during the first trimester or throughout gestation (Fortar & Nelson, 1973; Hill, Craig, & Chaney, 1977; Woodward, Brackbill, McManus et al., 1982). Women evidently do not view nonprescription drugs as drugs, even though they may be taking them for a physical complaint. Unnecessary drug ingestion is so much a part of our lives that it is equally common during pregnancy, so frequent that in most instances an association between a chemical agent consumed and a subtle congenital defect would never be recognized. Would anyone ever be able to relate aspirin, stomach preparations, or sleep aids with some subtle effect on the nervous system if it were manifested as a speech defect, a reading disability, a behavioral disorder, or a hyperactive child? Or, even more elusively, if it created the difference between a Phi Beta Kappa and a "C" student? With the current uncertainty concerning the effects of any environmental influence on the developing fetus, women should be conscious of everything that goes into their mouths or is in the air that they breathe from the time they miss their first menstrual periods until after delivery. They must take no drugs unnecessarily and must make certain that any pharmacological agent ingested is not only beneficial but essential.

Birth Defects and the Father

The general consensus is that 3% of newborn babies are affected with a congenital abnormality of prenatal origin. The cause may be genetic, that is, a mutant gene or a chromosomal abnormality, or it may be environmental, the result of maternal infection or other illness or maternal exposure to a teratogenic substance. There are hundreds of chemical agents that have demonstrated mutagenicity or teratogenicity when administered to pregnant animals; a logical question is, can a drug or toxic chemical be teratogenic through the male?

An overwhelming majority of human clinical and epidemiological studies concerned with the exposure of men to toxic substances have concluded that there is little or no evidence for an increased rate of malformation in the offspring. Although workplace hazards for women have been linked to birth defects, most studies of male workers exposed to toxic substances indicate that the reproductive effect in men is on themselves in the form of reduced fertility but does not directly affect the next generation in the form of congenital defects. Animal studies of drugs such as narcotics, thalidomide, anticonvulsants, and alcohol, and toxins such as lead, pesticides, or other kinds of contaminants and pollutants, show that reproductive toxicity, usually evidenced by temporary infertility, occurred in the male adults, but no malformation in the litters sired by the affected males resulted. Some human studies of men environmentally or occupationally exposed to various polychlorinated hydrocarbons (PCBs, PBBs, dioxin, Agent Orange) have shown an increased rate of spontaneous abortion in their wives, but other studies have found no increase in miscarriages or stillbirths, and none has demonstrated an increased rate of congenital malformations in their offspring as a result of exposure. But the absence of research evidence does not necessarily mean that no such effects occur. Reports indicating that fathers' exposure to therapeutic, environmental, or occupational agents may affect their genes in addition to affecting the quality and quantity of their sperm are beginning to appear in the scientific literature. Some studies have linked fathers' exposure to lead, various solvents, and wastewater materials with the size and development of their children. Esther John's research on the link between paternal smoking and children's cancer already has been mentioned. A 1990 report published in the *British Medical Journal* found an association between men working in a nuclear power station and leukemia in their children and suggested that the radiation could have caused a gene mutation in the sperm of the workers (Gardner et al., 1990). The hazards of environmental chemicals or drugs to which men, voluntarily or unwillingly, are exposed are certainly significant to their own health, since it is well known that they may develop liver problems or cancer or infertility. But although there are not very much data yet, it may be determined in the future that substances can act as teratogens via the father as well as the mother.

ℒABOR AND DELIVERY

Around the 40th week after the onset of the last menstrual period, pregnancy culminates in childbirth, or **parturition**. By this time, most women have difficulty remembering what not being pregnant was like, and the big event is fervently anticipated. All of the changes that have taken place during pregnancy have been in preparation for expelling the products of conception—the fetus, placenta, and membranes—from the inside of the uterus out into the world. The mechanism by which this happens is labor, aptly named because it is muscular work.

The labor process is a series of rhythmic, involuntary, usually quite uncomfortable uterine muscle contractions that bring about a shortening (effacement) and opening (dilatation) of the cervix, and a bursting of the fetal membranes. Then, accompanied by both reflex and voluntary contractions of the abdominal muscles (pushing), the uterine contractions result in the expulsion of the baby. The first stage of labor begins with the first true labor contraction and ends with the complete dilatation of the cervix, large enough to permit the passage of the infant. The second stage of labor ends with the delivery of the baby. The third stage is the period from the birth of the baby through delivery of the placenta and the membranes, and the fourth stage, a very critical period, is the first hour or two after labor is ended.

Exactly what happens during labor is well known; why it happens is still a mystery. Proposed hypotheses to explain the onset of labor range from the rather unscientific—"the baby outgrows the uterus," or "when the apple is ripe it falls from the tree"—to a group of theories that explains the control of parturition on an endocrine basis. The withdrawal of systemic progesterone, the oxytocin effect, the progesterone/estrogen ratio, the secretion of the fetal adrenals, and the role of prostaglandins have all been offered as suggested mechanisms. Current thinking assumes that many, perhaps all, of these factors are implicated in causing labor, that labor is initiated by a sequence of interacting endocrine events involving hormones from both fetal and maternal endocrine organs. One possibility being explored is that altered hormone levels stimulate the release of some agent from the fetal and maternal tissues that causes the formation of prostaglandins, perhaps by activating enzymes that can liberate arachidonic acid (the prostaglandin building block) from its storage site in cell membranes.

The position of the fetus and its relationship to the placenta and membranes during late pregnancy is illustrated in Figure 11–9. This is the position assumed by the fetus 95% of the time and is the one most favorable for normal labor and delivery. The head of the fetus is flexed so that the chin is down on the chest, and the presenting part, that which will descend first, is the top, occipital, or vertex part of the head. The presentation can be cephalic, that is, head first, but the presenting part may also be the face or the brow. A breech presentation means that the buttocks or the feet of the baby present first, and this occurs about once in 40 deliveries. Occasionally, the baby will lie in a transverse position, and the shoulder presents first.

Several changes take place in the uterus even before the start of actual labor. In most women who are having their first baby (primigravidas), lightening or dropping occurs. A few weeks before delivery, the presenting part of the fetus descends to settle into a position at the entrance of the true pelvis. Sometimes a first baby does not drop until labor begins, which is the usual situation in multiparas, women who have previously borne children. After lightening, the upper

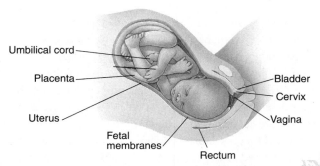

Figure 11–9 Cephalic presentation at the time of delivery.

abdomen becomes flatter and the lower abdomen becomes more prominent. Women notice they are able to breathe more easily again, but the urge to urinate frequently returns because of the increased pressure on the bladder. Pressure on the rectum and sacrum may also result in diarrhea and backache.

Another preliminary event is the taking up, shortening, or effacement of the cervix. During the first half of pregnancy, the uterine shape is the same as it is in the nonpregnant state. It consists of the upper corpus, or body, and the lower neck of the uterus or cervix, which extends into the vagina. As pregnancy advances, the corpus differentiates into two separate areas: an upper uterine segment that becomes the active muscular contracting part responsible for delivery, and the lower uterine segment—the thinner passive area located just above the internal os of the cervix. The demarcation between the upper and the lower segments is the physiologic retraction ring. During the last few weeks of pregnancy, the spontaneous, painless Braxton Hicks contractions that have been occurring all along become stronger. Each time the muscle fibers in the upper uterine segment contract and shorten, a very remarkable thing happens. Very unlike muscle in other parts of the body, these uterine muscle fibers never return to their former length when they relax. Instead they become progressively shorter and thicker, a property known as retraction or brachystasis. This continued shortening and thickening of the muscle fibers after contraction take place in the lower uterine segment as well but to a much lesser degree. As a result, the upper segment gradually increases in thickness, decreasing uterine volume, as the lower segment becomes thinner and elongated. The cervix softens, due to engorgement with blood, but remains closed, its canal plugged with mucus, until several weeks or even the last few days before labor begins. Eventually, however, the continual contraction and retraction of the upper segment causes the internal os to open and draws the entire cervix up from its position in the vagina. The cervix is thereby shortened, and the endocervical canal is obliterated as the cervix is pulled up around the fetal membranes and the presenting part and incorporated

into the lower uterine segment (Figure 11–10). The external cervical os then remains as a circular opening with extremely thin edges. Now, the further contractions of the uterus will bring about progressive cervical dilatation, or enlargement, of the external os.

With a first baby, complete cervical effacement usually occurs before there is any cervical dilatation. In women who have previously delivered a baby, dilatation takes place when effacement is incomplete or concurrently with effacement. Cervical effacement is measured by percentage. A cervix one-half of its normal length is 50% effaced.

The effacement and dilatation of the cervix cause the fetal membranes that are attached to the uterine wall at the region of the internal os to become loosened. As they pull away from the uterine wall, the little mucous plug that corks the endocervical canal is set free. Loss of the plug is painless, but a little blood escapes with it, and it constitutes the "bloody show." Increased vaginal discharge during the period of cervical effacement is not unusual, but when pink-tinged or blood-streaked mucus is expelled from the vagina, it is a sign that active labor has started or is imminent (Figure 11–11).

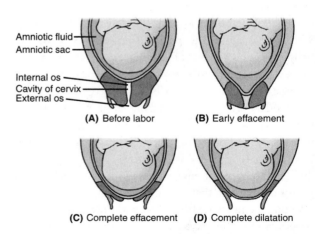

Figure 11–10 Effacement of the cervix in the first pregnancy. In a woman who has previously delivered a baby (multipara), effacement and dilation occur simultaneously. (A) Before any effacement. (B) Internal os is being drawn upward around the fetal membranes. (C) Complete effaced cervix. (D) Complete dilation.

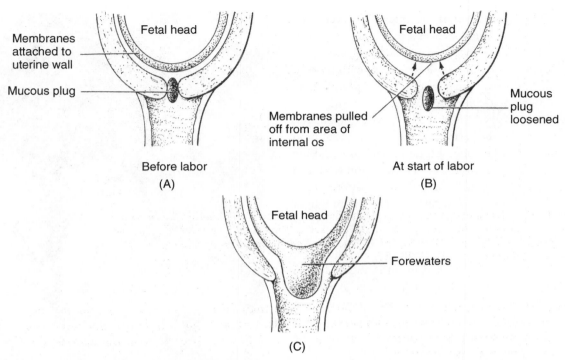

Figure 11–11   Cause of the bloody show. (A) Before the onset of labor, the membranes are attached to the uterine wall. A mucous plug, or operculum, blocks the endocervical canal. (B) With effacement and dilation of the cervix, the fetal membranes are pulled away from the internal os, and the mucous plug is set free along with a little bleeding. (C) After the plug is lost, the forewaters bulge in front of the fetal head.

First Stage

The criteria used to differentiate true labor contractions from the Braxton Hicks prelabor contractions are regularity and discomfort. When the contractions become painful, less than 10 minutes apart, last 30–90 seconds, and are regular in frequency, labor has begun. For a woman having her first baby, the average duration of the first stage of labor is about 12 hours, but there are wide variations. The length may be as short as 3 hours if contractions are strong and frequent.

The fetal membranes, or bag of waters, usually rupture during the first stage, but they may have burst earlier or may even remain intact until delivery. Actually, the part that ruptures is only a portion of the amniotic and chorionic sac, a little pocket of fluid called the forewaters that lies in front of the fetal head. The successive uterine contractions keep compressing the forewaters and even-

tually it breaks, permitting a little gush of amniotic fluid to exit. The rest of the fluid remains behind the baby's head as the hindwaters. If the membranes have not broken by the end of the first stage or early in the second stage of labor, they may be artificially ruptured with a sharp instrument during a vaginal exam.

In 10% of pregnancies, the fetal membranes burst before labor begins, and premature rupture is said to have occurred. Labor will usually start within the next 24 hours. If labor fails to ensue spontaneously, there may be an increased risk of fetal and maternal infection, and it is generally believed that infant mortality rate increases if more than 24 hours elapse between rupture and delivery. Many physicians, therefore, are of the opinion that labor should be induced with an oxytocin solution if it does not begin after 6 hours. A number of studies have evaluated the outcome of labor induction to shorten the interval between the premature rupture and delivery in women at term. The results indicate that such a procedure may be an unnecessary intervention because it appears to have no effect on newborn outcome and may result in more cesarean sections and more maternal infections.

When the cervix is dilated to 10 cm in diameter, it is large enough to permit the passage of a fetal head of average size (the baby's largest dimension), and the first stage of labor is over. Cervical dilatation is gauged subjectively by vaginal or rectal examination and is expressed in centimeters or finger widths. Throughout the first stage of labor, there are regular vaginal examinations to determine the degree of dilatation. They are performed under sterile conditions, and the index and second finger are inserted into the vagina to feel the extent of the cervical rim that remains. A woman hearing that she is "five fingers dilated" may envision the examiner's entire hand in the cervical os, but actually the subjective estimation is made by assessing the amount of spread between only the two fingers.

The last part of the first stage of labor, when the cervix is opening to complete dilatation, is called transition. It is the most difficult and, fortunately, the shortest phase for the woman, lasting approximately 1 hour in the first delivery and perhaps 15–30 minutes in successive births. At transition, the contractions are stronger, more painful, somewhat erratic, and last longer. Pressure on the rectum is great, and there is a strong desire to contract the abdominal muscles and push. Until the cervix is fully dilated, however, bearing down is not helpful. It will only intensify the discomfort and may cause cervical lacerations.

The techniques taught in prepared childbirth education classes are especially valuable in coping with the difficult physical and emotional aspects of the transition period (Figure 11–12).

Second Stage

The baby is completely passive throughout the entire progress of labor. With each succeeding uterine contraction, it is pushed lower and lower, and its position

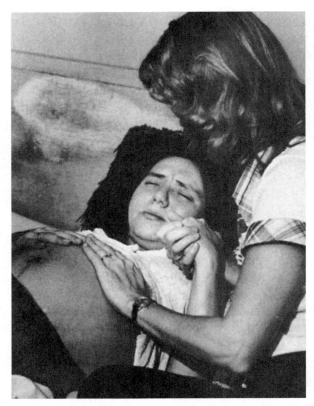

Figure 11–12 Transition stage during the first stage of labor. Coaching in the breathing techniques is being provided by a birthing attendant.

alters as it accommodates itself to passage through the different parts of the pelvis. At the beginning of the second stage of labor, the birth canal through which the baby descends is formed by the completely dilated cervix, the distended vagina, and the stretched and distended muscles of the pelvic floor. When the fetal head meets the resistance of the pelvic floor, it rotates 45° from its former oblique position. The face is now directed posteriorly, facing the mother's sacrum. As further descent continues, the anus dilates and the vagina begins to open with each contraction. The fetal scalp becomes apparent at the vaginal opening but disappears between contractions. When the top of the head no longer regresses between contractions, it is said to have crowned. The perineum bulges and thins out with each contraction as the fetal head continues to enlarge the vaginal opening. If an **episiotomy,** a small incision in the perineum that is performed to prevent tearing, is indicated, it is done at this time.

Episiotomies are neither routinely necessary, nor routinely unnecessary. When it is apparent that a small surgical cut is going to prevent a jagged laceration in the perineal skin and underlying levator ani muscles, it has to be done. Sometimes the procedure is necessary to protect the fetal head, especially in a premature baby, from consistent battering against an unyielding or slowly dilating vaginal opening. Even if tearing does not occur, it is possible that excessive stretching could cause enough damage to the connective tissue and muscles of the pelvic floor to result in problems years later.

The episiotomy may be midline and extend from the vagina directly down toward the anus, or it may be extended in a lateral direction at about a 45° angle to the left or to the right. The timing of the cut is important: if it is done too early, the normal blood loss will increase; if it is performed too late, lacerations may have already taken place. The episiotomy has to be sutured after the baby and the placenta are born. The perineum is still extremely sensitive, and, even with a local anesthetic, the repair is usually quite painful. As the stitches heal and are absorbed in the postpartum period, there is also considerable discomfort. Obviously, it is undesirable for episiotomy to be performed routinely, but it is virtually routine in American obstetrical practice. Doris Haire has pointed out the lack of scientific evidence to support the contention that episiotomy decreases pelvic floor relaxation or reduces the possibility of neurological damage to the infant. There also has been a suggestion that the lithotomy position in which a woman is placed during a traditional hospital delivery necessitates a greater need for episiotomies because of the increased tension on the pelvic floor. Alternative birth positions, such as those used in home deliveries or nontraditional hospitals, appear to lessen the strain on the perineum. Perineal massage practiced at home for a month before delivery and then performed by the birth attendant during the second stage of labor is advocated by some nurse-midwives. It is believed to help prevent lacerations. There is no way, however, to categorically decide ahead of time that an episiotomy will be unnecessary and should not be performed. It depends on the situation. If an episiotomy forestalls an imminent serious injury to the posterior wall of the vagina or the rectum, it has to be accepted with equanimity.

When the head crowns, the neck of the baby is no longer flexed forward but is extended backward. First the top of the head emerges, followed by the forehead, and then the brow and the face. When the head is born, it drops down over the perineum and rotates sideways to restore its natural position relative to the shoulders. This is called restitution of the head. Then the shoulders rotate to present their narrowest diameter for passage and the head is turned farther to the side (external rotation). The posterior or left shoulder is born first. It falls backward, the right shoulder slides out from underneath the pubic bone, and the rest of the body "squirts out" quickly and easily.

After delivery, the baby is kept below the level of the uterus. After a minute or so, when an adequate amount of placental blood has transfused to the infant, the umbilical cord is clamped and then cut about a half inch from the baby's abdomen. The other end of the cord still hangs from the vagina until the placenta is expelled.

Third Stage of Labor

Uterine contractions stop for a short time after delivery, but in a little while the relaxed uterus contracts again and causes the placenta, which has become partially separated from the maternal endometrial surface during expulsion of the baby, to become completely detached. At the same time, the upper segment of the uterus changes shape to become smaller, firmer, and rounder. There is a small gush of blood from the vagina, and the umbilical cord appears to lengthen as the placenta is forced downward. Continued uterine contractions cause the placenta to be expelled within 5–30 minutes. Most physicians prefer not to wait for the woman to expel the placenta herself, and they hurry it along by applying a little external pressure to speed up the first contraction. Once the uterus is firm and globular, it is further massaged to aid in expulsion of the placenta. The rationale behind the assistance is that in some women a significant amount of bleeding occurs if the placenta is allowed to be extruded spontaneously. Massaging the fundus of the uterus through the lower abdomen will probably be distinctly uncomfortable right after delivery, however. It is all the more unpleasant because, presumably, the hardest part—birth of the baby—is over. After the placenta is expelled, the uterus is still massaged to keep it contracting because contractions constrict the uterine blood vessels and minimize the possibility of hemorrhage (Figure 11–13 A–I).

The main case of postpartum hemorrhaging is uterine atony, or lack of contractions. Customarily, a uterotonic drug is given to stimulate firm contractions and reduce blood loss. An oxytocic solution may be used, but more often ergonovine maleate, the purified derivative of the rye fungus ergot, is administered intramuscularly or intravenously, after placental delivery. Both ergonovine maleate and the synthetic form, methylergonovine maleate, not only stimulate uterine muscle, but all smooth muscle as well and will elevate blood pressure. Oxytocin is, therefore, used in women with hypertension. Some doctors further prescribe oral tablets of ergonovine maleate every 6 hours until all danger of hemorrhage is past, about 48 hours.

If the newborn baby is permitted to nurse at the breast immediately after delivery and then at regular 3- to 4-hour intervals, pituitary oxytocin is released, which results in colostrum and later milk ejection from the breasts and which stimulates uterine contractions. Unless the mother has had little or no medication during delivery, however, the baby will generally be too sleepy to breastfeed right away.

Afterpains. Multiparas are frequently bothered by painful uterine contractions that may continue for as long as the first week after delivery. They get worse with each succeeding pregnancy, but almost never occur with a first baby. They last for a half hour or so

but are really uncomfortable for only the first 2 or 3 days and can be relieved with painkilling drugs. Afterpains are usually stronger during breastfeeding because the oxytocin released by the sucking reflex results in uterine contractions.

It also is not uncommon to have the "postpartum blues" set in within a week after the birth and to last for a while. The reason for the weepiness, irritability, and emotional lability is not known, but it happens to 50%–80% of new mothers and may have a hormonal basis. The term "postpartum depression" is often applied to this transitory state, but it actually denotes a postpartum psychiatric disorder of severe clinical depression that in some women involves a frankly psychotic state. Postpartum depression affects 8%–12% of new mothers and may last for months, although less than 1% become psychotic. The cause of postpartum depression is unknown, but Unterman, Posner, and Williams (1990) suggested risk factors for the disorder. These include having had a previous postpartum depression; the lack of parental emotional support in childhood or adulthood; a currently unstable life situation; inadequate financial resources; and the gap between a woman's expectations and the realities of being able to care for the baby and siblings, continue with her job, and keep up with the household duties.

Apgar Score. In 1960, American anesthesiologist Virginia Apgar introduced a method of assessing the well-being of the newborn within 1 minute and 5 minutes after delivery. The baby is scored at 0, 1, or 2 in each of five categories: heart rate (absent, slow, or fast); respiratory effort (absent, weak cry, or good strong yell); muscle tone (limp, or lively and active); response to irritating stimulus; and color. A score of 7–10 means the baby is in the best possible condition, while 3–6 means moderately depressed; any score below 2 indicates problems. The rating essentially is evaluating the functioning of the central nervous system. Babies born to mothers who have been heavily drugged for pain relief generally score around 5 or 6. The extent to which a moderately depressed **Apgar score** as a result of medication influences the future neurological and behavioral develop-

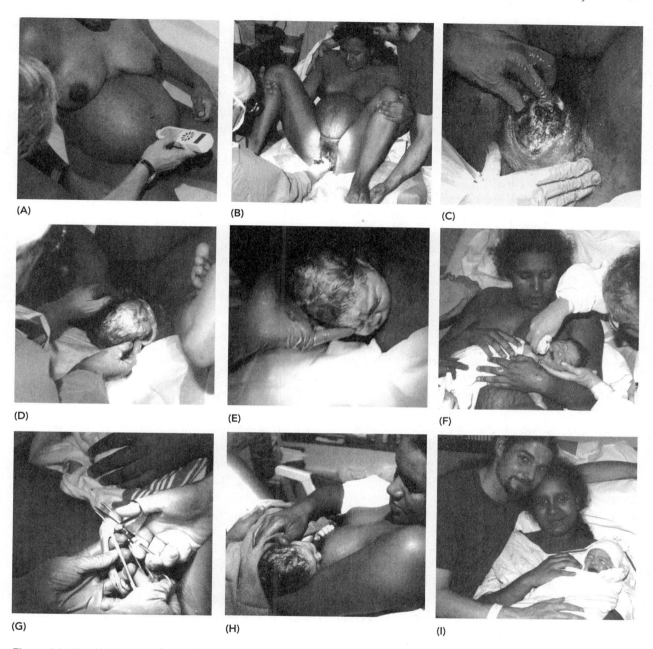

Figure 11–13 (A) Listening for the fetal heart tones. (B) Delivery takes place in a semireclining position. (C) Crowning of the head. The scalp is just visible. (D) Easing out the head. (E) The head is rotated. (F) Immediately after delivery, the baby is placed on the mother's abdomen. (G) The cord is clamped and cut. (H) Suckling of the breast immediately after delivery stimulates uterine contractions, stimulates milk production, and is beneficial for infant-mother bonding. (I) The happy family!

ment of the child is unknown, and it is assumed that there are no lasting effects.

The ability to predict developmental outcome and infant mortality on a long-term basis by use of the Apgar method is limited. Even very low scores at 1 and 5 minutes do not necessarily mean subsequent neurological dysfunction, illness, or mortality, particularly in low-birth-weight or premature infants. Similarly, high scores cannot guarantee that neurological development will be normal. Another problem with the Apgar system is its lack of objectivity. Assessment of the score is necessarily subjective, and Apgar believed that the emotional involvement of the delivery personnel could affect it. The general consensus is that the method can be used effectively if the limitations are understood and if an independent observer—not the obstetrician—does the scoring.

Group B Streptococcus Infection.

Group B streptococci are part of the strep family of bacteria, some of which cause strep throat, rheumatic fever and scarlet fever, and a type of pneumonia. Group B strep, however, are commonly found in the urogenital and digestive tracts of nearly a third of all healthy adults and normally cause neither symptoms nor harm. These bacteria are almost exclusively a life-threatening danger only to newborns. Ninety-eight percent of infected infants will have no problem, but if unrecognized and untreated in the other 2%, some babies will die or if they survive, will have permanent brain or lung damage. One in five pregnant women harbors Group B strep at the time of delivery and can pass the organism to the infant, but a carrier mother has a greater risk of delivering a baby with Group B strep infection under the following circumstances:

1. When there is premature rupture of membranes and labor does not start within 12 hours
2. When the newborn is premature or of low birth weight
3. When the mother has a fever before or during labor and delivery, or within 48 hours after delivery
4. If a woman has already delivered a baby with Group B strep

The symptoms of Group B infection—fever over 100°F, respiratory difficulty, irritability and then lethargy—mostly occur during the first week of life but also can happen to an infant up to 2 months of age.

The only protection against Group B strep infection is identification of the organisms in a pregnant women by a screening test. If she is found to be a carrier, she will be monitored and is likely to be treated with antibiotics if she is in a high-risk category. In view of the potentially devastating effects on newborns and infants, some obstetricians and pediatricians have recommended an aggressively active public education campaign and testing all pregnant women for carrier status. A group of parents whose babies died of the infection has formed a national organization to alert the public and health professionals to the disease and to spur research efforts and the development of a vaccine.

Childbirth Pain and Painless Childbirth

Only 8%–10% of all births are considered unusually difficult or abnormal. For the vast majority of women with normal labor, giving birth is not the acutely painful process we have been led to believe, but neither is it completely free from discomfort. To assert that ". . . the pain of delivery is the most intense that the human being can experience" (Niswander, 1976) is certainly an overstatement. But to claim that even for confident, calm, and totally prepared women, all parts of labor and delivery are comfortable and easy is an equal misrepresentation. Undeniably, smooth muscle contractions can hurt, as anyone who has experienced menstrual cramps or diarrhea will recognize. Uterine contractions are similar to menstrual and intestinal cramps, but they are also unlike them. The peak discomfort of labor contractions, even when they are coming very close together, only lasts a few seconds and completely disappears between contractions. The action of the uterine muscle, however, is not the only component of labor discomfort. Another is the result of cervical dilatation. The traction on the cervix that results in the enlargement of the cervical os stimulates nerve impulses that are transmitted along sacral nerves to the spinal cord. Those sensations in the sacral region result in the intense backache associated with labor experienced by some women. A third reason for discomfort during labor and delivery is the stretching of the vagina and the perineum. When a full-term baby's head, 10 cm in its widest dimension, starts its descent into the birth canal, it creates pressure on the bladder, rectum, and all the surrounding tissues. The sensations, carried along the pudendal nerve to the spinal cord, have been likened to the feeling of having a bowling ball move slowly through the pelvis. All of these feelings do not have to be interpreted as excruciating, but the brain is certain to recognize them as different and uncomfortable.

Some women need, or think they need, a great deal of pain relief. Others are able to manage with very minimal administration of medication, or none at all, depending to a certain extent on their attitude toward the event of giving birth. Unfortunately, the perfect painkiller, one that takes away all discomfort but does not hamper the progress of labor or present any danger to the mother or to the baby, does not exist. All drugs, whether they are given systemically, inhaled as gases, or injected for a local nerve block, have some risks and disadvantages. Any medication gets into the bloodstream, crosses the placenta, and, depending on the time of administration, the kind of drug, and the dosage, can affect the fetus and the newborn baby. Because a baby is unable to metabolize or excrete the drug as rapidly or effectively as an adult, the infant may be born with a varying amount of respiratory and nervous system depression.

Heavy medication can result in a sleepy baby for several days or even a week or longer after birth. Light medication produces an alert and active baby. There are no meaningful scientific data yet to prove a long-term deleterious effect as a result of a lethargic entry into the world, but common sense dictates that the least depressing drug in the lowest possible dosage is best.

Systemic analgesia (drugs) was once the main technique of pain relief and still is in those hospitals where the trained personnel needed to administer the currently popular lumbar epidural analgesia are unavailable. The drugs used to provide systemic painkillers include tranquilizers, narcotics, and barbiturates.

Systemic Analgesics.　Tranquilizers and sedatives have been used in early labor if a woman is particularly tense and anxious. They do not relieve pain but diminish anxiety. They also potentiate the effect of narcotic analgesics so that less pain reliever is needed. Sedatives and tranquilizers sedate—they can slow labor, cause drowsiness or sleep, and occasionally, dizziness or nausea and vomiting. In some women, their use results in paradoxical effects, and mood elevation, excitement, restlessness, or even delirium may occur. The closer to delivery the drugs are given, the more likely is central nervous system depression in the newborn.

Intramuscular meperidine (Demerol) is the most popular narcotic analgesic. Its action, the increasing of tolerance to pain, peaks at 1 to 1½ hours after injection. It easily crosses the placenta, so the amount and timing of administration are very important. If labor takes less time than expected, the adverse effects of the drug on the fetus/newborn are evidenced by respiratory depression. Adverse effects on the mother may include nausea, vomiting, and rapid heartbeat, so the drug should be used cautiously in women with cardiac disease. Butorphanol (Stadol) is a frequently used synthetic narcotic that appears to produce less incidence of infant respiratory distress than Demerol.

Inhaling gas through a mask to provide complete anesthesia or loss of consciousness is virtually nonexistent nowadays, but whiffs of low-concentration nitrous oxide-oxygen mixtures or trichloroethylene (Trilene) in a self-administered vaporizer may be used intermittently during the second stage of labor. Because there is a time lag of several seconds before the gas can get from the lungs into the bloodstream and to the brain, for maximum pain relief the inhalation has to be started before the contraction begins. Fetal depression is possible, but rare, with low concentrations of gas.

Maternal and fetal effects may not be the sole consideration in the use of inhalant analgesia. There is increasing concern about the effects of long-term exposure to trace amounts of the anesthetic gases on the health of delivery room personnel. Several studies have demonstrated that operating room nurses and anesthetists have a higher rate of miscarriage than the general population. Nitrous oxide, the most common anesthetic agent in a handheld vaporizer, may be a particular health hazard. A study of dental assistants and wives of dentists exposed to nitrous oxide, among other anesthetic gases, revealed that their rate of miscarriage was greater than that in the general population (Cohen et al., 1980).

Regional Blocks. Regional pain relief means that the sensory nerve impulses from the pelvic area are blocked by the injection of a local anesthetic in the same way that the dentist "freezes" a tooth before drilling. The most common techniques used are the paracervical, pudendal, and the "spinals"—subarachnoid saddle, continuous caudal, and continuous epidural blocks. All have advantages and disadvantages. In many parts of the country, epidural anesthesia has replaced the other types of local anesthetics.

A *paracervical block* is an injection that deadens the sensations arising from the dilating cervix during the first stage of labor. When the cervix has dilated to 4 or 5 cm, a local agent, such as Novocain, Xylocaine, or Carbocaine, is injected into the lateral fornix on either side. The anesthesia does not last very long and may have to be repeated after an hour or two. Transitory slowing of the fetal heart rate as a result of repeated injections has been known, so the total drug dosage must be kept at a minimum.

A *pudendal block* anesthetizes the nerve supply to the perineum, the vulva, and the vagina by an injection into the area surrounding the trunk of the pudendal nerve as it passes around the ischial spine. The injection can be made directly through the perineal tissue (transperineally) or, as is more frequent, through the vagina (transvaginally). The nerve block takes effect in 5 minutes and lasts about an hour. It is usually given late in the second stage of labor when the cervix is completely dilated, and it decreases the discomfort of the actual delivery. Pudendal block neither slows uterine contractions nor relieves their pain, so it is sometimes supplemented by another agent. With this kind of anesthesia

of the pudendal and perineal nerves, a woman can be fully conscious during delivery but have a minimum of pain. It is believed to have no adverse effect on the baby.

The other regional anesthetics are called spinals because the injections are made into the coverings around the spinal cord itself. The brain and spinal cord are protected by three complete coverings or meninges: the outermost tough dura mater, and thin and delicate arachnoid mater, and the even more delicate pia mater. Between the arachnoid mater and the pia mater is the subarachnoid space filled with cerebrospinal fluid that cushions the brain and cord. The sensory nerves that carry pain impulses from the pelvic organs enter the spinal cord at the level of the 11th and 12th thoracic vertebrae. The motor nerves that cause uterine contractions exit from the cord higher up, at the level of the 7th and 8th thoracic vertebrae. Therefore, injections of an anesthetic that are made below the 8th thoracic vertebra will block all sensations but will not interfere with uterine contractions.

Subarachnoid spinal anesthesia is performed by the introduction of a needle into the interspace between the third and fourth lumbar vertebrae until it enters the subarachnoid space below the arachnoid layer of the spinal cord. The injection is frequently made with the woman in a sitting position with her back rounded. A lumbar puncture sounds intimidating but is actually not that uncomfortable and does not take long to do.

The anesthetic solution is weighted with glucose or dextrose to make it heavier so that it settles in the lower spinal cord. The level of anesthesia up the back is controlled by positioning the woman or by tilting the table up or down following the injection. When the spinal block is kept very low, it is called a *saddle block* because the loss of sensation is in the part of the body that would sit on a saddle. A high spinal results in complete anesthesia from the waist down. Uterine contractions continue, but they may be slowed, and saddle block is performed when delivery is imminent during the second stage of labor. The effects last about an hour and alleviate the pain of episiotomy, delivery, and repair of episiotomy.

The administration of any type of spinal anesthetic requires the skill of an expert, and the subarachnoid injection is said to be safe and easy as long as it is properly performed. There is always the chance of nerve-root injury and possible neurological damage as a result, but the incidence is low. The major disadvantage to spinal injection is its tendency to cause a lowering of maternal blood pressure, which could impair the oxygen supply to the fetus. While there is a significant risk of such hypotension, it can be quickly alleviated by a change in the woman's position, either by elevating the legs or turning onto the left side.

Another drawback of this anesthetic is the chance of postspinal headache. Whenever cerebrospinal fluid is disturbed, either by injecting something into it or by removing some of it as in a spinal tap, a headache is likely to occur. Lying flat for 6–12 hours after a spinal may help to prevent a headache. The leakage of cerebrospinal fluid at the site of the injection may be a major factor in the cause of headaches, and the use of smaller gauge spinal needles is said to reduce their incidence. If the spinal headache does occur, it can be very severe and incapacitating, last for several days, and can be relieved only by lying flat in bed. For mother and infant, this is a less-than-optimal way to start postpartum life.

Epidural anesthesia is achieved by an injection into the epidural space, which lies between the dura mater of the spinal cord and the ligaments that connect the dura and the vertebrae. Lumbar epidural analgesia, as it is called, has become the most popular anesthetic during labor and delivery. It gives complete relief from pain with fewer effects on the mother and infant than most other types of medication. It may be given as a single dose just before delivery, but, more commonly, continuous administration is started during the first stage of labor. With the woman lying on her left side, a needle is introduced between the third and fourth lumbar vertebrae until it reaches the epidural space. A plastic catheter is then threaded through the needle, the needle is withdrawn, and the catheter is taped into place on the skin so that appropriate doses of the local anesthetic drug, usually bupivacaine, can be given at intervals.

Continuous epidural block is popular because of the high degree of pain relief and the absence of fetal depression. There are, however, several disadvantages to its use. It requires an experienced anesthesiologist to time it properly and perform it safely and effectively. It slows labor in the first stage and causes the bearing down or pushing reflex in the second stage to be reduced or lost so that the baby may have to be delivered by forceps. Maternal hypotension is an ever-present complication. Uncontrollable shaking of the legs or a temporary paralysis may occur. Neither is significant or lasts very long but can certainly be alarming if a woman is unprepared. And finally, if the dura mater is accidentally perforated, the result will be a subarachnoid anesthesia, which may not be desirable at the time and which increases the chance of a postspinal headache. For a cesarean section, a larger volume of drug is administered to produce greater blocking of pain higher up in the cord.

A *caudal block* is similar to an epidural in that it is made into a space outside the dura mater, but the site of the needle insertion is different. The injection is made through an opening or foramen in the sacrum into the caudal space, an area below the level of the dura mater in the lowest part of the spinal canal. The procedure requires a larger dose of anesthetic and somewhat more technical skill than does an epidural injection, and the risk of infection is slightly greater. The pain relief and the potential for complications are the same for both methods, and neither is thought to have much, if any, effect on the newborn unless maternal hypotension is prolonged and severe. Figure 11–14 shows the needle placement for three types of spinal anesthesia.

Relief of Pain without Medication

Childbirth educators, those who teach techniques of prepared childbirth, are reluctant to use the word *pain* at all. They refer only to "contractions" because of the negative connotation of the term *labor pains*. The fact that pain exists, however, is really not as significant as the way one feels about it and deals with it. There are mechanical and physical reasons for discomfort in childbirth; no one invents or imagines it. But there is a great deal of evidence from laboratory studies and from the way people have been observed to behave during pain-producing situations that suggests that while everyone

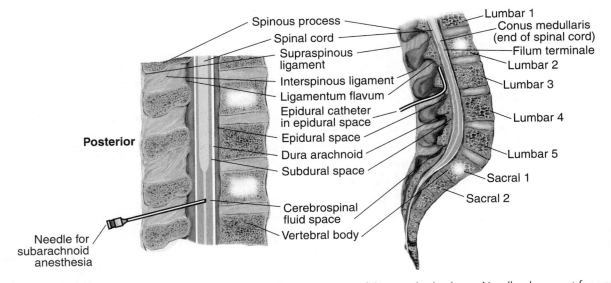

Figure 11–14 The spinal cord and its coverings in the lower portion of the vertebral column. Needle placement for a subarachnoid spinal block is shown. For an epidural block, the injection is made into the epidural space; in a caudal block the needle is placed in the caudal space.

probably feels pain in the same way physiologically, there is enormous variation in the way that different individuals perceive, interpret, and respond to pain. The degree and quality of pain during labor and delivery can be greatly influenced by a woman's attitudes and preconceived notions toward the birth process.

For centuries, women have been exposed to what Dr. Pierre Vellay, an associate of Dr. Lamaze, called psychological pollution. The traditional and destructive conditioning concerning childbirth pain is still being reinforced today by the motion picture and television portrayals of the agonies of laboring women, writhing and screaming in apparently intolerable torment. Such images have great dramatic impact and are difficult to dispel, even with the recognition that they are only cultural myths that exist in the minds of the film directors. When a woman learns to expect pain in childbirth and to fear it, she is likely to experience what she anxiously anticipates. The goal of prepared or natural childbirth is to reeducate and condition women to a positive attitude toward childbirth so that labor and delivery can be, if not actually painless, at least comfortable enough so that

they can experience the joy of the event. Prepared childbirth does not preclude the use of analgesic drugs, if a woman chooses to have them. Women who have been trained in its techniques, however, require far less medication. Not only can they actively participate in delivering the baby that they have carried for 9 months, but because lower doses of drugs can be administered, there is less risk for both mother and child.

The most widely used method of childbirth education in this country is the **Lamaze method,** also called psychoprophylaxis or prepared childbirth. Through the efforts of the American Society for Psychoprophylaxis in Obstetrics and the International Childbirth Education Association, increasing numbers of pregnant women are being prepared physically and mentally for the delivery of their children. First introduced in France in 1952 by obstetrician Fernand Lamaze, the method is based on the theories of the natural childbirth pioneer Grantly Dick-Read of England. Dick-Read emphasized the relationship of fear and tension to pain and stressed education to remove the fear, exercises to prepare muscles and joints for delivery, and muscle relaxation and breathing techniques to relieve the tension. Lamaze utilized the Dick-Read concepts, incorporating with them the Russian theory of psychoprophylactic preparation for birth.

The psychoprophylactic theory was based on the work of Russian physiologist Ivan Pavlov, who discovered conditioned reflexes. Pavlov conducted experiments to prove that dogs could be conditioned to respond to painful stimuli by salivating, as though the stimuli were actually food, instead of responding with howls of pain. Russian doctors, who had experimented with various methods of suggestion and hypnotism to alleviate childbirth pain, began to use a similar kind of conditioning training for pregnant women. Through stimulus-response conditioning, it was discovered that women could teach themselves to develop new responses to the stimuli of uterine contractions and could ease the progression of labor. During the last 2 months of pregnancy, women learned and practiced muscular and respiratory behaviors with which they would automatically respond during labor to eliminate or minimize the pain of childbirth.

The method, highly successful in Russia, was brought to France by Lamaze and spread to the United States in the early 1950s. As currently practiced, the technique is taught to pregnant women in the form of a series of lessons that begin at the end of the seventh month, although the orientation sessions may start as early as the second or third month. Various modifications of the method are taught, depending on the area of the country, or whether the classes are offered by a hospital, doctors for their patients, the Red Cross, the YWCA, or the Childbirth Education Association (Figure 11–15).

The basic principles of psychoprophylaxis are always the same:

1. Education about the anatomy and physiology of pregnancy, labor, and delivery, with positive information to replace the myths and superstitions
2. Physical exercises—squatting, tailor sits, pelvic rocks, various contraction and relaxation techniques—to strengthen, tone, and limber up the pelvic floor and abdominal muscles

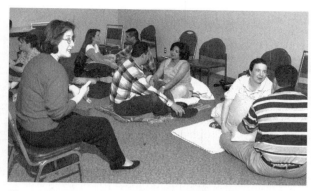

Figure 11–15 Prenatal conditioning exercises are taught in childbirth education classes.

3. Relaxation and breathing techniques for use during labor and delivery

The woman learns neuromuscular control techniques, the ability to differentially contract isolated muscle groups while simultaneously relaxing other muscles. During labor she will be able to consciously "release" or relax muscles upon direction. A further component of psychoprophylaxis is what appears to some to be "gimmicks." These are the distracting stimuli that give the woman something to concentrate and focus on to take her mind off labor and pain. The distractions take the form of various breathing patterns and *effleurage*, a light rhythmic stroking on the abdomen that is performed in time to the breathing. The more absorbed a woman can become in these additional activities, it is believed, the less the brain will perceive pelvic sensations as being painful.

The childbirth education classes are taught by trained and qualified childbirth educators. Strong elements of group dynamics and group therapy are involved in the course; a woman has a feeling of community with the other participants and is not isolated in her pregnancy. A labor coach—the father of the child, the mother of the woman, or a willing friend—accompanies the pregnant woman to the classes. The coach learns the physical exercises along with the woman and is able to provide the necessary reminders, encouragement, and support throughout the labor and delivery process.

Prepared childbirth works. Studies have shown that its techniques can effectively substitute for drugs in providing pain relief during labor and delivery. Many aspects of yoga, meditation, autosuggestion, and hypnosis are similar to the mental focusing components of psychoprophylaxis; there is nothing mysterious about it.

With childbirth education, the pain in a normal labor and delivery is quite bearable for many women. When it does become fairly intense, the discomfort also may be completely overshadowed by the exhilaration and joy of participation. The fantastic, incredible, miraculous experience of giving birth happens only a few times in a woman's life; she should be there to enjoy it and not be totally out of it as a result of medication.

The Lamaze method of psychological conditioning, while successful, cannot possibly be equally effective for all women. A woman should never feel that she has failed in some way, was not motivated enough, or have guilt feelings if she has to have some measure of chemical pain relief. People differ, and childbirth should never be viewed as an endurance contest. Medication is an option, available according to individual need, but psychoprophylaxis will reduce the need. Prepared childbirth will enable the woman to redirect her emphasis. Pain may no longer be significant in an atmosphere of full participation and encouraging support.

Leboyer Method

Another French physician, Frederick Leboyer, has advocated what has become known as the Leboyer delivery. Leboyer appears less interested in the mother than in the baby. In his 1975 book *Birth without Violence,* he sees the process of birth as "torture of the innocent," a perception gleaned from his own psychoanalytic recollection of birth. His concept, rooted in the concept of primal pain, is that the uterus is a prison, that contractions crush, stifle, and assault, and that, among other horrors, as the "monster" bears down, twisting the baby "in a refinement of cruelty," the baby,

"mad with agony and misery, alone, abandoned, fights with the strength of despair." To minimize this incredible trauma and pain associated with being born, Leboyer recommends a wide episiotomy for a controlled delivery, and gentle support of the head, neck, and sacrum as the baby emerges. The infant is then placed on the mother's abdomen, and its back is gently massaged by the obstetrician. While the cranial-sacral axis is continually supported, the baby is transferred to a warm water bath for several minutes, dried off, and diapered. All this time the room is kept very quiet and dimly lit to avoid overstimulation of the newborn.

Leboyer's attitude toward women in the process of birth is highly questionable, but his attitude toward establishing a more humane, gentle introduction to the world than that provided by the usual hospital practices is valid. Women could consider aspects of the Leboyer-type delivery that would be applicable to their labor and delivery. Most of Leboyer's suggestions are not new; they have been traditionally practiced by women and midwives.

Other Nonanalgesic Methods of Pain Relief.

Acupuncture, a thousand-year-old Chinese method of anesthesia performed by placing slender needles in acupuncture points on the body, has been used for cesarean deliveries in China and in labor and vaginal deliveries in the West. After the needles are inserted, they may be stimulated by rotation or electric current. Hypnosis, an altered state of consciousness, is reportedly effective when the woman has had previous training sessions with a skilled hypnotist who is, preferably, also skilled in obstetrics. Transcutaneous electrical nerve stimulation, also known as TENS, utilizes the application of a mild electric current to the skin to enhance the body's production of the pain-relieving endorphins. The device, about the size of a telephone beeper, is placed on the chest area at specific points. The frequency and intensity of the stimulation is ordinarily hand-controlled by the laboring mother, who increases the amount during contractions.

Another way of shortening labor, reducing the need for epidural anesthesia, and significantly reducing cesarean section rates could be a very old-fashioned method—the reliance on another woman as a birthing companion. Pediatricians Kennell and Klaus, the same researchers who earlier contributed to the recognition of the importance of parental–infant bonding after birth, did a controlled, randomized, clinical trial with 616 women who gave birth in a technologically sophisticated hospital in Texas. Of the women studied, one-third, or 216, received emotional support that included continuous talking and touching from a "doula," a Greek term that means an experienced woman who guides and helps a new mother in infant care. The doula met the laboring woman at the time of hospital admission and remained at her bedside—soothing, touching, and encouraging her throughout delivery. The doulas in the study were from 22–55 years of age, had each delivered at least one child vaginally, had taken 8 weeks of training, and were paid $200 per patient. The second group of 200 women in the study merely were observed in the delivery room, and the remaining women constituted the control group and received no special treatment. The researchers reported that the women with doulas had labors about 2 hours shorter than those who received no special care, that epidural block was used in 7.8% of the supported women as compared to 22.6% in the observed group and 55.3% of the control group, and that only 8% of the doula-attended women had cesarean deliveries compared with 13% of the observed and 18% of the control women (Kennell et al., 1991). Quoted in the *Chicago Tribune*, Kennell calculated that of the 4 million births annually, there could be more than $2 billion a year saved if every woman had a doula and the cesarean rate dropped accordingly. "I suspect some obstetricians are not wild about the idea of using doulas, but that could be because it may affect their fees," he said (Fowler, 1991).

Mother–Infant Bonding

The importance of the immediate period after birth for cementing the relationship between parent and child has been recognized. In a number of studies (1972, 1976), Marshall Klaus and his coworkers emphasized the importance of contact, both visual and tactile, between mother and baby in the first minutes, hours, and days after birth. Bonds of affection can be particularly strengthened if eye-to-eye and skin-to-skin contact take place. Klaus and Kennell advocate the value of mother, father, and infant togetherness for the first hour after birth in the delivery or recovery room. De Chateau reported that when mothers were given their naked babies for 1 hour within the first 3 hours after birth, such extra contact resulted in differences in maternal attachment behavior—smelling, kissing, close body contact—1 month, 1 year, and even 2 years after delivery (1980).

The necessity of such bonding or imprinting during a "sensitive period" after childbirth may be overemphasized. Not all parents, nor all children, will need such early extra contact to establish a loving relationship. If it has been denied as a result of a premature or otherwise high-risk delivery, a mother's attachment to her baby and the child's subsequent development can be just as positive as if the skin-to-skin contact had occurred. Klaus and Kennell, themselves, have become concerned about a too literal acceptance of the word bonding that suggests that "the speed of this reaction resembles that of epoxy materials" and produces feelings of guilt and failure if it does not take place (1983). The concept of the benefits of early contact, however, has helped to change the system that virtually excluded parents from the birthing process in most hospitals. The separation of mother and father from child during and after delivery is no longer routine and is unacceptable to many women who would choose to deliver at home if the hospital did not provide for parent–infant interaction.

INTERVENTION

The whole purpose of health care during pregnancy, labor, and delivery is directed toward achieving the outcome everyone wants—the birth of a normally functioning, healthy baby to a healthy and happy mother. About 85%–90% of pregnancies would terminate in spontaneous normal delivery, an uncomplicated labor that produces a healthy infant, even if the only birth attendant were Mother Nature. Few women would choose to deliver their babies alone and unattended, but most may be getting far more assistance than they require. "Normal delivery," as depicted in a medical teaching film by that name distributed under the auspices of the American Medical Association, is childbirth that is helped along by the following procedures:

1. 100 mg of meperidine (Demerol) administered to the mother during the first stage of labor
2. Paracervical block during the first stage
3. Artificial rupture of the membranes to hasten delivery
4. Bilateral pudendal block early in the second stage
5. Low forceps delivery when the head has crowned
6. Midline episiotomy
7. Oxytocin injection in the second stage to ensure uterine contractions in the third stage
8. Massage of the fundus of the uterus in the third stage to facilitate expulsion of the placenta
9. Manual removal of the placenta from the uterus if it is not spontaneously expelled within a few minutes
10. Repair of the episiotomy

One viewer, awed by all the injecting, cutting, sewing, and other maneuvers, commented that it certainly looks as though birth were impossible without that much help. The implication is clear: delivery is not a normal physiological process but a hospital illness that must be managed and technologically assisted. The normal delivery film is several years old, but revision today might be likely to show additional, rather than fewer, interventions. The laboring woman, for example, would probably be hooked up to a machine that electronically monitors fetal heart rate, maternal blood pressure, and uterine contractions through the entire birth process, and the climax of the film would more likely be a cesarean section rather than a vaginal delivery.

Many women and some doctors have questioned the need for and the value of such active obstetrical management of the normal spontaneous delivery. Birth is no longer the responsibility of the woman; it increasingly has become that of the attending physician. The substitution of a technically facilitated childbirth for letting nature take its course is being challenged, and there are doubts concerning the safety and the benefit of many of the interventions.

When it is indicated and necessary, an oxytocin infusion to start labor is a useful tool. How often is it done for convenience because the doctor wants to get back to an office full of patients, has a meeting to attend that night, or wants to leave on vacation the next day? Why is the incidence of use of forceps delivery or a vacuum extractor applied to the fetal scalp extremely limited in some hospitals but extremely frequent in others? There have been suggestions that a major factor may be the maintenance of the skills of the obstetrician. Critics of the American way of birth have alleged that high-tech procedures are used because normal delivery is too routine, too boring, and presents little challenge to the highly trained obstetrician. Intervention and management of labor, with all the technological gadgetry that accompanies current hospital obstetrics, may make the process more interesting as well as educational for the obstetrical residents.

Some deliveries do require every medical advantage to make certain that no tragedy occurs. Certain pregnancies are designated as high risk, and there is a significantly increased possibility of fetal or maternal mortality or morbidity. In that category are women with a history of previous obstetric difficulty, who have a major medical problem such as heart or kidney disease or diabetes, who have developed a hypertensive or a blood disorder, or who are having a multiple pregnancy. Along with the purely medical reasons, poverty, with its resulting social, nutritional, and emotional deprivation, is also seen as a major contributing factor to risky delivery.

Two-thirds of all complications in pregnancy and delivery occur in women who have been placed into a high-risk classification. These are the pregnancies for which all the tools of technology—the ultrasound scans, the contraction stress tests, the amniocentesis for fetal maturity determination, the continuous fetal heart-rate monitoring, the inductions to initiate labor, the cesarean sections to replace vaginal delivery—play an essential role in ensuring a favorable outcome. Although difficulty in delivery can occasionally occur without prior indication, the 10% of births that are abnormally complicated or unusual can almost always be predicted. But by some extrapolation of high risk to all risk, techniques formerly reserved for dangerous deliveries are now almost mandatory for all deliveries in most hospital-based obstetrical practices.

The usual medical controversy exists. An increasing number of doctors use maneuvers and techniques formerly reserved for the most exceptional of high-risk pregnancies as necessary and safe methods for all deliveries. Others view the liberal use of testing, monitoring, and management during labor and delivery, often culminating in cesarean section, as invasive and dangerous in itself. No one could argue that now, when birth rates in the United States are low and presumably most pregnancies (except in teenagers) are planned and wanted, every effort should be made to ensure the birth of a healthy, mentally and physically sound infant. Doctors who favor maximum interference imply that it is better to be safe than sorry and that new obstetrical techniques are responsible for a more favorable fetal outcome. Are they right?

After 30 years of increasingly medically managed births and expanded reasons for cesarean sections, the infant mortality rate in the United States, although still one of the worst in developed nations, declined from 29 deaths per 1,000 births in 1970 to 7.2 per 1,000 in 1996. Whether a cause-and-effect relationship exists is highly questionable, however. Approximately 60% of infant mortality occurs in newborns weighing less than 5½ lb. Perhaps improved techniques in neonatal intensive care units for premature and low-birth-weight infants have contributed to the mortality decline. Maybe the statistics are better because more women with greater education and understanding of the roles of smoking, drinking, and weight gain on birth weight are having babies. Besides, the improved figure reflects the total rate of infant deaths; there is a lower rate for white babies but still a higher rate for black and Hispanic babies, who are twice as likely to be of low birth weight and twice as likely to die in the first year of life. There is no reason to feel proud of a decrease in infant mortality unless it applies to all infants. High-technology intervention in normal deliveries may be affecting the health status of some children but may not be a significant component of the improved infant mortality statistics.

But another question persists. If interventions during prenatal care and parturition may not provide greater benefit to maternal and fetal outcome, do they present some inherent risks? That is, are there adverse effects of medical intercession that go beyond the psychological ones—the possible feeling of dissatisfaction and regret of a woman with the uneasy sense that it was the doctor, the hospital, and the machines that delivered her baby, and not she.

Chicago obstetrician Frederick Ettner maintains that "hospital technology breeds pathology" and that women should refuse to be part of hospital protocols that consider the extraordinary as routine. From the time a woman enters the hospital until she leaves with her baby, there are surely some aspects of obstetrical care that have become so institutionalized that they are performed almost ritualistically, with no real evidence that they have any effect on the improvement of maternal or fetal well-being. There are indications that some techniques may be not only unnecessary, but hazardous as well.

Induction of Labor

Labor can be induced or a slow labor can be enhanced by the administration of a solution of oxytocin. Usually the cervix has to be "ripe," defined as one that is soft, dilated, and effaced in order for induction to be successful, but labor can also be frequently induced in a woman whose cervix is "unripe." Induction is medically indicated when an early delivery is necessary, as in severe toxemias and hypertension, Rh incompatibility, and diabetes mellitus, or for a pregnancy that is considerably prolonged past the due date, or when the membranes have ruptured prematurely and infection could occur. The use of oxytocin should rarely be necessary in a normal pregnancy and delivery, but the hormone has been used for a planned delivery, that is, induction of labor at a predetermined date for convenience or to ensure an on-time birth. The safety of purely elective induction is questionable, and the FDA in 1978 required new labeling for oxytocin, restricting its use in inductions for medical reasons and warning that the hormone should not be used merely for convenience. Presumably, oxytocin is used today in normal deliveries after premature rupture of membranes or to enhance or accelerate what could be a very prolonged labor. The drug is highly potent and difficult to control and, for that reason, should only be administered intravenously so that it can be immediately stopped if there is evidence of uterine hyperactivity or fetal distress. Overdosage can result in uterine contractions that are too strong or too frequent, and if the uterus is hypersensitive, the results could be disastrous. Fetal heart rate abnormalities during labor and a significant increase in the incidence of neonatal hyperbilirubinemia (excessive levels of serum bilirubin with jaundice after delivery) have been directly attributed to the use of oxytocin induction (Conner & Seaton, 1982). Women should never be left alone after induction; they have to be observed constantly.

Unfortunately, hormonal induction of labor can be one component of a cascading series of interventions that turn a normal birth into a full-blown medically managed delivery. For example, the membranes may be artificially ruptured to start or hasten labor, a procedure called amniotomy. When such surgical induction is unsuccessful in initiating contractions and infection becomes a concern, an intravenous oxytocin infusion may be started. The fetus then must be electronically monitored to make certain it is getting all the oxygen it needs during the strong contractions, and the monitoring is likely to be internal, with electrodes attached to the fetal scalp—a procedure that can lead to

fetal complications. Also, few women are able to cope with the intense contractions produced by induction, so the Lamaze techniques they have practiced become ineffectual. They require some kind of analgesia or perhaps epidural anesthesia that then eliminates the ability to "push," so a forceps delivery becomes necessary. Or alternatively, indications of fetal distress on the monitor are interpreted as reason for a cesarean delivery.

Contraction Stress Test

Because blood flow to the uterus and placenta is slowed during uterine contractions, the **contraction stress test (CST)**, also called the oxytocin-challenge test (OCT), is a diagnostic procedure performed to determine the fetal heart response under stress, that is, when contractions are induced by oxytocin. The nipple stimulation test is a noninvasive contraction stress test in which the nipples are stimulated manually to cause the release of the woman's own oxytocin. The test tries to duplicate the stresses of labor in order to assess the condition of the placental-fetal circulation and the fetal ability to tolerate labor. The indications for performing a CST are in those pregnancies in which a placental insufficiency is suspected—preeclampsia, intrauterine growth retardation, diabetes mellitus, a previous stillbirth—or when an irregularity of fetal heart rate has been observed. The test takes place 5–6 weeks before term, but it is also used when the baby is past due, at 42 or 44 weeks of pregnancy. Oxytocin is administered, and fetal heart rate patterns and uterine contractions are recorded. The tracings are classified as positive or negative. A positive CST is one in which the fetal heart rate shows ominous changes in association with uterine contractions and is seen as an indication for cesarean rather than vaginal delivery. The test has serious limitations as is evidenced by the large percentage of false positives (35%–60%) and occasional false negatives. Originally prescribed solely for high-risk cases, there are indications that the CST is now widely used as a general screening for a successful labor and delivery, despite some of the inherent risks of the test itself.

There has been the suggestion that the kind and quality of uterine contractions that are stimulated by oxytocin during the stress tests can themselves compromise the oxygen supply of the fetus sufficiently to produce a "positive" interpretation of the results. The result may be an unnecessary cesarean section.

Nonstress Test

A fetal nonstress test (NST) that can be performed in the doctor's office or an outpatient clinic is based on the premise that fetal well-being can be assessed by the increase in fetal heart rate in response to fetal movement. After a meal or a sweet drink, because the fetus becomes more active following glucose ingestion, a woman is placed in a semireclining position and an external monitor to record fetal heartbeat during spontaneous movements is attached. If the fetus is sleeping, pressure on the abdomen or sounds may be used to awaken it. Manipulation of the fetal head or buttocks will also stimulate movement. After 20–40 minutes of recording, the results are classified as "reactive" or "nonreactive." A reactive or normal result is a baseline heart rate between 120 and 150 beats per minute with fluctuations of 10 beats per minute or greater and accelerations of heart rate of 15 beats above the normal baseline that accompany at least two fetal movements during a 10-minute period. A nonreactive result is absence of the preceding, that is, no heart rate accelerations with fetal movements, no response of the fetus to manipulation or stimulation, or fewer than two accelerations in the 10-minute period. A nonreactive test has been correlated to a higher incidence of fetal distress during labor, fetal mortality, and intrauterine growth retardation and is seen as an indication for a contraction stress test as a follow-up procedure. The nonstress test is noninvasive, safe, and a simple way to indicate fetal well-being in high-risk pregnancies. When fetal mortality from congenital abnormality, postnatal infection, or trauma at the time of delivery are excluded, a reactive NST is almost 100% predictive of fetal survival. The major disadvantage of the NST is the high rate of false-positive (nonreactive) and false-negative (reactive) results. In one series of tests, about half of the women showed an abnormal nonreactive result, but when they were retested, most of them turned out to be falsely abnormal (Hill, 1982). Decisions about the need for immediate delivery or other interventions should never be based on a nonstress test alone.

Fetal Heart Rate Monitoring

The use of continuous or intermittent electronic fetal heart rate monitoring (EFM) during labor is a part of the routine in almost all hospitals and has replaced the stethoscope as the primary method of observing changes that would indicate fetal distress. The normal fetal heart rate is between 120 and 140 beats per minute, although it is normal for the rate to slow during contractions. Prolonged slowing with irregularity, along with several other signs that include an abnormally low fetal blood pH, is an indication that the fetus is suffering from lack of oxygen, or hypoxia. Deprivation of oxygen results in asphyxia or suffocation. All tissues are affected by a lack of oxygen, but most cells can regain their function and regenerate even if damaged. When brain cells are deprived of oxygen, however, they undergo irreversible injury, and brain damage or death can be the result. Fetal heart rate monitoring is seen as a more precise and accurate way of identifying the fetus in acute distress so that stillbirth or brain damage can be prevented.

There are two methods of monitoring fetal heart rate patterns: externally and internally. In external monitoring, two electrodes are strapped around the woman's abdomen. One picks up the uterine contractions, and the other records the fetal heart rate. The electrodes are attached to a monitoring machine that produces a paper tracing of the recordings or a nonfading oscilloscope display. Because the tracings produced by external monitoring are subject to distortions from maternal movements, fetal movements, and other kinds of vibrations, this form of recording EFM is frequently used as a screening of women when they start labor. If there is any evidence of fetal distress, the internal monitoring technique is initiated. For internal EFM, two electrodes or leads are inserted through the cervix when it is 2–3 cm dilated and after the membranes are ruptured. One spiral electrode with a maximum penetration of 2 mm punctures the presenting part of the fetus, usually the scalp, to transmit the fetal electrocardiogram. The other lead is a catheter or very thin tube placed between the fetus and the uterus to record the changes in uterine pressure during contractions. Some machines permit simultaneous recordings of the fetal heart sounds by a cardiotachometer and a Doppler cardiogram, which records the heart beat signal obtained by ultrasound. Usually, an alarm device signals a deviation from the normal pattern, and, as the displays become more complex, greater skill is needed for their interpretation. Because it as been recognized that heart rate monitoring alone cannot provide an infallible guide to fetal distress, it is recommended that fetal scalp blood samples to analyze blood gas pressures and to determine the acid-base balance become a part of the procedure.

The criteria for the interpretation of the fetal heart rate were devised by one of the monitor's developers, Dr. Edward Hon of the University of Southern California Medical School. Hon described "innocuous" EFM patterns not associated with fetal asphyxia and "ominous" patterns that may indicate distress, acidosis, and ultimately death. After a baseline heart rate has been established, a marked decrease or deceleration is of significance.

A type I, or early deceleration, is evidenced by a dip in the shape of the baseline heart rate that occurs at a very early stage of uterine contraction and recovers before the contractions end. Early deceleration is considered benign and is associated with pressure on the fetal head. In a type II, or late deceleration, the dip comes toward the end of uterine contraction and may mean that the fetus is suffering from a lack of oxygen (hypoxia) or a reduced uterine-placental exchange. The variable deceleration, so called because it occurs in no uniform relationship with the uterine contractions, is associated with umbilical cord compression.

There is no evidence that variable decelerations indicate a lack of fetal oxygen when they occur in a moderate number. But frequent and prolonged variable decelerations are associated with fetal distress. Unless the cord compression is relieved, the fetus will suffer hypoxia and begin to suffocate. There will be a disturbance in the metabolic acid-base balance of the blood, and eventually, because neurons do not recover from damage, the possibility of brain injury. Most late and variable deceleration patterns can be restored to normal by changing the woman's position to relieve pressure on the cord or by giving oxygen. A sample of fetal blood obtained by scalp puncture should be taken to measure levels of oxygen in the blood and to determine the pH (acidity). If fetal hypoxia and acidosis are confirmed and all efforts to eliminate the lack of oxygen are unsuccessful, an urgent delivery by cesarean section is performed. But because fetal heart rate patterns that appear on the printout are not easy to interpret, an "innocuous" pattern may be misread as "ominous," and a deceleration pattern may result in overreaction. Variable deceleration patterns are known to appear in 80% of fetuses at the end of the first stage of labor, but only 30%–40% of them will actually be acidotic.

The benefits of continuous fetal monitoring seem obvious. Some studies have indicated a decrease in the number of stillbirths when all patients, both high risk and normal, are monitored. Other researchers maintain that fetal asphyxia during delivery, detectable by electronic fetal monitoring and fetal scalp blood sampling, is responsible for brain injury that results in mental retardation or cerebral palsy. Such contentions provide strong arguments for the use of EFM. Given that an ounce of prevention is worth a pound of cure, it would appear that routine application of monitoring to all pregnant women would be ideal. Or would it?

In a 1984 review of the possible relationship between fetal asphyxia and subsequent brain injury, Niswander and colleagues pointed out that according to the existing literature, the cause of cerebral palsy is still not known, that a brain injury cannot be predicted by abnormal EFM patterns, most fetal asphyxia during delivery does not lead to cerebral palsy, that both EFM and scalp blood sampling have resulted in false-positive rates of 20%–80% for a diagnosis of fetal asphyxia, and that "more randomized clinical trials desperately are needed to determine the usefulness of EFM." Another review of EFM by Haverkamp and Orleans (1983) reported similar findings: no beneficial effect of EFM on neonatal deaths, neurological outcome, or subsequent health of the child. Both reviews emphatically affirmed, however, that an increased cesarean section rate is associated with EFM. Subsequent studies came to similar conclusions. A randomized controlled trial showed a reduction in seizures in newborns with the use of EFM but no reduction in cerebral palsy (Grant et al., 1989). Shy and colleagues (1990) reported that the incidence of cerebral palsy actually was greater in the group that was electronically monitored than in the group monitored by auscultation (intermittent use of an abdominal stethoscope), the other principal method of assessing the fetal heart rate. Of course there are also advocates of the current practice of routine use of EFM. Shields and Schifrin (1988) reported a high correlation between abnormal fetal heart rate patterns and subsequent neurological anomalies. In a review of deliveries over a 12-year period, Erkolla and colleagues found a 40%–50% reduction in overall fetal mortality and an 80% reduction in fetal death during labor as the use of EFM became routine (1984). Schifrin (1990) thinks that because of medical malpractice cases, EFM should be "the medicolegal standard of care for both high- and low-risk patients in the current medicolegal climate." The preponderance of research, however, appears to indicate that the anticipated benefits of universal EFM have not materialized over the past two decades. The American College of Obstetricians and Gynecologists published a 1989 revision of their guidelines for fetal surveillance during labor and concluded that auscultation (listening to the heartbeat with a stethoscope) is an equivalent to EFM during normal labor.

Recent research on EFM has continued to provide somewhat ambiguous conclusions regarding its benefits, although it has now been very widely adopted. The debate remains about EFM's overall effectiveness, as well as the merits of its application in routine pregnancies or in high-risk pregnancies only. One study (Thacker & Stroup, 2000) showed a decrease in neonatal seizures with continuous use of EFM, but no other significant benefits. Another researcher argues the EFM does not reduce fetal mortality, morbidity, or cerebral palsy rates, and furthermore points out that EFM has a very high false-positive rate—resulting in a high cesarean rate. This author also argues that the widespread use of EFM is associated with obstetricians' belief "that they should use EFM because its status as the standard of care will protect them from liability"—not because it is actually effective in reducing fetal distress (Lent, 1999).

If universally applied EFM is not really an ounce of prevention, it may still constitute considerably more than an ounce of risk. The position necessary for EFM, lying flat on the back, is the worst possible position for labor and delivery. It adversely affects comfort, lowers uterine activity, and causes maternal hypotension. In some women, blood pressure falls by more than a third, and fetal oxygen deprivation results. Furthermore, to attach the electrodes for internal monitoring, the fetal membranes have to be artificially ruptured (amniotomy) early in labor. Because the protection afforded by the amniotic fluid is now lost, the fetal head is more vulnerable. The uneven pressure on the head produced by uterine contractions results in a decreased cerebral blood flow and a decrease in fetal heart rate. Both the position and the procedure for EFM, designed to indicate fetal distress, can actually cause fetal distress.

Additional adverse effects of fetal monitoring include an increased incidence of uterine infections as a result of the leads introduced into the uterus and the fetal complication of scalp abscess and infection. For the woman in labor, the electronic fetal heart rate monitor can be disconcerting, if not frightening. It may be impossible to concentrate on Lamaze techniques while hooked up to a machine with flashing lights, heartbeat sounds, and "innocuous" decelerations to watch (Figure 11–16). The few proven benefits of EFM must thus be carefully evaluated in the

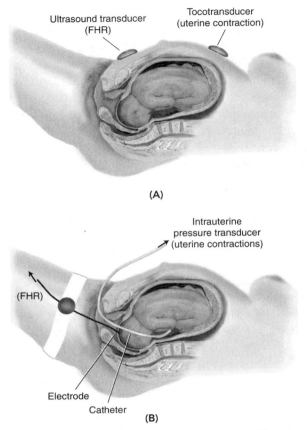

Ultrasound transducer
(FHR)

Tocotransducer
(uterine contraction)

(A)

Intrauterine
pressure transducer
(uterine contractions)

(FHR)

Electrode

Catheter

(B)

Figure 11–16 Fetal monitoring. (A) External (indirect). The top transducer picks up the uterine contraction and the lower transducer picks up the fetal heart rate and transmits the signals as electrical impulses to the monitor where they are recorded. (B) Internal (direct). The ECG electrode on the fetus's scalp picks up the fetal heart rate, and the intrauterine catheter picks up uterine contractions.

decision reached jointly by a pregnant woman and her obstetrician on whether to use continuous EFM.

Staying in the Hospital after Normal Delivery

Postpartum hospital stays lasting a week or 10 days were not uncommon during the 1950s and 1960s. But with an increased sensitivity toward what women wanted—less medicalized birth and more-natural

childbirth—the American College of Obstetricians and Gynecologists shortened the postpartum hospitalization with the intent of providing "a more family-centered birth experience." By 1970, 4 days in the hospital after delivery was average; by 1980, the average stay was 3.2 days.

As health insurance companies and managed care providers became more concerned with costs, however, the length of hospital stays for new mothers shortened. By the mid-1990s, many insurance companies would pay for only 24-hour hospital stays, and there was a public outcry over "drive-by deliveries." A number of states passed legislation mandating insurance coverage for a minimum stay, and in 1996, federal legislation, the Newborns and Mothers Health Protection Act, was passed and took effect in 1998. The law prohibits insurance companies from restricting postdelivery hospital stays after vaginal birth to fewer than 48 hours. According to a study released by the Centers for Disease Control and Prevention, 2.1 days was average by 1997 even before the federal law went into effect.

For healthy women with uncomplicated deliveries having their second or third baby, even 24-hour stays may be all they need or want, especially if the other children are well cared for at home. First-time mothers, however, with a longer labor and more questions concerning baby care and breastfeeding, may need more hospitalization than the minimum. The question of whether hospitalizing new mothers longer than the mandated minimum stay can be beneficial in terms of health of mother and infant and would be cost effective is being studied by researchers at the University of Chicago.

Cesarean Sections

In the past two decades the substitution of **cesarean section** (C-section), an abdominal and uterine incision to remove the fetus, for a vaginal delivery unquestionably has increased tremendously in association with electronic fetal heart rate monitoring, which is now considered to be routine obstetrical care.

In 1970, only 5% of deliveries nationwide were cesareans. By 1981, the number had nearly quadrupled to 18%, and a panel on cesarean childbirth convened by the National Institutes of Health expressed concern and called for a reduction of the cesarean rate. But despite efforts to counteract the trend, the C-section rate continued to climb throughout the 1980s, reaching nearly 25% by the end of the decade. It stabilized at about that rate for several years without significant change, but decreased to about 21% in 1999.

A number of explanations have been suggested for the precipitous increase. Fetal distress, as detected by means of increased electronic heart rate monitoring, is seen as a valid reason for emergency cesarean surgery, although some authorities claim that there is little need for the cesarean section rate to rise if EFM is used correctly and fetal blood sampling is done to confirm fetal distress. Currently, virtually all breech presentations are delivered by cesarean before labor starts to avoid any risk of fetal asphyxia. Although most older physicians were trained in the delivery of breech babies, many younger doctors, having been instructed during their medical education or residency to handle breech cases by cesarean, lack experience in vaginal delivery. Forceps deliveries, too, because of increased risk to the fetus, are often avoided in favor of surgical delivery.

An additional factor contributing to greater incidence of cesarean sections is the older age of first-time mothers, those who have delayed childbearing and, hence, are seen as being at greater risk for complications after age 30. The cesarean rate has increased even more for women under 30, however, and may lead to even greater numbers in the future because of the dictum, "once a cesarean, always a cesarean." Fortunately, that prevailing policy has been challenged, and vaginal delivery after cesarean section for selected cases has gained in popularity. A review of studies from 1950 to 1980 (Lavin, Stephens, Miodovnik, & Barden, 1982) presented data to show that vaginal delivery is a safe alternative to a C-section in 74.2% of women for whom there was no recurrent indication for a cesarean delivery after the first time and even a safe alternative in 33.3% of

women whose previous cesarean was the result of dystocia (fetal pelvic disproportion, difficult and prolonged labor). The national vaginal delivery after cesarean (VBAC) rates have risen from 3.4% in 1980 to 18.5% in 1989. Taffel, Placek, Moien, and Kasary (1991) explained why it is not even higher: (1) a hospital's inability to meet the American College of Obstetricians and Gynecologists guidelines for VBAC, which include 24-hour blood banking, continuous EFM, an anesthetist, and the on-site presence of a physician capable of performing a cesarean; (2) a woman's preference for a scheduled cesarean delivery or her reluctance to experience the pain of labor; (3) fear of malpractice suits by the obstetrician. A number of large studies and reviews now have conclusively demonstrated the safety of VBAC (Flamm et al., 1990; Rosen & Dickinson, 1990). The growing consensus is that the policy of routine repeat cesareans should be abandoned.

Whether the practicing obstetrician is paying attention to the scientific conclusions and recommendations is conjectural. More than one-third of all cesareans are performed on women who have had a previous cesarean, and fetal distress, dystocia, and breech presentation are the other major indications for cesarean delivery. But fear of malpractice is still the most frequently cited explanation for the increase in cesarean sections. A 1990 survey by the American College of Obstetricians and Gynecologists found that 78% of obstetricians had at least one claim of malpractice filed against them. Even though more than 50% of the cases are settled before trial, and doctors prevail in the vast majority of cases decided by trial, many obstetricians perform a C-section as a defensive measure if there is any indication of fetal distress.

Finally, that any financial considerations play a role in higher C-section incidence is lamentable, but the facts are that the number of obstetricians has increased while the birth rate has decreased, and the fee for surgical delivery is higher than that for vaginal delivery. As further evidence that monetary incentives may be a factor, a recent study reported that the rate of cesarean section delivery is highest in the Northeastern part of the United States, in hospitals larger than 500 beds, also in private for-profit hospitals, when insurance is the source of payment, and for mothers aged 35 years or over. The C-section rate is lowest in the North Central area of the country, in hospitals with fewer than 100 beds, in government nonprofit hospitals, for patients who lack health insurance, and for teenage mothers (Placek, Taffel, & Moien, 1983; Stafford, 1991). One Florida hospital, the University Medical Center in Jacksonville, saw the cesarean section rate fall from 27% to 8% with no adverse affects to mothers and babies after hospital officials put limits on the number of cesareans. Hoping to repeat that kind of success statewide, the state of Florida passed legislation applying to births paid for by Medicaid (state-funded deliveries). The law anticipated a saving of $10 million a year and required the establishment of guidelines for the performance of cesarean deliveries, mandated peer review of doctors who do them, and further required that vaginal birth be attempted before the cesarean.

There are circumstances under which a cesarean section is unquestionably necessary, but there is also evidence that the escalating trend is the result of somewhat less justifiable reasons—a situation not in the best interests of mother and babies. A C-section is significantly more risky than a vaginal delivery. The incision may be a cleverly placed "bikini cut" just above the pubic hairline, but it is nevertheless an abdominal incision. While many of the hazards of other abdominal surgery are quite minimal in a cesarean birth, the dangers of anesthesia, hemorrhage, and infection are still present. Almost half of the 4,000 cesarean patients in one 16-year study had one or more complications, some severe enough to compromise future pregnancies (Hibbard, 1976). Kettering and Wolter's 5-year study (1977) of 547 cases showed an overall complication rate of 22%, including urinary tract infections, pneumonia, and pulmonary embolism. And although cesarean sections are likely to have become safer in the past 20 years, particularly in view of all the practice physicians are getting in doing them, a conservative estimate of the risk of maternal mortality from a C-section is still that it is two to four times that of a vaginal delivery.

A decline in the infant mortality rate has paralleled the rise in the cesarean birth rate in the United States, a statistic that could encourage complacency with regard to the increased surgeries. But, as indicated previously, there is little evidence that the decrease can be attributed to the C-section rate. Similar declines in fetal mortality have taken place in Europe but without the accompanying increase in cesareans. O'Driscoll and Foley's study (1983) showed that at the National Maternity Hospital in Dublin between 1965 and 1980, the cesarean delivery rate remained virtually unchanged at about 4.5%, while perinatal mortality fell from 42.1 per 1,000 infants to 16.8 per 1,000 infants.

Because the reasons for a delivery by cesarean section have evidently expanded beyond their previous indications, the surgery is conceivably a possibility for every pregnant woman. It should, therefore, be discussed with the physician well in advance of delivery. A woman should know her doctor's criteria for emergency cesarean birth and should be aware of all the ramifications. She should get an explanation of the procedure that would be used, the anesthetic, the after-effects, whether she could have her husband or partner in the operating room with her, and whether subsequent pregnancies would also require abdominal surgery. It may be that women have little choice but to rely on the physician's professional judgment about the necessity for the operation, but they do have the right to participate in relevant decisions concerning the procedure (Figure 11–17).

Diagnostic Ultrasound in Obstetrics

Ordinary sound, the kind that sets our eardrums to vibrating, travels through space in the form of energy waves (actually compressions and rarefaction of air molecules). The number of times, or cycles per second, a wave is repeated is the frequency of sound, and the greater the frequency, the higher the pitch of the sound. Audible sound ranges in frequency from 16,000–20,000 cycles, or hertz. Ultrasound is similar to audible sound except that its frequency is

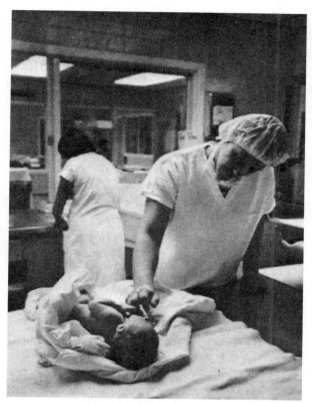

Figure 11–17 This infant was delivered by cesarean section, but the mother, under spinal anesthesia, was awake during the procedure. The father was present in the operating room; both parents were able to touch and hold the baby, and the father carried the infant to the nursery.

ultrahigh—in the millions of cycles or megahertz—and thus beyond the range of human hearing.

Ultrasound has had medical uses for many years. Ultrasound scalers are used by dentists to remove calculus from teeth, and, therapeutically, ultrasound waves of very high intensities (diathermy) produce a penetrating deep heat to treat muscle and joint injuries. But it is diagnostic ultrasound scanning for examination of all parts of the body that has become the greatest area of use in the past decade. The procedure can help detect abnormality or injury from head to toe, and ultrasound scan has joined computerized tomography (CT) and magnetic resonance imaging (MRI) scans for diagnostic visualization of internal organs.

Actually, ultrasound scanners are not particularly expensive or very sophisticated instruments and have, thus, become available to any physician; they are especially popular with obstetrician-gynecologists (OB/GYNs) for office use. The device consists of a small handheld transducer or scanner that converts electrical energy into sound waves that travel into the body of the person being scanned. As the waves, emitted in the form of pulses or short bursts, encounter blood, bones, and organs of different densities, they are reflected back toward the source. These bounced-back echoes of sound waves are shown as a pattern on a viewing screen where they can be "read" immediately or stored and photographed for interpretation. Two kinds of imaging devices are used: the static *B-scan*, which produces a two-dimensional cross section image of body structures, and the *real-time* or dynamic ultrasound scanner, which made its first appearance in 1978 and can display moving parts like a motion picture. The Doppler ultrasound scanner, used to detect fetal heart rate, employs a transducer that emits continuous, rather than pulsed, sound waves. The echoes from moving parts are then recorded as audio signals.

For OB/GYNs, ultrasound has dramatically increased diagnostic capabilities. It is a valuable adjunct to the detection of breast disease. In the pelvis, it reveals the presence or can confirm a suspected pelvic mass and can tell whether it is solid or cystic or how large it is. Ultrasonography can help detect ectopic pregnancy; show the number and extent of uterine myomas; localize an intrauterine device; evaluate the extent of inflammatory disease; and, by visualizing the follicles, determine the time of ovulation in an infertile woman who has been given ovulatory drugs. The applications to obstetrics are being perceived as even broader, and there is no doubt that when there are definite clinical indications for the use of ultrasound, the benefits are evident. A very significant advantage is that sonography, conducted at the appropriate time in gestation, can assist in accurately dating the age of the fetus. Knowledge of gestational age is important for amniocentesis, for determining whether preterm labor should be stopped with drugs or the delivery allowed to take place, and to assess the status of an alleged postdue-date fetus before induction of labor. Dating the fetus is absolutely essential when repeat cesarean is scheduled. Several studies have shown that a number of cases of respiratory distress syndrome, greater in premature infants, can be directly attributed to a too-early C-section, and that it is not unusual for babies delivered by surgical birth to weigh less than 5½ lb. Ultrasound can also confirm suspected multiple pregnancy; evaluate the reason for bleeding in pregnancy; guide the needle during amniocentesis; follow fetal growth patterns if intrauterine growth retardation is suspected; and determine fetal abnormalities, such as brain and spinal cord defects, heart, gastrointestinal, or skeletal anomalies, or kidney or bladder problems when there is suspicion that such defects may exist (Figure 11–18).

Although there are few arguments by physicians against sonography when there are definite indications for its use, it is the routine application of ultrasound during pregnancy that has become questionable. Each year there are 3.5 million pregnant women in the United States; currently, most of them receive at least one ultrasound examination. Increasingly, obstetricians have a real-time ultrasound scanner in the office that is used not only for appropriate indications in pregnancy but also defensively by the physician against malpractice and indiscriminately to "show the baby moving" to all their pregnant patients. It has even been suggested that ultrasound visualization of the unborn child enhances bonding, presumably on the shaky premise that the earlier the "adhesion," the firmer the attachment.

There are several difficulties with routine ultrasound screening of all pregnancies. Not all physicians are trained sonologists and even if they have the motivation to learn diagnostic ultrasonographic skills, they may not have the time and patient volume (Deutchman & Hahn, 1997). Acquiring the skill to use the machine appropriately and interpret the results accurately requires time and experience (and, as some have admitted, a great deal of imagination). Moreover, the potential for false-positive and false-negative diagnoses

is great. For example, at 20–24 weeks' gestation, more than one-third of all fetuses lie in abnormal positions; at term, only 3%–4% are breech presentations. Similarly, at 20–24 weeks, one out of five placentas is low lying or appears to be placenta previa; at term, the incidence of placenta previa is only 0.5%. Even gestational dating, one of the most frequent reasons for ultrasound, is subject to pitfalls. The correlation of the measurement of the fetal head, or the biparietal diameter (BPD), with fetal age is most precise only between 15 and 25 weeks of pregnancy, when the range of error is merely plus or minus 10 days. Before that time, between 8 and 13 weeks of pregnancy, a better dating can be obtained by measuring the fetal crown-rump length, which can pinpoint the age of the fetus back to the date of onset of the last menstrual period within 5 days. But beyond 26 weeks, a BPD measurement predicts fetal age with a range of error of about 3–5 weeks, with some small increase in accuracy with the addition of other measurements, such as long bone (femur) length and abdominal girth.

Another argument against routine ultrasound scans of all pregnancies is the lack of cost-effectiveness, except perhaps for the clinician who has paid for the machine and is effectively trying to recoup the cost.

By far, the major argument against prenatal diagnostic ultrasound in *all* pregnancies is the matter of safety. As yet, there is no evidence of any dangerous effects of ultrasound to humans, but neither is there sufficient evidence to state without qualification that it is completely harmless. Ultrasound energy is not ionizing radiation, like x-rays, with known harmful effects. There are, however, at least two mechanisms of action by which ultrasound could cause biological damage to tissues. One is the production of heat, but this is apparently minimal in diagnostic ultrasound equipment that has high frequency levels and low intensity (in contrast to ultrasound diathermy machines in which heat production is desirable and results from emission of low-frequency ultrasound waves with high intensity levels). A second mechanism is cavitation, a phenomenon that refers to the forma-

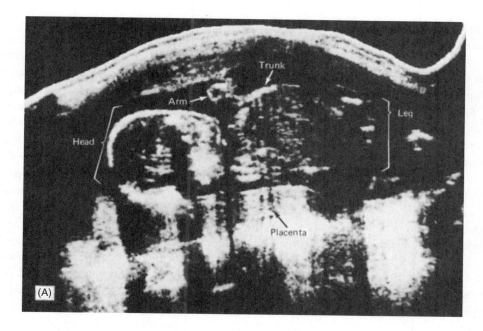

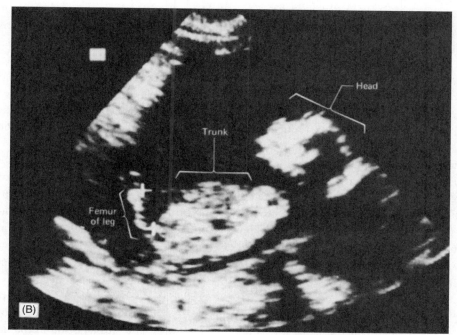

Figure 11–18 Ultrasonography of normal fetuses. (A) A B-mode scan of a 25-week fetus. The mother's abdomen is outlined at the top of the picture. (B) A real-time scan of a 15-week fetus. The distance between the two crosses at the left of the picture measures fetal femur length. The biparietal diameter of the head and the femur length are used to predict gestational age. Dating the fetus is most accurate between weeks 14 and 26. (Courtesy of Sinai-Samaritan Medical Center, Milwaukee, WI)

tion of gas microbubbles that form, increase in size, and burst in the tissue in response to sound waves. Although damage in insect eggs and some mammalian tissue has been produced by ultrasound-induced cavitation, the implications for human tissue are unknown.

One could worry about elusive effects on the developing nervous system produced by sound waves bouncing against immature neurons, for example, or be concerned about the gonads, especially in a female fetus, receiving radiation energy that could have disruptive intracellular effects. The ultrasound machines used in obstetrics are supposed to be low intensity, but the actual maximum output of an individual machine, or the attenuation effects on the intensity of focusing the ultrasound beam, is usually not known by the operator. As pointed out by Miller, Brayman, and Abramowicz (1998), there has been no discernible problem with fetal or maternal outcomes as a result of diagnostic ultrasound exposure, but data were collected using ultrasound machines whose outputs were low compared with what is now allowable and available. The power outputs have increased, and the potential for heat injury and mechanical injury, the two ways that ultrasonography is known to affect cells and tissues, necessarily has also increased.

Several long-term follow-up investigations of children exposed to prenatal diagnostic ultrasound, some initiated in the late 1970s, have produced reassuring results concerning detrimental consequences such as miscarriage, congenital abnormalities, communicative disorders, or cancer. There have been, however, several reports of a curious association between routine ultrasound screening in utero and subsequent left-handedness, especially in boys, but researchers found no evidence of impaired neurological development or attention deficit (Salvesen et al., 1993, Kieler et al., 1998).

Fetal Therapy

The two latest technological marvels are fetoscopy, or looking at the fetus through a special telescope, and fetal surgery, operating or in some way repairing the fetus before birth.

The first use of the term "fetoscopy" was in the early 1970s. It describes the technique of directly viewing the fetus within the uterus by means of a specially designed fiber-optic telescope. Although the field of vision through the fetoscope is not large, it is possible to see directly such anatomical abnormalities as limb and finger defects or facial clefts, undiagnosable by amniocentesis but suggested by an ultrasound examination. The procedure has also been used to provide fetal therapy, such as giving an intrauterine blood transfusion to a fetus with known erythroblastosis fetalis (severe Rh incompatibility)—treatment that has generally been given after birth. The other major use of fetoscopy is for fetal biopsy, the obtaining of samples of skin or blood from the umbilical cord for diagnosis of suspected various types of genetic defects that cannot be detected by analysis of amniotic fluid cells.

Fetoscopy is a risky business. There is a 5% chance of complications, including bleeding, amniotic fluid leakage, or pregnancy loss through infection or miscarriage. The technique is currently performed to confirm or exclude a genetic defect found through amniocentesis or a congenital anomaly picked up by ultrasonography. It is rarely employed as the primary prenatal diagnostic method.

The expansion of the ability to diagnose prenatally certain kinds of fetal abnormalities through such techniques as ultrasonography and fetoscopy also has expanded the possibilities of what to do with the information. Until the early 1980s, the only options after detection by amniocentesis of chromosomal or metabolic defects were abortion or continuing with the pregnancy. Not that such decisions are ever easy, but with the appropriate and necessary genetic counseling, women who choose to have amniocentesis do so with a full understanding and recognition of the potential consequences of the procedure. After it became possible to diagnose some kinds of anatomical malformations while the fetus was still in the uterus, the choices have become more complicated. If the anatomical defect is of the type that does not appear to compromise the continued growth and development of the fetus, surgical correction could be delayed until after delivery. But, in the opinion of the pediatric surgeons who have pioneered in the prenatal treatment of the fetus, there are some correctable structural anomalies that encroach on subsequent development and do not allow it to proceed normally. These defects, potential candidates for surgical correction while the fetus is still in the uterus, are diaphragmatic hernia, in which the intestines push up through a hole in the diaphragm and compress the lungs; hydronephrosis, in which a blockage in the fetal urinary tract causes a backup of urine into the abdomen; and hydrocephalus, or a buildup of cerebrospinal fluid in the fetal brain as a result of obstruction to the normal flow, which compresses the developing nerve cells and can cause severe mental retardation. In 1981, after 20 years of research in perfecting the techniques in sheep and monkeys, the first surgical correction of hydronephrosis was performed on a 24-week-old fetus by making an incision into the uterus, operating on the partially removed fetus to alleviate the urinary tract obstruction, and then replacing the fetus, who continued on to a nearly term delivery. Unfortunately, this medical milestone was a classic instance of "the surgery was successful, but the patient died." The baby died after birth because of other multiple abnormalities in addition to the kidney problem. The feasibility of prenatal treatment had been established, however, and a year later, Drs. Harrison, Filly, and Golbus of the University of California at San Francisco, who chaired a conference titled "Unborn: Management of the Fetus with a Correctable Congenital Defect," reported on experiences in fetal treatment derived from 13 centers in five countries. Correcting the obstructed urinary tract with a drainage catheter had been attempted in 21 fetuses, and placing a brain shunt to relieve hydrocephalus had been attempted in 8 fetuses, but the results were varied. Of the 21 fetuses with hydronephrosis, 10 survived with good kidney function. It has subsequently been determined that many fetuses with urinary tract blockages inexplicably undergo spontaneous correction on their own, so it is not known whether the interventionary treatment actually influenced the outcome. Of the 8 fetuses with hydrocephalus, 6 survived, but knowing for certain whether they have any evidence of retardation requires long-term follow-up. Correction of a diaphragmatic hernia is the most difficult of the procedures and at that point had not as yet been tried on a human fetus.

Several decades after the first surgery on an unborn human had been performed, it is evident that the initial expectations for prenatal treatment were overly optimistic. Surgical repair of prenatal defects currently remains a formidable technical challenge. Moreover, the ethical implications of the procedure regarding the autonomy and rights of the pregnant woman versus the interests of the fetus have become a moral quagmire to be explored by both physicians and philosophers. The future of fetal therapy is somewhat uncertain, but if past history can be relied upon, we can anticipate that medical marvels, even those in the dubious achievement category, will continue to be advanced.

BIRTHING ALTERNATIVES

Clearly, the original idea of a natural or prepared childbirth in a normal delivery, one in which the mother prepares physiologically and emotionally for a delivery that is relaxed, free of fear, and free of any medical intervention, has given way to another kind of prepared childbirth—one prepared for anything and everything, including surgery. But for many physicians, the combination of birth and technology is a major gain for women and their babies. In this view, increased technological intervention does not obstruct, but enhances, the outcome of the delivery. Moreover, lumbar epidural analgesia results in completely pain-free birth, an experience not really possible without medication. According to one director of an OB/GYN medical center, natural childbirth is a step backward, has never been scientifically substantiated to enhance the birth experience, and may even significantly contribute to maternal morbidity (Beecham, 1989).

But there are parents who are dissatisfied with the new, expanded forms of natural childbirth. To escape what they believe is unnecessary intervention in a normal physiological event, some couples prefer to avoid hospital delivery completely. As an alternative to what they perceive as the dehumanizing, impersonalizing, unnatural hospital setting, and possibly because of the expense or because they may already have had one unsatisfactory experience in the hospital, many women are choosing to deliver their babies at home. The birth attendant may be a lay midwife, trained through apprenticeship and currently sanctioned in 13 states; a registered nurse-midwife, one of the 2,000 nationwide and licensed in 47 states; or a physician. A woman who has a home birth is relaxed, in her own environment and in her own bed, in the birth position most comfortable for her, surrounded by friends, relatives, and, by family decision, older children who can see their brothers and sisters being born. Those who have experienced a home delivery are highly enthusiastic advocates; they believe that the participation of the entire family adds an invaluable psychological dimension to the birth process, which is ideal.

No matter how psychologically satisfying and advantageous home births can be, if they are medically more dangerous, they should not electively take place. Most traditional obstetricians take a dim view of home deliveries. They consider them an irresponsible risk to the lives and health of women and their babies, believing that only in a hospital setting can the necessary standards of safety be met. The American College of Gynecologists and Surgeons reported that it had compiled information from 11 states on babies born at home and had determined that the mortality rate was substantially higher. The College flatly categorized home births and the use of midwives as a form of child abuse.

Of course, the ACOG study was based on statistics on all births at home in those 11 states, including emergency deliveries and those not attended by any health professional at all. Owing to these inadequacies in data collection, it is probable that there is no real way of statistically determining the risks of home delivery or even how many out-of-hospital births are currently taking place. A more recent ACOG report claims that despite the vocal enthusiasm of home birth supporters and the publicity given to this alternative, the percentage of home deliveries has remained constant at about 1% in the United States since 1976. The Illinois-based American College of Home Obstetricians has denied that home deliveries are more dangerous than hospital deliveries when women are carefully selected for births and a professional attendant is present. They claim that when women classified as high risk are eliminated from the obstetrical population that participates in home deliveries and when a physician or a licensed midwife is present, home birth is just as safe as hospital birth, and probably safer.

Other Options

Obviously, a birth at home, attended by a midwife, is not for every woman even if she has a normal labor and delivery. With the uneasy sense that even low-risk or no-risk deliveries could suddenly become high-risk ones, some women would feel very uncomfortable unless they were in a hospital setting. Some women believe that they should have every advantage that modern medicine with its sophisticated technology can provide. There are some women, although the attitude is becoming more rare, who have little desire to participate or have more control in the childbirth process, and who are willing to have as much anesthesia as is necessary to have minimum discomfort, as long as it does not harm the baby.

For those who are dissatisfied with orthodox hospital-based obstetrics, but who may have some misgivings about delivering at home, some other options are beginning to be available. Not all obstetricians and hospitals have remained indifferent and inflexible to the not-unreasonable requests that women have made. Some hospitals have changed to provide, if not the complete warmth and comfort of the home, at least a more humane, personalized, family-centered kind of maternity care. Obstetric departments have made efforts to change existing procedures and staff attitudes. Routine preparations for delivery that were standard for so long, such as shaving the pubic area and giving enemas, have been eliminated. Fetal monitoring may be performed only when required, and only intermittently even then. Labor rooms have been converted to "birthing rooms," pleasant and bedroomlike, where the woman, supported by her husband, partner, close friend, or relative, can labor, deliver, and recover without being transferred to a delivery room. When the baby is born, it is placed on the mother's abdomen, and the parents can touch and handle the infant. Several hours can elapse before the family transfers to the postpartum area, rooms that contain rocking chairs and other homey comforts. There is no rigid schedule to which mother and infant must conform, and for the most part, the woman may choose the type of care for herself and the baby that she wants, getting the advice of the staff when necessary.

Of course, pretty paint and rocking chairs are no guarantee that the traditional hospital and doctor obstetrical practices have really undergone any change to make them a more positive experience. But it is possible in some hospitals to use a birthing chair or to give birth while squatting, avoid episiotomy, keep physician interventions to a minimum, and have a midwife delivery. Even warm-water immersion in a birthing pool during labor and delivery, a method familiar in Europe, has become an accepted alternative at some facilities, most of them freestanding birthing centers. There are a few innovative hospitals that allow and encourage sibling visitation after delivery, to see Mama and to touch and hold the baby.

There are some obstetricians who are willing to stand by and talk the prepared father through the delivery in much the same way that they would educate a first-year resident. And there are some doctors, although it may take some shopping around and word of mouth to find them, who are content to be birth attendants, not managers; who can be trusted to do, within the standards of medical safety, what the woman thinks is right for her; who see themselves not as central or authoritarian in the birth process, but as secondary to the main characters in the event, the mother and the child.

Right now, there are still too few alternatives to what some women and health professionals see as the highly interfering, invasive, technical hospital deliveries, and those alternatives are found only in certain areas of the country. As more women make their demands known, however, more doctors and hospitals may change their current all-risk pathological approach to a normal and individualized view of childbirth. Perhaps the change in many instances will not be out of any sense of real commitment. But the economic pinch that results from the low birth rate and the renewed interest in midwifery and home delivery are likely to mandate a different concept of obstetrical care that considers the needs of the 90% of women who have normal deliveries.

*B*REASTFEEDING

For several generations, breastfeeding an infant was seen as too restricting, inconvenient, lower class, and suitable only for poor and uneducated women. New mothers who may have wanted to try it received very little instruction (the ability to nurse successfully does not always come naturally) and even less encouragement. It was assumed that few women wanted to breastfeed, and so they virtually routinely received an injection to suppress lactation. Along with the movement toward natural birth and with the recognition of its value for the newborn, however, there was a resurgence of interest in breastfeeding (Figure 11–19). Fewer than 25% of women were breastfeeding their babies in 1971; currently, 60% of women leave the hospital breastfeeding, but only 21.6% are still nursing at 6 months. This falls far short of the goal established by the U.S. Surgeon General's office in 1990—for 75% of American women to be breastfeeding by the year 2000. And according to a 1999 report by the Centers for Disease Control and Prevention, among low-income children in federally funded programs in 42 states, breastfeeding rates were 46%, and only 30% of black children were breastfed.

Although breastfeeding has increased in the past decade in industrialized nations, it has declined in

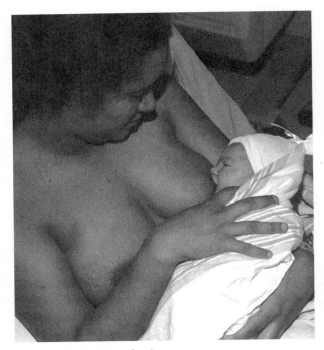

Figure 11–19 Breastfeeding.

Third World countries with tragic public health effects. The illness of 10 million infants and the death of possibly a million babies a year have been attributed to inadequate formula feeding. There is nothing wrong with infant formula when there is money to purchase enough of it, sufficient education to prepare it properly, and appropriate hygiene to keep in uncontaminated. But when overdiluted formula is prepared from filthy water supplies, the result is starvation and sickness in babies. The aggressive marketing techniques of certain infant formula manufacturers in underdeveloped countries have generated enormous controversy, and some critics have called for a consumer boycott of all the products of one major infant formula company.

The American Academy of Pediatrics advocates breastfeeding for all full-term newborns, maintaining that ideally, breast milk should be the sole nutrient for the first 4–6 months of life. All available scientific evidence, and there have been scores of papers published in the past decade, overwhelmingly attests to the superiority of human milk for human babies. Cow's milk is undoubtedly ideal for calves, but as more is becoming known about the biochemical properties of human milk, it is becoming more evident that nature has designed it to be particularly suitable for the human species. Formulas made from cow's milk have been modified to make them more like breast milk, but even when cow's milk is made more "human," there are still some significant differences.

In comparison with cow's milk proteins, human milk proteins are completely digestible, provide all the essential amino acids, and are generally of greater biological value than the proteins in formula. Moreover, the proteins in cow's milk can cause allergic reactions, and circulating antibodies have been found in a majority of formula-fed babies even when they show no evidence of allergy, such as asthma, eczema, and diarrhea. Instances of unexplained crib deaths have been linked to anaphylactic, or very severe, allergic reactions to cow's milk.

The fat content in human milk is more digestible and allows greater uptake of fat-soluble vitamins A and D from the intestine. Human milk is unique in containing lactose as the principal carbohydrate. Lactose is the least sweet of sugars and is less likely to program the child for a future sweet tooth. The mineral content of human milk is less than that of cow's milk, which is not a disadvantage because the infant's kidneys are not equipped to handle large loads of salt. Breast milk is always ready, at the right temperature, does not have to be pasteurized, and is not subject to the bacterial contamination highly probable in formulas. Breastfed newborns have a greater resistance to gastrointestinal disorders and to respiratory and ear infections than do formula-fed infants. The mechanisms that underlie the protective functions of human milk that result in the lowered infection rate are not completely known. Most antibodies to infectious diseases, such as scarlet fever, measles, and diphtheria, are transferable from the mother to the infant across the placenta before birth. How and to what extent the large molecule maternal antibodies contained in breast milk are able to survive digestion and pass through the infant's intestinal cells to get into the bloodstream to immunize the baby has not been determined. It is possible that maternal antibodies may function to inactivate organisms in the baby's intestinal tract so that they cannot cause infection. Whatever the mechanism, the anti-infective properties of human milk exist and are a major advantage that cannot be matched by cow's milk. The level of immune factors is highest in colostrum and milk produced in the first weeks of nursing.

Breastfed babies are not likely to be as fat as formula-fed babies. The correlation between early obesity and overweight adults has not been proved, but there is some evidence that the seeds may be laid in infancy and childhood.

For the past five decades, researchers have attempted to measure the effects of breastfeeding on later intelligence, learning abilities, activity levels, personality, and adjustment of infants, but results have been inconclusive. Some data indicate an apparent behavioral advantage from breastfeeding, but there is equal evidence to indicate that no overall benefit exists. For many women, however, the successful breastfeeding of their babies provides a secure, gratifying, and satisfying experience that contributes to the quality of mother–child interaction. There are some definite maternal physical benefits as well. The uterus involutes to its normal size more easily and rapidly, and there are fewer problems with uterine infection. It is much easier to reattain prepregnancy weight if a woman is nursing; the calories expended to produce milk help in shedding unwanted pounds. Nursing mothers are relatively infertile, since menstruation and ovulation return more slowly in women who lactate. The frequency and amount of nursing prolongs the amenorrhea, but it is also affected by body weight, being of shorter duration in heavier women. In many parts of the world where women are poorly nourished, breastfeeding is thus able to prevent a significant number of pregnancies. Half of the women who breastfeed are able to conceive within the first 6 months postpartum, while the other half seem to be protected, but because there is no way of knowing in which 50% a woman may fall, lactation is no substitute for contraception.

The only possible health disadvantages to breastfeeding occur when breast milk contains substances that may adversely affect the infant. Although the levels of some substances smoked, drunk, breathed, or otherwise ingested by a woman may appear in breast milk in minuscule quantities, generally speaking, whatever she has in her bloodstream can get to the infant through the milk supply. The baby, smaller in size and with immature kidneys and liver, is not as well able to handle or detoxify substances that are harmless to an adult. Some drugs are definitely known to cause health problems (Table 11–3); others, such as alcohol and caffeine, are considered safe in moderate amounts, but large quantities could result in responses in babies similar to those in adults. Few mothers would want the possible nervousness, wakefulness, and irritability from excessive caffeine intake to be present in their infants. A lactating woman, like a pregnant woman, has to be careful of what she takes into her body.

One source of contamination of mother's milk over which women have little or no control is environmental pollutants. Pesticides, heavy metals, antibiotics, and all sorts of organic industrial wastes eventually find their way into food, and a woman has to eat. Industrial pollutants, such as polybrominated biphenyls (PBBs), polychlorinated biphenyls (PCBs), pentachlorophenols (PCPs), and dioxins, a contaminant of PCPs, are so ubiquitous in the food and water supply that it is impossible to avoid them no matter where one resides, although higher levels have been found in breast milk from women who regularly consume fish from contaminated waters. These organic toxic chemicals are stored in the body fat, resist breakdown by usual body detoxifying enzymes, and are excreted only through breast milk. That means that nursing mothers would have lower body levels of contaminants than other people, but their babies are exposed—a no-win situation. The role of such environmental contaminants in

TABLE 11–3 Some Maternal Drugs Known to Pose Potential Health Problems for the Breastfeeding Infant[a]

Drug	Possible Symptoms or Effects on Infant
Anticoagulant	
Ethyl biscoumacetate	Bleeding problems
Phenindione	Bleeding problems
Anticonvulsant	
Mysoline	Drowsiness
Phenobarbital	Hypnotic effect
Phenytoin (diphenyl-hydantoin)	Methemoglobinemia
Carbamazepine	Long-term effect unknown
Antidepressant	
Lithium	Loss of muscle tone, lowered body temperature, bluish skin
Antihypertension	
Reserpine	Nasal congestion, weight loss, bluish skin
Antimetabolite	
Cyclophosphamide	Bone marrow depression
Methotrexate	Bone marrow depression
Antimicrobial	
Chloramphenicol (Chloromycetin)	Refusal to nurse, sleepiness, vomiting
Metronidazole (Flagyl)	Causes cancer in test animals
Nalidixic acid	Hemolytic anemia
Nitrofurantoin[b]	
Sulfonamides[b]	Hemolytic anemia
Antithyroid	
Iodide	Altered thyroid synthesis and release
Thiouracil	Altered thyroid synthesis and release
Radioactive iodine	Cancer, loss of thyroid activity
Autonomic drugs	
Atropine	Constipation
Laxative	
Anthraquinone derivatives: (Danthron, Dialose Plus, Dorbane, Dorbantyl, Doxidan, Peri-Colace)	Bowel problems

(continues)

TABLE 11–3 *(continued)*

Drug	Possible Symptoms or Effects on Infant
Aloe	Bowel problems
Calomel	Bowel problems
Cascara	Bowel problems
Narcotic	
Heroin	Addiction
Methadone	One death recorded
Oral contraceptives	Gynecomastia, long-term effects unknown
Painkiller	
Propoxyphene (Darvon)	Addiction
Sedative	
Barbiturates	Drowsiness
Bromides	Drowsiness
Chloral hydrate	Drowsiness
Diazepam (Valium)	Lethargy, jaundice, weight loss
Steroid	
Prednisone	Poor growth
Prednisolone	Poor growth
Miscellaneous	
Dihydrotachysterol	Renal calcification
Ergot alkaloids	Ergotism
Gold thioglucose	Rash, hepatitis, hematologic alteration

Source: From *Human Milk and Infant Formula,* by V. S. Packard, 1982, New York: Academic Press. Used with permission.

[a]For a more complete list of drugs and chemicals that can be transferred into human milk, see American Academy of Pediatrics. (1994). The transfer of drugs and other chemicals into human milk. *Pediatrics, 93*(1), 137–150.

[b]This drug causes problems mainly in infants suffering the inherited enzyme deficiency glucose-6-phosphate dehydrogenase.

producing harmful effects in children is unknown, but that is primarily because it is virtually unstudied. Lactating women have been advised to have their breast milk analyzed for PCBs and PBBs if they work on a farm, have frequently eaten large quantities of fish from contaminated waters such as Lake Michigan and Lake Superior, or are otherwise exposed occupationally. Some states provide free testing; private laboratories may charge $60 and up for the analysis. Although some advisory "tolerance" levels for the contaminants in milk have been adopted, the results of breast milk analysis actually mean little because the long-term effects of "high," "moderate," or "low" levels of the chemicals, if any, are still unknown. Besides, it can take weeks before the test analysis is returned, and what is a woman to do in the meantime? Lactation cannot be turned off and on again like a faucet. Breast milk analysis would appear to be of very limited value.

No woman should avoid breastfeeding solely because our food and water supply contains toxic hydrocarbons. Cow's milk has them, too, although in lesser amounts. It does make sense to avoid the only major dietary source of PCBs—sport fish from the Great Lakes—and to avoid making a concerted effort to lose a lot of weight quickly, which could release the chemicals suddenly from their storage site in fat tissue. What we all can and must do is persist in our efforts to have these potential poisons, as well as all other pollutants, eliminated from our environment.

All in all, there are economic, biochemical, psychological, and physiological advantages to breastfeeding, and a woman could at least try it. It is important to remember, however, that the emotional benefits are highly subjective and that the physiological benefits are based on statistics. The decreased incidence of infection, disease, and allergy for babies fed with breast milk is not necessarily going to be evident for any individual infant on human milk or on formula. It should be remembered that much of the back-to-breastfeeding movement has been promoted by white, affluent, educated, and for the most part, nonworking mothers who are in a position to nurse their infants for the better part of a year. Continuing to nurse while going back to work is an enormous challenge. Mothers have to express their milk with a breast pump before they leave or use one at the workplace and may have to get the milk back home to the baby during the day. And even if women are not working outside the home, they frequently face public humiliation and harassment when attempting to breastfeed in public even though public breastfeeding has always been legal. Twenty states have passed legislation protecting a woman's right to breastfeed in public and indicating that breastfeeding is not considered a lewd or indecent act. But women who, by choice or necessity, are unable to breastfeed—if, for example, they have to return to work right after delivery, or have a medical problem that requires taking large doses of drugs—should never feel that they have shortchanged their babies by bottle-feeding. Human milk is ideal for human infants, but if a baby must be fed with formula, there are commercial preparations that have been modified until they resemble human milk as closely as possible. Certainly a woman who chooses to or has to formula-feed her infant can develop a mother–child relationship that is just as close as if she breastfed.

Many women who are highly motivated to breastfeed can still have trouble with lactation unless they get the instruction, skill, and encouragement necessary for success. If they have initial difficulty in getting the baby started, or run into a problem with engorged breasts, leaking, or sore nipples, they may give up too easily and switch to formula. An inability to breastfeed is sometimes the result of anxiety and stress, which inhibit the milk-ejection reflex. Ordinarily, the stimulus of sucking at the breast causes the release of oxytocin, which results in the contraction of the alveoli of the glands and the ejection or "letting down" of the milk into the milk ducts. Oxytocin, released from the neurohypophysis, is under direct neural control. Anxiety about breastfeeding, especially when accompanied by inadequate instruction and lack of encouragement, can readily inhibit the ejection reflex.

The support and information that many nursing mothers need can be provided by the La Leche League. Founded in 1956 by two women who had the idea of forming an organization where nursing mothers would inform and advise other nursing mothers, the League today has grown to more than 3,000 chapters throughout the world. In its manual, *The Womanly Art of Breastfeeding,* interested women can obtain the practical knowledge that is usually unavailable elsewhere. If there is a chapter in the area, La Leche League is listed in the telephone directory, and group meetings and individual counseling are provided.

Induced Lactation

Induced lactation, also called relactation, is the ability to produce breast milk in response to sucking stimulation when there has been no preceding pregnancy. Elizabeth Hormann (1977), a pioneer of the relactation movement, reported the results of a survey of 65 women who wanted to provide the psychological and physiological benefits of breastfeeding to their adopted babies. Eighteen of the women had never been pregnant, seven had been pregnant but had not nursed, and forty had been pregnant and had lactated before. The majority of infants received by the adoptive mothers were under 1 month of age, but some of them were already receiving some type of solid food as well as formula when they arrived. All 65 women were successful in producing milk, although all but one had to supplement with formula because in most of the women the mammary gland production was not enough to fully sustain the baby. The act of nursing was evidently seen as having as much or greater value as the nourishment derived from breastfeeding (http://medicalreporter.health.org).

Producing breast milk without a pregnancy seems amazing to most people. It does require an inordinate amount of preparation and motivation but is not that mysterious physiologically. It is known that it is possible to induce lactation in nonpregnant farm animals by milking. In humans, it has been shown that when the breasts and nipples are manually stimulated, or sometimes as a result of chest injury, surgery, or shingles (herpes zoster), lactation can result. Sensory nerve impulses from the breasts are relayed to the spinal cord and then up to the hypothalamus of the brain. The prolactin-inhibiting factor of the hypothalamus that ordinarily keeps lactation from occurring is suppressed, and the prolactin from the anterior pituitary gland can then be released to result in milk synthesis and production by the alveoli of the mammary glands

(Chapter 7). Women who want to nurse adopted babies require a month or more of preparation through breast stimulation to increase serum prolactin levels, which can be accomplished by self-stimulation or regular use of a breast pump. Waterson (1995) suggests that the baby be put to the breast frequently and that a supply line or "Lact-aid," which supplies formula milk through a feeding tube, be placed alongside the nipple to supplement the breast milk. The baby suckles at the breast and also obtains nutrition through the tube. The tube is attached to a pack on the chest so the baby does not become accustomed to a bottle. As the woman's own supply builds up, the supplementation can gradually be reduced.

Although nursing an adopted baby took a great deal of preparation beforehand and a great deal of time since a large part of each day must be spent in nursing, the women in Hormann's study indicated that they felt it was well worth the trouble.

As a further indication that with enough motivation, hormones, and help, *anyone* can nurse a baby, a Brooklyn doctor reported that his treatment of a 40-year-old male enabled that man to successfully breastfeed his infant daughter. The unidentified individual, a married transvestite who shared everything with his wife, including clothing and makeup, wanted to share equally in the raising of their child. The man received estrogen to develop his breasts before the birth of the baby, and after the birth, the physician administered oxytocin to result in prolactin secretion. The man was then able to split the breastfeeding duties with his wife for 3 months. But probably not in public.

ℛEFERENCES

Aladjem, S. (Ed.). (1980). *Obstetrical practice.* St. Louis, MO: C. V. Mosby.

American College of Obstetricians and Gynecologists. (1989). *Intrapartum fetal heart rate monitoring.* (ACOG Technical Bulletin No. 132). Washington, D.C.

Aselton, P. J., & Jick, H. (1983). Additional follow-up of congenital limb disorders in relation to Bendectin use. *Journal of the American Medical Association, 250,* 33–34.

Barker, D. J. (1997). Fetal nutrition and cardiovascular disease in later life. *British Medical Bulletin, 53*(1), 96–108.

Beecham, C. T. (1989). Natural childbirth—A step backward? *Female Patient, 14,* 37–43.

Beernink, F. J., & Ericsson, R. J. (1982). Male sex preselection through sperm isolation. *Fertility and Sterility, 38*(4), 493–496.

Chasnoff, I. J., Griffith, D. R., McGregor, S., et al. (1989). Temporal patterns of cocaine use in pregnancy. Perinatal outcome. *Journal of the American Medical Association, 261*(12), 1741–1744.

Cohen, E. N., Gift, H. C., Brown, B. W., et al. (1980). Occupational disease in dentistry and chronic exposure to trace anesthetic gases. *Journal of the American Dental Association, 101,* 21–31.

Conner, B. H., & Seaton, P. G. (1982). Birth weight and use of oxytocin and analgesic agents in labour in relation to neonatal jaundice. *Medical Journal of Australia, 2,* 466–469.

De Chateau, P. (1980). Parent–neonate interaction and its long-term effects. In E. G. Simmel (Ed.), *Early experience and early behavior.* New York: Academic Press.

Deutchman, M. E., & Hahn, R. (1997). Office procedures. Obstetric ultrasonography. *Primary Care, 24*(2), 407–431.

Dermer, A., & Montgomery, A. (1997). Breastfeeding: Good for babies, mothers, and the planet. *Medical Reporter.* Retrieved from the World Wide Web: http://medicalreporter.health.org.

Dunnihoo, D. R. (1990). *Fundamentals of gynecology & obstetrics* (p. 445). Philadelphia: J. B. Lippincott.

Erkolla, R., Gronroos, M., Punnonen, R., et al. (1984). Analysis of intrapartum fetal deaths: Their decline with increasing electronic fetal monitoring. *Acta Obstetrica et Gynaecologica Scandinavica, 63,* 459.

Eskanazi, B., & Bracken, M. B. (1982). Bendectin (Debendox) as a risk factor for pyloric stenosis. *American Journal of Obstetrics and Gynecology, 144*(8), 919–924.

Eskanazi, B., Fenster, L., & Sidney, S. (1991). A multivariate analysis of risk factors for preeclampsia. *Journal of the American Medical Association, 266*(2), 237–241.

Ettner, F. M. (1977). Hospital technology breeds pathology. *Women and Health, 2*(2), 17–22.

Fabro, S., & Sieber, S. M. (1969). Caffeine and nicotine penetrate the pre-implantation blastocyst. *Nature, 223*(204): 410–411.

Flamm, B. L., Newman, L. A., Thomas, S. J., et al. (1990). Vaginal birth after cesarean delivery: Results of a 5-year multicenter collaborative study. *Obstetrics and Gynecology, 76*(5), 750–754.

Forfar, J., & Nelson, M. M. (1973). Epidemiology of drugs taken by pregnant women: Drugs that may affect the fetus

adversely. *Clinical Pharmacologies and Therapeutics, 14,* 632.

Fowler, S. (1991, June 23). Coach makes birth easier and reduces caesarean rate. *Chicago Tribune.*

Gardner, M. J., Snee, M. P., Hall, A. J., et al. (1990). Results of case-control study of leukemia and lymphoma among young people near Sellafield nuclear plant in West Cumbria. *British Medical Journal, 300*(6722), 423–429.

Golding, J., Vivian, S., & Baldwin, J. A. (1983). Maternal antinauseants and clefts of lip and palate. *Human Toxicology, 2,* 63–73.

Grant, A., O'Brien, N., Joy, M., et al. (1989). Cerebral palsy among children born during the Dublin randomized trial of intrapartum monitoring. *Lancet, ii,* 1233–1236.

Grantham-McGregor, S. M., & Fernald, L. C. (1997). Nutritional deficiencies and subsequent effects on mental and behavioral development in children. *Southeast Asian Journal of Tropical Medicine and Public Health, 28* (Suppl. 2), 50–68.

Haire, D. (1977). *The cultural warping of childbirth.* Seattle: International Childbirth Education Association (rev.).

Harrison, M. R., Filly, R. A., Golbus, M. S., et al. (1982). Fetal treatment. *New England Journal of Medicine, 307*(26), 1651–1652.

Haverkamp, A. D., & Orleans, M. (1983). An assessment of electronic fetal monitoring. *Women's Health, 7*(3), 115–133.

Hibbard, L. T. (1976). Changing trends in cesarean section. *American Journal of Obstetrics and Gynecology, 125,* 798–804.

Hill, R. M., Craig, J. P., & Chaney, M. D. (1977). Utilization of over-the-counter drugs during pregnancy. *Clinical Obstetrics and Gynecology, 20*(2), 381–394.

Hill, W. C. (1982). How to interpret antepartum monitoring, *Female Patient, 7*(1), 32/1–32/13.

Hormann, E. (1977). Breast feeding the adopted baby. *Birth and the Family Journal, 4*(4), 65–173.

Imperiale, T. F., & Petrulis, A. S. (1991). A meta-analysis of low-dose aspirin for the prevention of pregnancy-induced hypertensive disease. *Journal of the American Medical Association, 266*(2), 260–264.

John, E. M., Savitz, D. A., & Sandler, D. P. (1991). Prenatal exposure to parents' smoking and childhood cancer. *American Journal of Epidemiology, 133*(2), 123–132.

Kennell, J., Klaus, M., McGrath, S., et al. (1991). Continuous emotional support during labor in a US hospital. *Journal of the American Medical Association, 265*(17), 2197–2201.

Kettering, H. S., & Wolter, D. F. (1977). Complications of cesarean section. Transactions of the Pacific Coast Obstetrical and Gynecological Society, 44, 29–34.

Kieler, H., Axellson, O., Haglund, B., et al. (1998). Routine ultrasound screening in pregnancy and the children's subsequent handedness. *Early Human Development, 50*(2), 233–245.

King, J. C., & Fabro, S. (1982). Alcohol consumption and cigarette smoking: Effect on pregnancy. *Clinical Obstetrics and Gynecology, 26*(2), 437–448.

Klaus, M., & Kennell, J. (1983). Parent to infant bonding: Setting the record straight. *Journal of Pediatrics, 102*(4), 575–576.

Klaus, M., & Kennell, J. H. (1976). *Maternal-infant bonding*. St. Louis, MO: C. V. Mosby.

Klaus, M., Jerauld, R., & Kreger, N. (1972). Maternal attachment. *New England Journal of Medicine, 286*(9), 460–463.

Lavin, J. P., Stephens, R. F., Miodovnik, M., & Barden, T. P. (1982). Vaginal delivery in patients with a prior cesarean section. *Obstetrics and Gynecology, 59*(2), 135–148.

Leboyer, F. (1975). *Birth without violence*. New York: Knopf.

Lent, M. (1999). The medical and legal risks of the electronic fetal monitor. *Stanford Law Review, 51*(4), 807–837.

Linn, S., Schoenbaum, S. C., Monson, R. R., et al. (1982). No association between coffee consumption and adverse outcomes of pregnancy. *New England Journal of Medicine, 306*(3), 141–145.

Michaelis, J., Michaelis, H., Gluck, E., & Koller, S. (1983). Prospective study of suspected associations between certain drugs administered during early pregnancy and congenital malformations. *Teratology, 27*, 57–64.

Miller, M. W., Brayman, A. A., & Abramowicz, J. S. (1998). Obstetric ultrasonography: A biophysical consideration of patient safety—The "rules" have changed. *American Journal of Obstetrics and Gynecology, 179*(1), 241–254.

Milunsky, A., Jick, H., Jick, S., et al. (1989). Multivitamin/folic acid supplementation in early pregnancy reduces the prevalence of neural tube defects. *Journal of the American Medical Association, 262*(20), 2847–2852.

Mitchell, A. A., Schwingl, P. J., Rosenberg, L., et al. (1983). Birth defects in relation to Bendectin use in pregnancy. *American Journal of Obstetrics and Gynecology, 147*(7), 737–742.

Mulinare, J., Cordereo, J. F., Erickson, J. D., & Berry, R. J. (1988). Periconceptional use of multivitamins and the occurrence of neural tube defects. *Journal of the American Medical Association, 260*(21), 3141–3145.

Niebyl, J. R. (1990). Teratology and drugs in pregnancy and lactation. In J. R. Scott, et al. (Eds.), *Danforth's obstetrics and gynecology* (6th ed.). Boston: J. B. Lippincott.

Niswander, K. (1976). *Obstetrics: Essentials of clinical practice* (p. 267). Boston: Little, Brown.

Niswander, K., Henson, G., Elbourne, D., et al. (1984). Adverse outcome of pregnancy and the quality of obstetric care. *Lancet, ii*, 827–831.

O'Driscoll, K., & Foley, M. (1983). Correction of decrease in perinatal mortality and increase in cesarean section rates. *Obstetrics and Gynecology, 61*(1), 1–5.

Page, E. W., Villee, C. A., & Villee, D. B. (1976). *Human reproduction* (2nd ed.). Philadelphia: W. B. Saunders.

Pitkin, R. M. (1977). Diet advice for the expectant mother. *Female Patient, 2*(1), 38–41.

Pitkin, R. M. (1976). Nutritional support in obstetrics and gynecology. *Clinical Obstetrics and Gynecology, 19*(3), 489–513.

Placek, P. J., Taffel, S., & Moien, M. (1983). Cesarean section delivery rates: United States, 1981. *American Journal of Public Health, 73*(8), 861–862.

Ralt, D., Goldenberg, M., Fetterolf, P., et al. (1991). Sperm attraction to a follicular factor(s) correlates with human egg fertilizability. *Proceedings of the National Academy of Sciences, 88*, 2840–2844.

Rosen, M. G., & Dickinson, J. C. (1990). Vaginal birth after cesarean: A meta-analysis of indicators for success. *Obstetrics and Gynecology, 76*(5), 865–869.

Rosenberg, L., Mitchell, A. A., Shapiro, S., & Slone, D. (1982). Selected birth defects in relation to caffeine-containing beverages. *Journal of the American Medical Association, 247*, 1429–1432.

Ross, P. (1989, August 31). Drug did not cause birth defects, court says. *The New York Times*.

Rossett, H., Quellette, E. M., Weiner, L., & Owens, E. (1978). Therapy of heavy drinking during pregnancy. *Obstetrics and Gynecology, 51*(1), 41–46.

Russell, M. (1991). Clinical implications of recent research on the fetal alcohol syndrome. *Bulletin of the New York Academy of Medicine, 67*(3), 207–222.

Salvesen, K. A., Vatten, L. J., Eik-Nes, S. H., et al. (1993). Routine ultrasonography in utero and subsequent handedness and neurological development. *British Medical Journal, 307*(6897), 159–164.

Schieve, L. A., Coqswell, M. E., & Scanlon, K. S. (1998, June). Trends in pregnancy weight gain within and outside ranges recommended by the Institute of Medicine in a WIC population. *Maternal and Child Health Journal, 2*(2), 111–116.

Schifrin, B. S. (1990). Electronic fetal monitoring and malpractice. *Female Patient, 15*, 79–82.

Seidman, D. S., Ever-Hadani, P., & Gale, R. (1990). Effect of maternal smoking and age on congenital anomalies. *Obstetrics and Gynecology, 76*(6), 1046–1049.

Shields, J. R., & Schifrin, B. S. (1988). Perinatal antecedents of cerebral palsy. *Obstetrics and Gynecology, 71*, 899.

Shy, K., Luthy, D., Bennett, F., et al. (1990). Effects of electronic fetal-heart-rate monitoring, as compared with periodic auscultation, on the neurologic development of premature infants. *New England Journal of Medicine, 322,* 588–593.

Stafford, R. S. (1991). The impact of nonclinical factors on repeat cesarean section. *Journal of the American Medical Association, 265*(1), 59–63.

Streissguth, A. P., Aase, J. M., Clarren, S. K., et al. (1991). Fetal alcohol syndrome in adolescents and adults. *Journal of the American Medical Association, 265*(15), 1961–1967.

Streissguth, A. P., Barr, H. M., & Sampson, P. D. (1990). Moderate prenatal alcohol exposure: Effects on child IQ and learning problems at age 7 and 1/2 years. *Alcoholism, 14*(5), 662–669.

Taffel, S. M., Placek, P. J., Moien, M., & Kasary, C. L. (1991). 1989 U.S. cesarean section rate steadies—VBAC rate rises to nearly one in five. *Birth, 18*(2), 73–77.

Thacker, S. B., & Stroup, D. F. (2000). Continuous electronic heart rate monitoring for fetal assessment during labor. *Cochrane Database Systems Review 2000, 2,* CD 000063.

Unterman, R. R., Posner, N. A., & Williams, K. N. (1990). Postpartum depressive disorders: Changing trends. *Birth, 17*(3), 131–137.

Waterson, T. (1995). Any questions. *British Medical Journal, 310*(6982), 780–781.

Woodward, L., Brackbill, Y., McManus, K., et al. (1982). Exposure to drugs with possible adverse effects during pregnancy and birth. *Birth, 9*(3), 165–171.

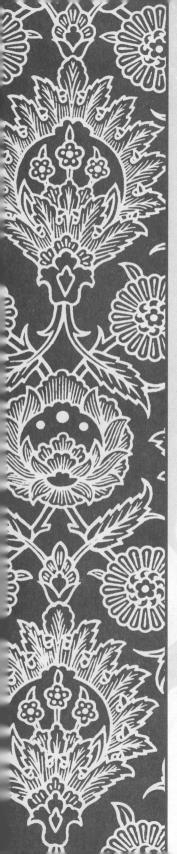

PROBLEMS OF INFERTILITY

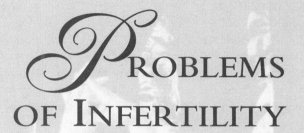

KEY TERMS

Anovulation

Gamete intrafallopian
transfer (GIFT)

Infertility

Intercytoplasmic sperm
injection

In vitro fertilization

Oligoovulation

Superovulation

Zygote intrafallopian
transfer (ZIFT)

Fertility or fecundity is the ability to conceive and produce a child. Most people take this capacity for granted. If anything, they are concerned about too much fertility, and this is a reasonable assumption. It is easy to make a baby.

Culturally, people have long regarded their own capability for baby making as a measure of power in this world; it is a rare man who doubts his capacity to father a child, and just as rare is the adult woman who would ignore the possibility of pregnancy by thinking herself infertile. From menarche to menopause, a 40-year span, women live with the ever-present possibility of pregnancy. And it is obvious that there is much more effort and anxiety expended in trying to avoid conception than in trying to conceive. Parenthood is not necessarily being ruled out, but it is probably being delayed until the time is right. "Not now," says the single woman, "who needs the hassle?" "Not now," say the newly married couple, "we're not ready to make that commitment," or "we can't afford it yet," or "we want to get ahead professionally first," or "we want to buy a house," "travel," "get to know each other better first." For some couples who want to replace "not now" with "now," however, an unsuspected and frustrating situation may emerge. Fertility cannot always be taken for granted. Until a man and a woman actually achieve a successful pregnancy, there is no way of knowing whether or not there is any problem. While most couples experience no difficulty in producing a baby, an estimated 15%–18%, or one out of every seven couples in the United States, remains involuntarily childless. Couples, after practicing birth control for years, ironically may discover that they are infertile.

There is a prevailing belief that the incidence of infertility in the United States is becoming greater, and several reasons have been suggested for the apparent rise in the problem. Undeniably, the epidemic rise in the incidence of sexually transmitted disease has increased the prevalence of infertility in both men and women. Moreover, while little is known about the long-range effect of environmental pollutants on fertility, there is a growing awareness that both males and females could be exposed to a variety of chemicals such as polychlorinated hydrocarbons in the workplace or in the environment that may adversely affect their reproductive processes. But according to demographic statisticians, there really have been no dramatic changes in the incidence of infertility. The reason there currently are more infertile couples is primarily because there are more couples wanting to have children. The youngest of the baby boomers, the generation born between 1946 and 1964, have reached the age range where they now want to have children. Apparently many of them deferred marriage and postponed childbearing well into their 30s and early 40s,

past the age of maximum fertility. Also, there has been extensive media coverage of infertility treatment, which leads more people to seek help. Moreover, there are many more doctors trained to treat infertility, which has necessarily resulted in more couples who have received treatment or advice for infertility. According to data from the National Center for Health Statistics, any perception of an infertility epidemic is erroneous. Birth and fertility rates declined very slightly in 1998 from 1997, the most recent year for which information is available. Rates for women in their 20s did not change, whereas rates for women in their 30s rose 2% (Ventura et al., 1999).

Pointing to an already overpopulated world and the enormous cost, both financial and psychological, of raising a family, some would minimize infertility as a problem or might even consider it a blessing. Many couples are choosing to be child free, guaranteeing it with a vasectomy or a tubal ligation. It is one thing to choose not to be parents as a result of mutual decision, but it is a very different and painful situation when a man and a woman have decided to have a baby and discover that their right to choice has been biologically denied. Just a few years ago there was little recourse for couples who did not want to remain childless. Today, advances in infertility research have made it possible with medical assistance for two-thirds of infertile couples to conceive and produce a baby.

WHAT IS INFERTILITY?

Infertility is defined as the inability to conceive a child during the course of 1 year of regular sexual intercourse unprotected by contraception. Data indicate that without birth control, 25% of couples conceive in 1 month, 60% within 6 months, 80% after a year, and that 90% have initiated a pregnancy by 18–24 months. Statistically, however, if a couple has not conceived by the end of a year, the chances of becoming pregnant decrease. The age of the couple is also a factor, and the older they are the more difficulty they have. A woman's peak fertility occurs between the ages of 20 and 25; fertility is less optimal after 30 and is at its lowest after 40. Similarly, male fertility is greatest in the mid-20s, decreases in the 30s, declines markedly after 40, but never terminates completely as it does in a woman after menopause. Until the age of 30, men and women should probably wait a year or even longer before seeking medical help, but older couples should go for an evaluation if they have been unsuccessful after 6 months. If a couple has decided to postpone their childbearing until their 30s, they should at least start trying for a pregnancy early in that decade, giving themselves enough time to be helped, if necessary.

That human infertility in men and women decreases with age is nothing new. Biological factors associated with the normal aging process are responsible, and there may be additional environmental reasons in the sense that the infectious agents or pollutants to which we are exposed throughout life have had a longer time to act. Most women have always recognized that their chances of getting pregnant decreased with age, but increased anxiety about possible infertility was generated by a report in 1982 by French researchers Schwartz and Mayaux of the Federation CECOS. The study, evaluating the success rate for pregnancy in 2,193 women receiving artificial insemination because their husbands were sterile, reported that the percent of women conceiving after 1 year of attempted inseminations was 73% for women under age 25, 74% between 26 and 30, dropped to 61% between ages 31 and 35, and went down another 5 percentage points between 36 and 40. What these findings mean to an individual woman not having artificial insemination is debatable, but the heightened concern about age and infertility was probably fueled by overreaction to the study in the press and an editorial accompanying the report that actually suggested that, in light of the study, women may want to reevaluate their priorities and devote their 20s to childbearing and their 30s to career development, reversing the current trend. Some women were justifiably skeptical, but others viewed these conclusions with apprehension, believing that their biological clocks were not only ticking away, but somehow running down.

The greater risk of infertility with age is real, but the outlook for getting pregnant in the fourth decade of life is obviously not that bleak. The number of first births to women in their 30s has risen dramatically in the past 15 years, surpassing by a wide margin the modest increase in first births to women in their 20s. In fact, the largest rise in childbearing is occurring among women in their 30s. These are women whose greater educational achievement and desire to get their careers established led them to put off having a family and resulted in fewer adverse effects on their offspring than in those of younger women. For example, there was less incidence of low-birth-weight infants born to women in their 30s than in any other age group. The French study was alarming to many women, but needlessly. Demographer John Bongaarts, who called it a "false alarm," questioned the validity of the conclusions and pointed out that the French findings of lower fertility with artificial insemination should present little cause for concern. The data from long-term studies of the general population indicate that the figures from France do not even approximate the considerably greater fertility of women over 30 when insemination occurs in the usual way, rather than artificially. Another study of 751 women trying to get pregnant through artificial insemination at fertility clinics in the Netherlands found, like the French study, that the probability of conception declined in women as young as 31, but emphasized that the decrease could be compensated for by continuing insemination for a longer period. That is, women in their 30s will conceive, but at a slower rate (van Noord-Zaadstra et al., 1991). Women 40 years old and beyond also will conceive but perhaps can anticipate a higher risk of complications with the pregnancy and delivery. A study of more than 24,000 women who delivered their first child at age 40 or over, when compared with women who delivered between age 20 and 29, found a higher cesarean rate, greater use of forceps during vaginal delivery, a higher incidence of gestational diabetes, and lower birth weight of the infants among the older women (Gilbert et al., 1999). Obviously not all women having their first child at age 40 or over will

396 • CHAPTER 12

have complications, but given the larger number of women who are delaying childbirth until the fifth decade of life because of career choices, they should be aware of what they might expect with their pregnancy and delivery.

Traditionally, infertility has been seen as a "female problem." Even the words "barren" and "unfruitful" are feminine—who ever heard of a barren male? For this reason, all infertility research until recently focused on the female. Women, too, accepting the old beliefs and assuming responsibility in a childless marriage, have always been the first to seek help and become the more willing patients. Currently, the chances for correcting female infertility are still better than the possibilities for correcting male infertility, but now there is the general recognition that it takes both a man and a woman to make a baby, and it also takes the two to share responsibility for an inability to conceive. Some factor in the male is at fault 40% of the time, but because research on male infertility is in its infancy, treatment is not as successful. Actually, infertility is rarely the sole fault of either partner but is more usually the result of several minor dysfunctions in both. Together, they may be incapable of conceiving a child, but with another partner of greater fertility, there might be little difficulty.

Occasionally, there is no physiological reason for the infertility in either the man or the woman, but their inability to produce an offspring is the result of not knowing the best way or the best time to go about it. Not that there is anything wrong with their sexual technique—many people have read the manuals—but they may inadvertently be deterring rather than enhancing the possibility of conception. Perhaps the couple is having intercourse twice a day in an attempt to conceive, but increasing the frequency of coitus beyond four times a week may actually be lowering the sperm count to the point where pregnancy is unlikely. Even in a very fertile male, 12–24 hours should elapse between ejaculations for the sperm quality to have good fertilizing capacity. If a man is somewhat less than optimally fertile, it could take at least 48 hours to regain an appropriate sperm concentration.

Sometimes, conception is hampered because the couple is using a commercial vaginal lubricant that is lethal to sperm. Even saliva, usually the only lubricant recommended, has been found to be deleterious to sperm motility and activity (Tulandi, Plouffe, & McInnes, 1982). All such aids are somewhat spermicidal, but if couples really need the help of a lubricant, petroleum jelly, glycerine, and raw egg white have been tested and found to have minimal effects on sperm. Another mistake may be that the woman is getting out of bed too soon after coitus. She should lie on her back for an hour before arising, giving the sperm every opportunity to ascend through the cervix. And, because there is a strong likelihood of conception only 1 or perhaps 2 days a month, a couple could theoretically be missing the right time for years if they attempt pregnancy in a kind of random, hit-or-miss fashion. The simplest way of knowing when ovulation—the optimal time for conception—occurs is to keep a daily basal body temperature chart.

Basal Body Temperature (BBT) Curve

If the body temperature is taken daily under basal conditions—that is, after a period of rest and before any regular activity, daily work, or meals—it will fluctuate daily over a very small range. This is true for all individuals, male or female, young or old. If the daily recordings are plotted on a chart in a healthy adult ovulating woman, however, the BBT pattern will show not only the daily variation in the period between two menstruations but also a definite elevation in temperature that occurs within 1–3 days of ovulation. This elevation of temperature remains until 3–0 days before the onset of the next menstruation, when the curve again deflects back to the postmenstrual level. The morning temperature generally varies from about 97.2°F before ovulation to about 98.6°F–98.8°F after ovulation. Women before menarche or after menopause, anovulatory women, and men do not show this biphasic basal body temperature curve.

If a woman is having menstrual periods at relatively regular monthly intervals and the periods produce some premenstrual symptoms, such as a little puffiness, breast tenderness, or complexion trouble, she can be reasonably certain that she is ovulatory. Another useful sign, although not every woman has them, is the presence of intermenstrual ovulatory pains. Regular examination of cervical mucus would also indicate the occurrence of ovulation. All of these criteria can be confirmed by keeping a basal body temperature chart for a number of months. While the actual day of ovulation cannot be accurately predicted, it can certainly be approximated after the chart has been kept through several cycles, and intercourse to produce a pregnancy can be timed around it. Waiting for the increase in temperature before trying to conceive is a mistake, however. The actual release of the ovum from the ovary probably occurs 24–38 hours before the temperature elevation. The most favorable schedule for conception would be coitus every other day for the 3–4 days before the rise, including the 2 days after it. After the basal body temperature has been elevated for 2 days, conception is biologically impossible. BBT charts are, therefore, useful for both infertility and fertility control.

Printed charts on which to record the BBT are available from a physician, but it is easy enough to make one using graph paper. Figure 12–1 illustrates the normal morning temperature curve and the optimal days for conception. Each morning before getting out of bed, after at least 5 hours of sleep and before eating, drinking, or any extensive conversation, a thermometer is placed in the mouth for 3 minutes, read, and the temperature recorded on the chart. The rectal temperature has been determined to be more reliable and the most accurate measure of the actual basal body temperature, but the temperature taken orally or even under the armpit, as long as the same method is always used, will be accurate enough in most instances. Because the actual temperature in degrees is not as significant as the difference that occurs between successive recordings at the time of the elevation, it is possible to use a regular thermometer, but reading it may be more difficult. Special and more expensive thermometers that show a range of only a few degrees can be purchased (see Figure 12–2).

The temperature is marked on the chart for the appropriate day, and the mark is joined to the one for the previous day, thereby charting the curve for the month. The days of menstruation should be noted. Obviously any illness or infection that could cause a rise in temperature and be falsely interpreted as an ovulation elevation should also be noted.

A basal body temperature chart, recorded over five to six cycles, is easy to do and to interpret, requires only 5 minutes a day, and provides invaluable information to a woman interested in knowing her body's rhythms. It can tell her whether she ovulates every month, when ovulation occurs, when the best time is to get pregnant, and when the best time is not to get pregnant, although its reliability in this regard is more suspect. If the temperature elevation remains, and no menstrual period occurs, she can assume that a pregnancy has occurred. If a couple is having difficulty conceiving, they will certainly be ahead if the BBT has been charted when they consult a physician. The first thing the doctor is likely to do is hand the woman a basal body temperature chart to keep through several cycles.

Home Ovulation Predictor Kits

Ovulation predictor kits have been on the market since the mid-1980s. They contain monoclonal antibodies specific for luteinizing hormone and use the ELISA test to determine the amount of LH present in the urine. A significant color change from baseline indicates the LH surge and presumably the most fertile day of the month for the woman. Different kits contain supplies for five to nine tests and are used most effectively when a woman knows the time frame for her ovulation from the BBT method. Some medications may interfere with test results, and, of course, there will be no LH surge during an anovulatory cycle.

When All Systems Are "Go"

Fertilization, and thus conception, occurs when a normal sperm unites with a normal ovum at just the right time. A man's testes must have produced a sufficient

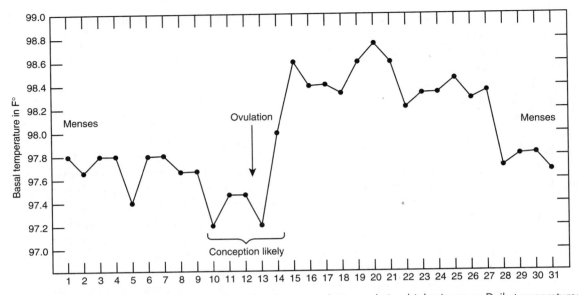

Figure 12–1   Basal body temperature (BBT) plotted during an ovulatory cycle is a biphasic curve. Daily temperatures tend to fluctuate in a pattern that is specific for every woman. Ovulation porbably occurs the day before the elevation, which may be preceded by a drop of the lowest temperature of the cycle. Sperm retain fertilizing capacity for 24–48 hours, and eggs are able to be fertilized for 12–24 hours. Coitus every other day for about 3–4 days before and 2–3 days afterward would increase the probability of conception. Unfortunately, not all charts are as easily interpreted as this one.

number of mature active sperm that move through unobstructed ducts so that they can be ejaculated in the appropriate concentration. He must be potent so that the sperm can be deposited in the woman's vagina, reach and penetrate the cervical mucus, and ascend into the uterus and up to the fallopian tubes.

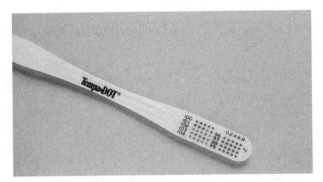

Figure 12–2   Thin strips of plastic with chemically impregnated dots that change color to reflect temperature can be purchased as disposable single-use thermometers.

The likelihood of sperm ascent is greatest when intercourse takes place in "missionary" position, with the woman on her back with her thighs flexed. Insemination is favored by this arrangement because the cervix will then lie in the pool of ejaculated semen that collects in the posterior fornix of the vagina.

The woman has to have produced a normal, fertilizable egg that has entered the fallopian tube so that it can be fertilized by a sperm within a period of several hours after ovulation. The resulting conceptus must move down the tube and implant in the previously prepared endometrium of the uterus so that it can continue its development. In both sexes, there must be appropriate levels of secretion of pituitary gonadotropins and gonadal sex steroids to sustain the reproductive processes. Any restriction or impairment of these basic events, even very slight, can cause a problem of infertility. Investigations of infertility are geared to systematic assessment of all the factors involved in the passage of the sperm and ova toward each other. They include five main tests aimed at diagnosing the possible defects that may be present and include an evaluation of the (1) male factor, (2) the vaginal and cervical factor, (3) the uterine factor, (4) the tubal factor, and (5) the ovarian factor.

$\mathscr{E}$VALUATION OF INFERTILITY

Ideally, each couple seeking a diagnostic evaluation would be able to go together to an infertility clinic where a gynecologist, an andrologist (the counterpart for men to a gynecologist), a reproductive endocrinologist, and perhaps an immunologist and geneticist form an infertility team that uses the latest diagnostic tools and offers treatments unknown just a few years ago. Unfortunately, these advantages are available only in major urban areas or at centers associated with university medical schools. But at least a doctor who specializes in infertility diagnosis and treatment should be sought. All gynecologists do not automatically qualify. It would also be wise, if possible, to find a physician whose practice is limited to infertility problems. The investigation will take 3 or 4 months, and some of the procedures would require immediate access to the doctor. Ovulation, for example, occurs any day of the week, including Saturday, Sunday, and holidays, and the availability of a physician who also maintains an obstetrical practice and performs gynecological surgery is obviously going to be limited.

It is logical to begin an evaluation of a couple's infertility by conducting the simplest, least complicated laboratory test—a semen analysis or sperm count. Knowing the extent to which the man is implicated in the couple's childlessness can direct the nature of the further tests to be performed on both partners. If he is completely normal, his part in the investigation may be finished. If he is completely sterile and the woman is subsequently determined to be normal, the couple may want to think about artificial insemination, adoption, or a childless existence. If the male is somewhat subfertile, he may be contributing to but

not solely responsible for the infertility. The evaluation would then continue on the woman while further investigation and possible treatment could be initiated on the man. But obviously, a woman should not agree to having a complete diagnostic workup, which may involve invasive tests or even surgical procedures, until the role played by her partner has been determined.

The Male Factor

Male infertility can have many causes—nutritional, endocrinological, developmental, pharmacological, occupational, immunological, anatomical—but they are generally expressed and recognizable in the semen analysis. For a semen examination, a man is asked to produce a specimen by ejaculation into a glass jar after 2–3 days of sexual abstinence. The ejaculate then has to be delivered to the laboratory for analysis within 1–2 hours. For religious or other reasons, some men find this method of providing a semen sample objectionable. Other methods of collecting sperm are by coitus interruptus (withdrawal before ejaculation during intercourse) or the semen can be aspirated from the woman's vagina immediately after coitus. It should not be collected in a condom, which may contain spermicidal chemicals.

When the specimen is brought to the laboratory, it is analyzed for volume, viscosity, number of sperm, sperm viability, motility, and sperm shape. The average volume of ejaculate is 3.5 ml, but it can normally vary from 2–10 ml. A low volume (1 ml or less) can be significant because it may not be enough to come in contact with the cervix when it is deposited into the vagina. For unknown reasons, a volume higher than 8 ml is also associated with infertility. After determining volume, the specimen is diluted and the numbers of sperm in a sample are counted under the microscope. To be considered normal, the specimen should contain at least 20 million sperm per milliliter, but experts in male fertility believe that the number of live and active sperm in the semen is a better correlate to fertility than their actual numbers. For there to be a strong probability of pregnancy, the semen should contain

50%–70% live sperm that move rapidly forward across the microscopic field and that retain their motility for several hours. A low sperm count with highly motile sperm usually represents greater fertility than a high sperm count with poor motility.

The shape and configuration of the sperm are also important. It is generally agreed that the chances for pregnancy are greatest when not more than 40% of the sperm in the specimen are considered to have abnormal morphology—too large, too small, too tapered, immature, or doubleheaded.

There are so many variables that can affect seminal quality and quantity that several analyses have to be performed before a diagnosis of fertile, subfertile, or sterile can be made. During the past decade, a number of tests to aid diagnosis of male infertility have been developed. The bovine cervical mucus penetration test is an evaluation of the ability of the sperm to pass through the mucus of the cervical canal. Since human cervical mucus necessary for the test is produced only around the time of ovulation, cow cervical mucus is substituted. A kit containing bovine mucus is commercially available in order to perform the assay in the laboratory. The zona-free hamster egg penetration test determines the ability of a given male's sperm to penetrate, and thus fertilize, oocytes. In 1976, Yanagimachi and colleagues discovered that when the zona pellucida of the hamster ovum is removed, the species specificity for penetration by sperm is also lost and that any animal's sperm including human, can then enter a hamster egg. For this assay, a number of hamster oocytes, collected from golden hamsters given gonadotropins to stimulate ovulation, are treated enzymatically to remove the outer layers of the eggs, including the zona pellucida. Then the eggs are incubated with human sperm cells. If fertilization (penetration of sperm) occurs, it suggests that the individual is fertile. Additional diagnostic laboratory tests may include the sperm antibody assay, which tests the woman's cervical mucus or blood serum, or the man's semen or blood serum, for the presence of antibodies directed against the sperm. These kinds of tests, in addition to semen analyses—now performed with the aid of computer software—have value in diagnosing male infertility, but unfortunately may not be able to define the cause.

Some factors are known to have a temporary effect on male fertility. Virus diseases, such as infectious mononucleosis or hepatitis, or actually any illness that produces a fever, can depress sperm production for several months. Certain tranquilizers or mood-elevating drugs may not only produce impotence but also suppress growth and production of sperm. Heavy marijuana smoking depresses sperm counts and testosterone production; smoking tobacco has also been associated with a depression of sperm motility. A number of therapeutic drugs such as cimetidine (Tagamet, used in treatment of ulcers) and nitrofurantoin (Macrodantin, an antibiotic used in urinary tract infections) are known to produce a temporary infertility. Testicular heating also adversely affects sperm production. Scrotal temperature is ordinarily 2.2°C less than body temperature and optimum for sperm. Exposing the testes to heat by taking a sauna or steam baths; wearing tight pants, thermal underwear, or jockey shorts; or even having the kind of occupation (truck driver on cross-country hauls) that results in scrotal heating can reduce fertility.

It has been found that about 25% of infertile males have a condition called *varicocele,* a varicosity of the left internal spermatic vein that drains the testes. A simple surgical procedure that ties off the vein has been found to improve fertility in the majority of men with the disorder.

When no reason for the poor semen quality can be determined, medical opinions vary as to whether there is any really effective way of treating the deficiency. Various hormones have been administered, but there is general consensus that their efficacy is questionable unless there is some definite indication for their use. Clomiphene citrate, a drug used to induce ovulation in women, has been tried in men in various dosage regimens. Some doctors report improvement in sperm concentration and motility; others have given the same medication with little or no beneficial effect.

$\mathscr{A}$RTIFICIAL INSEMINATION

When the sperm count has been determined to be only moderately deficient, artificial insemination using the male partner's own semen may be possible. The procedure—called AIH for artificial insemination, husband—may involve different techniques. In intracervical insemination, the semen is placed into the cervical mucus. When the semen is placed through the cervix into the uterine cavity by means of a sterile transcervical catheter, it is called intrauterine insemination, or IUI. Intratubal insemination is more complicated. It involves placing the semen in a catheter that is passed through the cervix, through the uterine cavity, and into the fallopian tube. The catheter is guided appropriately with ultrasound. Intratubal insemination was developed to improve the success of pregnancy but thus far does not seem to have demonstrated any significant improvement over IUI.

In intracervical insemination, the entire ejaculate of semen is transported to the doctor's office and then placed into the cervical mucus. A cervical cap or specially designed tampon is used to hold the semen against the cervix. In intrauterine insemination, the sperm are capacitated and washed to eliminate the seminal fluid and concentrate the sperm. Capacitation, or the changes in the sperm plasma membrane that allow interaction with the egg, normally occurs in the female genital tract but can also take place when the sperm are incubated in an artificial culture medium. Ejaculated spermatozoa are first washed in a special kind of insemination medium and centrifuged to eliminate the rest of the seminal fluid and increase the sperm concentration. In the "swim-up" technique, the sperm pellet is then overlaid with fresh culture media and the most motile and vigorous spermatozoa swim up into it. The processed sperm are then placed into the uterus near the tubal openings with a catheter directed by ultrasound. The insemination is timed to ovulation in the woman, who has been given fertility drugs to stimulate follicular development. Studies have indicated an overall pregnancy rate of about 25% using IUI in couples who had been infertile for 5 years. A recent clinical trial with 932 couples compared intracervical insemination alone, intrauterine insemination alone, **superovulation** (giving fertility drugs to the woman to increase follicle production and ovulation) and intrauterine insemination, and superovulation and intracervical insemination. The couples treated with superovulation and intrauterine insemination had a higher rate of pregnancy (33%) than the couples who had not been treated with fertility drugs prior to intrauterine insemination (18%) or those that had intracervical insemination only (10%). The rate of pregnancy was higher (19%) in couples who had been treated with superovulation and intracervical insemination (Guzick et al., 1999).

Sometimes several ejaculates of the subfertile male's semen are frozen and stored so they can be combined to increase the number of sperm. Sperm can be successfully frozen and thawed without damaging them genetically, but their efficacy in producing pregnancy is not as great as that of fresh semen.

Artificial insemination using donor semen can be performed when the husband is considered clinically sterile. More than 70,000 American babies per year are born via assisted reproduction techniques; of those, 25,000 were conceived by artificial insemination. Artificial insemination, donor (or AID) is an alternative to irreversible male infertility. It has become increasingly more acceptable, performed not only for infertile heterosexual couples but also for single women who are homosexual or who expect to remain unmarried and want a child.

Not all physicians are equally enthusiastic about performing AID. It involves ethical and legal considerations for the doctor, who must select the donor, preserve his anonymity, and worry about the threat of future litigation should anything go wrong. The latter possibility is circumvented by strongly worded consent forms. The donors are usually medical students, interns, and residents who provide sperm specimens for a fee. It is claimed that these men are preferred as donors because of their availability and their greater awareness of their own and their family's medical history. It can also be assumed that many doctors reason that the best source of sperm of high genetic quality should be from healthy stable men of superior intelligence—other doctors, naturally.

For the couple or the single woman, there are similar ethical and legal difficulties. There are unanswered questions about the legitimacy of the child and the rights and responsibilities of the parents. In some states, the husband must legally adopt the wife's child after birth. In others, some specific measures have to be taken to protect the child's right to the husband's estate. The considerable emotional and psychological ramifications of the procedure also must be confronted. Generally, it is recommended that the insemination be kept a completely private matter between the physician and the couple. Some have even suggested that the obstetrician who delivers the baby be different from the physician who did the insemination so that as few people as possible know how the pregnancy was established. Eventually, a single parent or couple has to deal with disclosure of AID status to the child, or risk the possibility of accidental discovery. The anonymous donors, who may have provided semen for a number of inseminations, are emotionally uninvolved, but where does that leave the child who wants to know the identity of the biological father? Some physicians routinely mix the donor's semen with the husband's sperm as a means of blurring paternity—a practice of better legal than medical value. For couples who are able to adjust to the idea of artificial insemination, it can be a method of achieving a pregnancy, but there are no guarantees. After a year of artificial inseminations, the reported national success rate averages 57%–70%, with the majority of pregnancies occurring in less than 6 months.

But even beyond the ethical and legal concerns of sperm donation and insemination, there could be a risk for the woman of acquiring a sexually transmitted disease or the possibility of transmission of a hereditary defect to the child unless the physician or sperm bank follows the guidelines on AID, established in 1986 by the American Society for Reproductive Medicine, for-

merly the American Fertility Society (the group of M.D. and Ph.D. specialists in infertility and reproductive physiology and technology). Unfortunately, the guidelines are not binding and not every practitioner follows them. According to the society, semen donors should be tested for infectious diseases such as AIDS, syphilis, gonorrhea, or hepatitis. Also, given the threat of acquiring an AIDS infection through an AID insemination, the society recommended that donated fresh semen should not be used even though it is associated with a better pregnancy rate. Semen should be frozen for 6 months. Freezing specimen will not destroy human immunodeficiency virus, but it provides the opportunity to screen the donor *twice*—3 months apart—to make certain that virus-infected semen will not be inseminated. Reputable sperm banks screen donors for HIV, hepatitis, and other sexually transmitted diseases and will test donors for genetic diseases such as cystic fibrosis, donors with African-American ancestry for sickle cell carrier status, and donors with Jewish ancestry for Tay-Sachs carrier status. There is no formal policy in most states, however, that requires testing donors or even taking a medical history or keeping accurate records. Women considering donor insemination have to choose their practitioner or clinic carefully and ask the right questions. They may not need or want to know the identity of the donor but should be able to review the donor's medical history and insist that the sperm bank or infertility clinic keep accurate records of the individual's name and address should they subsequently be needed.

Most of the major sperm banks are able to honor requests for sperm from men of specific racial or ethnic background. A California businessman had an even "better" idea about 20 years ago—to found a sperm bank and also contribute to the nation's intelligence by soliciting and accepting donor sperm only from Nobel Prize winners in science. The Herman Muller Repository for Germinal Choice, named after geneticist Muller, whose death in 1967 eliminated *him* from the donors, provides supposedly intelligent (but aged, given the usually advanced years of Nobel laureates) sperm for a price. More recently, college-aged women and men recruited for egg and sperm donations are screened for SAT scores and GPAs, with high payments reported in the national press for "top-quality" reproductive material.

VAGINAL AND CERVICAL FACTORS

The uterine cervix is a gateway—it permits the entry of sperm to the uterus. The unique properties of the cervical mucus determine whether the gate is opened or closed. Around the time of ovulation, the cervical mucus is clear, watery and less viscous, more alkaline, and most receptive to sperm penetration. Within a day or two after ovulation, the cervical mucus, now influenced by progesterone, becomes thick, viscous, and opaque, and it impedes sperm passage. The cervix and its mucus have an obvious significance in problems of infertility.

Vaginitis is not known to cause infertility, but neither is it likely to encourage fertility. Semen is alkaline, the vaginal secretion is acid, and the combination is optimal for sperm survival. If a vaginal infection changes vaginal pH, sperm motility may be hampered. Even if there are no symptoms or clinical signs of vaginitis, a microscopic examination of vaginal discharge is a necessary part of an infertility investigation. Any foreign microorganisms present should be eliminated to ensure a normal vaginal pH.

There is some evidence that mycoplasma infections are associated with infertility. Mycoplasmas bear similarities to both viruses and bacteria. One of the organisms belonging to this group, T-mycoplasma or *Ureaplasma urealyticum,* is believed to account for about half of the cases of nongonococcal urethritis in men and is frequently found in the vaginas of women where it produces no apparent symptoms. *Ureaplasma urealyticum* has been implicated by a number of investigators as the cause of repeated spontaneous abortion, stillbirths, and unexplained infertility, but its actual contribution is still unproved. When the infection has been discovered in the male partner of an involuntarily infertile couple, however, and the man was treated with a tetracycline derivative, pregnancy was achieved in a number of cases. Witkin and Toth (1983) noted that conception occurred in 60% of previously infertile couples once the *Ureaplasma urealyticum* infection was eradicated by doxycycline therapy for both partners. These authors suggested that this kind of hidden but prevalent infection may play a significant role in infertility.

The postcoital or Sims-Hühner test is an evaluation of both partners, routinely performed in any infertility evaluation. The test, first reported by Sims more than 100 years ago, is made at the time of ovulation and consists of a microscopic examination of vaginal secretion and cervical mucus for the presence of motile sperm within some hours after sexual intercourse. It provides information concerning sperm quality and cervical mucus quality and is, therefore, an evaluation of both partners.

If a sample from the endocervix taken 4–6 hours after intercourse shows 10 or more motile and active sperm per high-power microscopic field that are progressing forward in a clear and plentiful watery mucus, it is taken as evidence that semen is normal and that no block to fertility exists at the level of the vagina or cervix. If there are sperm in the vaginal secretion but not in the cervix, the assumption is that the cervical mucus is blocking their entry, but the bovine mucus test could determine whether the problem is cervical mucus or some defect in the sperm. If the semen analysis has been previously determined to be normal, but there are few or dead sperm in the vagina and cervix, it may mean that the cervical mucus is hostile or even lethal to the sperm. If there are no sperm or semen present in the vagina or the cervix, it may mean either that there was something wrong with the test and it should be repeated, or that there should be some tactful investigation of why there were no sperm deposited when intercourse presumably took place a few hours before. There could be some problem, possibly unrecognized by the couple, of incomplete penetration or even total lack of intravaginal penetration.

Mucus that is "poor," that is, thick and impenetrable, may have an endocrinological basis or be the result of infection and can frequently be successfully treated by endocrine or antibiotic therapy. If the cervical mucus remains a barrier despite treatment, the previously described washed intrauterine insemination method, which bypasses the barrier, may result in pregnancy.

IMMUNOLOGICAL FACTORS

There is little doubt that immunological factors play a role in infertility, but the actual mechanism and the site of action are poorly understood. Rare cases have been reported in which women have suffered strong allergic reactions to semen—hives, hay fever symptoms, vulvovaginal swelling—and, in isolated instances, even anaphylactic shock, an acute, severe response. Less dramatically, it has also been reported that a variety of sperm-immobilizing antibodies can be detected in the blood serum and/or the cervical-vaginal secretions of a proportion of infertile women. Their significance for otherwise unexplained infertility is unknown, however, because fertile women have also been found to have sperm antibodies circulating in their blood.

The presence of an unfavorable immune response to sperm can be demonstrated by a simple agglutination test in which a solution of diluted sperm is mixed with a sample of the woman's serum and observed for agglutination, or clumping. A positive test indicates that sperm-agglutinating antibodies are present in her blood that may be interfering with fertility. A more sophisticated test is the sperm antibody assay, in which the sperm are first mixed with the woman's serum or cervical mucus. If she has antisperm antibodies, they will bind to the sperm. Then the sperm are mixed with immunoglobulin-coated beads. Any bound sperm will now bind to the beads, which appear microscopically as motile sperm with beads attached. By altering the type of immunoglobulin attached to the bead, the antisperm antibodies can even be localized to the sperm head or

tail. Head-directed antibodies can mean interference with the ability of the head of the sperm to enter the egg and result in fertilization. Tail-directed antibodies may indicate an interference with sperm motility.

It is assumed that once sensitization of the woman to her partner's sperm has occurred, continued and frequent intercourse will maintain a high level of antibodies in her blood. The condition, therefore, is treated by occlusion or "condom therapy." The woman is protected from contact with the sperm by the use of a condom for several months in order to cause enough of a drop in the antibody level so that sperm motility and, thus, pregnancy can take place. Some doctors have reported great success with this form of treatment; others believe the method to have doubtful value. It could take 9–12 months of protected intercourse before an antibody test becomes negative, and sometimes the antibodies to sperm persist even in the absence of exposure to sperm.

Sperm-agglutinating antibodies also have been demonstrated in the serum of infertile men as well as in two-thirds of vasectomized men. This kind of autoimmune response—a man is allergic to his own sperm—has not been shown in the serum of husbands of pregnant women. A similar autoimmune response in women, that of developing an allergic reaction to their own ova, has been suggested for some cases of unexplained infertility. Antibodies might bind to the zona pellucida, for example, and make it impossible for the sperm to penetrate the ovum. Treatment with high-dose corticosteroids (prednisolone) to reduce the level of antibodies in both men and women has been used with mixed results regarding pregnancy rates. The side effects of the prednisolone also are a deterrent to its use.

Any kind of treatment for men or women who show autoimmune responses to their own gametes is as yet unknown. Research on the immunological aspects of infertility is still in its earliest stages. The work that is exciting the most interest deals with the problem from another angle—the development of a vaccine to *prevent* pregnancy. When the exact nature of the antigens, the agents that cause the production of antibodies, can be identified and isolated, it may be possible to find a way of suppressing those antigens in the infertile and to prevent their effect on fertility reduction—and also to develop a way to immunize women against sperm or against their own ova and thus reduce fertility.

$\mathcal{U}$TERINE AND TUBAL FACTORS

The uterus alone seldom interferes with fertility. A small uterus (the so-called infantile uterus) has successfully carried many pregnancies, and a "tipped" uterus, as long as it remains mobile and not fixed or bound down by adhesions, is rarely significant. Only if the retroversion and retroflexion (Chapter 2) is very severe is it possible, but not likely, that the cervix is displaced enough to impair entry or passage of sperm through the endocervical canal. Fibroids are important only if they obstruct the fallopian tubes or interfere with the implantation of the fertilized egg. Endometriosis, even when the fallopian tubes and ovaries are unaffected, for elusive reasons does have an effect on infertility, however, and women who are aware that they have the disease should probably start to have their children early and space them close together before the endometriosis becomes further advanced.

A tubal disorder is the causal factor in 30% of couples with a failure to conceive. If the fallopian tubes are completely or even partially occluded, the egg may not be able to get into the tube from the ovary, the sperm may not be able to get to the egg to fertilize it, and, even if it does, the larger fertilized egg may not be able to pass down the tube to the uterus. Any bout with bacteria in the pelvis—either secondary to chlamydia, gonorrhea, abortion, miscarriage, normal delivery, an intrauterine contraceptive, a D and C, or a ruptured appendix—can cause scar tissue and result in tubal obstruction.

The patency, or openness, of the fallopian tubes can be determined by a relatively low-risk test that can be performed in the gynecologist's office. The Rubin, or uterotubal insufflation test, is a procedure by which carbon dioxide gas under pressure is injected through a cannula into the uterus so that it can flow out of the tubes into the peritoneal cavity. If one or both tubes are patent, only a normal amount of carbon dioxide pressure will be needed to produce the endpoint of the test—the experiencing of pain referred to the left shoulder when sitting up. The pain results from the gas passing into the peritoneal cavity to collect under the diaphragm.

When the carbon dioxide pressure has to be higher than normal to produce the shoulder pain, it probably means that the tubes are partially obstructed. If there is an absence of shoulder pain, the tubes are blocked. The pain is acute and unmistakable if it is present, but it is temporary and subsides as the woman lies down again and the gas is slowly absorbed. Usually, there is little or no discomfort after the test is over, but occasionally a diaphragmatic irritation will persist.

If the Rubin test is normal, that is, normal pressure to produce shoulder pain, some doctors will forgo any further tubal evaluation at that point in order to proceed to investigate other factors. The test is uncomplicated, produces some discomfort but no other side effects, does not expose a woman to radiation, is not expensive, and occasionally is even therapeutic. It is evidently not unusual for a pregnancy to occur after the Rubin test has been used for diagnosis, perhaps because, as Rubin claimed, a clearing or flushing out of the tubes occurs.

The information provided by the Rubin test is limited, however, because all it can really determine is whether at least one fallopian tube is open. For this reason, and because technical problems with the Rubin apparatus can cause false normal and false abnormal test results, it is rarely used today, having been replaced by hysterosalpingography. In this test, 3–10 ml of an opaque contrast medium, either an oil-soluble or water-soluble dye, are slowly injected through a catheter into the endocervical canal so that the uterus and tubes can be visualized during fluoroscopy and on x-ray film. If the fallopian tubes are patent, the dye will ascend upward to distend the uterus and tubes and spill out into the peritoneal cavity.

The disadvantages are that hysterosalpingography is very painful for many women (somewhat alleviated if a prostaglandin inhibitor is taken 30 minutes prior to the procedure), it must be performed in the hospital or in a radiologist's office, and it exposes a woman to pelvic irradiation. In its favor, the test provides information concerning the actual site of a tubal obstruction or uterine abnormality and seems to have equal fertility-enhancing properties as the Rubin test, especially when an oil-based dye is used. Some physicians maintain that in addition to possibly enhancing fertility, an oil dye produces a better film image and causes less pain on injection than does a water-soluble dye. Although a hysterosalpingogram can pinpoint the level of obstruction in a tube, it cannot indicate anything about the nature of the problem. Further tests of tubal structure before treatment may include direct visualization of the pelvic anatomy by pelvic laparoscopy; the use of an endoscope inserted into the abdominopelvic cavity to examine the pelvic anatomy; or hysteroscopy, the insertion of a cystoscope into the uterus through the cervical os.

When it has been determined that the infertility is the result of some kind of tubal factor, the current prospects for successful treatment are still meager. Various kinds of surgical procedures have been developed, but oviduct tissue is extremely delicate, difficult to handle, and easily traumatized. Surgery on it is similar to operating on a thin, short strand of spaghetti. Even in the hands of the most experienced infertility surgeons, using the smallest of instruments and sutures thinner than hairs, the results in terms of postoperative pregnancies are not that encouraging. A further reason for a general reluctance to attempt tube repair is its association with a high rate of subsequent ectopic pregnancies. Continued refinements of the tools and techniques of microsurgery may produce more positive results in the future. Balloon tuboplasty has been used to dilate the wall of the tube with some success.

ᴛHE OVARIAN FACTOR

The two basic functions of the ovary are to produce an ovum and to produce estrogens and progesterone. Both are equally important to pregnancy. It is estimated that 10%–15% of fertility problems are the result of some disorder of ovulation. Either the woman does not ovulate at all, ovulates very irregularly and infrequently, or ovulates and produces a corpus luteum that inadequately secretes progesterone and fails to sufficiently prepare the endometrium for implantation. The easiest profile of ovulatory function is provided by the basal body temperature chart. As previously described, a normal biphasic ovulatory pattern shows lower temperatures in the first half of the cycle, a dip to the lowest point before ovulation, and a sustained rise in temperature in the second half of the cycle until it falls again premenstrually. Another confirmatory test of ovulation that indicates whether the secretion of progesterone is adequate is an endometrial biopsy, a strip of tissue removed from the lining of the uterus, just before menstruation. Since the histological appearance of the endometrium during the entire menstrual cycle is well known and standardized, the sample of endometrium is dated to see whether it corresponds to the estimated date of ovulation that has been ascertained by the basal body temperature. An endometrium that does not conform to the normal histological pattern indicates a defect in the luteal phase. This relatively rare problem, estimated to occur in 3%–10% of infertile women, is treated with human chorionic gonadotropin or by progesterone administered through intramuscular injection or vaginal suppository. Progestational agents other than progesterone should not be used. Not only have they been proved ineffective for luteal phase defect, but they have been implicated in birth defects if pregnancy occurs during their administration.

Endometrial biopsy is performed in the doctor's office, usually without anesthesia or with only a local numbing of the cervix. Thus, it may be painful for many women, rivaling, as Barbara Eck Menning (1988) observed, the hysterosalpingogram in discomfort.*

Other tests of ovulatory function include daily observations of cervical mucus and daily vaginal

---

*Menning is the founder of Resolve, Inc., a support organization for the infertile. See web site directory for the address.

smears, which are stained and examined to indicate estrogen and progesterone secretion. Because ovulatory dysfunction may also be the result of hyperprolactinemia (elevated circulating levels of prolactin that could interfere with the synthesis or release of GnRH or progesterone) or a disturbance of the hypothalamic-pituitary-ovarian axis because of increased androgen production secondary to an adrenal disorder, daily measurements of the amounts of steroids and gonadotropins in the blood or of hormone metabolites in the urine can be made. Daily ultrasound examinations can follow the growth of follicles, watch for the emergence of a dominant follicle, and see whether it disappears, suggesting follicular rupture and ovulation. All of the preceding techniques are expensive and time consuming; they require a woman to go to the doctor's office or hospital lab daily. Ovulation detection kits that check for urinary luteinizing hormone (LH) are available for home use and are an option.

*F*ERTILITY DRUGS

Lack of ovulation **(anovulation)** or irregular ovulation **(oligoovulation)** has been treated in the past by various methods—thyroid medication, adrenocortical hormones, estrogen, progesterone, x-irradiation of the ovaries, surgical removal of a wedge of ovarian tissue—that were sometimes successful and sometimes not. In the past 25 years or so, the biggest breakthrough in the field of infertility research has been the development of the only really effective treatment available for ovulatory dysfunction. The use of fertility drugs to induce ovulation has made it possible for many women who would formerly have remained childless to become pregnant and bear children.

The preparations used most often, either singly or in combination are clomiphene citrate (Clomid, Serophene), a nonsteroid synthetic antiestrogen chemically related to diethylstilbestrol and tamoxifen; bromocriptine (Parlodel), an orally effective dopamine agonist that inhibits prolactin release from the anterior

pituitary when ovulatory dysfunction is associated with hyperprolactinemia; human menopausal gonadotropins (HMG) or Pergonal, obtained from the urine of postmenopausal women and containing equal amounts of FSH and LH; purified FSH (Metrodin), separated from LH and also extracted from the urine of postmenopausal women; human chorionic gonadotropin (HCG), obtained from the urine of pregnant women; and gonadotropin-releasing hormone (GnRH), intravenously administered in pulsatile fashion via a portable, automated pump, or synthetic GnRH agonists (Buserilin, Lupron) given subcutaneously or by nasal spray.

The only indications for treatment with fertility drugs are absent or infrequent ovulation when other reasons for the couple's inability to conceive are lacking. Only after it has been determined that her tubes are patent; that she has ovaries capable of producing ova; that her partner is fertile; and that there is no thyroid, adrenal, or pituitary disorder responsible for anovulation does a woman become a likely candidate for ovulation induction.

Clomiphene citrate in low doses is the safest and least expensive method of ovulation induction and is generally used first if conditions warrant it. Human menopausal gonadotropin is reserved for women who do not respond to this drug. Structurally, clomiphene is a distant relative to diethylstilbestrol, but it has very weak estrogenic effects in humans. Because the compound inhibited ovulation in laboratory rats, it was originally believed to have promise as a contraceptive and was tested on women in a clinical trial in 1961. An unexpected result, and probably even more surprising to the women subjects, was that clomiphene citrate turned out to induce rather than suppress ovulation. Its action is still not completely understood, but it is now believed to be antiestrogenic at the level of the hypothalamus. It apparently blocks the negative feedback effect of estrogen on the hypothalamus by occupying the estrogen receptor sites in the nuclei of hypothalamic cells for long periods of time. As a result, the estrogen receptors are not replenished as usual by the hypothalamus and are unavailable to be occupied by the estrogen in the circulation. The hypothalamus is deceived into thinking that the endogenous estrogen level is low and produces GnRH to signal the pituitary production of FSH and LH and to ensure the ovarian follicle production that ultimately results in ovulation. According to several sources, 80%–90% of women who meet the criteria for clomiphene therapy can be expected to ovulate, and about half will get pregnant (Speroff, Glass, & Kase, 1989; Hutchinson-Williams, 1990).

The usual starting dose of clomiphene is 50 mg daily for 5 days, starting on the fifth day of the cycle. If ovulation does not occur that month within 5–12 days after the last pill, the dose is doubled in subsequent cycles to a maximum of 150–200 mg until the desired effect of ovulation, and happily, pregnancy takes place. Treatment plans vary. Some doctors will give HCG to increase the chances of successful ovulation after a few days of initial clomiphene therapy; others wait until the maximum dose proves ineffective. In some women, clomiphene's antiestrogenic properties tend to cause the production of a less receptive cervical mucus. Even if ovulation occurs, conception may be hampered. Small doses of estrogen started on day 9 and continued through expected ovulation may be successful in counteracting poor cervical mucus.

There are a few major hazards and several side effects associated with clomiphene citrate therapy, but they are fewer with this drug than with the other ovulation inducers and are relatively infrequent at the lower doses. When treatment is prolonged and large amounts are being taken, the ovaries may be overly stimulated to result in enlargement and cyst formation. If treatment is discontinued, spontaneous regression of ovarian enlargement will usually occur within several weeks. About 7%–10% of the pregnancies after clomiphene are multiple, primarily twins, but triplets may occur as frequently as 1 in 400 live births and quadruplets as frequently a 1 in 800. Since prematurity frequently accompanies multiple birth, there is some fetal risk involved. No evidence of a greater incidence of birth defects following ovulation induction has been documented. Some side effects include hot flashes, breast soreness, nausea and vomiting, abdominal pain or soreness, visual disturbances such as blurring or spots in front of the eyes, and temporary dryness or loss of hair. All of these symptoms occur infrequently and are reversible within a few days of discontinuation of the drug.

Bromocriptine may be added to clomiphene citrate to increase the sensitivity to clomiphene. Bromocriptine, acting as a pituitary prolactin inhibitor, can induce ovulation in a woman with hyperprolactinemia and galactorrhea (milky secretion from the breasts not related to pregnancy or breastfeeding) but apparently also can enhance ovarian responsiveness to clomiphene when prolactin levels are normal.

Clomiphene citrate functions by the domino effect; it acts on the hypothalamus, which acts on the pituitary, which produces gonadotropins, which act on the ovaries. Chorionic gonadotropins and human menopausal gonadotropins bypass the hypothalamus and pituitary and act directly on the ovaries to cause follicular maturation and ovum release. Human menopausal gonadotropin (HMG) was originally obtained from the urine of Italian nuns, who are still a major source of the drug. Marketed in this country as Pergonal, HMG contains FSH and LH activity in a 1-to-1 ratio. Pituitary FSH and LH are chemically different from urinary gonadotropins, but they seem to have the same clinical effect on the ovaries. Pergonal is administered by daily muscular injection to cause follicular growth and development. When appropriate follicular maturation has been achieved, as measured by ultrasound and daily determination of blood or urinary estrogen levels, an injection of HCG (trade names Antuitrin-S, A. P. L., Pregnyl, or Follutein), which is biologically similar to LH, is given to create the LH surge that precedes ovulation. The couple is advised to have intercourse on the day of the HCG injection and for the next 2 days.

The use of human gonadotropins to induce ovulation has a high cost and high risk and is used only for women who do not respond to clomiphene citrate. The average multiple-birth rate is 25%, but more of the births are greater than twins after HMG, and this adds to increased fetal mortality. The incidence of ovarian enlargement is also considerably higher. The ovarian hyperstimulation syndrome, which includes enlarged tender and painful ovaries, distension of the abdomen by fluid, and weight gain, can be a life-threatening problem in its severe form. Serious hyperstimulation occurs in 1% of women treated with HMG.

HMG is a highly potent preparation, the last resort for the fewer than 5% of women who need gonadotropins because all other treatment plans for ovulatory dysfunction have failed. It should be administered only by a skilled and experienced fertility specialist who will do the intensive daily monitoring that is required. It should be taken only with full knowledge of the expense of the treatment, the willingness and time to undergo the daily therapy, and the full recognition of the potential hazards, both maternal and fetal, of the treatment.

Purified FSH may be used to achieve pregnancy in women with polycystic ovary syndrome, a chronic state of anovulation characterized by excessive androgen and estrogen production with increased LH and reduced FSH secretion. Administration of GnRH and the synthetic GnRH agonists has been effective in women with amenorrhea of hypothalamic origin (exercise-induced, severe weight loss, anorexia nervosa) and in some women with polycystic ovaries. The advantages of using GnRH are its lesser side effects and the general absence of ovarian hyperstimulation and multiple pregnancy. Polycystic ovaries affect from 5%–10% of American women and are a common cause of infertility. It has been suggested that the condition may result from a failure to use insulin properly. A recent small study with an investigational drug, D-chiro-inositol, which helps insulin to function more efficiently, showed that the drug appears to improve ovulation in women with polycystic ovary syndrome (Nestler et al., 1999). A clinical trial, involving a large number of women, is taking place to determine the safety and effectiveness of the drug.

High-Order Multiple Births

The incidence of high-order multiple gestations, defined as giving birth to three or more infants induced by fertility drugs, is fortunately still relatively small but has quadrupled since the mid-1980s. Recent "miracles" are exemplified by the Texas sextuplets (five survived), the Iowa septuplets (all survived), and the extraordinary Texas octuplets (seven of whom survived). The media went wild, reporting in detail the struggles of the tiny premature infants to make it. The reality of multiple births is far from a miracle, however, and is viewed by many as a disaster, not a success. The babies are at risk for a range of devastating defects and problems. Inevitably born prematurely, they have increased possibilities of lung and intestinal infection. If they survive, the infants may face cerebral palsy and developmental and physical disabilities. For the parents, these problems are in addition to an astounding food and formula bill; unimaginable sleep deprivation; and, more often than not, living in a small house with singleton children that they produced prior to giving birth to the multiples.

The risk of multiple births after fertility drugs depends on a number of factors, including the woman's age, the quality of the sperm, and the dosage and duration of treatment, but it is generally 10%–20%. One option to prevent a high-order multiple gestation is "selective reduction," or removal of one or more fetuses in the uterus, leaving others to develop normally. Because selective reduction could imperil the entire pregnancy, it is generally viewed as a last resort. Another possibility is to remove some follicles before fertilization if an ultrasound reveals many mature follicles. Or the physician could cancel the cycle by withholding the final injection of HCG, a procedure that is heart wrenching for the couple wanting a pregnancy. Control of multiple births also can be accomplished by removing the follicles from the ovaries, fertilizing them outside of the body (in vitro fertilization), and returning only two or three to the uterus. These options are expensive, costing thousands of dollars, and most frequently are not covered by insurance.

Dealing with multiple births has become a fertility debate. That fertility drugs, which can be prescribed by any primary care doctor, are effective in producing a pregnancy was assessed in a 1999 study carried out on 932 couples at 10 fertility centers. The couples had no known physical bars to fertility and had tried to get pregnant for an average of 3.5 years (Guzick et al.). Using fertility drugs to induce "superovulation" and injecting the partner's sperm directly into the woman's uterus was the most effective method and produced a pregnancy in 33% of the women. Intrauterine insemination was three times as likely to result in pregnancy than intracervical insemination. Multiple pregnancies—three sets of quadruplets and four sets of triplets—occurred in 24 of 72 women who took fertility drugs and got pregnant. It should be noted that two of the authors of the study were paid consultants for Serono, a company that makes fertility drugs.

*U*NEXPLAINED INFERTILITY

In 10% of the couples who are looking for an answer to their problem of infertility, no physical or physiological reasons for the difficulty can be detected. After all the tests are over, after the two people have willingly endured the indignities engendered by an infertility investigation, they are now subjected to a final indignity. They are told their infertility is idiopathic with no discernible cause.

As if coping and adjusting to the situation were not difficult enough, everyone, from well-meaning relatives and friends to members of the medical profession, believes they do have an answer. No physiological reason is apparent, so the problem is obviously psychological. The couple is tense and anxious because they want a baby so badly, and it is hampering their fertility. All they really have to do is to stop worrying, to take it easy, and a pregnancy will occur. Some doctors are convinced that all these young people really need is a little calm reassurance from their friendly physician, and they relate stories about the couples that came just once to the office and then conceived with no further treatment. It is also commonly accepted that pregnancy frequently occurs after adoption, when the stress that precipitated the infertility is presumably relieved.

While there is no dearth of anecdotal folklore to bolster the hypothesis that there are psychogenic factors in infertility, scientific substantiation is absent. Even the generally accepted notion that adoption leads to pregnancy in apparently normal infertile parents has not been supported by statistical studies. Pregnancy rates for infertile couples who adopt children are the same as for infertile couples who do not adopt children. A certain number of spontaneous pregnancies do occur in couples presumed sterile, but their association with a single visit to the doctor, with a Caribbean cruise, or with any other relaxing change in the environment is likely to be coincidental.

In the absence of any organic reason for the infertility—at least one discernible by current techniques—it is tempting to categorize it as emotionally induced. Not unexpectedly, the diagnosis of psychosomatic infertility is more frequently applied to women. It has been theorized that infertile women may consciously verbalize their wish to have a baby, but that they are masking their underlying rejection of pregnancy, childbirth, and motherhood. As previously noted, this subconscious-rejection-of-the-female-role theory has been used to explain many disorders—among them menstrual difficulties, spontaneous abortion, and the nausea and vomiting of pregnancy. Some psychiatric theories speculate that the women's movement has been responsible for a higher incidence of psychological infertility, that the career-oriented woman may suffer even greater psychic trauma than before as her biological role conflicts further with her personal goals.

Given that the hypothalamus is integral to the function of the reproductive tracts in both males and females, a psychological basis for infertility in men and women that could be mediated through some neuroendocrinological pathway is certainly a possibility that cannot be ruled out. But what are the mechanisms involved in the unconscious prevention of conception? If psychogenic infertility, rooted in conflict and anxiety, actually exists, it still would have to be manifested physically and physiologically on the cells, tissues, tubes, and secretions of the reproductive tract. In other conditions presumed to have a psychosomatic origin—stomach ulcers, colitis, asthma, tension headaches—there is also little real proof linking the disorder to the psyche, but at least there are visible signs of dysfunction. In the normally infertile woman, however, there are no visible abnormalities. It would appear, then, that there is even less reason to presume that the infertility is psychogenic.

For unknown reasons, a small percentage of evidently normal couples fail to conceive. Under such circumstances, any woman can be expected to react with feelings of frustration and depression. She should not also have to deal with the implication that no matter how much she may protest that she wants a baby, the reason that she cannot is her underlying subconscious wish not to be pregnant. There has been no meaningful documentation to support the hypothesis that psychogenic factors cause nonphysiological female infertility. Furthermore, there is no evidence, other than isolated case reports, that psychotherapy has ever been effective in causing previously infertile women to conceive. If they can afford it, today a couple with the diagnosis of idiopathic infertility is far more likely to be offered the option of entering the brave new world of high-tech fertility techniques.

ASSISTED REPRODUCTIVE TECHNOLOGY: IVF AND OTHER ACRONYMS

The birth of a baby girl in mid-1978 to a British woman whose tubes were irreparably obstructed signaled the beginning of a new era in infertility therapy, that of "assisted reproductive technology." Although the successful transfer of early embryos from one animal to another had been done before the turn of the century and millions of cattle have been produced by a combination of artificial insemination with embryo transfer, this was the first time the scientific feat of conceiving a human child outside of the mother's body and then placing it in the uterus to complete its embryonic development had occurred. After 12 years of research and many unsuccessful attempts, British gynecologist Patrick Steptoe and Cambridge University physiologist Robert Edwards successfully established a pregnancy in 30-year-old Lesley Brown through **in vitro** (outside the body) **fertilization** (IVF). Just prior to ovulation, an oocyte was removed from Mrs. Brown's ovary by laparoscopic surgery. The ripe ovum was combined for fertilization with her husband's sperm in what the newspapers called a "test tube"—actually a sterile petri dish. The fertilized egg was cultured in appropriate nutrient media until it reached the eight-cell stage, when it was reintroduced for implantation into Mrs. Brown's hormonally prepared uterus. The embryo burrowed into the endometrial lining and survived. Nine months later, heralded by banner headlines, the first "test-tube baby" was delivered by cesarean section.

Since Louise Joy Brown was born, IVF has become an accepted method of infertility therapy throughout the world. The success rate, initially very low and still not that good, has improved. By 2000, 60,000 American children and 300,000 worldwide had been conceived through in vitro fertilization. There are more than 300 IVF programs in the United States alone. Infertility treatment has become a major medical industry.

Originally, IVF treatment was limited to women with tubal obstruction or destruction, but during the 1980s the therapy (although different programs have different selection criteria) was extended to include unexplained infertility, endometriosis, pelvic adhesions, congenital or DES–induced anomalies of the reproductive tract, immunologic causes for infertility, women whose partners have low sperm count, and women age 40 or older (at about half of the fertility centers).

The IVF Procedure

Even including the technological advancements of the past decades, the fundamentals of IVF appear straightforward and simple: the ovaries are hyperstimulated with agents to induce follicle formation, follicle development is monitored daily, the ovum is removed from the ovary just prior to ovulation, it is fertilized in vitro, and then it is placed into the uterine cavity for implantation. In actual practice, however, the procedure is medically complex and far from simple. Although different IVF programs vary in their protocols, the basic steps of IVF are described as follows.

Ovulation Induction and Monitoring. Originally, IVF procedures were done without stimulating ovulation. Currently, the use of drugs is routine, although a few reports indicate that the success rate for unstimulated cycles is virtually equal to that for stimulated cycles. The fertility drugs to cause superovulation may be clomiphene alone; HMG and clomiphene, either in combination or sequentially; HMG alone; purified FSH in combination with HMG; or GnRH followed by HMG. Whichever regimen is used, the follicular development is monitored by the daily measurement of serum estradiol levels and ultrasound imaging of the growing follicles. When several follicles are at least 14 mm or greater in diameter and the estradiol level is 300 picograms/ml per follicle, a single injection of human chorionic gonadotropin (HCG) is given to mimic the LH surge and induce the final maturation of the follicles.

Oocyte Retrieval

The next step is to retrieve the oocytes from the ovary through aspiration, a procedure often called harvesting the ova. Ovum recovery was formerly performed by laparoscopy under general anesthesia, but ultrasound-guided techniques have largely replaced the laparoscopic method at most IVF centers. The routes for oocyte aspiration may be through the abdomen and the urinary bladder (transabdominal-transvesical), through the urethra and the urinary bladder (transurethral), or into the body cavity through the vagina (transvaginal). In the transvaginal approach, preferred by many IVF programs, a needle with a bore large enough to aspirate all the mature follicles is attached to a real-time ultrasound scanner in the vagina. Guided by the ultrasound image, the needle is passed through the posterior cul-de-sac into the ovary to remove the oocytes by suction. The recovered oocytes quickly are identified under the microscope by an embryologist and are evaluated for their maturation. Any that are assessed as mature (identified by a loose and expanded cumulus oöphorus and evidence of the first polar body) are incubated in culture medium for 4–6 hours before the sperm are added; immature oocytes are incubated for a minimum of 24 hours to ensure full fertilizability.

Fertilization

While the oocytes are incubating, the partner provides a semen specimen. The spermatozoa are prepared by washing, centrifugation, and the "swim-up" technique to isolate the most motile sperm. About 50,000–100,000 of the prepared and now capacitated sperm are added to each dish of culture medium that contains an oocyte. Sixteen to 17 hours later (usually timed for the next morning after insemination), each oocyte is examined for signs of fertilization. Once a sperm enters an oocyte, it completes its second meiotic division, so the presence of a second polar body and two pronuclei indicates that fertilization has occurred. When the sperm count is very low, micromanipulation of the oocyte to ease the path of a sperm is likely to be done. The zona pellucida may be slit, partially dissected, or lasered, or the sperm may be microinjected into the oocyte (Hill et al., 1991).

Embryo Transfer

Fertilization is followed by the first cleavage division to the two-celled stage (31–43 hours, average 37 hours); the second cleavage to the four-celled stage occurs several hours later (37–51 hours, average 44 hours). Embryos are most often transferred between 48 and 80 hours after fertilization when they are four to eight cells. Although the transfer of more than one embryo increases the chances of implantation and pregnancy, generally no more than four, or possibly five, embryos are placed in the uterus to decrease the risk of multiple pregnancies. The embryos are loaded into a catheter and transferred through the cervical os into the woman's uterus without anesthesia. When more than four embryos exist, most programs offer the option of cryopreserving (freezing) them, although the survival rate of frozen embryos is estimated at about 50%. The woman remains flat for the next 6 hours, is discharged, and is told to remain at rest as much as possible for the next 2–3 days. Frequent pregnancy tests may begin in 10 days; it will be 2 weeks—likely to be an agonizing wait for the woman—before rising HCG levels can confirm a positive diagnosis of pregnancy. Because the drugs used to stimulate superovulation are believed to alter the estrogen-progesterone ratio, progesterone suppositories or injections beginning on the days of transfer are usually given to supplement the luteal phase of the uterine endometrium. The actual value of such supplementation to endometrial support has not been proven.

Results of IVF

The success rate for IVF programs should be easy to measure: what is the percentage of live babies that result from treatment? Each year, the Centers for Disease Control prepares a national report and a national summary table based on data provided by the 300 fertility clinics in operation in that year. Most of the clinics are members of the Society for Assisted Reproductive Technology. This group's data make up the 1997 national summary table for cycles started in 1997. (Given that the data for final outcomes of pregnancies conceived in December of 1997 were not known until late 1998 and additional time was then required to collect and analyze the data and prepare the report, the success or nonsuccess rates may have changed since 1997.) According to the 1997 summary, in women under 35, the number of live births was about 30%, about 26% in women between 35 and 37, 17% in women 38–40, and about 8% in women over 40. The live birth rate using frozen embryos was 16%, and the success rate using donated eggs, usually from a young and healthy woman, was about the same as when nondonated eggs were transferred. The fertility clinic tables displayed in the CDC national report provide information by state, city, and clinic. Comparisons between clinics should be made with caution, however. The data are self-reports, and a clinic could report and advertise rates many times greater by using different criteria for what constitutes a pregnancy than the "take-home baby" rate. For example, some programs would count a transient and unsustained rise in ICG as a "preclinical" or "biochemical" pregnancy, although the pregnancy is resorbed or lost (miscarried) prior to 4 weeks, when ultrasound can identify the gestational sac and fetal heartbeat of a true "clinical" pregnancy. Both preclinical and clinical pregnancies (a quarter of which are also spontaneously aborted) may be counted in the clinic's statistics as pregnancy success. Or, an IVF center could inflate its pregnancy rates because it selected as patients only the cases with the best possibility for success and screened out all the difficult ones. Conversely, a clinic could have lower rates because it specialized in the cases with little hope of success. Before starting an IVF program, an infertile couple should get an explanation of how the clinic's figures are derived. They also should ask about the credentials of its practitioners, who should be board certified in reproductive endocrinology, and find out how many oocyte retrievals and embryo transfers they already have done.

The bottom line is that IVF, even with all its current advances and permutations, is a gamble. The odds of success of IVF treatment are set not only by the clinic's record but also by a number of additional factors—the couple's age; the man's fertility; the experience and skill of the clinic's physicians, embryologist, and other staff; the quality control in the laboratory culture media and apparatus; and a huge measure of pure luck. Even when human reproduction takes place without technological assistance—the natural way—it is not particularly efficient. There are estimates that in any given cycle, only 20%–30% of fertilized eggs from normally fertile couples will actually continue on to produce a live baby. All of the rest become preimplantation losses of the embryo, never even recognized by the woman because her menstrual period arrives at the normal time. Given that Mother Nature only has a 20%–30% success rate, failure to achieve a viable pregnancy through IVF, even after two or three attempts, *is not a personal failure* (although it is frequently seen that way by the woman) but realistically could be viewed as a very expensive way to have a miscarriage. Starting from the beginning of the menstrual cycle to the results of the pregnancy tests 2 weeks after embryo transfer, each attempt costs $8,000–$12,000, with many parts of the procedure uninsured.

If a couple is able to undergo more than three attempts, there is evidence that the chances of achieving a pregnancy increase. The group at the Jones Institute for Reproductive Medicine of the Eastern Virginia Medical School, one of the nation's oldest, largest, and most respected IVF programs, has reported that their cumulative pregnancy rates were 32.75% after one cycle of treatment, 50.75% after two cycles, and 63.75% after three cycles. IVF, however, carries physical risks for the woman, high anxiety levels and stress for the couple, and constitutes a huge financial burden. Few couples would have the stamina to go through it six times.

Additional Techniques of "Assisted Reproduction"

Not very long ago, the last chance for an infertile couple to make a baby was through in vitro fertilization as described previously. Now, to assist in the pursuit of a baby, a myriad of IVF technological spin-offs have been developed. Today the infertility business is a multimillion dollar international growth industry. Eggs can be donated from one woman to another, menopausal women can deliver a baby conceived with the egg of a younger woman, embryos can be flushed out of the uterus of one woman to be transferred to another woman's uterus, frozen for later use, and when multiple gestations occur, several can be selectively aborted. The technology of reproductive manipulation has progressed with amazing speed.

GIFT and ZIFT. When the sperm count is low or there may be a problem with sperm motility and the woman has at least one open fallopian tube, **gamete intrafallopian transfer (GIFT)** is an alternative to IVF. GIFT is similar to IVF in that superovulation induction and the aspiration of oocytes take place, but fertilization by the sperm does not take place in vitro in the laboratory. Instead, the mixture of sperm and the oocytes are loaded into a catheter and, through laparoscopy, two oocytes and about 100,000 motile sperm are introduced for a short distance into the fimbriated end of each fallopian tube. Thus, fertilization takes place in the body *(in vivo),* which distinguishes the procedure from IVF. The advantage of GIFT is that it is less complicated; there is less need for embryologists and sophisticated laboratory apparatus and no need for embryo transfer, so the procedure is less expensive. Also, it appears to be more "natural" in that fertilization occurs where it normally takes place. A major disadvantage is the necessity for laparoscopy under general anesthesia, which increases risk, potential complications, and discomfort.

Zygote intrafallopian transfer (ZIFT) is similar to GIFT in that the transfer is made into the fallopian tubes, but fertilization takes place in vitro as in IVF and it is the fertilized eggs, or zygotes, that are transferred. ZIFT is a variation used when it is deemed important to get direct evidence of the fertilizing capacity of the oocytes and sperm. ICSI (pronounced ick-see) is **intercytoplasmic sperm injection,** in which a single sperm is injected into a single egg to fertilize it. The technique, which has been in use since the early 1990s, enables any man who produces sperm, even though the sperm have not been ejaculated and have been removed from the testes by the physician, to father a child if the procedure works. The method costs about at least $10,000 per attempt. Some infertility researchers have raised questions about the popular technique, citing concerns about the possibility of chromosomal defects in the ICSI babies (Kolata, 1999). Beyond ZIFT are two other modifications of the combination of outside-body fertilization and intrafallopian transfer designated as tubal pre-embryo transfer (TPET) and pronuclear stage tubal transfer (PROST). "Pre-embryo" is a term recently coined to encompass the developmental stages of the fertilized egg—zygote, morula, blastocyst—that occur prior to implantation, although there is no biological justification for its use. Once the oocyte has been fertilized, it is not pre-anything, but is an "embryo" until the beginning of the ninth week of gestation, when it is termed a "fetus" until delivery.

Wombs for Rent. A more controversial method of obtaining a child when the husband is fertile but the wife cannot conceive is through the use of a hired ovary and uterus, or surrogate mother. A healthy fertile woman is paid by the couple to undergo a pregnancy achieved by artificial insemination with the husband's semen. The baby thus conceived would have half its genetic makeup from the husband of the couple and the other half from the woman who is donating her body for 9 months, generally for a fee paid by the infertile couple who also pay the broker who found the surrogate. After delivery, the baby is relinquished by the surrogate to the couple and the wife files for adoption. The practice is condemned by those who find the notion of women as incubators unacceptable. It also has become a legal dilemma, since few states have passed laws to regulate any of the reproductive technologies, let alone surrogacy. Nevertheless, since the late 1970s, there are said to be 4,000 babies born in the United States as a result of the "traditional" surrogate using a husband's sperm and a surrogate's egg. The newer form of surrogacy is the "gestational" type, offered to women who have functional ovaries but nonfunctional uteri or for whom pregnancy would be too great a health risk. In gestational surrogacy, the infertile couple creates embryos from their own oocytes and sperm and then hires another woman to carry the transferred embryo(s) to term. In contrast to the traditional surrogate, the gestational surrogate is genetically unrelated to the fetus.

Maybe many people have adjusted to these kinds of transactions, but the questions persist. Does "commercial" surrogacy—paying one woman to carry someone else's fetus—amount to buying a baby, and should such contracts be banned? What happens if a surrogate mother wants to keep the child; does the contract she signed to give it up have legal standing? And what about the gestational surrogate who wants custody of the child? Does her lack of a biological tie to the child she bore lessen her claim? Suppose the couple who contracted with the surrogate back out and change their minds because of illness or death? If the child is born with physical or mental defects, what then? What if the contracting couple divorce, the biological father wants to raise the child alone, the surrogate says she wants a stable, two-parent home for the child, and all three "parents" battle for custody? Each of these situations is real and has occurred; courts and judges already have had to decide the answers and are likely to be faced with more complicated cases in the future.

Another twist is the altruistic surrogate—a woman who is not paid for surrogacy. The surrogate could be unrelated or could be a close relative or sibling who bears the child and complicates the usual patterns of kinship. But surrogacy, even without a financial reward, still is troubling to many, especially because of several unusual cases. In a small U.S. city in 1991, a 42-year-old school librarian gave birth to twins conceived from her daughter's oocytes, fertilized in vitro by her son-in-law's sperm. A similar case occurred in South Africa in 1987, when a 48-year-old woman gave birth to her daughter's triplets. Both these women were surrogates for their own grandchildren. In Italy, a 20-year-old daughter loaned her uterus for the fetus produced by the ovum of her 48-year-old mother and the sperm of her 35-year-old stepfather. She gave birth to her own half brother—a situation termed "unacceptable experimentation" by the Vatican.

A variation of surrogacy is nonsurgical embryo transfer, a procedure in which a woman who acts as an ovum donor is artificially inseminated by the sperm of the husband of an infertile woman. Four days later, assuming fertilization has occurred in vivo, the surrogate's uterus is flushed out with saline (uterine lavage), and the conceptus is recovered and transferred by catheter into the uterus of the infertile wife. This technique, exactly the same as the one extensively used by cattle breeders to allow ordinary cows to bear the calves of the most expensive purebred supercows, was first used in 1983. Although it has the advantage of avoiding surgery to aspirate oocytes, uterine lavage largely has been replaced by the use of egg donors and in vitro fertilization. This eliminates the possibility of a failed uterine lavage and a retained pregnancy in the donor.

Oocyte Donation.

If a woman has a uterus but dysfunctional or nonfunctional ovaries, oocyte donation is yet another option for a woman wanting a baby to carry through pregnancy and deliver.

There are about 30 firms nationwide with a database of healthy young women, allegedly screened for health, intelligence, education, and medical history, who will go through the process of ovulation induction and oocyte retrieval to donate their oocytes for the going rate of $2,500–$3,000. Some of them are college students who say they need the money to continue their education. There are also web sites that advertise ova for sale. But in an echo of the "Repository for Germinal Choice" that offered Nobel prize winners' sperm for artificial insemination so that brilliant children with a high IQ could be fathered, in 1999 an enterprising fashion photographer (and Arabian horse breeder) placed pictures of beautiful models on the Internet and offered their eggs for sale on auction for up to $150,000. The web site received millions of hits immediately, and, according to a newspaper report, one bid for $42,000 appeared to be legitimate. Although federal law does not allow the purchase and sale of human organs, sperm and egg sales are legal. And evidently there are prospective parents who would actually purchase donor eggs from a web site with pictures of glamorous women. They should be aware of basic genetics. An ovum from a beautiful woman or a sperm from a "smart" man guarantees neither beauty nor intelligence in the offspring.

Oocyte donation by younger women provides a possibility for the older, less fertile woman to carry and bear children. The donation technique thus has, in addition, enabled the dubious achievement of establishing pregnancy in menopausal women—to several of them in their late 40s, to a few in their 50s, and at least to one woman in her 60s. The "biological clock" has not only been slowed by reproductive technology, but to some extent, appears to have become irrelevant.

Frozen Embryos.

Early in IVF technology, there was objection to the practice of removing as many oocytes from the woman's ovary as possible to be inseminated and incubated because of concern for the unused and possibly discarded embryos. But some of that concern was allayed by the ability, pioneered in Australia in 1984, to successfully store embryos through cryopreservation. An Australian research team, led by Alan O. Trounson, director of the Center for Early Human Development in Melbourne, reported on the birth of a healthy baby after an eight-cell embryo had been frozen for 6 months, thawed, and transferred to the mother's uterus. The ability to successfully freeze and thaw viable embryos (at least 50% of the time) so that they may be implanted at a later, perhaps more propitious time has removed the need for the physical ordeal and the expense of successive superovulation and oocyte retrieval in follow-up embryo transfer attempts when the first one fails. With current techniques, only zygotes in the pronuclear stage or embryos can be frozen because freezing and thawing disrupts the fragile cytoplasmic membrane of an unfertilized egg. But researchers are developing techniques for freezing unfertilized oocytes. It is now possible to extract a woman's immature oocytes when she is in her prime of fertility and "bank" them for her future use. Or oocyte banks, along with sperm banks, could be utilized by infertile couples to make an embryo.

Embryo freezing has raised thorny issues. If the parents die, what should be done with the stored "orphans"? Who has the rights to the embryos after a divorce if the wife wants them implanted and the husband refuses? Are the embryos joint property, or should they be subjects for a custody decision? What should be done with the embryos if the center storing them goes out of business? These cases, too, are real and have turned into court battles.

Obviously, the problems generated by the techniques of assisted reproduction can get very complicated. Using current technology, a pregnancy could have as many as five participants: the sperm donor, the egg donor, the surrogate who bears and delivers the child, and the couple who has paid for the other three and will raise the child. Even forgetting for the moment the potential legalities that might have to be sorted out, what consequences might this have for the child? On the positive side, a very happy, healthy, loving family may be the result. On the other hand, as bioethicist Ruth Macklin points out, we have been forced to rethink the concepts of "mother," "father," and "family." Adjustment to adoption has been shown

to be psychologically difficult for children, and adopted children often seek to find their biological parents despite being in a loving family. Although it might be easier to keep the circumstances of artificial insemination, surrogacy, or ovum donation secret from a child, the results of having such secrets revealed could be emotionally devastating for everyone involved. But would it be reasonable, asks Macklin, to abolish these practices, which have changed our traditional concept of the family, because they have potentially negative consequences?

It is clear that as one remarkable advance of assisted conception has followed another, the accompanying ethical, social, and legal problems have lagged behind. The questions remain. Perhaps one final question should be asked: merely because a medical technique *can* be done, *should* it be done?

REFERENCES

Fédération CECOS, Schwartz, D., & Mayaux, M. (1982). Female fecundity as a function of age. *New England Journal of Medicine, 306*(7), 404–406.

Gilbert, W. M., Nesbitt, T. S., & Danielsen, B. (1999). Childbearing beyond age 40: Pregnancy outcome in 24,032 cases. *Obstetrics and Gynecology, 93*(1), 9–14.

Guzick, D. S., Carson, S. A., Contifaris, C., et al. (1999). Efficacy of superovulation and intrauterine insemination in the treatment of infertility. *New England Journal of Medicine, 340*(3), 177–183.

Guzick, D. S., Wilkes, C., & Jones, H. W., Jr. (1986). Cumulative pregnancy rates for in vitro fertilization. *Fertility and Sterility, 46,* 663.

Hill, D. L., Adler, D., Rothman, C., et al. (1991). Micromanipulation in a center for reproductive medicine. *Fertility and Sterility, 55*(1), 36–38.

Hutchinson-Williams, K. A. (1990). Induction of ovulation. In N. G. Kase, A. B. Weingold, & D. M. Gershenson (Eds.), *Principles and practice of clinical gynecology* (2nd ed.). New York: Churchill Livingstone.

Kolata, G. (1999, March 30). New questions about popular fertilization technique. *The New York Times,* D10.

Macklin, R. (1991, January/February). Artificial means of reproduction and our understanding of the family. *Hastings Center Report, 1,* 5–11.

Menning, B. E. (1988). *Infertility: A guide for the childless couple* (2nd ed.). Englewood Cliffs, NJ: Prentice-Hall.

Nestler, J. E., Jakubowicz, D. J., Reamer, P., et al. (1999). Ovulatory and metabolic effects of D-chiro-inositol in the polycystic ovary syndrome. *New England Journal of Medicine, 340*(17), 1314–1320.

Speroff, L., Glass, R. H., & Kase, N. G. (1989). *Clinical gynecologic endocrinology and infertility* (4th ed.). Baltimore: Williams & Wilkins.

Trounson, A. (1985). *Clinical progress and new research developments in embryo and egg cryopreservation*. Abstract presented at the Fourth World Congress on In Vitro Fertilization, Melbourne, Australia.

Tulandi, T., Plouffe, L., & McInnes, R. (1982). Effect of saliva on sperm motility and activity. *Fertility and Sterility, 38*(6), 581–589.

van Noord-Zaadstra, B. M., Looman, C. W. N., Alsbach, H., et al. (1991). Delaying childbearing: Effect of age on fecundity and outcome of pregnancy. *British Medical Journal, 302,* 1361–1365.

Ventura, S. J., Martin, J. A., Curtin, S. C., Mathews, T. J., &

Park, M. M. (2000). Births: Final data for 1998. *National Vital Statistics Report, 48*(3), 1–100.

Witkin, S. S., & Toth, A. (1983). Relationship between genital tract infections, sperm antibodies in seminal fluid, and infertility. *Fertility and Sterility, 40*(6), 805–808.

Yanagimachi, R., Yanagimachi, H., & Roberts, F. J. (1976). The use of zona-free animal ova as a test system for the assessment of the fertilizing capacity of the human spermatozoa. *Biology of Reproduction, 15,* 471–476.

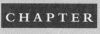

13

PROBLEMS OF FERTILITY—CONTRACEPTION

KEY TERMS

Abortion

Basal body temperature
  (BBT)

Cervical cap

Coitus interruptus

Condom

Depo-Provera

Intrauterine device (IUD)

Minipill

Oral contraceptive

Thrombus

Tubal ligation

VACTERL syndrome

Vaginal diaphragm

Vasectomy

There are more than 6 billion people on earth and at the rate the population is growing, the United Nations projects that the world population could reach 10.7 billion in 50 years. If we think there are problems on the planet now with worldwide malnutrition, starvation, environmental pollution, and a myriad of additional economic and social ills, we have but to wait. For many years the United States led the world in contraceptive research and development and provided aid in family planning to lesser developed countries. Unless it suddenly became in the national interest to focus a massive research effort on contraception, genuine improvements in contraceptive methods are not likely to be available in the near, or even the distant, future. Our options in birth control are currently limited and even fewer than they were several decades ago. It is possible to find a means of preventing pregnancy that is, if not ideal at least fairly compatible with the different needs of different people.

We have learned to be skeptical about scientific "breakthroughs" in contraceptive technology, particularly concerning claims of increased effectiveness and safety. When oral contraceptives were developed in the early 1960s, it was believed that the ideal method of birth control had indeed been discovered. The pill was said to be totally effective, completely safe, easy to take, inexpensive, reversible, and did not interfere in any way with the sex act. All other methods suddenly became outmoded as millions of women went "on the pill." After a few years, the bubble burst. The oral contraceptive turned out to have only some of its presumed qualities. The combined pill is unquestionably effective and easy to use and has been studied extensively for safety, effectiveness, advantages, and disadvantages. Its complete safety and reversibility are still suspect, however, and pills are not currently covered by most health insurance, making them costly to use.

Then, the **intrauterine device (IUD)** was described as the ideal contraceptive: it, too, was unrelated to intercourse, and it had an added advantage—once inserted it could be totally ignored. So easy—there was not even a daily pill to take. The side effects and complications associated with IUD usage, however, made this method less than ideal for many women. Now Norplant, a device implanted under the skin of the upper arm that lasts for up to 5 years, is touted as the most effective contraceptive ever marketed. The presence of this device, like an IUD, can be ignored and forgotten, and no major adverse complications have as yet been attributed to it. Severe problems with Norplant do not occur in most women, but common side effects such as menstrual irregularities, headache, weight gain, nausea, acne, and breast tenderness remove this contraceptive, too, from ideal status.

The truly ideal contraceptive method would not seesaw between safety and effectiveness but would be both completely free of any present or future health hazard and completely effective in preventing an unwanted pregnancy. It would be completely reversible; fertility would be fully restored when the method was discontinued. It would be cheap enough for anyone to afford, distributed and marketed so that anyone could easily obtain it, and it would require no medical intervention or prescription. It would be so convenient to use that it would require a minimum of motivation, and it would be unrelated to the act of sexual intercourse—there would be nothing to put in or put on to interfere with lovemaking. The responsibility for using the method would be shared by both men and women, and it would meet everyone's cultural, religious, political, and philosophical requirements for controlling fertility. Not only does this paragon of pregnancy prevention not exist, but it should be obvious that no single method of contraception could biologically or sociologically ever have all the above attributes. What we really need, and could settle for, are a variety of new and improved methods of contraception that fulfill more of the criteria or at least strike a better balance among them. The choice between safety and effectiveness should not have to be made by any woman or man. Currently, there are a rather limited number of contraceptive techniques, all with advantages and disadvantages, and none that is free of potential side effects or complications, either medical or emotional. No method except sexual abstinence is 100% effective and reversible. No method that is highly effective, convenient, and unrelated to intercourse is completely safe. No technique that is completely safe is that easy to use. The choice of which method to use depends on the kind of trade-offs an individual is prepared to make. Every woman has to decide, based on her lifestyle, her experiences, her personal preferences, and her right to do what she wants with her body, which attributes of a particular method are most important. There is no best way of birth control. The only best method is the one that is chosen and is consistently used—the technique that a woman feels is right, natural, and comfortable for her and her partner.

A woman should not feel chained to a particular method throughout her reproductive lifetime. As circumstances and attitudes change, so will the requirements for a contraceptive. When intercourse is infrequent or unexpected, it may not be necessary to use a method that provides constant daily protection. A married couple who is delaying or spacing their family may be more concerned about reversibility than effectiveness; a woman who does not ever want children or couples who have completed their families could decide on sterilization. Not infrequently, the choice of a contraceptive method depends on the availability. For adolescents or many unmarried young women, ambivalent and anxious about "planning" for sex, the psychological costs of obtaining and using birth control are already very high. Unless there is a family planning agency in the community, their access to medical contraception is limited, and getting drugstore methods can be embarrassing.

But the bottom line of birth control is the irrefutable fact that unprotected sexual intercourse, sooner or later, causes pregnancy. Engaging in sex carries the assumption of risk of pregnancy and the responsibility for preventing it. Each woman knows how she alone would be able to cope with the consequences of an unplanned pregnancy or the alternatives of abortion or childbirth. If the prevention of pregnancy is important, she has to take the necessary steps to avoid it.

It is not possible to choose a preferred method in the absence of complete and accurate information about all existing techniques. In the past, when oral contraceptives and IUDs were prescribed more often than any other methods, women who relied on their physicians for advice resentfully claimed that they were never told that anything more than "nuisance" side effects accompanied their usage. All of the emphasis was placed on the convenience and effectiveness of those two methods, while any considerations of risk were soft-pedaled. Some doctors rarely recommended use of or provided information about any other types of contraception. Although much more is known today about the benefits and the risks of hormonal contraceptives and IUDs, women still may be steered away from other methods because of the personal preferences or biases of their physicians or health professionals.

Oral contraceptives, Norplant, and intrauterine devices all are undeniably highly effective in preventing pregnancy. What proves most surprising to many people is that *all major contraceptive methods* (that is, legitimate means of fertility control rather than hope and prayer) can be *approximately equally effective in avoiding an accidental pregnancy*. The major difference is that the effectiveness of methods other than pills, Norplant, and IUDs requires more *effort* on the part of the user to achieve the same success.

THEORETICAL EFFECTIVENESS AND USE-EFFECTIVENESS

The effectiveness of any method of birth control refers to its ability to prevent pregnancy. Oral contraceptives are known to be highly effective. All that is required of a woman to achieve this high efficacy is to swallow one every day. As long as she remembers to do that, the chances of her conceiving are extremely small. If she forgets to take her pills, however, or runs out of them without another pack handy, or for any other reason neglects taking them, she is not going to be as well protected by the pill. The *theoretical effectiveness* of a method is its maximum success rate when it is used correctly, perfectly, and without error. The actual *use-effectiveness* of a method refers to all the possible ways it is used by everyone—not only properly, but also incorrectly, carelessly, and not according to instructions.

Any ranking of contraceptive effectiveness generally places hormonal contraceptives and IUDs up at the top of the list along with sterilization and abstinence. Such methods as the diaphragm, the condom, and vaginal foam, while rated above rhythm, douching, and jumping up and down after intercourse, are usually considered well below the pill and IUD in effectiveness. Diaphragms have long been called "baby makers"; condoms are said to burst, leak, or otherwise prove untrustworthy; and spermicides are said to have a failure rate that makes them virtually useless for women who must not become pregnant. Such quantitative comparisons between common methods of birth control can be very misleading, however, because what is usually being quoted is the theoretical effectiveness of the pill and IUDs, and the use-effectiveness of all the other methods.

Measurements of contraceptive effectiveness are based on statistics gathered from major studies published in scientific literature over the past 40 years or so. These studies have been conducted at various times in many different countries on groups of people who varied in age, marital status, income, education, and in motivation to use the method. When all the results are lumped together, obviously a very wide range of effectiveness for a contraceptive technique or device is possible. The diaphragm, for example, is often said to be only about 80% effective. This could mean that if 100 fertile women get a diaphragm and use it for a year, at the end of that period, 20 of them may be pregnant—a statistic that would discourage almost anyone from using a diaphragm. But this takes into account all the ways in which a diaphragm is used—well fitted, properly, and consistently or poorly fitted, forgotten, and neglected.

Table 13–1 illustrates the theoretical effectiveness and the use-effectiveness of the various methods of birth control. Note the great latitude in effectiveness for most techniques. The ability of almost all contraceptives (omitting only Norplant and the IUD) to prevent pregnancy is dependent on the person using the method. With motivation and consistency, the success of a diaphragm or condom in avoiding conception compares very favorably with the pill or IUD. Using two methods together, such as the diaphragm and a condom, or a condom with spermicidal jelly or foam, dramatically reduces the failure rate. Even vaginal spermicides, long believed to be disastrously ineffective, have an equivalent success rate when used properly and have been used by many couples for long periods of time without a problem.

ORAL CONTRACEPTIVES

In June 1960, the Food and Drug Administration (FDA) approved for safety and efficacy a little pink pill called Enovid-10, produced by Searle & Company. Enovid had actually been on the market for several years, prescribed for threatened spontaneous abortion and menstrual disorders, but its introduction as an **oral contraceptive** was the start of a new era in birth control—chemical contraception. Other brands soon appeared, and what generically became known as "The Pill" rapidly achieved enormous popularity. The social impact of what was hailed as a breakthrough in effective, easy, and safe contraception was so far-reaching that people began to speak of a "pill revolution" and then later of a "sexual revolution."

Never before in history has a drug treatment been so widely prescribed on a continuing basis to so many people who were normal and healthy. There were some scientists who had misgivings about the prolonged administration of sex steroids and questioned the wisdom of a daily hormonal onslaught on the basic female endocrine mechanisms. There were some doctors who were reluctant or refused to advise the use of oral contraceptives. Almost everyone else, however, was extraordinarily pleased with the pills—the drug companies that produced them at a substantial profit, the federal agencies that sanctioned their use, the doctors who prescribed them, and the women who took them as if Swallow Me were written on every tablet. By 1962, 2 million American women were on the pill; by 1965, oral contraceptives were being ingested in this country alone at the annual rate of more than 2,000 tons. Pharmaceutical company stocks rose as "buy birth control" became the watchword on Wall Street. And society at large was gratified by continued progress toward a currently popular goal, the slowing of the population rate.

Table 13–1 Contraceptive Effectiveness: Theoretical and Actual Use Rates[a]

Method	Theoretical Effectiveness	Use-Effectiveness (range)
Abstinence (total)	0	0
Tubal ligation	0.04–0.2	0.4
Norplant and Norplant-2 implant	0.04	0.04
Vasectomy	0.15	0.15
Oral contraceptive (combined) (all types)	0.34–1.2	3–10
Progestin-only pill	0.5	5–10
IUD		
Progestasert	2.0	3.0
Copper T380A	0.8	3.0
Condom	2	14
Condom plus spermicide	1	5
Female condom	5	21
Diaphragm with jelly or cream	3	2–20
Cervical cap	3	2–20
Spermicidal foam or cream	3	2–30
Sponge	9–11[b]	18–28
Coitus interruptus (withdrawal)	4	18–25
Rhythm (calendar only)	13	21
Natural family planning (symptothermal)	2.5	5–40
Chance	85	85

Sources: Trussell & Kowal, 1998

[a]Number of pregnancies per 100 women during the first year of use

[b]More effective for nulliparous women

It is not surprising that women needed little encouragement to go on the pill. The rewards were many. For centuries the idea of swallowing something to prevent or eradicate pregnancy had caused women to dose themselves with ineffective and often dangerous potions and nostrums. Now the magic pill had really been found. For young single women, it was such a nice, tidy, guilt-free way of avoiding pregnancy. The pill was completed dissociated from sexual activity, so there was no need to plan ahead for sex—no diaphragm and big tube of jelly in the purse, no other equipment to carry—to destroy the illusion of, or somehow mess up, a completely spontaneous encounter. It was true that there appeared to be some minor side effects associated with usage, but the biological advantage of almost perfect effectiveness plus the added benefit of the elimination of menstrual pain and bleeding for many users outweighed any disadvantages. Younger women, both single and married, took to the pill with alacrity, and a new kind of social ideology arose—that the entire responsibility for birth control belonged to women. But even that seemed to be liberating. A woman, after all, is the one who bears the burden of an unwanted pregnancy, and she should have complete control of her reproductive capacity without needing assurances that her partner would "take care of her."

Any anxieties about safety were relieved not only by women's physicians but also by numerous articles in popular magazines and newspapers. With titles such as "What You Should Know about Birth Control Pills," "How Safe Are the Birth Control Pills?" and "Birth Control Pills: The Full Story," *Vogue, Redbook, Ladies' Home Journal,* and *Good Housekeeping* reassured readers that no adverse effects had as yet become apparent in the years of clinical trials since 1956. Later, the popular media were to sensationalize the risks of oral contraception; originally, the media were instrumental in allaying women's fears about it.

By the mid-1960s, it had become apparent that not only nuisance effects but also serious complications were possible for pill users. Reports that oral contraceptives were related to clotting disorders, strokes, and a number of other serious complications resulted in a decline in usage. Congressional hearings were held to determine the safety of oral contraceptives, and there were warnings and speculations concerning the possible risks to health. It also became evident that the adverse affects were estrogen related. When new formulations containing less estrogen came on the market, renewed confidence in the pill's safety resulted in a regaining of popularity. In time, the pre-warning levels of pill usage were again reached and exceeded (Figure 13–1).

Sales of the pill in the United States climbed until 1976 when, in response to additional evidence of health hazards associated with usage, a sharp decrease

occurred. Concern for safety was illustrated by a Gallup poll taken in July 1977, when the pill was believed to be unsafe by 62% of the women and 43% of the men surveyed. But the drop in pill sales ended in the early 1980s coinciding, not unexpectedly, with several studies that reported the noncontraceptive health benefits of pill taking and claiming that the risks were exaggerated. With the publicity and wide dissemination given to the studies as well as the introduction of lower-dose formulations, pill usage underwent a revival. The number of women taking oral contraceptives in the United States rose from 8.4 million in 1982 to more than 18 million in 1995 (Rosenberg, Waugh, & Long, 1995). Women are remaining on oral contraceptives for longer periods of time, with an average duration of use of 5 years. Birth control pills are the leading form of contraception for unmarried women, and next to sterilization, the favored method for married women as well. Worldwide, an estimated 70 million women are on the pill.

Mechanisms of Action of Oral Contraceptives

Although hormonal contraceptives are commonly referred to as "the pill," they are not all alike. They differ in their composition, their potency, and the side

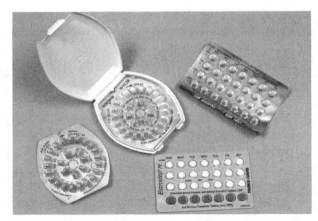

Figure 13–1   Some of the various brands of birth control pills.

effects that they produce. Depending on the amounts and kinds of steroids they contain, the pills even differ in their contraceptive effectiveness. All combination pills are composed of a synthetic estrogen and one of nine synthetic progestational agents, or progestins. Most are available in both 21- and 28-tablet packages. The progestin-only, or minipills, contain a low dose of one of the progestins, have a lower theoretical effectiveness rate than the combined pills, and are supplied in 28- and 42-tablet packages. There have been no real changes in oral contraceptives since their introduction in 1960, but most of the manufacturers believe there is a marketing advantage in being able to provide a variety of pills, so they keep introducing combinations of different strengths and potencies. The low-dose and ultralow-dose pills became available in the late 1970s, and more recent entries in the production line are the "biphasic" and "triphasic" combinations that step up the dose of the progestin at intervals through the pill-taking cycle and provide a multicolor assortment of tablets during the month. Sales of Ortho Tri-Cyclen, on the market as a birth control pill since 1992, were approved by the FDA in 1996 for treatment of moderate acne. Although other pills are known to be just as successful in prevention of acne, only Ortho-McNeil, the manufacturer of Tri-Cyclen, has done the research to get FDA approval. When this triphasic was introduced, it was the seventh most popular pill. Intensive advertising on television shows and in teen magazines in 1998 created interest for the "pill for acne" and sales of the drug skyrocketed. By 2000, Ortho Tri-Cyclen was the number one birth control pill in popularity. It can have the same side effects—weight gain, headaches, irregular bleeding, and nausea—as other birth control pills. Currently, the most commonly used pills have about one-fifth the amount of estrogen that was present in the pills of the 1960s and about one-twentieth the dose of progestin.

When the combined estrogen and progestin pills are taken daily, they are believed to function primarily by suppressing the production of the releasing hormone from the hypothalamus. Because pituitary production of FSH and LH is then altered, normal follicle growth, maturation, and ovulation of an oocyte cannot occur. The synthetic steroids in the pills provide a constant amount of hormones, which are metabolized within 24 hours and which replace the normal cyclic production of a woman's own ovarian estrogen and progesterone. If for some reason the midcycle surge of LH is not completely inhibited, it is possible that an "escape" ovulation may occur. Secondary contraceptive mechanisms are then available from the progestational activity in the pills. Sperm penetration into the uterus is prevented by an alteration in cervical mucus, tubal transport of the ovum is slowed, and the endometrium undergoes changes that inhibit implantation. Progestin-only pills—the minipills—probably rarely prevent ovulation and exert their function primarily through these secondary effects.

The monthly bleeding that occurs while taking oral contraceptives is a false menstruation produced by estrogen and progesterone stimulation of the endometrium, followed by withdrawal of the hormones 7 days before the onset of bleeding. On a 21-day pill, no hormones and no pills are taken for 7 days, and on a 28-day regimen, the last 7 pills are of a different color and contain no hormones. Menstruation is provided by the pills so that a woman feels more natural and comfortable about taking them. If a woman wants to avoid menstruating while on vacation or during some special occasion, all she has to do is to take some extra pills from a different package—the menstruation offered by pills is so fabricated that it can be avoided completely.

Since ovulation and menstruation do not occur during pregnancy because of the inhibitory effect of the estrogen and progesterone from the placenta on the hypothalamus, it has been suggested that a woman who takes oral contraceptives and also does not ovulate is in a state of pseudopregnancy and can thus be physiologically equated with a pregnant woman. In this view, held by many including John Rock, a developer of oral contraceptives, the pills are the most "natural" form of birth control. After all, proponents of this notion suggest, early in human history, primitive women were likely to experience 10 or more pregnancies during their fertile years. In the absence of any contraception, all those pregnancies, plus the lack of menstruation as a result of breastfeeding afterward, probably meant that early women had only rare intervals of regular menstrual cycles. In contrast, this argument continues, contemporary women using any contraceptive other than the pill are having years of true menstrual cycles that could, in an evolutionary sense, be more unnatural. Biologically speaking, women may be intended to gestate and lactate more and menstruate less. The specious supposition is that oral contraceptives are more nearly in accord with Mother Nature's wishes because they suppress the many true menstruations that women were not meant to have anyway.

Even if one accepts the theory that under primitive conditions women spent the greater part of their reproductive lives in a state of amenorrhea, the major fallacy in this reasoning is that contraceptive steroids are not natural at all—they are synthetic. They do not produce the same effect as the hormones of pregnancy, and they function similarly, but not identically, to the estrogen and progesterone produced by a woman's own ovaries and adrenal glands. They have metabolic effects in addition to, and different from, their contraceptive effects. When oral contraceptives are taken in a constant daily dose, they do not produce a physiologically natural state; they produce a pharmacologically hormonally-induced state. The endocrine balance in a woman on oral contraceptives is not the same as it is in a pregnant woman or in a woman not taking synthetic hormones, but this may or may not be harmful to an individual woman's health. Some women do develop serious complications associated with taking oral contraceptives. Unfortunately, it is difficult, and in many instances impossible, to predict which women will be affected.

Natural ovarian estrogens and progesterone are inactivated when they are taken orally. More than 40 years ago, it was discovered that if estradiol were chemically changed by the addition of an ethinyl group at the 17 position (Figure 13–2), the estrogen became orally active. *Ethinyl estradiol* is, therefore, one of the two forms of estrogen in every combined oral contraceptive. The other form is *mestranol,* the 3-methyl ether

of ethinyl estradiol. Mestranol has less estrogenic activity when tested in animals than ethinyl estradiol.

The progestational agents, or progestins, in oral contraceptives are all synthesized from testosterone or hydroxyprogesterone. Some of them retain their androgenic activity in addition to their estrogenic and progestation potency. Some are also variously antiestrogenic and antiandrogenic. Norethynodrel is a highly estrogenic progestin, but it has no androgenic ability. Norgestrel has no estrogenic ability but has the strongest androgen effect of all the progestins as well as a strong antiestrogen effect. Norethindrone, norethindrone acetate, and ethynodiol diacetate are weakly estrogenic and androgenic at low doses but can become relatively antiestrogenic at higher doses. Thus, every pill on the market has its own profile of estrogenicity, androgenicity, and progestational potency. It is believed that the occurrence of minor and major side effects is correlated to the differences in the various hormonal activities in different pills (Table 13–2).

Disadvantages Associated with Oral Contraceptive Use

A brochure that accompanies any package of oral contraceptives to be dispensed to a prospective user warns of more than 50 side effects, some merely unpleasant but minor and tolerable, others serious enough to be life threatening or fatal. Such detailed labeling was first mandated by the FDA in 1978 and has not been changed.

According to the information given to both physicians and women, the absolute contraindications to pill usage are pregnancy, current or past history of blood clotting disorders, current or past history of cerebrovascular or coronary artery disease, known or suspected estrogen-dependent malignancies, any undiagnosed vaginal bleeding, or any current or past liver disease. There are also a substantial number of women who *should* not take oral contraceptives—women whose age, health, family history, heredity, and/or behavior is such that for them, taking the pill is too chancy. When, for example, a woman already has an

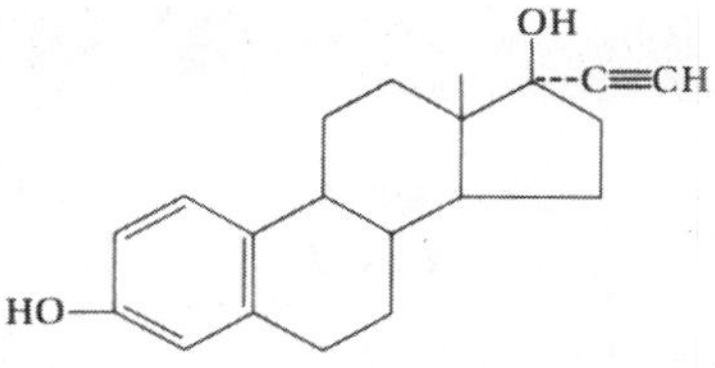

Ethinyl estradiol

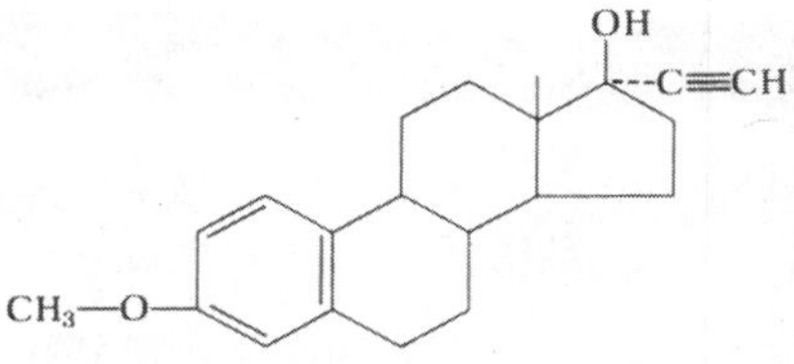

Mestranol

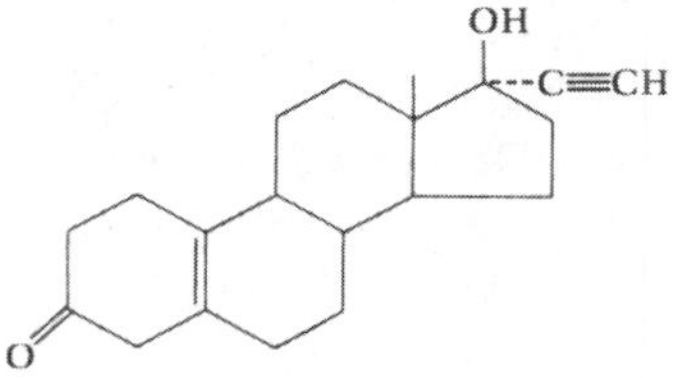

Norethynodrel
(Enovid)

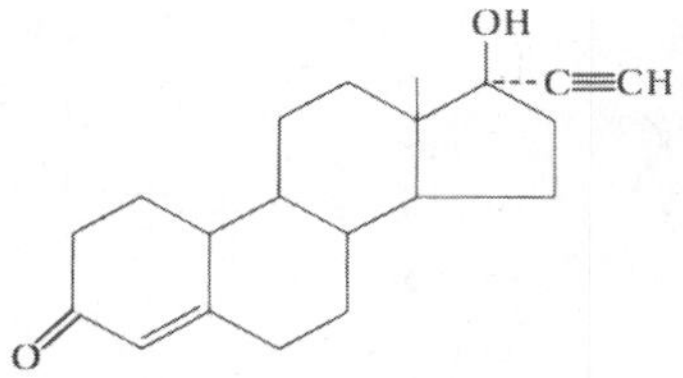

Norethindrone
(Ortho-Novum, Norinyl, Norlutin)

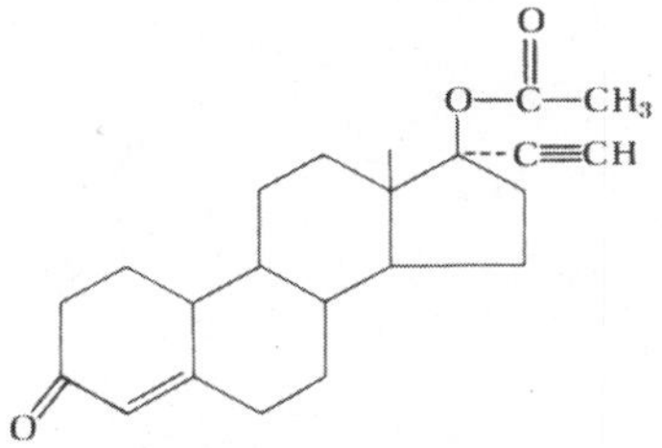

Norethindrone acetate
(Norlestrin, Norlutate)

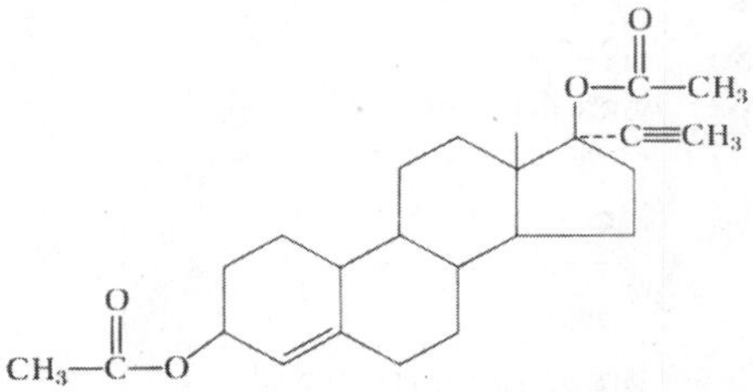

Ethynodiol diacetate (Ovulen, Demulen)

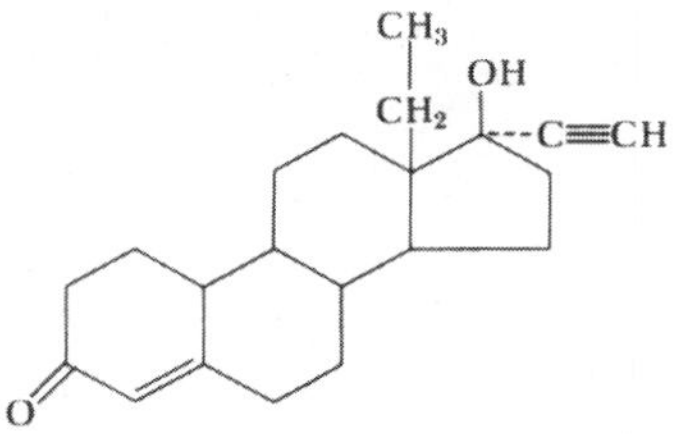

Norgestrel (Ovral)

Figure 13–2 Chemical structure of some oral contraceptive agents.

underlying risk of developing heart disease or cancer, the superimposition of oral contraceptives on those predisposing factors could increase her odds of developing pill-associated problems.

When a woman has none of the conditions or predisposing factors that precludes oral contraceptive use, is not a smoker, and has no minor problems that might worsen as a result of taking pills, the risks of developing

Table 13–2 Pill Side Effects: Hormone Etiology

Estrogen Excess	Progestin Excess	Androgen Excess	Estrogen Deficiency	Progestin Deficiency
Nausea, dizziness	Increased appetite and weight gain (noncyclic)	Increased appetite and weight gain	Irritability, nervousness	Late breakthrough bleeding
Edema and abdominal or leg pain with cyclic weight gain	Tiredness and fatigue and feeling weak	Hirsutism	Hot flashes	Heavy menstrual flow and clots
Leukorrhea	Depression and decrease in libido	Acne	Uterine prolapse	Delayed onset of menses following last pill
Increase in leiomyoma size	Oily scalp, acne	Oily skin, rash	Early and mid-cycle spotting	Dysmenorrhea
Chloasma	Loss of hair	Increased libido	Decreased amount of menstrual flow	Weight loss
Uterine cramps	Cholestatic jaundice	Cholestatic jaundice	No withdrawal bleeding	
Irritability	Decreased length of menstrual flow	Pruritus (itching)	Decreased libido	
Increased female fat deposition	Hypertension (?)		Dry vaginal mucosa and dyspareunia	
Cervical ectropia	Headaches		Headaches	
Contact lenses do not fit	Candida vaginitis cervicitis		Depression	
Telangiectasia (vascular "spiders")	Increase in breast size (alveolar tissue)			
Vascular-type headaches	Breast tenderness without fluid retention			
Hypertension (?)	Decreased carbohydrate tolerance			
Lactation suppression	Pelvic congestion syndrome			
Headaches while taking pills				
Cystic breast changes				
Breast tenderness with fluid retention				
Thrombophlebitis				
Cerebrovascular accidents				
Myocardial infarction				
Hepatic adenoma				

Adapted from Hatcher et al., 1998

major or minor complications should be small. It should be kept in mind, however, that research continues on possible long-term risks associated with use of oral contraceptives. This research has been conducted for more than 30 years, producing a wealth of data. These studies have caused modifications in formulations of oral contraceptives, such that today's lower-dose pills in general carry lower risks for complications. Nonetheless, oral contraceptives challenge the body's physiological resources, and some women by nature are probably better equipped to handle the challenge.

Thromboembolic and Other Cardiovascular Disorders.

A *thrombus* is an abnormal blood clot that forms in an unbroken blood vessel. When a thrombus occurs in a vein *(phleb)* secondary to inflammation of the vein *(phlebitis),* the condition is called thrombophlebitis. Thrombophlebitis most frequently occurs in the superficial and deep veins of the pelvis and legs, sometimes for no apparent reason, sometimes because of injury or trauma, sometimes postoperatively as a result of immobilization of patients in bed. Once a thrombus or clot forms, it may spontaneously dissolve, but more often it remains intact and grows to interfere with the oxygen supply to the surrounding tissues, resulting in tissue damage and swelling. When a piece of thrombus breaks off from its attachment to be carried in the bloodstream, it becomes a traveling clot, or *embolus.* Emboli are dangerous because they flow freely in the circulation, stopping only when they become stuck somewhere, and then they block the blood supply to a vital organ, such as the lungs, brain, or heart. A clot large enough to completely occlude the pulmonary arteries causes massive pulmonary embolism and instant death. A clot in one of the brain arteries could occlude circulation to a part of the brain and cause cerebral thrombotic stroke. Strokes can also occur as a result of cerebral aneurysm, a ballooning out and bursting of an artery to cause hemorrhage.

It has been established that oral contraceptives affect clotting factors in blood and somehow produce alterations in blood vessel walls to create an increased risk of pulmonary embolism, cerebral thrombotic stroke, and cerebral hemorrhagic stroke. Women who use pills for birth control are more likely to develop these conditions than nonusers.

Any factor in a pill user that increases the likelihood of the development of thromboembolic disorders will obviously increase the risk. Women who have high blood pressure or diabetes or who have any past history of phlebitis have predisposing conditions and should not take oral contraceptives. Because deep vein blood clots in the legs have a greater tendency to form after surgery, a woman must not initiate taking oral contraceptives or must discontinue their use if elective surgery is planned within the next 4 weeks.

The abnormal vascular changes induced by oral contraceptives can also increase the chances of a fatal heart attack (myocardial infarction). The danger is much greater for women who already have some of the risk factors associated with heart disease—age over 40; high blood pressure; high cholesterol levels; diabetes; and of major importance, cigarette smoking. Smoking plus oral contraceptives can be a lethal combination not only because the risk of heart attack is increased but also because of a greater incidence of other circulatory diseases. Cigarette smoking adds to the risks of oral contraceptives to such an extent that a woman must decide whether she wants to smoke or to take the pill; *she must not do both.*

In fact, smoking interacts with oral contraceptive use and age to the extent that a woman of 25 who takes oral contraceptives and smokes ages her heart and blood vessels by 10 years; that is, she faces the same risk of death from cardiovascular disease as a non-smoking pill user who is 35 years old.

Major epidemiological studies linking pill use to increased mortality from cardiovascular disease were done 15–20 years ago when women were taking the 50-microgram estrogen pill. The low-dose formulations are believed to have substantially reduced the circulatory system effects. Recent data suggest there is some incidence of cardiovascular disease in healthy women currently taking the low-dose pills, and that there is no increased risk of heart attack in former users of the pill after 10 years (Mishell, 1989; Beral et al., 1999).

The development of *high blood pressure* is another cardiovascular effect that occurs in a small number of women on the pill (Laragh, 1976; Guillebaud, 1985). Women who previously have developed hypertension, black women, or women with a family history of hypertension are more likely to develop high blood pressure when taking oral contraceptives. Slight to moderate elevations of systolic blood pressure, still within the normal range, occur in almost all women after 3 years of continuous pill use. Most of the women in the epidemiological studies cited previously were taking the high-dose estrogen formulations, but evidence showed that the low-estrogen combination and progestin-only pills also resulted in increased blood pressure readings (Khaw & Peart, 1982). In a study of women with oral contraceptive-induced hypertension, Weir (1982) found that changing from a high- to low-dose pill resulted in a marked decline in blood pressure, but the pressure never went back down to pre-pill-taking levels. The hypertension as a result of pill usage appears to be reversible when the contraceptives are discontinued, but the long-term effect of even "normal" induced high blood pressure is unknown.

The incidence of excessive bleeding and "dry sockets" is reportedly higher in women who have tooth extractions while on the pill. The vascular changes that accompany pill usage can also occur in the blood vessels that supply the eye. There have been some reports of visual loss as a result of retinal artery blockage, retinal swelling, and optic nerve damage, but the incidence is rare. But when a woman on oral contraceptives has blurring of vision or double vision, sees flashing lights, or has a sudden loss or diminishing of sight, it may mean a vascular spasm and an impending stroke. Such symptoms require an immediate cessation of pill taking and a medical consultation.

Because estrogen causes fluid retention, some visual changes may occur as a result of swelling or steepening of the cornea. Blurring or difficulty in focusing, the need for a new contact lens prescription, or the inability to wear contacts at all are side effects of pill taking that can sometimes be relieved by switching to an even lower-dose estrogen pill. Those who wear contacts may view this as more than merely a small annoyance; lenses are expensive to change, and most women would be reluctant to give them up completely.

Migraine headaches are a vascular phenomenon. They may, therefore, be intensified by oral contraceptives, and women who are subject to migraines should not take the pill. A vascular headache that signals a cerebral thrombosis often has the same symptoms and may be indistinguishable from a severe migraine headache.

For years, women on the pill have been advised to find another form of contraception after the age of 35 if they smoked and 40 if they were nonsmokers. Women at risk for cardiovascular disease are also advised against using oral contraceptives. It is this advice, gleaned from epidemiological research, that has lowered the risk of cardiovascular disease associated with oral contraceptives (La Vecchia, 1990).

Carbohydrate and Fat Metabolism Effects.

In a significant number of women, combined oral contraceptives produce an abnormal response to the glucose tolerance test, a measure of a fasting individual's ability to handle the ingestion of 1 g of glucose per kilogram of body weight. Such a disturbance in carbohydrate metabolism is a pill-produced diabetes-like effect and makes it unwise for women with prediabetes as yet clinically undetected or women with a strong family history of diabetes to take combined oral contraceptives. The change is reversible when pills are discontinued. Diabetic women on oral contraceptives do not get worse or need more insulin, but diabetics have an increased risk of developing cardiovascular disease, and the pills may augment their danger. The progestin-only pill (minipills) has no effect on carbohydrate metabolism.

The lipid content of the blood—neutral fats or triglycerides, phospholipids, cholesterol, high- and low-density lipoproteins—is influenced by oral contraceptive use. An elevation in blood triglyceride and cholesterol levels, reported in some pill users, may be a predisposing factor for heart disease. Studies have shown that women using oral contraceptives have reduced blood levels of high-density lipoproteins (HDL). High levels of high-density lipoproteins are believed to be protective against heart disease; low or reduced HDL levels are considered a major risk factor. This alteration in the high-density lipoprotein fraction of the blood in older women pill users may be significant in the reported increase of mortality from circulatory disease. Low-dose oral contraceptives also have been shown to alter lipoprotein concentrations in the direction consistent with the development of coronary heart disease, but the greatest effects were seen with formulations containing levonorgestrel (Godsland, Crook, & Wynn, 1991).

The relationship between hyperlipidemia (high lipid levels in the blood) and heart attacks is well recognized. Even a young woman who has a family history of heart disease and high cholesterol and triglyceride levels should have a complete blood chemistry analysis before initiating oral contraceptives.

Liver and Gallbladder Disease. A number of sources reported that the incidence of gallstones (cholelithiasis) and inflammation of the gallbladder (cholecystitis) is higher in pill takers than it is in women who are not on oral contraceptives. This association appears to be greater only in the first few years of pill use, but women who have had previous gallbladder disease or who have had their gallbladders removed should choose another form of contraception.

There are three studies in the literature that distinctly associate cancer of the liver with the long-term use of oral contraceptives (Henderson et al., 1983; Forman, Vincent, & Doll, 1986; Neuberger, Forman, Doll, & Williams, 1986). This could not be shown in a more recent analysis of studies (Rabe, Feldmann, Grunwald, & Runnebaum, 1995). The risk of developing benign tumors of the liver (hepatic adenomas) with the current low-dose pills is much less than with the previously high-dose pills. For women on the pill in the United States, the incidence of liver adenoma does not appear to be a large risk. But even though the tumors are benign, death as a result of rupture and hemorrhage can occur. Women taking the pill should

always have an abdominal palpation to check for liver enlargement at their annual physical examination. If at any time they experience pain under the right rib cage along with loss of appetite or nausea and vomiting, the pills should be discontinued immediately and medical treatment sought as soon as possible.

Oral Contraceptives and Cancer

A woman's risk of developing breast cancer is influenced by many factors, one of which is the length of time she is exposed to estrogen, whether her own or synthetic estrogen taken to prevent conception or to moderate menopause. It follows that oral estrogens would be suspect in affecting a woman's risk for breast cancer. Evidence of this risk, however, is inconsistent. For example, before 1990 nearly all published epidemiological studies failed to find an association between cancer and pill usage, but much of the data had been accumulated within 10–15 years of the introduction of oral contraception. If, as is believed by many researchers, some forms of breast cancer could take as long as 30 years to develop after being exposed to a carcinogen, it would take that long before anyone could say with certainty that pills do or do not cause breast cancer.

Suggestions that a woman's risk of breast cancer could be increased by taking oral contraceptives began to emerge in the early 1980s. Researchers discovered that there was an increased risk of breast cancer in women on the pill, and that women who had taken oral contraceptives for 2–4 years before having their first pregnancy had almost twice the chance of developing breast cancer than a control group (Pike et al., 1981; Harris, Weiss, Francis, & Polissar, 1983; Pike et al., 1983). Clearly and consistently, these researchers demonstrated that there was an association of breast cancer with oral contraceptives when they were taken before ever giving birth. In the latter investigation, Pike and his colleagues specifically related the increased risk to long-term use of certain combination oral contraceptives with a high progestin content. This study, which appeared in the British journal *Lancet*, was widely publicized and widely criticized for its methodology but created considerable public concern. Another dimension had now been added to the question of whether to take the Pill—which pill to take?

In 1980, the Centers for Disease Control (CDC) in Atlanta had begun the Cancer and Steroid Hormone Study (CASH), an investigation of the relationship of long-term oral contraceptive use to breast, endometrial, and ovarian cancer. Data were accumulated on study participants, women with cancer and their matched controls, aged 20–54 years, in eight geographic areas of the United States. The first report to emerge from this investigation, based on analyses of information collected after 6 months, was published in 1983. The findings of a study of 689 women with breast cancer and 1,077 control women showed that neither short- nor long-term use of oral contraceptives appeared to increase significantly the risk of developing breast cancer. With respect to pill usage before the first pregnancy, the risk of developing breast cancer appeared to be increased, and additional research on that issue, as well as on the influence of specific brands and doses of oral contraceptives, was planned.

Reports from CASH published in 1986 and 1988 (Stadel) suggested an increased risk of breast cancer before the age of 45 and a decreased risk after 45 in nulliparous women who had used the pill for more than 8 years and had started menstruating before the age of 13.

More recent studies are summarized in "Cancer Facts," published on-line and updated in February 2000 by the National Cancer Institute (NCI). In June 1995, NCI investigations reported an increased risk of breast cancer development among women under age 35 who had used birth control pills for at least 6 months, compared with women who had never used oral contraceptives. They also noted a slightly elevated risk among women ages 35–44 using birth control pills, and a higher risk among long-term users, especially those who began taking oral contraceptives before the age of 18 (Brinton et al., 1995). In 1996, the Collaborative Group on Hormonal Factors in Breast Cancer used metanalysis to examine worldwide

epidemiological evidence on the relationship between breast cancer and oral contraceptives and analyzed 54 studies that included 53,297 women with breast cancer and 100,239 women without breast cancer. Its main conclusions were that while women are taking combined oral contraceptives and in the 10 years after stopping, there is a small increase in the risk of breast cancer, but the resulting tumors were localized and less likely to have spread aggressively beyond the breast. Second, 10 years after stopping use of oral contraceptives, there was no increased significant risk. This conclusion was reiterated by Westhoff in 1999.

The data concerning cervical cancer also are equivocal. Thirteen large epidemiological studies have produced conflicting results. Seven of them found that oral contraceptives did not appear to be associated with an increased risk of cervical cancer, but one common finding emerged in five of them—that long-term use of oral contraceptives appeared to be related to an increased incidence of cervical cancer. Still, investigators have been reluctant to assume that the pill was causing cervical cancer because sexual activity and a number of other factors also are believed to contribute to the development of cancer of the cervix. In 1983, Vessey, Lawless, McPherson, and Yeates's 10-year follow-up study of more than 10,000 women in Great Britain strengthened the link between oral contraceptive use and cervical cancer. The authors recommended that all long-term users (more than 4 years) have regular and more frequent Pap smears. A number of years later, the same British researchers believed that the effects of the pill on cervical cancer still are inconclusive and need more evaluation. Vessey et al. suggests that taking oral contraceptives for more than 6 years may increase the risk of cervical cancer by 50% (from 1.0 to 1.5), and that the risk may persist after the pill is stopped (1989). The National Cancer Institute, in a February 2000 update of its on-line "Cancer Facts," notes that research supports a relationship between extended use of the pill (5 or more years) and a slightly increased risk of cervical cancer.

The link between oral contraceptives and uterine cancer is more propitious. Taking the combination pill appears to offer some protection against the development of uterine cancer. Although an increased risk of uterine cancer had previously been shown to be associated with the sequential pills that had been discontinued in 1975, in 1980, and thereafter, epidemiological studies, including the preliminary results from the CDC study, have provided evidence that the risk of endometrial cancer developing in women who had ever taken combination oral contraceptives was less than that in women who had never used them. The mechanism for the protective effect is believed to result from the progestin component of the pill ("Cancer Facts," National Cancer Institute, updated February 2000). As yet, however, the influence of other known risk factors for endometrial cancer, such as obesity and use of estrogen replacement therapy, on the presumptive protective effect of the pill, has not been determined.

The other good news concerns the association between oral contraceptives and cancer of the ovaries. A number of studies, starting with those published in the early 1980s, demonstrate that taking oral contraceptives appears to decrease the risk of developing ovarian cancer, and the CDC investigation confirmed that the small but significant decreased risk persisted even after cessation of pill usage. Four years of use results in a 50% reduction in risk, and 7 or more years confers a 60%–80% reduction in the risk of ovarian cancer (Schlesselman, 1989).

But back on the negative side of the ledger, long-term use of oral contraceptives appears to be correlated with a quick-spreading type of skin cancer. Whereas some earlier studies had suggested a very weak or no link at all between pill use and malignant melanoma, a study by epidemiologist Elizabeth Holly and her colleagues (1983) of 87 women with malignant melanoma and 863 control women residing in the same county in the Seattle area did find an association. The researchers showed that pill usage for 4 years or less resulted in no increase in risk; 5–9 years of use produced a 2.4 times increased risk of developing the cancer; and more than 10 years on the pill caused the risk to increase almost fourfold. In contrast, the largest epidemiological study to date found no association

between malignant melanoma and oral contraceptive use (Helmrich et al., 1984). The incidence of malignant melanoma has increased in the past 15 years in both women and men for unknown reasons, but increased exposure to sunlight and the depletion of the protective layers of the atmosphere have been suggested. Studies of the relationship between oral contraceptives and skin cancer have to take such factors into consideration.

The Pill and Pregnancy

The danger to the developing embryo of prenatal exposure to sex hormones used for pregnancy tests or to ward off threatened abortion is recognized and has been discussed previously. The inadvertent taking of oral contraceptives in early pregnancy is a possibility, and a number of years after the introduction of the pill, Nora and Nora (1975) reported that exposure to oral contraceptives during pregnancy resulted in a combination of abnormalities called **VACTERL syndrome**—vertebral, anal, cardiac, tracheal, esophageal, renal, and limb defects. Other large-scale studies published shortly thereafter provided additional evidence that the risk of congenital heart defects appears to be greater when hormones, including oral contraceptives, were taken during the first months of pregnancy. But by now, a number of additional surveys, reanalyses of data, and reviews of the medical literature have minimized the connection between oral contraceptives and certain congenital malformations. The current view is that, if it exists at all, the potential of inadvertent oral contraceptive use in early pregnancy for causing heart, limb, and central nervous system defects is very small. A technical bulletin issued by the American College of Obstetricians and Gynecologists (ACOG) concluded that "there is no evidence that there is an increased risk of fetal anomalies for previous pill users, from inadvertent exposure early in pregnancy, or in pregnancies occurring immediately after discontinuation of oral contraceptives" (1987). The possibility of genital abnormalities—sexual ambiguities as seen in fetuses exposed to DES—as a result of continued contraceptive use when pregnant has not been

434 • CHAPTER 13

discounted, however, and should still be a concern. A 1999 Finnish study (Hemminki, Gissler, & Toukomaa) supports the hypothesis that exposure to female hormones during pregnancy can cause a higher rate of malformations in exposed children, including genital malformations in male infants, but there was no evidence of increased incidence of cancer in offspring or their mothers.

Also of concern is the suggestion that there is a greater incidence of abortuses showing chromosomal defects when conception occurred soon after discontinuation of oral contraceptives. There is no evidence that more miscarriages occur after a period of pill taking, but only that when they did take place, chromosomal abnormalities were greater. For this reason, before trying to conceive, women are advised to discontinue use of the pill and use another method of contraception until they have had two spontaneous cycles.

According to evidence from the Royal College of General Practitioners, many women experience a delay in the return of ovulation and fertility for a varying period of time after discontinuation of the pill. This is another good reason to stop taking the pills for several months before an anticipated pregnancy. A small percentage of pill users, about 2–3 out of every 100 women, develop a postpill amenorrhea, and fertility may be delayed for a prolonged period or even permanently impaired. Postpill amenorrhea evidently is unrelated to duration of pill use, type of pill, or dosage but is strongly correlated with a previous history of menstrual irregularity, late onset of menarche, and low body weight. A young, very slender woman who has always had infrequent, irregular, and scanty periods is a prime target for postpill amenorrhea and perhaps should not take oral contraceptives if she wants to become pregnant at some future date.

If one or two pills are accidentally skipped during a cycle and the expected withdrawal bleeding does not occur at the end of the cycle, pregnancy is a possibility. If the pregnancy is to be retained rather than terminated, it is important to get a pregnancy test before starting a new package of pills to avoid any teratogenic potential of the pills during the next cycle. If no pills

have been missed and the period is skipped, there is no reason to worry; the chances of pregnancy are slim. Each pill should be taken at the same time every day to maintain a constant level of hormones in the body; they are most effective that way. Following are instructions for what a woman should do if she fails to take some of her birth control pills.

> If one pill is forgotten, *it should be taken as soon as remembered and the next one should be taken at the regular time, even if two are then taken on the same day or at the same time. A backup method or abstention should be used in addition to the pill for 7 days (some say a full 14 days) even if menstruation occurs.*
>
> If two pills in a row are missed, *two pills each day for the next two days should be taken and the chances of pregnancy will be reduced. If the missed pills were from the first 14 pills in the packet, a backup method (condom plus foam) or abstention should be used for the next 7 (or 14) days for extra protection. If the 2 missed pills were from the last 7 active pills (out of the 21), the rest of the packet should be discarded and a new packet started. In a 28-pill packet, the last 7 pills are inactive. If any of those are missed, a backup method is not needed. The missed pills should be discarded, the remaining ones taken each day as usual, and a new packet started on time.*
>
> If 3 or more pills, 1 after the other, are missed, *there is a significantly increased risk of pregnancy, and another form of birth control should be used for the rest of the month if sexual intercourse takes place. A new cycle of pills can be started when menstruation occurs. If the menstrual period is late, a pregnancy test should be taken before starting a new packet.*

If all of these instructions about missing pills sound inordinately complicated, a fallback method could be to keep taking the pills, 1 a day, use backup birth control for the next 14 days, and not to worry if some bleeding irregularities occur. It is not unusual to have intermenstrual bleeding take place when women miss a pill, even if they make it up the next day. In practice, while the chance does exist, the risk of pregnancy occurring if 1 pill is missed is low, according to several studies, and may depend on when in the cycle the omission takes place. But a woman who misses 3 pills in a row or consistently misses 1 each month might ask herself whether she really wants to take oral contraceptives. She will be better off with another method of birth control.

Nutritional Effects of Oral Contraceptives

The steroid hormones in oral contraceptives affect not only carbohydrate and lipid metabolism but produce alterations in the metabolism and/or absorption of certain vitamins and minerals as well. Thus, women on the pill appear to have an increased need for vitamin B_6 and folic acid and, to a lesser extent, B_1, B_2, and vitamin C. In contrast, the blood serum levels of some nutrients increase, and women appear to have a lesser need for vitamin A, iron, copper, and zinc.

Table 13–3 illustrates the nutritional aberrations that can occur when oral contraceptives are used. These changes may not be induced in all women taking oral contraceptives because much depends on their prior and current nutritional status. Certain women, because of an inadequate diet, may be more vulnerable to a vitamin depletion, but the symptoms of actual deficiency have occurred rarely.

The most markedly increased requirement appears to be vitamin B_6. As measured by an observable alteration in the metabolism of the amino acid tryptophan, vitamin B_6 is depleted in 80% of pill users while the other 20% have an absolute deficiency. The clinical significance of the altered tryptophan metabolism is unclear, but this biochemical change is reversed when oral contraceptives are discontinued or when a vitamin supplement is taken.

While 20%–30% of oral contraceptive users have abnormally low folic acid levels, clinical signs rarely appear. Fewer than 30 cases of megaloblastic anemia (abnormal red blood cell production) produced by folate deficiency have been recorded in the medical literature. On the basis of several studies, nutritionist Daphne Roe of Cornell University concluded that the risk of a serious folic acid depletion developing in women taking oral contraceptives is related to their dietary intake of the vitamin. Raw leafy vegetables, whole grain cereals, organ meats, nuts, legumes, and yeast are excellent sources of folic acid. A woman who has a bowl of fortified cereal for breakfast and a salad during the day is not likely to develop a folic acid deficiency while taking the pill. Roe suggests that a vitamin supplement of 35 μg of folic acid daily would more than compensate for any difference in folic acid status in women taking oral contraceptives. If a state of vitamin depletion exists, she advocates 100-μg supplementation.

There are several multivitamin-mineral preparations on the market that contain greater amounts of B vitamins and C than the usual cheaper multivitamin tablet. They also contain vitamin A. As Roe pointed out, vitamin A levels are increased in women on the pill; additional supplementation is not helpful and could even be hazardous with possible hypervitaminosis developing in women consuming large amounts of dietary vitamin A.

Much of the evidence that oral contraceptives have an adverse effect on a woman's nutritional status is incomplete, and many of the studies are inconclusive and contradictory. There is no real proof that supplemental vitamin and mineral tablets are necessary or useful for women on the pill who eat a balanced, nutritious diet. Any supplementation should be confined to the B vitamins, especially B_6 and folic acid, and possibly to vitamin C. A moderate extra intake of water-soluble vitamins is not going to be harmful.

There are a number of drugs that interact with oral contraceptives and may reduce the efficacy or increase the side effects of either the oral contraceptives or the drugs taken. Drugs known to decrease the contraceptive effects of oral contraceptives are anticonvulsants such as phenytoin (Dilantin); antibiotics and antifungal agents; clofibrate, a cholesterol-lowering drug; and sedatives and tranquilizers such as barbiturates, benzodiazepines, and some preparations taken for migraines. Because oral contraceptives may modify the activity of the additional drug taken, the 1998 edition of Dickey's *Managing Contraceptive Pill Patients* says

Table 13–3 Nutritional Alterations Attributed to Oral Contraceptives

Nutrient	Function	Effect of Oral Contraceptives
Vitamin B_6 (pyridoxine)	Enzymatic reactions necessary for protein metabolism	Reduced serum levels Depression (?)
Folic acid	Metabolism of nucleic acids; normal blood cell production	Reduced serum levels Reduced erythrocyte levels Megaloblastic anemia (very rarely) Reduced serum levels
Vitamin B_{12}	Metabolism of nucleic acids; normal blood cell production	Reduced serum levels
Vitamin B_1 (thiamine)	General metabolism; cellular respiration	Reduced serum levels
Vitamin B_2 (riboflavin)	General metabolism; cellular respiration	Reduced serum levels Glossitis (when diet is inadequate)
Vitamin C (ascorbic acid)	General metabolism, especially in connective tissue	Reduced serum levels
Vitamin A	Normal vision, growth, reproduction; normal epithelial tissue	Increased serum levels
Iron	Oxygen transport; cellular respiration	Increased serum levels
Copper	Enzyme component in cellular respiration	Increased serum levels
Zinc	Enzyme component in cellular respiration	Increased serum levels

that oral contraceptives should not be used if a woman is taking anticoagulants, anticonvulsants, or antibiotics.

Minipills

Because so many adverse effects appeared to be associated with the estrogen content of the combined oral contraceptives, attempts were made during the mid-1960s to develop a progestin-only pill that could prevent pregnancy but would have less effect on the body's metabolism. The **minipill** or small-dose progestin pill, has been available since 1973. Nor-QD and Micronor contain norethindrone; Ovrette contains norgestrel. None of these contains any estrogen, although assays have shown some weak estrogenic potency.

Minipills are taken every single day with no interruption right through the menstrual period. They may prevent ovulation during some cycles, but that is not the primary basis for their contraceptive action. It is believed that one effect of microdose progestin-only pills is to slow the movement of the ovum down the fallopian tube, delaying it to the point where implantation is not likely to occur. The endometrium is also altered by the progestin to further inhibit implantation. Sperm motility and penetration through the cervix are impaired or prevented because minipills cause the formation of a thick and hostile cervical mucus.

Minipills are said to have a somewhat lower theoretical effectiveness rate than combined pills, in the area of 98.5%–99%, or as low as 97%, according to some sources. The additional number of pregnancies per 100 woman-years of use may be attributed to the fact that in contrast to the combined pills, missing 1 day of minipills can result in pregnancy.

When a pill is missed, two should be taken the next day and another contraceptive method used until the next menstrual period. Because pregnancies are more likely to occur during the first 6 months of use, it is recommended that a second method be used during that period.

Progestin-only pills are very effective in preventing pregnancy in older women, however. At age 40 or older, the rate is 0.3 pregnancies per 100 woman-years (Vessey, Lawless, Yeates, & McPherson, 1985). In breastfeeding women, in whom ovulation is irregular even if menstruation has resumed, progestin-only pills also are highly effective and have the additional benefit of not altering the quantity or quality of breast milk.

Because minipills contain no estrogen, they tend to produce less frequent menstrual bleeding, cause spotting or breakthrough bleeding, or result in changes in the volume of menstrual flow. When after 23–30 days menstruation does occur, it probably means that ovulation is taking place each month. Many women, however, experience some regular cycles but can also have intervals between bleeding that may last up to 45 days or more. There are women taking minipills who menstruate very infrequently—perhaps once or twice a year. The known lesser effectiveness of minipills along with the irregular bleeding can make women on the longer cycles very nervous about a possible pregnancy.

It seems reasonable to question whether taking an oral contraceptive, even one containing only a micro-dose of progestin, is worthwhile if menstrual irregularities cause anxiety about pregnancy and the necessity for a second method of contraception. A substantial number of women on progestin-only pills do have some kind of disturbance of duration or amount of menstrual flow, and many of them discontinue use as a result.

If one is willing to accept the possibility of irregular withdrawal bleeding and the probability of slightly lower effectiveness, are there any other advantages of minipills over a low-estrogen combined pill? Progestin-only pills have been shown in laboratory and clinical studies to produce fewer metabolic effects than combined low-estrogen oral contraceptives. The side effects associated with estrogen excess would not be expected to occur with minipills, and many of the progestin-excess miseries—because minipills contain less progestin than any of the combined oral contraceptives—also should not take place. It has not been proven that minipills increase the risk of blood-clotting disorders as much as combined oral contraceptives, but neither has it been shown that they do not. The FDA mandates that manufacturers of the minipills include a package insert that warns of the same health hazards that are associated with the combined orals. There is no present evidence to indicate that minipills, while theoretically safer, are actually less harmful or different in their adverse effects than other oral contraceptives.

The use of the minipill is not particularly widespread, and it accounts for only 0.2% of the total oral contraceptive market in the United States. Many pharmacies do not even stock the minipill and have to special-order the pills when they are prescribed. Even the manufacturers—Syntex, Ortho and Wyeth—apparently prefer to promote the use of low-dose combined pills and seemingly never advertise the minipills in medical journals.

Pills—Pro and Con

To be able to take one pill a day and then completely ignore the possibility of pregnancy is a very positive benefit of oral contraception, probably the main one for most women. There are, in addition, a number of noncontraceptive benefits that should be considered in making a decision about oral contraceptive usage.

They include a decrease in menstrual discomfort and a decrease in the possibility of ovarian retention cysts, since follicular development does not take place. A woman who uses the pill for at least a year has only half the risk of developing pelvic inflammatory disease (PID) as women who use no contraception at all and has more protection against PID than that offered by barrier contraception. Less incidence of PID would necessarily affect the incidence of ectopic pregnancy, and current pill users are, therefore, protected against ectopics as well. Oral contraceptives do *not* provide any protection against HIV, and oral contraceptive users at risk for sexual exposure to HIV should insist that their sexual partners use condoms.

A report from the RCGP said that current users were only one-half as likely to develop rheumatoid arthritis as nonusers. A woman taking pills is not likely to develop iron-deficiency anemia because her volume of bleeding is less, and there is evidence that the possibility of developing uterine fibroid tumors is decreased. Her menses will be regular, and there may be reduced premenstrual tension. And, for what it is worth, there is a 25% reduction in the amount of earwax formed.

On the other side of the scale are the intimidating number of possible side effects associated with pill use. Assuming that a woman meets the medical criteria for oral contraceptive use—under age 35, neither underweight nor obese, regular menstrual cycles, no high blood pressure, no family history of cardiovascular problems, no diabetes or family history of diabetes, no breast disease or family history of breast cancer, no migraines, no previous gallbladder disease, a nonsmoker, and is willing to put up with minor side effects that may or may not become worse with continued pill use, she still has to answer the question, "Am I going to be better off or worse off if I use birth control pills?"

Only a woman herself knows what the potential benefits of using this form of contraception mean to her. If pregnancy at this time in her life would be an absolute disaster and abortion as a backup is out of the question, the peace of mind concerning the effective-

ness of pill use may outweigh the annoyance of minor side effects and the back-of-the-mind anxiety concerning the possible hazards. A 1999 report by Beral et al. that tracked 46,000 women for 25 years demonstrated that oral contraceptives have no long-term effects, although there are increased risks of previously mentioned diseases while taking them. Also reassuring is that most of the women in the study were taking high-dose pills, common in the 1960s and 1970s. The low-dose pills used currently are believed to be safer. A fatalist could point out that life itself is a risk, that the risk of walking across the street and getting hit by a car is likely to be greater than the probability of mortality from oral contraceptives. Moreover, it is recognized that more women die from pregnancy and childbirth than from pill usage (unless they are over 40 and smokers).

Oral contraceptives provide an effective and convenient method of birth control. If a woman elects to use them, she must recognize that there are certain responsibilities associated with their use. It is essential that she have an initial examination by a private physician or a nurse-practitioner that includes a medical history, a physical examination that includes a pelvic exam, a Pap smear, a VD culture for gonorrhea and a blood test for syphilis, a urinalysis, blood pressure determination, blood chemistry analysis, and a breast examination. She should be aware that possible drug interactions with other medications may occur while she is taking oral contraceptives, and she must be certain to tell any other physician she consults that she is using birth control pills. She must return annually for a similar examination and must be constantly alert for indications of trouble. *Virtually none of the major complications of pill use occurs without some prior warning.* The authors of *Contraceptive Technology* (Hatcher, Trussel, Stewardt, et al., 1998) have listed five symptoms with the acronym ACHES: Abdominal pain that is severe, Chest pain or shortness of breath, Headaches, Eye problems, Severe leg pain in the calf or thigh. These are symptoms that must not be ignored nor accepted as a matter of course, nor expected to just go away. Delay could be fatal. As would be true with any potent drug, it is possible to minimize the serious complications of usage when informed and aware users are alert to the warning signs.

NORPLANT IMPLANT

The first significantly new technique of hormonal contraception in the United States in 25 years was introduced in January 1991. Norplant, a hormonal subdermal implant, was developed by embryologist Sheldon Segal of the Rockefeller Foundation. In the past decade, as American pharmaceutical companies virtually withdrew from the expensive and potentially nonprofitable research and development necessary to market a new contraceptive, it was left to the New York–based Population Council, a small nonprofit group concerned with population problems, to bring Norplant to the FDA for approval—a process that took 24 years. Before it was available in the United States, Norplant had been tested in 46 other countries, approved in 17, and had been used by more than half a million women.

The hormone in Norplant was not new; the method of delivery—by subdermal implant—was what makes it unique. The device consists of an implant of six silastic (silicone rubber) capsules, each filled with 36 mg of the synthetic progestin, levonorgestrel, also found in many oral contraceptives. The six soft and flexible tubes, each about the size of a matchstick (34 mm long by 2.4 mm wide), are inserted in a fan-shaped distribution, one after the other, with a large-bore needle under the skin of the inside of the woman's upper arm (Figure 13–3). The procedure requires local anesthesia, takes about 10 minutes, and no stitches are needed for the incision. Although they can be felt, the capsules are invisible after implantation in most women. Over a period of 5 years, the Norplant capsules release 30 micrograms of levonorgestrel per day into the body by diffusion. An oral contraceptive containing levonorgestrel usually releases about 150 micrograms daily, and not in a constant low dose. A two-rod implant, Norplant-2, was approved by the

FDA in 1996 but is yet to be marketed by Wyeth-Ayerst in the United States. It is to be sold as Jadelle in Europe.

Norplant, like progestin-only pills, acts by thickening cervical mucus so sperm cannot enter the cervical os, affecting the movement of the cilia lining the fallopian tubes thus limiting egg transport, and by decreasing the thickness of the endometrial lining of the uterus to make it unreceptive to implantation. Although it inhibits ovulation only about 50% of the time, the device is still very effective. The 5-year cumulative pregnancy rate is 1.1 per 100, and the 7-year rate is 1.9 per 100 for thin women. The capsules have to be removed after the end of the fifth year because the failure rates significantly increase in the sixth year after implantation. The risk of ectopic pregnancy is about the same as it is with intrauterine device users. Like other hormonal contraceptives, the efficacy of Norplant may be decreased by its interaction with other drugs.

The reversibility of Norplant is evidently not a problem. After removal of the device, 20% of women trying to get pregnant succeed the first month, 49% by the fourth month, 73% after the sixth month, and 86% by the end of a year (Shoupe & Mishell, 1989). In terms of effectiveness, Norplant is surpassed only by sterilization. For both effectiveness and reversibility, Norplant is ahead of any other currently available contraceptive, but it loses points on side effects.

Like the progestin-only pills, the most frequent side effect is irregular bleeding, occurring in 60%–70% of women. The irregularity tends to decline after the first year, but 10% continue to have irregular bleeding for the entire 5 years. Usually the number of days of menstruation increase while the amount of bleeding per day decreases, but 25% of the women who have Norplant inserted have amenorrhea for up to 3 months. Other side effects include the increased development of ovarian cysts, headaches (sometimes severe enough to require removal of the implants), weight gain or weight loss, breast tenderness, nausea, dizziness, nervousness, acne, excessive hair growth or hair loss, pain or itching at the implant site, anemia, depression, or high blood

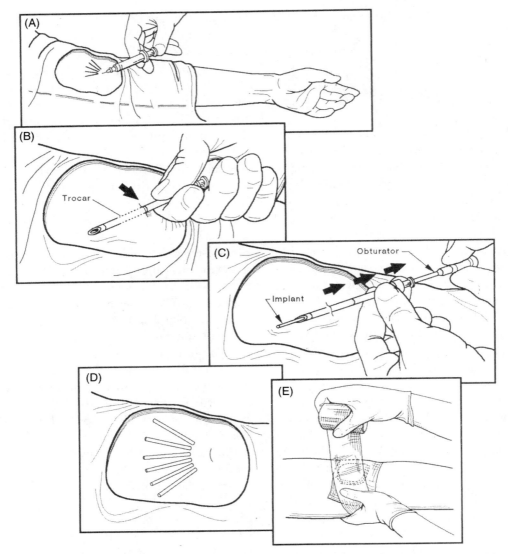

Figure 13–3 Insertion of Norplant. (A) A local anesthetic is injected in a fan-shaped area on the inside of the upper arm. (B) A trocar, a metal tube into which a rod (obturator) fits, is inserted under the skin up to a special mark. (C) The first Norplant capsule is loaded and pushed out by the obturator, which is then withdrawn, leaving the trocar in place. (D) The same process is repeated until the remaining five implants are inserted in a fan shape. (E) After removal of the trocar, the incision is closed with a bandage.

pressure. There is conflicting evidence as yet for Norplant's effects on lipoprotein levels. Some studies have reported a 10%–15% decrease in "good" cholesterol (HDL) levels but found that they returned to preinsertion levels after the first year. Other studies found that HDL increased rather than decreased. As with oral contraceptives, the use of Norplant is contraindicated in women with acute liver disease, a history of breast cancer, heart attacks, blood clots, stroke, or unexplained vaginal bleeding. Smokers should not use Norplant.

Clearly, Norplant has advantages: it is long lasting, provides very effective protection for 5 years, is unrelated to sexual intercourse, and is reversible. A woman who chooses hormonal contraception with Norplant has to make that decision only once rather than daily as with oral contraceptives. In the clinical trials that preceded its release, up to 7% of Norplant users had the device removed in the first year because of bleeding, but 90% of the women users said they were very satisfied. The disadvantages of Norplant are its side effects, that insertion and removal must be done by clinical practitioners, and that the initial expense of insertion and removal of the device—about $500–$700 in 1998—is high, although Medicaid covers the cost for poor women in almost all states. Norplant suffered a slight setback in the late summer of 2000. Certain lots of the product were discovered to be low in levonorgestrel. As a result, women who received Norplant insertions between October 1999 and September 2000 were urged to use an additional, and nonhormonal, backup contraceptive (http://www.safetyalerts.com).

THE DEPO-PROVERA INJECTABLE

Even the controversy surrounding the safety of oral contraceptives paled beside the great debate on **Depo-Provera,** the injectable contraceptive manufactured by the Upjohn Company. Depo-Provera is the trade name for the synthetic progestin medroxyprogesterone in depot form and is known internationally as "the shot" or "the jab" because a single injection of 150 mg into the buttocks or upper arm prevents ovulation or acts like other progestin-only preparations to prevent pregnancy for 3 months. The drug is currently used in nearly 80 developing and developed countries by an estimated 2 million women but was initially denied for use as a contraceptive in the United States by the FDA in 1978, primarily because animal studies conducted by Upjohn's own scientists had suggested a link between Depo-Provera and benign and malignant breast tumors in beagle dogs and endometrial cancer in monkeys. Subsequently, and at Upjohn's request, a special board of inquiry consisting of three scientists was convened to reconsider the agency's decision. In January 1983, the board held a public hearing for testimony concerning the issues surrounding Depo-Provera's use. Supporters of the drug include the WHO, International Planned Parenthood Federation and many other family planning organizations and population groups, and the ACOG. A longtime foe of approval for the injectable contraceptive in this country is Sidney Wolfe of the Health Research Group, joined by a number of other opponents, including the National Women's Health Network and, in an unusual alliance, highly conservative right-to-life groups who are against Upjohn because the company sells products that cause abortion.

The proponents of Depo-Provera claim that its benefits outweigh any potential and as-yet-unproven risks. They allege that epidemiological studies and 25 years of use have demonstrated no serious effects of medroxyprogesterone.

The opponents, however, criticized the existing epidemiological studies that showed no harmful effects as flawed because of small sample size, insufficient exposure and follow-up, lack of appropriate controls, and other methodological problems. They remained unconvinced that these studies in humans have provided evidence for the long-term safety of the drug. One report from New Zealand by Skegg and Spears (1989) suggested that Depo-Provera may increase the risk of breast cancer in young women, probably acting as a promoter after the cancer has already occurred rather than as an initiator.

There are other concerns about Depo-Provera that extend beyond its possible carcinogenicity. The drug, unlike oral contraceptives, does not suppress lactation and can be used during breastfeeding, but there is little information about the effects of depo medroxyprogesterone acetate transmitted to the nursing infant. Moreover, almost all women on Depo-Provera have menstrual irregularities ranging from spotting and staining to occasional episodes of very heavy vaginal bleeding. Fifty percent become amenorrheic. Women who lose their periods do not know if they are pregnant or not, and possible prenatal exposure to the drug poses a risk of congenital abnormalities or masculinization of female fetuses. Also, the amenorrhea is apt to continue after cessation of Depo-Provera injections, so the return of fertility is frequently delayed, sometimes by as much as 2 years. Other side effects associated with Depo-Provera use are unsurprisingly those associated with hormonal contraception—headaches, weight gain, abdominal bloating, depression, dizziness, and fatigue.

Although the British government in mid-1984 approved its use as an injectable contraceptive, the board of inquiry in October 1984 recommended against the release of Depo-Provera for marketing in the United States. But in 1991, yet another panel of scientists convened by the FDA unanimously recommended that it be approved as a contraceptive. In late 1992, after nearly two decades of dispute concerning both its safety and its potential for coercive use, the FDA approved Depo-Provera for birth control.

Long before its release as a contraceptive, medroxyprogesterone acetate had been approved for other therapeutic purposes. It often is used in the treatment of dysfunctional bleeding, habitual miscarriage, hormonally sensitive malignancies, and for endometriosis. It is generally considered both safe and effective by gynecologists when used for those health problems. The drug also has been sanctioned by the government for use on sex offenders to create "chemical castration." Several treatment clinics and some state prisons in the country are empowered, under strict guidelines, to administer 500 mg weekly injections of Depo-Provera to sex crime offenders who volunteer, sometimes in lieu of conviction and sentence, for the program. In those doses, the hormone inhibits the production of testosterone, thus sometimes, but not always, reducing the sex drive and causing testicular atrophy and impotence. But when the massive doses of hormones are stopped, so are the effects, and there is reversion back to the original sexual urges that resulted in the criminal acts. The question of how it can be guaranteed that the rapist who has been paroled or the child molester who has been released will continue to come back for the weekly expensive injections has not been answered. Obviously, any expanded use of the chemical castration program has become highly controversial. It is opposed for different reasons by such groups as the American Civil Liberties Union and Women Against Violence Against Women.

INTRAUTERINE DEVICES

That the presence of a small object in the uterus prevents pregnancy may have been known since ancient times. One frequently told story concerns the Arabian practice of inserting a small pebble into the uteri of camels to make certain that pregnancy was avoided on long caravan journeys—a procedure, considering the nature of camels, that must have required extraordinary tact on the part of the camel drivers. The writings of Hippocrates, the Greek physician who is called the father of medicine, describe the use of a hollow tube passed into a human uterus through which medication or a small device would be inserted. Whether the method was actually used for contraception is not clear.

For several thousand years after Hippocrates and ancient camel drivers, there was no further historical mention of intrauterine devices, although intravaginal suppositories or pessaries were widely used as a method of birth control. The forerunners of the modern IUDs were most likely the stem pessaries of the late 19th and early 20th centuries. Placed into the vagina ostensibly to correct a displaced uterus or other "female disorders," stem pessaries were small caps or buttons made of wood, ivory, pewter, or even precious metals. They fit over the cervix and were attached to little stems that led into the cervical canal or even farther into the uterine cavity. Little reference was made to their contraceptive ability, but they were probably quite effective. In 1909, a German doctor, Richard Richter, published his description of the first completely intrauterine device, a ring made of dried silkworm gut. In the 1920s, another German doctor named Pust combined Richter's silkworm ring with the older pessary idea of a glass disc that fit over the external os. He inserted this device into hundreds of women, claiming that no pregnancies or serious complications occurred. The idea never caught on with other physicians, however, who feared that the use of the device would cause pelvic infections. More attention was paid to the work of Ernst Grafenberg, still another German doctor, who began using completely intrauterine silkworm gut rings for contraception and later developed a silver ring device. The *Grafenberg ring* was very popular in Germany and elsewhere for several years, but enthusiasm waned in the middle 1930s as the devices were almost universally condemned by the medical profession as dangerous and ineffective. Although Grafenberg's most vociferous critics had little or no practical experience with his ring, they opposed it on the theoretical supposition that it might cause serious complications from pelvic infections. The Grafenberg ring fell into complete disrepute, and no more was heard about IUDs for the next 25 years.

In the early 1960s, two independent workers, Oppenheimer in Israel and Ishihama in Japan, who had earlier rediscovered the Grafenberg rings, published their reports of the successful use of intrauterine devices at approximately the same time. There was a sudden and renewed interest in IUDs, occurring, perhaps not coincidentally, with the recognition of a worldwide population explosion. Many clinical trials in various countries were initiated, and when the successful and favorable results of these trials were reported at two international conferences on IUDs held in New York in 1962 and 1964, it became evident that medical opinion had undergone a reversal. The IUDs became established as a medically acceptable contraceptive, and 10% of American women were using them in the 1970s.

Intrauterine devices were originally believed to be closest to the "ideal" contraceptive. Although they had the drawback of requiring a clinical procedure for insertion, once in place IUDs could be ignored except for periodic checking by the woman, and they provided long-term protection against pregnancy that was

completely reversible once the device was removed. There were believed to be no serious systemic side effects associated with their use. After a decade and a half, it became apparent that IUDs did not fulfill their expectations. Problems of accidental pregnancy, spontaneous abortion, involuntary expulsion, perforation, pelvic infection, pain, and excessive menstrual bleeding have made IUDs far less than ideal for many women.

Approximately half of the accidental pregnancies that occur when a woman is wearing an IUD will terminate in a spontaneous abortion if she decides to continue the pregnancy. And approximately half of those miscarriages may be accompanied by infection and be preceded by a fever, a combination that is very rare when spontaneous abortion occurs in non-IUD wearers. Some of the infections, called septic abortions, spread with incredible rapidity and were severe enough to be fatal. A greater incidence of septic abortions and associated mortality occurred when the IUD was a Dalkon Shield. This device, crab shaped with little "feet" that clung to the uterine lining, was especially favored in the early 1970s because it appeared to tenaciously resist expulsion, a particular problem in young nulliparous women.

After it had been implicated in a high rate of pelvic infections, 14 deaths, and 223 septic abortions, the Dalkon Shield was voluntarily withdrawn from the market by its manufacturer, A. H. Robins Company, in 1974. There was subsequent disagreement among doctors as to whether the nearly 3 million women who were already wearing the Dalkon Shields should have them removed. While a kind of recall for removal did take place as a result of newspaper and television publicity, there were unknown numbers of women, many of whom had no idea what kind of device had been inserted, wearing a Dalkon Shield. Moreover, because Robins had removed the IUD only from domestic distribution, about 2 million more shields were inserted abroad before sales were completely halted. Finally, in 1980, the A. H. Robins Company, which by then had thousands of lawsuits filed against it, wrote to physicians in the United States recommending removal of the device because of the risk of infection. How many women were "recalled" by their doctors is unknown, but an estimated 80,000 women in this country (and probably hundreds of thousands worldwide) could still have had them in place.

Although initially the pharmaceutical company's earnings were not affected by the Dalkon Shield's withdrawal, eventually claims were filed against the company, and it was ordered to pay compensatory and punitive damages. In 1985, A. H. Robins filed for Chapter 11 bankruptcy. As part of the company's reorganization under federal bankruptcy law after it was purchased by American Home Products, the Dalkon Shield Claimants Trust was established. This trust paid out nearly $3 billion in claims by the time it closed on April 30, 2000 (http://www.law.harvard.edu/news/librarydalkon.html).

After the manufacturer experienced the Dalkon Shield disaster, "guilt by association" occurred for other IUDs. Most of them on the U.S. market were withdrawn, not because of proven adverse effects, but because profits were low as a result of bad publicity, and the costs of liability insurance and litigation were high. Subsequent attempts to improve the safety, effectiveness, and acceptance of IUDs were only somewhat successful. Their contraceptive action was enhanced and some of the side effects were reduced by the addition of bioactive substances such as copper or progesterone, but by 1991 only two types of IUDs were available in the United States (although a number of different IUDs continued to be the most widely used reversible form of contraception in other countries such as China, for example). The two remaining types are the Copper T 380A and the IUD that releases progesterone. The levonorgestrel-releasing IUD, widely available in Europe and Asia as Mirena IUS, is anticipated to be approved by the FDA by 2002. Mirena is said to combine the best features of hormonal contraceptives and IUDs and is effective for up to 5 years.

Mode of Action

IUDs function to prevent pregnancy, but exactly how they accomplish this contraceptive action is not clearly understood. The most widely accepted theory is that the IUD makes the endometrium of the uterus hostile to implantation of the fertilized egg, probably by causing a nonspecific inflammatory reaction—which sounds much worse than it is. Inflammation is a normal body defense against foreign material; it does not mean infection, although a similar kind of foreign body reaction would occur against bacteria. The presence of an IUD in the uterus evokes a kind of "sterile" inflammation—the release of large numbers of phagocytic white blood cells that have the ability to engulf and devour cells or to disrupt them through release of toxic products. These phagocytic leukocytes may kill some of the sperm, may attack the embryo, or may change the endometrium so that it is no longer an ideal medium for implantation. Other mechanisms thought to contribute to the IUD's action may be an increased intrauterine prostaglandin level, an alteration in total motility so that fertilized ova reach the uterine cavity prematurely, or possibly an immunological change. IUDs evidently have no effect on ovulation or the function of the corpus luteum. Their antifertility effect is confined to the uterus, and it presumably disappears when the device is removed.

The addition of copper to an IUD increases its contraceptive ability. How this works probably involves a series of intracellular biochemical reactions, which are not clearly understood. In some fashion, copper ions enhance the prevention of implantation, perhaps by interfering with estrogen receptors on endometrial cells or in other ways inhibiting intracellular enzyme activities; but they may also be toxic to sperm or inhibit their transport. It is known that the contraceptive effect is related to the amount of copper that is released into the endometrial cavity. The Copper T 380A is a plastic device with total surface area of 380 mm^2 of copper on the vertical stem and the two horizontal arms, which releases a very small amount of copper daily. Data indicate that it is effective for 8–10 years. This IUD has the lowest failure rate of any intrauterine device yet developed. Research efforts to improve the design of the copper-releasing mechanism are presently under way.

Copper IUDs have been in use for a relatively short period of time, and the long-term effects of constant exposure to copper are obviously unknown. Most of the copper released from the IUD remains in the uterus and is expelled with the menstrual fluid, but the rest of it is presumed to be absorbed into the bloodstream. The amount of copper that gets into the general systemic circulation has been calculated as being only 5% of that which is normally absorbed from the diet (Hasson, 1978). This small amount would ordinarily be expected to have no effect, but there have been several reported allergic reactions. Skin rash developed in one woman, and another got hives as a result of wearing a copper IUD (Barkhoff, 1976). Product information provided by Ortho-McNeil, manufacturer of the ParaGard T 380A intrauterine copper contraceptive, warns that "additional amounts of copper available to the body from the ParaGard T 380A may precipitate symptoms in women with Wilson's disease" (http://www.ama-assn.org/special/contra/ortho/paragard.htm).

Wilson's disease is a genetic disorder causing excessive copper accumulation and can be fatal unless detected and treated before serious illness develops from copper poisoning. Wilson's disease affects 1 in 30,000 people worldwide.

As yet there has been no evidence of a greater risk of cervical or endometrial cancer as a result of wearing a copper IUD. Should a woman become pregnant while using one, there is also thus far no evidence to indicate that exposure to intrauterine copper until the device is removed has any teratogenic effect on the fetus.

The other available IUD is the Progestasert, a vinyl T with a reservoir of 38 mg of progesterone in a silicone oil base. The quantity of progesterone released daily is 65 μg. The manufacturer claims that this amount, a total of 35 mg in a year, is less than the amount of progesterone produced in 1 day by a woman's own postovulatory corpus luteum. Theoretically, then, the dose levels of progesterone contained in Progestasert should not interfere with any normal body function, suppress ovulation, or have any damaging effect on the fetus should pregnancy occur. Subsequent studies of hormone levels of FSH, LH, progesterone, and estrogen in women wearing the Progestasert have confirmed that this IUD does not appear to affect hypothalamic, pituitary, or ovarian function and, like nonmedicated types, exerts its contraceptive effect only locally. The current version of the progesterone IUD requires removal and reinsertion of a new device every year, which tends to provide a deterrent to its use. Other models with an anticipated life expectancy of 2 years were discontinued when pregnancy rates increased after they were left in that long.

Adverse Effects of the IUD

Pregnancy. A paramount factor in choosing a contraceptive method is its reliability. *Population Reports* (1982) summarized the rates of failure to prevent pregnancy of the most commonly used intrauterine devices. For all IUDs, net pregnancy rates in the first year after insertion range from 0.0 to 5.6 per 100 women. The variation depends on which studies and follow-ups were included and can also be attributed to different IUD characteristics in size and shape. The rate of pregnancy is similar to that of oral contraceptives and proves that, unquestionably, IUDs are highly effective. Failure rates are highest in the first few months after insertion, and some have recommended the use of additional protection, such as foam or cream, at least during ovulation in the first few cycles.

Ectopic Pregnancy. While IUDs prevent uterine pregnancies quite well, they have little or no effect in preventing ectopic pregnancies. The IUD wearer, therefore, unprotected from ovarian conception or tubal implantation, is going to exhibit nonuterine pregnancy in greater numbers than the general population. The diagnosis of ectopic pregnancy, never easy anyway, is more difficult in IUD wearers. Some of the side effects commonly associated with IUD use— episodes of bleeding and pelvic pain—are similar to the symptoms of an ectopic pregnancy.

Spontaneous Abortion. The problem of spontaneous abortion associated with infection and fatality appeared to be greater with the Dalkon Shield, but it was not really determined that this IUD was any worse than the others in causing septic abortion. It is now recommended that if a woman decides to continue a pregnancy that accidentally occurs when any IUD is in the uterus, the device should be removed as soon as possible. The chances of spontaneous abortion as the result of removal, however, are 25%.

Even those pregnancies with an IUD present that proceed to term without miscarriage may not be entirely uneventful at the time of delivery. Problems of premature labor, excessive bleeding, and stillbirths have been reported.

Pregnancy in the presence of an IUD is rare because this method is an effective way of preventing it. When other contraceptives fail, however, a woman has to cope only with the pregnancy—not with life-threatening complications caused by the contraceptive. *Any woman wearing an IUD whose period is delayed by 1 week or more must have an immediate evaluation for pregnancy.* If she is pregnant, her IUD must be removed.

Expulsion, Pain, and Bleeding. A woman may choose to rely on an intrauterine device as a contraceptive, but her uterus may not agree with her decision. In the first year after insertion, the expulsion rate for the Copper T 380A IUD is 2.3% and the occurrence of pain and bleeding is 3.4% (http://www.ama-assn.org/special/contra/ortho/paragard.htm). This means that one out of every four to five women will either spontaneously expel the IUD or need to have it removed for intolerable side effects within a year after insertion.

Retaining the device is a real problem for some women and may be particularly difficult if they are young and nulliparous. Older women who have delivered one or more children are less likely to expel the IUD. Age may actually be a more important factor than parity.

Spontaneous expulsion is also most frequent in the first few months after insertion and usually occurs during menstruation. If a woman notices that the IUD has been ejected, she might fare better upon reinsertion. More than half of the women who have experienced one expulsion are ultimately able to retain an IUD (Tietze, 1973). But a 1995 study (Bahamondes et al.) reported that a woman who has expelled one IUD has a 30% chance of expelling subsequent insertions. A woman could have a more serious problem—pregnancy—if she has not recognized the expulsion. One-third of the pregnancies in IUD wearers are the result of unsuspected loss of the device. It is important to always look for the IUD on tampons or pads during menstruation and to check for its presence after each period by palpating for the end of the string that hangs out of the cervix. If it is not there, or if the string appears to be longer than it was originally, an office or clinic visit to check its location is necessary.

A missing string could mean that the IUD has been expelled, but it could also mean that it has migrated in the other direction. Embedding of the IUD into the uterine wall or perforation through it to end in the peritoneal cavity is infrequent but possible. An examiner must then probe the endocervical canal to look for the string or must use an IUD "hook" to fish around in the uterine cavity for the device. If it still cannot be found, x-ray hysterography or ultrasound can be used to localize the IUD.

Pain on Insertion. Some discomfort may occur when the IUD is inserted, but most women find it tolerable, and an anesthetic or analgesic is rarely necessary. Women can expect to feel a pinch from the tenaculum, the instrument used to grasp and steady the cervix, then perhaps a sudden stinging sensation as the cervix is dilated by the introduction of the IUD inserter barrel, and finally a slight cramping when the device is placed into the uterine cavity. In a few women, there will be a severe pain on insertion. A paracervical block can be used to numb the cervix to eliminate discomfort on insertion, but the cramps that most women feel afterward will not be relieved by this form of anesthesia. The paracervical block cannot eliminate uterine pain. Very infrequently, the procedure of insertion causes women to experience changes in heart rate, cold sweats, nausea, and even fainting. The overall incidence of one or more of these kinds of responses has been reported as ranging from 1%–10%.

Problems Persisting after Insertion.   Virtually all women can expect some cramping pain after an IUD is inserted. In women who have had children, the pain is usually minimal, lasts a few minutes to an hour at most, and requires only a couple of aspirin for relief. Very young or nulliparous women usually have moderate to severe menstrual-type cramps that last for hours or for several days. They need something stronger than aspirin to feel comfortable.

After insertion, almost all women will have some vaginal bleeding accompanying the pelvic pain. The bleeding, too, lasts several hours to several days. Most women will also experience a change in their menstrual periods. The period is likely to start earlier, last longer, and be characterized by a heavier flow. In many instances, the presence of an IUD will also increase the incidence and severity of menstrual cramps, or at least change their character. Dysmenorrhea may appear throughout the entire period instead of merely on the first day, for example.

The reason for increased pain and blood loss during menstruation in women using IUDs is speculative. Perhaps there are increased levels of prostaglandins that trigger muscle irritability. It may also be possible that the pelvic pain is caused by the uterus attempting to adjust its size and shape to the size and shape of the foreign object within it.

When the muscular wall of the uterus periodically contracts, the movement of the IUD over the endometrial lining may cause abrasions that result in pain and bleeding. Howard Tatum, inventor of the T-shaped model, concluded that the pain and bleeding were the result of compression of the endometrial lining and distension of the muscle by the large, stiff devices. His smaller T-shaped IUD was shown to decrease pain and bleeding, but it was less effective in

preventing pregnancy. Addition of copper or progesterone to the T enhanced the contraceptive ability and resulted in fewer problems of pain and blood loss.

Excessive blood loss during menstruation, even in the absence of pelvic pain, can be uncomfortable and restricting. Depending on a woman's diet, it could even increase the risk of iron-deficiency anemia and require iron supplementation if blood tests indicate a low hemoglobin concentration. A woman has to decide for herself how much discomfort and inconvenience she is willing to tolerate for the sake of the IUD. A menstrual period that lasts longer, is twice as heavy as before, and is accompanied by dysmenorrhea that may not have been a prior problem could make many women ask themselves, "Do I really need this grief?" and request removal.

Because a certain amount of additional monthly bleeding and pain is so commonplace in IUD wearers, there is a tendency for doctors and women themselves to ascribe these symptoms only to the IUD. The excessive blood loss has been found to persist with time, but *excessive* (this is the key word) pain that continues past the first couple of months after insertion should not be accepted and requires an examination and a reevaluation.

Decreasing the Problems with IUDs

It has been recognized by authorities that one of the most important factors affecting failure and expulsion of IUDs is the skill and experience of the person who does the insertion. The only correct placement of the device is high up in the uterine fundus, but proper positioning is not always achieved. If the IUD is placed insufficiently high to begin with, the device is more likely to be displaced, dislodged, or spontaneously expelled. What has not been indicated by the experts is how women can evaluate the competence of the person doing the insertion. Other than asking around to determine who does a lot of them, one might assume that a gynecologist who is cautious, considerate, and takes time with all procedures would be careful and meticulous with insertions. It would be wise, if possible, to go to a family planning clinic or a university medical center where the IUD insertion is regularly done by trained personnel.

Placing the IUD high up in the fundus of the uterus does not mean *through* it, but perforation of the uterus that unknowingly places the IUD into the pelvic cavity is a frequent complication of IUD insertion. Perforations that occur at a later date may also be related to original faulty insertion techniques. It has been claimed, although proof is lacking, that an IUD in the uterine cavity is not capable of penetrating through the uterine wall by itself. It has to have been aided by a trauma to the uterine wall at the time of insertion. A uterine cavity less than the average 6.5 cm in length is a contraindication for IUD insertion. According to the recommendations of the ACOG, placing an IUD into a smaller-than-average uterine cavity is an invitation to complications.

Any history of excessive menstrual bleeding or significant dysmenorrhea would also exclude a woman as a candidate for IUD insertion. Another major reason to rule out the use of an IUD is the presence of any pelvic infection or even having once had a pelvic infection.

Pelvic Infection

An infection of the upper reproductive tract is generally referred to as pelvic inflammatory disease (PID). The term PID can be used to describe any bacterial infection involving the uterus (endometritis), the fallopian tubes (salpingitis), and the ovaries (oophoritis). Widespread, acute PID usually refers to a salpingitis that has spilled over into the peritoneum to infect the adjacent pelvic structures. As noted in Chapter 9, an untreated gonorrhea can progress to the upper genital tract as gonococcal salpingo-oophoritis, but other bacteria, such as staphylococci and streptococci, can also invade the tubes, ovaries, and peritoneum and cause acute PID. One symptom of an acute pelvic infection is lower abdominal tenderness or pain, usually localized in an area above the pubic bone. Originally the pain may come and go, but it can also progress to a constant discomfort. It is accompanied by fever, sometimes by nausea and vomiting, and a general feeling of really being sick. There may be symptoms of urinary tract infection—frequency and burning. PID tends to occur more frequently after a menstrual period because the sloughed-off endometrial tissue forms a good growth medium for bacteria.

In 1968, a report from an Advisory Committee on Obstetrics and Gynecology of the FDA conceded that it was probably impossible to insert an IUD without some bacterial contamination. No matter how careful and aseptic the technique, several species of organisms normally found in cervical mucus are likely to ride along into the uterine cavity with the IUD insertion device. In most instances, the normal body defenses in the uterus are able to counteract this minimal infection. Mishell, Moyer, and others have shown in separate studies that uterine cultures taken within the first 24 hours after insertion were positive for bacteria, but that the infection was completely gone and the uterus was again sterile a month later. Depending on a variety of factors, however (the technique of insertion, the number of bacteria introduced, their virulence, possibly the kind of IUD, the resistance of the woman, and most important, the presence of a preexisting infection that is aggravated by the insertion), the bacteria are not destroyed by uterine mechanisms. Instead, they survive, multiply, and cause pelvic inflammatory disease. A study by Tietze found that 2%–3% of women had symptoms of PID in the first year following insertion, but that the incidence was substantially higher (7.7%) in the first 15 days than during later periods. According to Tietze, it is questionable whether insertion of an IUD can cause infection unless a minimal chronic or subchronic infection is present. Any woman with past episodes of PID is not a good candidate for IUD insertion.

Pelvic infection that occurs months or even years after insertion has been recognized as a serious complication in IUD wearers, but there has been a general reluctance to admit to the causal relationship between the IUD and an increased risk of PID. It seemed reasonable to suggest that at least part of the incidence of

PID in IUD users could be related to the loss of protection against infection provided by condoms, diaphragms, and spermicides. It also was evident that it was difficult to attribute an increased risk of PID to the IUD because there were so few valid statistics concerning the incidence of PID in the general population. The exact figures were hard to obtain because different doctors tend to apply different criteria to the diagnosis of the disease. Furthermore, the majority of women who received IUDs from clinics during the 1960s were from the group referred to as "lower socioeconomic status"—poor, black, and other minority women. It is stereotypically accepted that the incidence of venereal or other intercourse-related PID is much higher in this group of IUD users.

Subsequently, however, there were enough large-scale controlled epidemiological studies to indicate that while factors such as socioeconomic level or sexual activity could contribute to the increased incidence of pelvic inflammatory disease in IUD users, one of the major reasons for a higher rate of PID in IUD users is the very fact that they were IUD users. Overall, there appeared to be a relative risk of PID that was 1.5 to 10 times greater than it was in non-IUD users (Eschebach, Harnish, & Holmes, 1977; Westrom, 1980; Vessey, Yeates, Flavel, & McPherson, 1981; Lee et al., 1983). Vessey and coworkers showed that the higher rate of PID for IUD users was not the result of differences in age, parity, social class, or smoking and suggested that the link between PID and the IUD was one of cause and effect. Lee and her colleagues used data from the National Institutes of Health–sponsored Women's Health Study, a multicenter, hospital-based study of PID, and concluded that IUDs increased the risk of pelvic infections in general and that the Dalkon Shield carried a substantially higher risk compared with other IUDs and with using no method of contraception.

Pelvic infection can be dangerous and even life threatening without treatment, but with antibiotic therapy, the infection clears up and the fever and abdominal tenderness will disappear. The real problem with IUD-related PID is the effect it may have on a woman's ultimate fertility. Even a mild infection in the fallopian tubes can contribute to infertility by causing the development of scar tissue or adhesions that block tubal transport of ova or sperm. Although a reanalysis of the Women's Health Study data by Kronmal and colleagues has cast doubt on some of the earlier findings on pelvic infections and resulted in a resurgence of interest in the devices, women who have thoughts of becoming pregnant in the future may want to think about the risk, no matter how small, of jeopardizing their fertility.

On the other hand, the disease risk and the threat to fertility may not be the same for all IUD users. When the data from the Womens Health Study were reanalyzed by Lee, Rubin, and Robucki a decade after the end of the study, the researchers found that married women in a stable, monogamous relationship had no higher risk of developing PID when they use an IUD (1988). The chances of contracting a sexually transmitted disease, which may lead to gonococcal or chlamydial PID, are greater for those who tend to be sexually active with many partners or who change partners frequently. IUD use is not a good option for such women at risk, but monogamous women who want to space their children by an effective and reversible contraceptive method that has the benefit of being unrelated to intercourse may want to consider one of the currently marketed types.

BARRIER CONTRACEPTIVES

Barrier contraceptives are forms of birth control that prevent pregnancy by preventing the sperm from getting to the egg. They include the diaphragm and the condom, which physically obstruct the passage of sperm throughout the cervix, and the contraceptive foams, sponges, jellies, creams, and suppositories, which chemically destroy the sperm in the vagina. Barrier contraceptives were very popular and widely used until the 1960s. After the introduction of oral contraceptives and IUDs, the use of diaphragms, condoms, and vaginal contraceptives declined, and they acquired a poor image. These methods were seen as aesthetically inferior and far less effective, and they were considered old-fashioned, somehow suitable only for older couples. But with the disillusioning recognition of the shortcomings of hormonal contraception and the protection against sexually transmitted diseases afforded by barriers, there has been a recent new respect for the old reliables.

Barrier contraceptives, unlike oral contraceptives, implants, injections, and IUDs, are used only when they are needed. This is a major advantage since the body is not subjected to a daily dose of hormones or the constant presence of a foreign object. It can also be viewed as a major disadvantage because the barrier must be present each and every time there is sexual intercourse and obviously requires more effort to use than methods nonrelated to coitus. But, except for an occasional allergy to a particular product, the barrier contraceptives present no health risk; they may, in fact, provide some health benefits to be mentioned later. Their drawbacks include less reliability when compared with sterilization or oral contraception and what some perceive as their nuisance or inconvenience factors.

Condoms

A **condom**, probably the most widely used contraceptive in the world, is also the only kind of birth control mechanical device used by the male. Also known as a "rubber," "safety," or "prophylactic," a condom is a thin, usually transparent, and flexible sheath made of latex or animal membrane that is closed on one end and open at the other. The condom is rolled over an erect penis to fit tightly during intercourse in order to trap the ejaculate and prevent semen from entering the vagina.

The origin of the condom is unknown. As soon as people recognized that intercourse was related to pregnancy 9 months later, there must have been some clever individuals who figured out that covering the penis might help to prevent pregnancy. The first recorded account of a condom appeared in 1564 in the writings of Italian anatomist Gabrielli Fallopius, who claimed that he invented it. Fallopius described a linen sheath to cover the penis in order to protect males from syphilis, and no mention of its use as a contraceptive was made. Condoms of fabric, fish skin, and intestinal membranes were used as prophylactics (the term is still in use today) against venereal disease for many years thereafter and were common in the brothels of the 18th century. Their value as contraceptives was always secondary to their protective function and only came to be appreciated gradually. It could be that because of the connotations of condoms to VD, prostitution, and illicit sex—a throwback to war-training films and furloughs—older couples had a bias against their use. According to the 1975 National Fertility Study, the condom was the preferred method of contraception for only 11% of married couples. But an upswing in condom use took place after 1988, and sales skyrocketed for the very reasons they had previously been disdained—the recognition of their protective as well as contraceptive benefits. Evidence that condoms exert a preventive effect not only on gonorrhea and syphilis but also on HIV, herpes, chlamydia, PID, amniotic fluid infections during pregnancy, and cervical cancer has revived interest in their use. Condoms rank third in preference among all women, after sterilization and oral contraceptives. Apparently more people are willing to accept a little loss of spontaneity in lovemaking to obtain the protection afforded by condom use.

Condoms today are of two basic kinds—those made of latex rubber and the natural membrane or skin condoms. Skin condoms, actually made from the intestine of a young lamb, are now manufactured only in the United States and cost more than double the price of the most expensive latex condoms. It is claimed that the skin type stimulates the "feel" of the vaginal mucosa better and permits greater sensitivity during intercourse. Whether or not this is true, skin condoms are status items perceived as luxury or "classier" condoms. In contrast to latex condoms, which have no pores or openings, membrane condoms have numerous pores of various sizes. *They are, therefore, unable to prevent the passage of hepatitis B virus or HIV.* Neither of these viruses can pass through latex condoms. Any type of condom will protect against herpes virus particles and bacterial or parasitic agents (those that cause gonorrhea, trichomonas, syphilis, or chlamydia infections).

Modern condoms are quality controlled, free of defects, prerolled, and sterilely packed in aluminum foil or paper envelopes. It is possible to buy them one at a time, but they are usually sold in a pack of three or in boxes of a dozen. Until the introduction of the "Magnum Condom," 20% larger than the standard latex condom, American condoms came in only one size—7 in. long. This size accommodates the erect penis length of virtually all men, especially since the condom can be unrolled to a greater or lesser extent until the entire penis is covered. Larger condoms, however, are available.

Condoms can be purchased with a plain tip or a reservoir end to collect the ejaculate, which is a better idea. Without the reservoir, the ejaculate could be pushed down along the sides of the condom to escape at the bottom during intercourse. Condoms also come smooth or textured, straight sided or contoured, dry or prelubricated with a water-soluble or a silicone substance. Some are lubricated with a spermicide-containing gel. Most condoms are transparent, but they may also be opaque and colored red, green, yellow, black, or any other color. Some of the varieties, openly aimed at increasing pleasurable sensations, are rippled or flocked with a rough rubber surface (Figure 13–4).

A condom that is used correctly is put on over an erect penis before it enters the vagina and is worn throughout sexual intercourse. An objection to condom use has been that it requires having to interrupt loving sex play in order to roll it on. Some couples have found that a condom need not detract from, but can actually enhance, sexual enjoyment by incorporating the activity of putting on the condom as part of their foreplay. If the condom has no reservoir to hold the semen, the first half inch should be pinched with the fingers while unrolling to keep out the air and leave a space to catch the ejaculate. Breakage or tearing of a

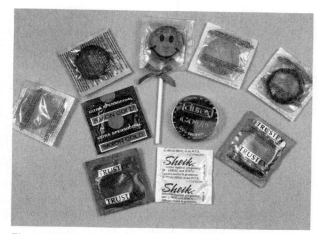

Figure 13–4 The variety of types of condoms should make it possible for couples to find a brand that is mutually pleasing.

condom is rare, but when it happens, it may be the result of friction or lack of lubrication, even in a prelubricated condom. Contraceptive foam is an excellent lubricant, and when used with a condom, the *combination is virtually 100% effective in preventing pregnancy.*

Soon after ejaculation and orgasm, the condom should be held tightly by the rim at the base while the penis is withdrawn from the vagina. If the penis becomes flaccid in the vagina, it might be possible for the sperm to spill over or swim out of the open end. If the condom tears or comes off in the vagina, contraceptive foam or jelly should immediately be inserted.

When condoms are used correctly with every act of sexual intercourse, their effectiveness in preventing pregnancy is generally regarded as fair. According to Reproductive Health Online, a web site affiliated with Johns Hopkins University, condoms are "fair" in actual use, resulting in 15%–21% pregnancy rates, but are "good" with perfect use, resulting in 2%–12% pregnancy rates (http://www.reproline.jhu.edu).

The major argument against the use of the condom, aside from its presumed failure rate, is that it interferes with sexual satisfaction. This disadvantage may be more psychological than physiological. Most women who have sufficient lubrication for an unsheathed penis would not be able to notice any difference in a sheathed one. An unlubricated vagina will make penetration difficult or painful whether or not a condom is used. Contraceptive jellies or foams, K-Y Jelly, saliva—anything but petroleum jelly or oil that affects latex—can be used to ease entrance. Men have been known to complain that using a condom thwarts their enjoyment of the sex act and is indeed a hindrance, somewhat equivalent to "taking a shower with a raincoat on." Condoms are very thin—they range from 0.4–0.9 mm in thickness—and they transmit body heat and touch sensations with no problem. Some men who have difficulty with premature ejaculation may find that their belief in the reduction of sensation provided by a condom may actually help them to retain their erections for a longer period of time. The rim of the condom may also help by providing a slight tourniquet effect.

The simple condom is reliable; relatively cheap or at least comparable in price to other methods; compact and easily disposable; completely safe; and needs no medical examination, supervision, or prescription to obtain. It provides excellent protection against pregnancy when used properly, approaching 100% when used with contraceptive foam. It gives the male a chance to participate in the responsibility for birth control, and it has the added advantage of protecting both partners against HIV and other sexually transmitted diseases and the woman against most types of vaginitis. With so much going for them, condoms should not be ignored.

But even with the current emphasis on the ability of condoms to protect against HIV, an obstacle to condom use is their limited availability in some areas of the country in which coming to terms with sexuality, especially adolescent sexuality, is difficult. Because of the misguided notion that ready availability of contraceptives leads to increased sexual activity, condoms may be neither easy nor convenient for young people to obtain. There has never been any evidence that withholding information or contraceptives prevents teenagers from engaging in sex. It only makes the sex they engage in more dangerous to them. Although strong opposition to the plan had previously been voiced by religious and other groups, with little fanfare New York City schools

began distributing condoms to junior high and high school students as early as 1991 as a way of combating teenage pregnancies and the spread of HIV.

Several alternatives to the traditional male condom are under development or under review by the FDA. The microcondom or glans condom is a miniature version of the standard condom that fits over the tip of the penis and is held on by a special adhesive. Another variant of male condom that is being tested is a loose sheath made of durable polyurethane plastic instead of latex. A condom that a woman can wear was approved by the FDA in 1993. The condom is a polyurethane sheath that resembles a sock with a flexible ring at both ends (Figure 13–5). When inserted like a diaphragm, the inner ring fits behind the pubic bone, and the outer ring surrounds and covers the labia.

Diaphragm

A **vaginal diaphragm** is another highly effective and safe method of contraception that has suffered from distrust fostered by misleading statistics on the use-effectiveness rates. Studies have demonstrated that with thorough education about the diaphragm, careful fitting, motivation, and encouragement in an atmosphere free of negative bias, the use-effectiveness rate of the diaphragm can actually be less than the theoretical effectiveness rate quoted in the beginning of this chapter.

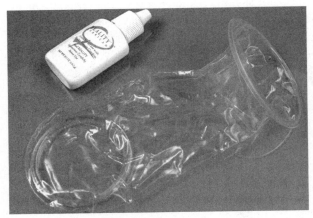

Figure 13–5 "Reality," the female condom. (Courtesy of Wisconsin Pharmacal Company, Jackson, WI.)

On its most recently updated web site, Planned Parenthood reports that of 100 women using diaphrams, 18 will become pregnant in 1 year. Of 100 women correctly using diaphragms, 6 will become pregnant in 1 year (http://www.plannedparenthood.org/birth-control/diaphragms.htm).

A vaginal diaphragm is a soft rubber dome surrounded by a metal spring. Used in conjunction with a spermicidal jelly or cream, it is inserted into the vagina to fit between the nooks of the anterior and posterior fornices to cover the cervix. The diaphragm itself is a good mechanical barrier to sperm, but it alone cannot completely bar the passage of sperm that might be able to get around its rim. The diaphragm must always be used with *liberal* amounts of a spermicide. It has been suggested that the diaphragm be viewed as a cup to hold the real contraceptive—the jelly, cream, or cream-gel—against the cervix (Figure 13–6).

Diaphragms vary in both type and size. A woman must be properly fitted with the specific type and size suited especially for her. They are available in rim sizes of 50 mm–110 mm, increasing in increments of 5 mm. Most women need a 70 mm–80 mm diaphragm. There are four basic rim types:

1. The coil-spring diaphragm, with a rim that is flexible all the way around, is particularly appropriate for a woman with strong vaginal muscles and no relaxation of the pelvic floor, a uterus that is not tipped, and a vagina that is average in size and contour.

2. An arcing-spring diaphragm, which has a firmer rim and forms an arc when compressed, makes insertion easier. It is designed for women who have less than normal vaginal muscular support and those with a mild or moderate cystocele (bladder bulges into anterior vaginal wall) or rectocele (rectum bulges into posterior vaginal wall), or a tipped uterus. The firm ring may be uncomfortable for some women, however.

3. The flat-spring diaphragm, less frequently used, is soft and flexible with a flat metal band in the anterior rim. It is especially suited for women whose anterior fornix forms a shallow niche in front of the pubic bone and who, therefore, need a thinner rim in that location.

4. The wide-seal rim diaphragm is unavailable from a pharmacy with prescription and must be obtained directly from a clinician. It comes in both arcing- and coil-spring styles and has a flexible flange rim attached to the inner rim of the diaphragm. The purpose of the additional rim is to create an improved seal and hold the spermicide in place inside the diaphragm.

There should be a diaphragm from among these types to fit every woman, but there are some contraindications to use. Occasionally, a woman is sensitive to the spermicidal agent, but switching to another one usually solves that problem. Infrequently, there is an allergy to the latex rubber that prevents use. Rarely, there is an anatomical problem that makes it impossible to achieve a proper fitting. Sometimes a combination of short fingers and a deep vagina prevent a woman from inserting the diaphragm herself—a difficulty that can be circumvented by a properly instructed partner or the purchase of an inserter.

Proper fitting, in an unhurried and unharried positive manner, by someone who knows how and who is willing to take the time to instruct the woman in the

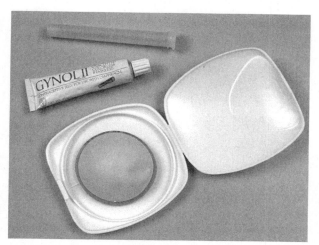

Figure 13–6 Diaphragm kits with applicator for insertion of additional contraceptive jelly or cream.

techniques of insertion, removal, and use is the answer to successful use of the diaphragm. A properly fitted diaphragm is the largest size that can be tolerated without being noticed by the woman or her partner. Fitted too small, a diaphragm may become dislodged during intercourse and leave the cervix uncovered. A too large diaphragm may cause problems with vaginal or abdominal discomfort or recurrent bladder infections, or may slip out of place to lie lengthwise in the vaginal canal. An inexperienced diaphragm fitter may not recognize that the size originally selected for a woman who is nervous about the fitting—and almost everyone feels somewhat awkward with the device at first—may be too small when she and her vaginal muscles are more relaxed. Other factors that affect diaphragm size besides the degree of tenseness at the time of fitting are those that occur during sexual activity. The vaginal barrel is known to expand during the sexual excitement phase of the female response cycle, so the presumed correct size in the sexually unstimulated state may be too small and slip out of position during intercourse. The frequency and intensity of intercourse and the position during intercourse can also affect the diaphragm if it does not fit snugly enough. All of these possibilities must be considered in the selection of the appropriate size.

Fitting should be done with sample diaphragms rather than with a set of fitting rims. Otherwise, a woman has no opportunity to practice putting in and taking out the diaphragm. Aside from getting the proper size, a most important part of the procedure is the chance for a woman to learn to comfortably insert and remove her diaphragm herself without aggravation or frustration. No woman should have to leave the office after a fitting with only a prescription for the pharmacist and a printed set of instructions. She must have been shown proper techniques of insertion and placement and have practiced until she feels confident.

Successful use of the diaphragm as a contraceptive requires use of the diaphragm. Trouble getting it in, trouble getting it out, and negative attitudes about using the diaphragm are reasons why it ends up in a drawer instead of over the cervix. The diaphragm's undeserved reputation as a baby maker may have its origins in the kind of climate prevalent in the initial fitting procedure. If a woman does not feel good and positive about using a diaphragm after the fitting, then she should express this to her OB/GYN and/or a nurse-practitioner at a family planning association.

Using the Diaphragm. Inserting and wearing the diaphragm will be more comfortable if both the bladder and bowel are empty before putting it in. Step one in insertion is the application of the spermicide to the diaphragm. Jelly, cream, or cream-gel preparations are made for use with the diaphragm. Any of them can be used, depending on personal preference, but foam is not recommended, and Vaseline, cold cream, or any other makeshift should never be used. Some women find that jelly leaks and that they like the consistency of the more viscous cream or cream-gel better. A teaspoon or more (more is better) of spermicide is placed in the bottom of the cup of the diaphragm and spread around the inside and the rim with the fingers. Keep in mind that diaphragms with spermicide are slippery and can zing out of the hand if not held tightly. Diaphragms are not and need not be messy to use, but there may be occasions when lack of privacy for insertion and cleaning present problems that may temporarily favor the use of another barrier method. Using one hand, the rims of the diaphragm are squeezed tightly together, jellied-side up, allowing half or two-thirds of the diaphragm to protrude from the grasping hand. While standing with one leg elevated, squatting, sitting, or lying down—actually any position that is convenient—the labia are spread apart with the other hand and the diaphragm is pushed into the vagina in the same way that a tampon is inserted—upward and backward—as far as it will go. It should then be checked for position by feeling for the cervix through the diaphragm and the rim just behind the pubic bone. If the finger cannot get by under the rim, neither can the penis (Figure 13–7).

The diaphragm, unlike the other barrier contraceptives, does not have to be coitus related. It can routinely be inserted daily or nightly and left in place for hours. Intercourse can take place immediately after

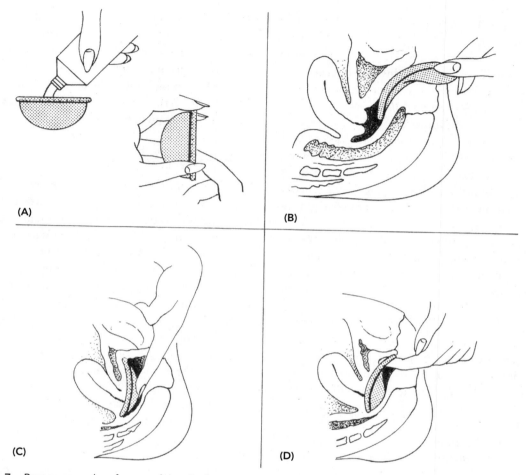

Figure 13–7 Proper procedure for use of the diaphragm. (A) Jelly or cream specific for diaphragm use is applied to the cup and the rim. (B) Diaphragm is inserted into place. (C) Diaphragm is checked for position by feeling for the cervix through the dome. (D) To remove, the finger is hooked under or over the rim of the diaphragm, and it then can be pulled out.

insertion or within 4 hours without needing the protection of additional jelly or cream. If more than 4 hours elapses, an additional applicatorful of spermicide should be inserted. After intercourse, the diaphragm *must not* be removed for a minimum of 6 hours. Normal activities—urinating, bowel movements, bathing, working—can all take place, but the position of the diaphragm should be checked after a bowel movement. Should intercourse take place again during the waiting period, more jelly or cream must be applied to the outer part of the diaphragm without disturbing it. Some spermicides come with applicators for inserting

the cream or jelly into the vagina. It may be that the additional loads of jelly provide too much lubrication, and some women may prefer the use of a condom.

Most women like to take the diaphragm out for washing every 24–36 hours to avoid the development of any discharge or odor or the possible risk of toxic shock syndrome. For removal, the finger is hooked under the rim of the diaphragm, and it is pulled down and out. Should removal ever be difficult because of the suction that forms under the diaphragm, squatting and bearing down with the abdominal muscles will dislodge it enough so it can be taken out.

After removal, the diaphragm should be washed with warm soapy water, rinsed, and dried with a towel. It may be dusted with cornstarch to help keep the rubber from corroding, but this is not necessary. It should be stored in its plastic container away from heat and not in the same drawer with nail-polish remover or perfume because the fumes can cause deterioration of the latex rubber. A diaphragm may discolor with time, but it should last for several years with proper care. It should be checked frequently for tears or holes, particularly around the rim. Refitting may be necessary after pregnancy, pelvic surgery, or any weight loss or gain of 10–20 lb.

A well-fitting diaphragm should not produce any discomfort, back pain, or difficulty in urination. Any irritation or itching may mean a mild allergy to the spermicidal perfume, and changing brands will eliminate the reaction.

The jellies and creams used with a diaphragm are not only spermicidal but also toxic to bacteria. Use of a diaphragm, therefore, may offer some protection against venereal disease and some forms of vaginitis. It has also been claimed that the diaphragm may be a protection against the development of cervical cancer. Another advantage to diaphragm use is that it can be used during menstruation to hold the menstrual flow. This may be convenient for sexual intercourse during the period.

One disadvantage of diaphragm use is its association in epidemiological studies with urinary tract infections (UTIs). The reasons for the increased risk of UTI in some diaphragm users is essentially unknown but may have a mechanical basis. It could be that the pressure on the neck of the bladder from a too-large diaphragm hampers the flow of urine and increases the chance of recurring UTIs. Refitting with a smaller size or different rim type may alleviate the problem. But there may be other factors that contribute to the link. Several studies have shown that a mild and transient increase in the number of *Escherichia coli* (normal colon bacteria) in the urine and in the vagina normally occurs as a result of sexual intercourse. Hooten and colleagues (1991) found, however, that while the increase in bacteria disappears within 24 hours in oral contraceptive users, both the prevalence and the persistence of these bacteria in the urine and the vagina is significantly increased in diaphragm with spermicide users as well as in condom with spermicidal foam users. These workers suggest that barrier contraceptives used with spermicidal foam or jelly predispose users to UTIs.

Cervical Cap

In contrast to the diaphragm, which covers the entire upper part of the vaginal canal between the pubic bone and the posterior fornix, a **cervical cap** as indicated by its name, is thimble shaped and covers only the cervix. The caps are made of rubber and are used with spermicide in the same way diaphragms are. They must be fitted to an individual woman so that the rim of the cap surrounds the base of the cervix while the dome of the cap does not actually touch the cervical os. The device remains in place through suction and is removed by tilting the rim away from the cervix with the index finger to break the suction.

Fifty years ago, cervical caps were considered an excellent method of contraception and rivaled the diaphragm in popularity both in the United States and in Europe, but their appeal waned with the introduction of oral contraceptives and IUDs. The only U.S. manufacturer of the caps ceased production in the early 1960s because there was little demand for the devices. Fifteen years later, when increased awareness of the adverse effects of hormonal and intrauterine contraception revived interest in barrier methods of birth control, the cervical cap was rediscovered. Feminist health centers imported the caps from Lamberts, Ltd., a British firm that currently is the only company manufacturing them, and distributed them to thousands of American women. In 1980, however, the FDA limited distribution and use of the cervical caps by classifying them as medical devices that could not be marketed until sufficient data had been accumulated to establish their safety and efficacy. Today, because their safety and efficacy have been demonstrated, they are available under prescription, just like diaphragms.

The Prentif Cavity-Rim type, available in four inside diameter sizes, has a firm rim with a groove running around the circumference to enhance the suction at the base of the cervix. The Vimule style is rimless and has a shallower dome; its flaring sides adhere with strong suction to the vaginal vault rather than to the cervix, and it is useful when the cervix is short.

One disadvantage of the cervical cap is that it may be somewhat more difficult to learn the proper technique of self-insertion and removal because the cap must be placed deep in the vaginal canal. Because the cap can stick by suction to any part of the vaginal walls or to the side of the cervix, it must be checked with the finger to make certain the cervix is covered. Another problem may be dislodgement during intercourse, although it is less likely than with a diaphragm. Difficulty with dislodgment may result from cervical changes in size or position that normally occur during the month or take place during sexual excitement. The cap could also be knocked off position by a different sex partner. Use of an alternate cap of a different size will frequently solve problems of periodic dislodgement, and women who are fitted with caps are told to use condoms as a backup for the first month of use and check for cap position after each intercourse.

Although there are mechanical drawbacks to cap use, there are many women who prefer this method to a diaphragm. For one thing, the tube of spermicide appears to last forever. The amount of cream or jelly required to fill one-third to one-half way up the cap is a tiny fraction of that needed for proper diaphragm use. Like the diaphragm, the cap must remain in place for at least 6 hours after the last intercourse. Unlike the diaphragm, additional spermicide does not have to be added to the vagina if multiple intercourse occurs unless the cap is accidentally dislodged. The cap is thus less messy, and for many, more convenient.

The effectiveness of the cap appears to be about the same as the diaphragm, which seems reasonable, given the similarities between the two devices.

The safety of the cap also is similar to that of the diaphragm. Although several cases of toxic shock syndrome (TSS) have been reported in diaphragm users, there have been no occurrences of TSS as a result of using a cap. One matter of concern has been the possibility of cervical changes. A study by Bernstein and coworkers (1986) found that 4% of cap users had abnormal Class III Pap smears after 3 months of use compared with only 1.7% of diaphragm users, a result that was unsubstantiated by other cap researchers (Gollub & Sivin, 1989; Richwald et al., 1989). Bernstein et al. had also reported cervical ulcerations as a result of Vimule cap use (1982), but no such damage has been associated with the Prentif cap. In approving the Prentif cap, the FDA mandated that a Pap smear be done before fitting and recommended a repeat Pap smear after 3 months.

An additional safety issue concerns the amount of time the cap can stay in place. In the past, when caps were made of rigid materials such as silver, ivory, aluminum, or plastic, women were advised that they could safely leave them inserted for the entire month, removing them only at the menstrual period. Current recommendations are far more conservative. The cap should be inserted for a maximum of 48 hours to minimize any possibility of irritation, vaginal infection, or cervical abrasion and also to reduce the chances for developing an unpleasant odor. A cervical cap should not be worn during menstruation because it can obstruct the menstrual flow and cause an upward reflux that may, according to some theories, result in endometriosis.

All in all, the cervical cap can be viewed as an improved, less messy, miniature diaphragm. It provides greater comfort, can be left in place longer, requires no additional applications of spermicide with repeated sexual intercourse, and may be a better option for a diaphragm user who gets frequent UTIs. It is perhaps a little trickier to insert and remove (Figure 13–8).

Contraceptive Foam

Foam preparations look, feel, and smell something like shaving cream. Foam consists of two ingredients: an oil-in-water emulsion medium to provide a mechanical cervical barrier, and a chemical spermicide, usually

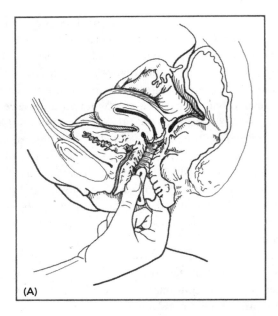

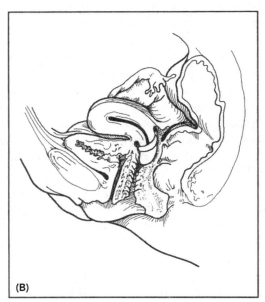

Figure 13–8 Insertion of the cervical cap. (A) The cap is filled halfway with spermicide and lubricated around the rim. The rim is compressed, the cap is inserted into the vagina with the dome pointing downward. (B) Once the cap is in the vagina, two fingers are used to push the open end inward until it complete covers the cervix. It is removed by breaking the seal around the rim with one or two fingers and pulling the cap out of the vagina.

nonylphenoxypolyethoxyethanol (nonoxynol-9), that immobilizes and kills sperm. The foam is packaged in a pressurized container propelled by chlorofluorocarbons. It may be released into an applicator from the can or may be purchased in packets of disposable applicators for direct discharge into the vagina. Although contraceptive creams and jellies for use without diaphragms are also available, they are not recommended because they are less likely to spread out rapidly and evenly. Foam preparations are the most effective of the spermicidal contraceptives (Figure 13–9).

With spermicidal foam, as with other barrier contraceptives, consistent use, each and every time there is sexual intercourse, is the main factor in effectiveness. Many couples have very successfully used foam as the only method of contraception for years. The effectiveness indicated by clinical trials shows such a wide variation that is virtually impossible to assess the actual success of foam in preventing pregnancy. *Population Reports* reported failure rates of 1.75–29.25 pregnancies per 100 woman-years of use occurring in trials conducted between 1961 and 1974. It is more than likely that with belief and confidence in foam, consis-

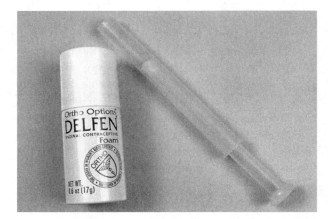

Figure 13–9 Spermicides. Packages tend to be close together on the pharmacy shelves, and care must be taken to choose the right preparation. The creams and jellies are specifically designated for use with the diaphragm and should not be used alone. Foam preparations are not meant to be used inside the diaphragm cup but may be used after the diaphragm is in place for repeated intercourse.

tent use according to directions, and use with every intercourse, foam can be highly effective. A fatalistic it's-not-going-to-work-anyway attitude will cause careless use and a high failure rate. Of course, foam and a condom used together result in supersafe and supereffective contraception.

The authors of *Contraceptive Technology* point out that even a conscientious foam user can make mistakes in the use of the method. Errors that can be made include not using enough of the foam in the right place. The manufacturers indicate that foam can be inserted up to 1 hour before intercourse, but vaginal secretions may interfere with dispersal after a while. It is recommended that application take place just before intercourse or not longer than a half hour before intercourse.

Other considerations important to effective use include making certain that the foam container still contains the material. With most of the brands there is no way to recognize when it is almost empty. Also, the foam container must be shaken vigorously at least 20 times to ensure mixing of the spermicide and the vehicle. It is also important not to douche after intercourse. Foam does not usually drip out, but a tampon can be inserted if an annoying wetness becomes a problem.

Other than an occasional allergy, there are no adverse side effects from using a foam. A noncontraceptive benefit is the decreased incidence of vaginal infections and sexually transmitted disease.

Spermicidal Suppositories

Encare Oval was the first product of its type—a vaginal suppository that melts and then effervesces into a foam for dispersal—and was introduced in late 1977 amid claims of very high efficacy (99%). The claims turned out to be based on studies of rather questionable and unconventional design in West Germany. The manufacturer revised its original promotional advertising, and the Ovals, along with subsequent market entries, are to be considered no more or less effective than any other foam preparation—about 97% if used properly and consistently, 85% in typical use.

The various tablets and suppositories have to be inserted 10–30 minutes before intercourse to give them time to dissolve, melt, or fizz to form a barrier. If intercourse does not take place within 2 hours, another one must be inserted. Some women have found that the suppository or tablet does not dissolve within the appropriate time; others have complained, perhaps because they have more natural lubrication, that the preparations are messy and drippy. For some women, Encare's effervescence releases a small amount of heat that burns and feels unpleasant to the vagina and penis. Others find the sensation unnoticeable or pleasant. Trying the method out is the only way to find out whether it is satisfactory. In concept, suppositories are attractive, providing the efficacy of foam in a small, convenient, and for many, more aesthetic form.

Vaginal Contraceptive Film. A contraceptive film, originally available only in Europe, is now sold in the United States. It consists of a 2-by-2-in. thin sheet of film containing 72 mg of nonoxynol-9. The little square must be inserted into or near the cervix not less than 5 minutes before intercourse to allow enough time for the sheet to dissolve and release the spermicide. It is effective for about 2 hours and has failure rates equivalent to other spermicide barrier preparations.

Vaginal Sponge

In April 1983, the FDA approved a polyurethane foam vaginal sponge that can be worn for up to 24 hours as a nonprescription contraceptive. The sponge, marketed as *Today,* is approximately 2 in. in diameter and 1½ in. thick. It is saturated with 1 g of nonoxynol-9 that has to be activated with water before inserting and also contains small amounts of benzoic, citric, and sorbic acids to adjust it to the vaginal pH. The sponge has a small depression on one surface to aid in positioning it over the cervix and a string loop on the other surface to help in its removal.

Although the *Today* sponge was the most popular over-the-counter female contraceptive for the 12 years it was in production, it has been unavailable since

1995, when it was used annually by more than a million women. The FDA had informed the manufacturer, Whitehall-Robins, that unacceptable high levels of bacteria in the air and water were found in the production plant, although the product itself was safe and did not warrant a recall. The manufacturer decided it was too expensive to upgrade the plant and discontinued manufacture of the sponge. This had little impact on Whitehall-Robins's profits but major impact on the women who used this low-tech, inexpensive contraceptive method. In 1998, Allendale Pharmaceuticals Inc. bought the manufacturing rights from Whitehall-Robins and anticipates that the sponge will be available for purchase in late 2000 or early 2001.

CONTRACEPTION WITHOUT CONTRACEPTIVES—RHYTHM

Rhythm is an older term for a method of birth control based on periodic abstinence from sexual intercourse. It is also called variously "natural birth control," "natural family planning," "BBT," "Billings Method," or "sympto-thermal method." No contraceptive devices are used. Instead, certain observations, techniques, and calculations are used to determine the "fertile" and the "safe " periods of the menstrual cycle.

Paul Ehrlich, professor of biology at Stanford University and founder of Zero Population Growth, said that people who practice rhythm are called parents. This assessment of the method's effectiveness is probably unjustifiably severe. Currently, in its most sophisticated form, using a combination of several procedures along with the skills necessary for their proper interpretation and with motivation and cooperation of the man and the woman, certain couples are very successfully able to plan, delay, or avoid pregnancy.

Techniques for the use of periodic abstinence for contraception are based on several assumptions:

1. That ovulation occurs once per cycle about 14 days before the onset of the next menstrual period

2. That the ovum is viable and capable of being fertilized for about 72 hours

3. That sperm are able to survive in the female reproductive tract to fertilize an ovum for about 72 hours

Calendar Rhythm

The calendar method of calculating the fertile period during which sexual intercourse cannot take place requires keeping track of the length of each of the menstrual cycles over an 8-month span. With the first day of bleeding as day 1, the number of days until the first day of bleeding of the next menstrual period is recorded. When she gets into the ninth cycle, a woman can calculate her fertile or unsafe days as follows: subtract 18 days from the length of the shortest cycle, and subtract 11 days from the length of the longest cycle. For example, if during the eight cycles the shortest period was 24 days and the longest was 33 days, the first fertile day during which intercourse must not take place is the 6th day after the onset of her period (24 − 18) and the last fertile day is the 22nd day (33 − 11). This method of calculation presumes that ovulation occurred 14 days before menstruation in both the shortest and the longest cycles but takes into account a possibly earlier or later ovulation, the life span of the egg, and the life span of the sperm.

Calendar rhythm works better, psychologically and physiologically, if a woman has regular 28-day cycles. With that cycle length, the period of abstinence can be shorter, and the likelihood of accuracy in estimating the period of greatest fertility is better. Cycle lengths in young women; in premenopausal women; and in women after childbirth, miscarriage, and abortion are likely to be irregular. Therefore, calendar rhythm alone is really a nonmethod of contraception and is now considered obsolete. Even with luck, its effectiveness is only about 60%–80%.

Basal Body Temperature

The use of the **basal body temperature (BBT)** chart is a way to enhance the effectiveness of periodic abstinence. Unlike calendar rhythm, which is mostly dependent on a regular cycle, BBT relies on a visible, measurable indication of ovulation—the elevation of the body temperature under basal conditions that occurs at the time of or shortly before the egg is released from the ovary. The use of the BBT chart has been described in Chapter 12 as a technique for couples who want to become pregnant. To use BBT to avoid pregnancy, a woman must have cycles in which an obvious rise in temperature occurs—only then can this method be used to determine ovulation. When sexual intercourse is restricted until three consecutive days after the elevation of temperature has occurred—that is, until the postovulatory phase when conception is biologically impossible—the BBT method can be a virtually infallible means of birth control.

The BBT of an adult, healthy, ovulatory woman throughout the month characteristically describes a biphasic curve between two menstruations. If the body temperature is taken orally or rectally under basal conditions (after at least 3 hours of sleep, at rest, and before engaging in any activity) starting from day 1 of the cycle, the daily variations are in the range of 0.1°–0.2°, until just before ovulation. The BBT then shows a slight drop—small and sometimes unnoticeable—followed by a sustained rise called the *thermal shift*. An elevation in temperature of at least 0.4° that continues for at least 3 days means that ovulation has occurred. After the shift, unprotected sexual intercourse can take place until the onset of the next menstrual period, when the preovulatory phase of the next cycle is entered. Strict adherence to the BBT method in this fashion is highly effective.

In practice, a woman may have shifts in body temperature that are difficult to recognize. The elevation may not occur during 1 day but may take place gradually over 5 or 6 days, may rise stepwise with several plateaus in between, or may zigzag up and down but with a progressive rise that can take as long as a week to level off. Illness, a night of insomnia, or even sleeping under an electric blanket may make interpretation of the chart puzzling. Although the same variation may not appear each month, a woman tends to have a consistent pattern that is unique and distinctive to her, and she has to learn to recognize her own graph (Figure 13–10).

During an anovulatory cycle, there will be no temperature rise. Under those circumstances, waiting until it is safe to have intercourse will frustratingly take the entire month, but there is no way of knowing for certain whether ovulation is merely being delayed or is completely absent. In some instances, ovulation may be occurring even though the temperature elevation is absent. Moghissi reported (1976) on one study of 30 healthy menstruating women who recorded their BBT daily while their levels of estrogen, progesterone, and luteinizing hormone were also being measured. As indicated by changes in hormone levels, ovulation occurred in 27 of the 30 women, but a rise in BBT occurred at the time of ovulation in only 21 women. Evidently, the absence of a rise in BBT may not necessarily mean an anovulatory cycle.

A major drawback to the BBT method is that it does not predict ovulation. It merely indicates when it has occurred. For complete safety, sexual intercourse is limited to the 10 or 12 days before the next menstrual period. To extend the range of days for unprotected intercourse, other techniques must be used in addition to BBT to try to define the safe or infertile days that occur before ovulation.

Sympto-Thermal Method

The sympto-thermal method is the most recent refinement of the rhythm method. It relies on a combination of techniques to recognize ovulation, including basal body temperature; changes in the quality of cervical mucus; alterations in the position and firmness of the cervix; the openness of the cervical os; and other symptoms of ovulation, such as ovulatory pains, breast tenderness, and edema, that can be subjectively interpreted by the woman.

The cervical mucus produced by the endocervical glands undergoes changes during the menstrual cycle. Reliance solely on these mucus changes has been promoted as a separate method of contraception by John

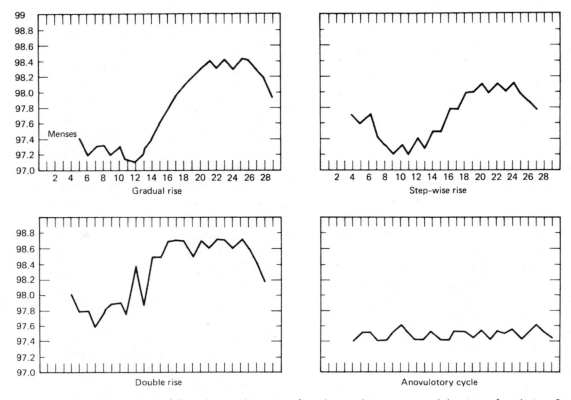

Figure 13–10 Not all BBT curves follow the usual pattern of an abrupt elevation around the time of ovulation. Some curves show a gradual rise, some a stepwise elevation, and others a double thermal shift or rise. Abstinence is always necessary until there have been 3 consecutive days of temperature elevation recorded at the highest point.

and Evelyn Billings in Australia and is called the ovulation method or the Billings method. Presumably, the Billings method eliminates thermometers, charts, and calendars, but unfortunately not all women experience easily discernible changes in cervical mucus or may have them in some cycles and not in others.

The cervical mucus method is not difficult to practice. A woman has to learn to recognize sensations of dryness and wetness of the vaginal discharge and be able to distinguish between feelings of stickiness or tackiness and of slipperiness or lubrication.

It may be possible to make some of these differentiations on the cervical mucus merely by noticing what appears on the underwear, but to gather the information properly, it is necessary to check the mucus as it appears at the vaginal opening, or even better, by a two-finger digital examination inside the vagina. The following patterns of mucus production in response to changing levels of hormone secretion occur:

1. Dry days, also called the early safe days, that occur immediately after menstruation. The vagina is moist inside, but the vulva is definitely dry. There is no sensation of wetness or lubrication or slipperiness and no staining in the panties.

2. Early preovulatory mucus. Mucus is opaque white or yellow, and its consistency is described as tacky, gummy, pasty. A woman has a sensation of stickiness, an awareness of mucus in contrast to the dry days. The less fertile mucus continues unchanged from day to day until it becomes wet mucus.

3. Wet mucus—thin, watery, more profuse. Estrogen levels are high, and the cervical discharge increases in amount, becomes clear, and has a high salt content. At the time of ovulation, the mucus becomes very profuse, has the consistency of egg white, and at the peak production during the time of ovulation, has *spinnbarkeit*. This is the ability of the mucus to be stretched between the thumb and forefinger into a long, clear, thin strand. If this clear mucus is smeared onto a glass slide and permitted to dry, it can be seen under the microscope to fern, forming a highly branched pattern because of the salt content. These signs indicate very fertile mucus—a very unsafe time—and persist for several days after ovulation.

4. Postovulatory mucus—again sticky and thick under the influence of progesterone. This viscous mucus may again become clear and watery just before menstruation, but this stage occurs inconsistently.

Approaching ovulation can also be gauged by changes in the cervix itself. Right after menstruation, the cervix is easy to reach and feels firm and almost dry. As the early preovulatory mucus develops, the cervix remains easy to reach in the vagina and is still firm. When the wet fertile mucus days appear, the cervix begins to feel slippery, softer, and is harder to reach. The os gets larger and begins to open. On the peak mucus day when spinnbarkeit and ferning are greatest, the cervix is virtually out of reach of the fingers, and the os is definitely open. In the dry, postovulatory days, the cervix again descends, is easy to reach, and the os is closed.

The sympto-thermal method of birth control requires a daily charting of the BBT, the cervical mucus, the cervical os, and any other subjective signs of ovulation—pain, spotting, pelvic pressure, and breast tenderness. The first 5 days of the cycle are considered safe, as long as cycles are never less than 26 days. Then the rule is no intercourse on dry days until mucus begins because semen may obscure the signs a woman is looking for during the day. Nighttime coitus is permissible. After the wet mucus begins, no intercourse or any genital contact is allowed until 3 days after BBT rise has occurred, the cervix has closed and lowered, and the mucus is again reduced and "dry."

Many people might justifiably feel that practicing this method is too involved and complicated considering that a barrier method can be used with equal safety, less psychological difficulty from abstinence, and probably greater effectiveness in preventing pregnancy. For couples whose religious beliefs prevent the use of other contraceptives, however, the sympto-thermal method can be acceptable and successful, especially when forms of sexual expression other than intercourse are used during the fertile period. In its favor, the method is a cooperative form of birth control; both partners must be equally committed to its use. If a woman has had little experience in exploring her own body, use of the sympto-thermal method creates a new and healthy body awareness.

There are few studies that have evaluated the success of the sympto-thermal method. In the largest trial to date, of 1,022 couples, conducted between 1970 and 1973 in five different countries, there were 7.2 pregnancies per 100 women in the first year of use; most of the women were over 30 and were well experienced in the method (Rice, Lanetot, & Garcia-Devesa, 1977). The study of 590 U.S. users by Wade et al. (1981) reported 16.6 pregnancies per 100 woman-years. Another 1980 report of a clinical trial sponsored by the World Health Organization among new users in Colombia found a much higher pregnancy rate— 34.4 per 100 woman-years in the first year of use (Medina et al.). More recent data from a WHO clinical trial indicate that the probabilities of perfect use are 3.1%, but the imperfect use, that is, user failure, results in a pregnancy rate of 86.4%—virtually higher than if the couples were using no contraception at all (Trussell & Grummer-Strawn, 1990). Hatcher and coauthors (1998) suggest that perfect users of the sympto-thermal method really should have a first-year failure rate of about 2%. Clearly, unplanned pregnancies are more likely the result of risk taking (intercourse) during fertile days than an inability to understand and use the method.

Coitus Interruptus

The withdrawal of the penis from the vagina before ejaculation occurs is called by the refined Latin term, **coitus interruptus.** It is better known colloquially as "pulling out in time" or "don't worry, I'll be *careful*!" As a method of contraception, it is the oldest, best known, and most widely used means of preventing pregnancy in the world. It requires no device or preparation, it is cheap and always available, safe and reversible, but it does have one obvious disadvantage—for most couples it is less effective than other methods.

The method requires that the male withdraw his penis completely from the vagina before orgasm and ejaculate well away from the vaginal orifice. The first few drops of the true ejaculate contain the greatest concentration of sperm, and if some preejaculatory fluid escapes from the urethra before orgasm, conception may result. (As Margaret Nofziger has commented, "A man is like a basketball player—he dribbles a little before he shoots.")

Obviously, this technique of contraception is not as desirable as some others, but it is probably underrated for its effectiveness and overrated concerning the potential physical and psychological problems. Psychiatrists, urologists, and sex therapists have warned of dire consequences as a result of habitual practice of withdrawal. There is no substantiated proof, however, that it causes premature ejaculation, pelvic congestion in the female, or any other inevitable difficulties.

When a couple uses coitus interruptus consistently, they are likely to have developed their own techniques to make the method mutually satisfactory. It does require rather rigid self-control during an activity in which loss of control is usually conceded to be more pleasurable. A woman may find it more difficult to relax and let go when she is concerned about the man's ability to withdraw in time. If a couple prefers that the male have complete charge of birth control, as he does with this method, it would seem that less "interruptus" and more peace of mind would occur when the man uses a condom.

STERILIZATION

Sterilization is a very attractive method of contraception for those who are certain that they do not want children. It is a one-time process, providing almost perfect protection against pregnancy (nothing is 100% except abstinence), and after it is over, it never requires any further action, thought, or worry about which method to use and the possible side effects. This can be a tremendous emotional relief. Sex is bound to be a lot more fun when the constant burden of birth control has been removed.

Sterilization is the most popular method of contraception in the United States for couples married 10 years or more. Nearly one-third of all married couples, and millions of adults, married and single, have undergone voluntary sterilization. While the number of male sterilizations, or vasectomies, exceeded the female sterilizations, or tubal ligations, in the early 1970s, the popularity of the female procedure increased rapidly after 1973, partly because of the introduction of newer and similar techniques, partly because the Supreme Court's ruling on abortion, giving women the right to control their own bodies, extended to voluntary sterilization and made the dictatorial formulas and criteria for sterilization used by doctors and hospitals obsolete.★

For the married couple who has all the children they want or who choose to be childless, the decision

---

★The "120 Rule" was standardly used by the medical profession. A woman's age times the number of her children had to equal 120 before she could have a sterilization unless she could come up with a psychiatric evaluation or enough symptoms of pain and bleeding to justify a hysterectomy. Part of the alarming increase in "unnecessary hysterectomies" during the 1960s and early 1970s may have been initiated by women themselves, who had little choice about sterilization except by removal of the uterus.

about which of them is to be sterilized can be influenced by many factors unique to their particular relationship. **Vasectomy** is the simpler operation, a 10-minute office procedure that ordinarily requires no general anesthetic. It is not expensive, and although both male and female surgeries are covered by many group health insurance plans, some policies may not provide complete coverage and expense may be a factor. The present physical condition and the medical history of both partners have to be considered. Of equal importance is their emotional status—their feelings about each other, about their future together, and about the surgical procedure itself. A woman may have a very happy monogamous relationship but still choose a **tubal ligation** because she wants to retain control over her reproduction. The final decision about which one is sterilized, or whether sterilization should take place at all, should be a mutual decision. There is no legal requirement for the consent of the partner, but if one has to sell the other one on the idea, there may be later recriminations.

Obviously, voluntary sterilization is not only for the married. Single men and women who are certain that they will never want any children in the future have also chosen sterilization for contraception. Those using Medicaid funds for sterilization may find that there are some federal and state regulations governing age and competence and some requirements for waiting periods or counseling. But anyone, married or single, who makes the decision must recognize that the result of the surgery is permanent infertility. Although various claims are made for the reversibility of vasectomy and tubal ligation, the operation has to be considered irreversible. What has been removed or cut cannot be expected to be replaced or put back together. Men or women who believe there is any possibility that they may change their minds should continue to use another form of contraception.

Vasectomy

The vasa (ductuli) deferentia are paired muscular tubes, about 35 cm long, that lead from the testes to the prostate gland where each joins with the ducts of the seminal vesicles to form the ejaculatory ducts. During orgasm, muscular contractions in each vas deferens propel the sperm from the epididymis of the testis to the urethra where they are expelled from the body along with the seminal fluid. The portion of the vas deferens that is located in the scrotum is surrounded by a sheath of connective tissue called the spermatic cord, which contains pain nerves and blood vessels. In a vasectomy, local anesthetic is injected into the scrotum and a small incision, either single in the midline or on either side, is made. The spermatic cord is drawn out, opened, and the vas deferens is exposed. A small segment of the vas deferens is removed on both sides, and the two ends are tied or clipped and coagulated by cautery with an electric needle. The incision is then sutured and after a short recovery period, the man walks out of the office—rather carefully—and goes home.

There is some minimal postoperative discomfort. An ice pack to the scrotum helps to reduce swelling and pain. A scrotal support is worn for several days, and strenuous physical exertion is avoided until there is no further discomfort. Because some viable sperm remain in the tubes of the reproductive tract, sterility is not immediate, and contraceptive precaution must be taken until about 10 ejaculations have taken place. The man then takes a sperm specimen to the laboratory to see whether it is negative. After two negative sperm counts, sterility is complete.

A no-scalpel vasectomy technique developed in China and introduced in the United States in 1988 promises less discomfort and fewer complications (http://www.nich.nih.gov/publications/pubs/vasect.htm). Under local anesthetic, a unique kind of clamp is used to encircle the vas deferens without penetrating the skin, and then a special sharp-tipped dissecting forceps is used to make a small midline puncture in the skin of the scrotum. Each vas in turn is lifted out through the one punctured area and occluded as in the usual vasectomy technique, and no sutures are needed to close the tiny wound. This technique was introduced in the United States in 1988, and many doctors now use it here.

There is no statistical evidence for any long-term clinical effects resulting from vasectomy, although considerable publicity has been given to scare stories concerning the relationship of the surgery to virility as well as all kinds of pathological conditions from arteriosclerosis to thrombophlebitis. More than 11 studies have now reconfirmed the lack of association to any illness, and a large epidemiological study—a federally funded look at 10,590 vasectomized men and 10,590 controls followed for 5–10 years—showed that the incidence of heart disease, cancer, or immune system diseases in vasectomized men was the same or lower than the incidence in nonvasectomized men (Massey et al., 1984). About one-half to two-thirds of vasectomized men develop antibodies to their own sperm, a condition that has been found, but less commonly, in both normally fertile and infertile men as well. No association between such sperm antibodies and any systemic condition has yet been established.

Despite overwhelming confirmation that vasectomy is one of the safest, easiest, and most effective, albeit permanent, methods of contraception known, occasionally reports of adverse effects continue to receive inordinate attention. One small study in Scotland raised the question of a cancer-vasectomy link when the researchers found that 8 of 3,079 vasectomized men developed testicular cancer from 3 months to 4 years after having the procedure. In a group that size, only about two cases statistically would be expected (Cale et al., 1990). The authors urged that doctors carefully check their patients' testes for any small tumors that already may be present but overlooked at the time of the surgery. Larger studies thus far have found no association between testicular cancer and vasectomy, so the validity of the link remains unproven. Previously, another small study had reported an association between vasectomy and impotence in 14 men over 50 years of age. Despite issues such as the tiny sample size, the fact that some of the men had been sterilized as much as 20 years before, the numerous other factors that could have contributed to the impotence, and the absence of any prior or subsequent corroboration, this study, like the one concerned with the link to cancer, generated, unsurprisingly, the usual media publicity. For some men who would have considered vasectomy as a method of birth control, the damage probably has been done.

Although half a million U.S. males already elect this procedure annually, reversible rather than permanent sterilization probably would have greater appeal to younger men. The procedure, called *vas anastomosis,* uses microsurgical techniques to reconnect the two stumps of the cut vas deferens. The surgery is very delicate and time consuming and has been successful only by the efforts of highly skilled and experienced microsurgeons. The reversibility of vasectomy is too unpredictable to make the possibility of changing one's mind a factor in the decision to be sterilized. Besides, the presence of sperm antibodies in the blood plasma of many vasectomized males makes the restoration of full fertility through reversal surgery even more chancy. Preliminary results using a *vas valve,* a device that is inserted into the vas deferens and can be turned on or off, permitting or restricting sperm passage, look promising.

Tubal Ligation

Ligation means tying, and tubal ligation has long been the classic operation for female sterilization and is the origin of the expression "having her tubes tied." Simple ligation, or tying a suture around the loop of the fallopian tube without cutting it, is rarely performed today because of its high failure rate. The tie had a great tendency to slip off the loop. Today surgeons doing tubal ligation may electrically cauterize the tube in several places (fulguration), use a plastic clip or a silicone rubber band (the Falope Ring, Figure 13–11), a silastic plug to occlude the tube, or simply remove a piece of the tube (resection). A popular, frequently performed operation uses the Pomeroy technique. In this method, a loop of the fallopian tube is elevated, the base of the loop is tied off with absorbable suture, and the loop is cut off or resected. When the suture absorbs several weeks later, the ends of the tube pull apart and leave a gap in between (Figure 13–12).

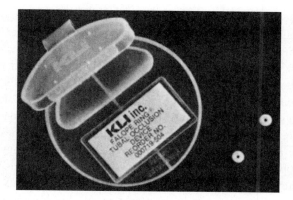

Figure 13–11 The Falope Ring, a silicone plastic band that fits over the fallopian tube for sterilization.

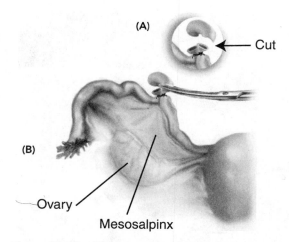

Figure 13–12 The Pomeroy technique for tubal ligation. (A) The fallopian tube is drawn up into a loop, tied with a dissolving suture, and cut. (B) Appearance of the fallopian tube a short while after surgery.

Colpotomy. Several methods may be used to expose the fallopian tubes. In the vaginal approach, performed by colpotomy, there is no visible scar. The cul-de-sac, or pouch of Douglas, located between the front of the rectum and the back of the uterus, is entered via a small incision into the posterior fornix of the vagina. Each oviduct is brought into view, tied and cut, and the incision is closed. This form of tubal ligation is very popular in India but not performed that much in Europe or the United States because surgeons have not been trained in the procedure. In skilled hands, the vaginal approach is safe, effective, quick, and easy. The incidence of complications from infection and hemorrhage is known to be higher, however, when the physician is inexperienced.

Endoscopic Methods. Laparoscopic sterilization, also known as the Band-Aid or the belly button operation, is the preferred technique of tubal ligation most frequently used in this country. A laparoscope is a form of endoscope or internal telescope that is used to visualize the abdominal organs. It consists of a long, slender tube that has a fiber-optic light source—cold, nonburning light conducted through a bundle of glass or plastic fibers—and a lens system that permits a viewer to look at the internal structures. The laparoscope is inserted through a tiny incision in the lower

edge of the navel, which is why the procedure has been called belly button surgery. Because the abdominal viscera are very close together and difficult to see, before introducing the laparoscope, several liters of gas, usually carbon dioxide or nitrous oxide, are pumped into the abdominal cavity via a Veres needle inserted through the same small incision (Figure 13–13). When the abdomen is distended to the point where it appears that the patient is in the second trimester of pregnancy, the organs have been spread far enough apart so that the instruments can be placed without doing any internal damage. During the procedure, the operating table is tilted so that the head of the woman is lowered (Trendelenburg position), which allows the larger intestine to fall away from the reproductive organs. A trocar, a sharp instrument encased in a metal sleeve or sheath, is placed into the abdominal cavity through the umbilical incision. The trocar is then removed, leaving the sleeve in place, and the laparoscope is inserted through the sleeve. A second small incision along the pubic hairline is made for the cauterizing forceps, or the forceps may be introduced right alongside the laparoscope (Figure 13–14).

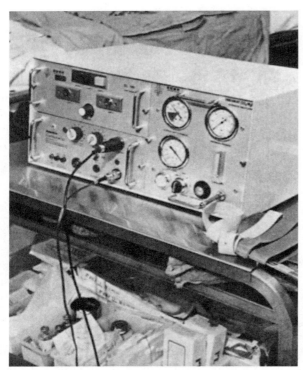

Figure 13–13   The automatic insufflator for distending the abdomen with gas and electrocoagulator for tubal sterilization.

About 2 cm of each tube is then electrically cauterized to coagulate the tissue and seal it. Some surgeons also cut or remove a piece of tube. Newer techniques that avoid electrocautery use plastic clips or rings to ligate the tubes. When the operation is completed, the laparoscope and the instruments are removed, the gas is allowed to escape, and the incision is closed by a stitch or two covered with a small bandage.

A woman who has had a tubal ligation by laparoscopic surgery can expect to feel a little discomfort around the incision, but the greater source of pain may be in the shoulders and chest as a result of the gas distension. This may last a few hours or a day or two until all the gas is absorbed. The amount of pain, the aftereffects of the surgery, and the resumption of normal activities vary in different women; some recover much more rapidly than others. If a local anesthetic has been used, the whole procedure from admittance to dismissal will take just a few hours in the hospital. A general anesthetic usually requires an overnight stay. The vast majority of laparoscopic sterilizations are performed under general anesthetic, despite the risks associated with the anesthesia itself. Use of a general anesthetic may result in some postoperative nausea and probably a sore throat because of the tube that has been placed in the trachea as an airway. Most doctors who perform laparoscopy appear to prefer that the patient be completely "out" during surgery, perhaps because they are not accustomed or have not been trained to do the procedure under local anesthetic. When local anesthesia is used, a tranquilizing or sedative premedication is injected into a vein, and the area of the incision is numbed with procaine or a derivative. Because the woman is sedated and feels nothing, there is no danger of her moving at the critical moment of cautery, although some doctors claim this as a reason for general anesthesia. Howard Shapiro, a physician and author of *The Birth Control Book,* contends that for him, an advantage of general anesthetic is the avoidance of a "distracting conversation with an inquisitive or apprehensive patient while laparoscopy is being performed." One would hardly disagree that nothing should be permitted to detract from the surgeon's utmost concentration to the task at hand, but, in practice, most operating rooms rarely lack irrelevant conversation. There is a great deal of casual, jocular, and presumably distracting conversation in the OR, frequently emanating from the surgeon, especially when a patient is totally anesthetized.

Obviously, no one kind of anesthetic is going to be appropriate for all women undergoing laparoscopic sterilization, but it is worth looking for a physician who is experienced at doing them under local anesthesia. Because the cost of the procedure itself from the surgeon may be high, the added expense of the anesthesiologist and the overnight hospitalization can price the surgery beyond the capability of a woman whose insurance does not cover it.

Minilaparotomy.   A laparotomy means an incision into the abdominal cavity. A minilaparotomy is the

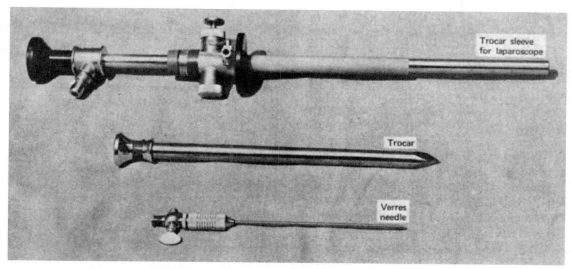

Figure 13–14   Instruments used in laparoscopic tubal sterilization.

term applied to a laparotomy through a very minimal incision in order to ligate the fallopian tubes. In the "minilap," a 1-in. incision is made just above the pubic hairline, the skin and muscle layers are retracted, and the fallopian tubes are brought to the surface and ligated, usually by means of the Pomeroy technique. Electrocautery may also be used, but because the oviducts can be brought out through the incision and directly ligated, the possible hazard associated with cautery can be avoided. No gas is needed or used to distend the abdomen, and the entire procedure usually takes 20 minutes or less.

Minilaparotomy is a safe, simple, and inexpensive procedure, but it is more common abroad. In the United States, most gynecologists appear to prefer the laparoscopic method. Minilaparotomy can be performed under local anesthesia in an outpatient clinic, or it may also be done in a hospital under local, general, or spinal anesthesia.

The complications of the laparoscopic tubal ligation are infection, hemorrhage, or cautery burns to the bowel or surrounding organs. A survey of 1,452 respondent members of the American Association of Gynecological Laparoscopists (AAGL) revealed that of the 89,492 sterilizations performed, the major complication rate was 1.8 per 1,000 women, and the death rate was 2 per 100,000 women. A pregnancy rate of 6 per 1,000 women was also shown, indicating that even sterilization is not perfect contraception (Phillips et al., 1981). As surgeons gain experience with the techniques of sterilization, the incidence of complications becomes more rare, but when adverse consequences of the procedure occur, they appear to be related to the skill and experience of the laparoscopist. A previous AAGL survey provided evidence that surgeons who performed fewer than 100 sterilizations a year had a complication rate four times that of the more experienced doctors. A woman considering a tubal ligation by laparoscopy must make certain that her doctor is thoroughly familiar with the technique and regularly performs sterilizations by that method. This appears to present the usual difficulty—how is a prospective patient to evaluate the expertise of the physician? In this instance, the best way is to conduct a telephone survey—to call the physician's office, to speak to the doctor, and to *ask*. The gynecologist should be asked what kind of training in the procedure has been taken and where; how many laparoscopic sterilizations have been performed annually; what kind of anesthetic is preferred by the doctor, and has there been experience in using a local anesthetic; and would the physician consider using a nonelectrical form of sterilization? These are reasonable and valid questions. A doctor who refuses to answer them on the telephone or makes a woman uncomfortable about asking is not the right doctor to use.

Obviously, physicians disagree concerning methods of female sterilization, and there are lengthy debates in the medical literature on laparoscopic tubal ligation versus minilaparotomy, epidural spinal anesthesia versus general anesthesia versus local anesthesia, and whether the gas infusion into the abdominal cavity is essential. In the same way that any one method of anesthesia cannot be appropriate for all operations, no one method of sterilization is suitable for all women. If a woman has uterine fibroids or any other condition of the reproductive organs that would make it advisable for the surgeon to be able to look in and around the pelvic cavity, then a laparoscopy is the more sensible operation. Under ordinary circumstances, when there are no abnormalities, a minilaparotomy under local anesthetic is less traumatic for a woman because it is simpler, but both procedures have their pros and cons. Neither minilap nor laparoscopy is recommended for women who have a lot of subcutaneous fat under the abdominal skin. Obesity prolongs the operating time, creates a problem in getting to the oviducts, and makes the operation more hazardous; but obese women usually can be sterilized by laparoscopy with a lower complication rate.

Theoretically, one form of sterilization may be better than another; pragmatically, the best and safest operation in any local community is the one performed by a skilled and experienced surgeon who has done a lot of them. There is no point in demanding a vaginal approach or the minilap in preference to the Band-Aid operation if the doctor is unfamiliar with the technique.

Even sterilization is not 100% effective, so a woman who misses a period or has any reason to suspect she is pregnant should check out the possibility without delay.

EMERGENCY CONTRACEPTION

No one really knows for certain what the risk of pregnancy is from one instance of unprotected intercourse. Some researchers have estimated that the chances are 2%–4%; others think that it may be as high as 20%–30%. In theory, this means that one can get away with playing the just-this-once game of unpremeditated sex at least 70% of the time, or possibly 98% of the time. Even those kinds of odds are not likely to be comforting to a worried woman waiting for her menstrual period. Emergency contraception, or "morning-after" contraception, reduces the risk of pregnancy after unexpected or unprotected intercourse, from failure to use a contraceptive at all, or from contraceptive failure such as condom breakage. Various methods are available in different parts of the world. The most commonly used in this country is ingestion of oral contraceptives containing ethinyl estradiol and levonorgestrel in higher doses than usual, within 72 hours of intercourse and then again 12 hours later. As originally described and tested by Yuzpe (1979) on 1,500 women and by Schilling (1979) on 115 college women, what became known as the Yuzpe regimen had a nearly 100% success rate in preventing pregnancy. After many subsequent studies, today the Yuzpe regimen is known to reduce the chance of becoming pregnant by 75%.

The mechanism of action of morning-after contraception is *not* as an abortion pill. The major action of the Yuzpe regimen of four pills is interference with ovulation, fertilization, or implantation. There is no evidence that oral contraceptives have any effect on an already-implanted ovum. The side effects of the Yuzpe method are nausea and vomiting and, in some women, abdominal pain, headache, dizziness, and breast tenderness. Obviously, this approach to pregnancy prevention is for emergency, one-time use only and is *not* a birth control method.

Although any oral contraceptive containing ethinyl estradiol and levonorgestrel given via the Yuzpe method will function as a morning-after contraceptive, a dedicated emergency contraceptive kit, containing four pills, was developed by Gynetics Inc., a pharmaceutical company, and marketed as Preven after FDA approval. One of the nation's leading pharmacy chains, Wal-Mart, perhaps under the erroneous impression that the kit was an abortifacient and would antagonize its customers, announced in mid-1999 that it would not sell Preven in its pharmacies, giving no explanation other than it was a "business decision."

A new emergency contraceptive technique was approved by the FDA in 1999. It causes less nausea and vomiting than the Yuzpe method and will be marketed under the brand name Plan B. It consists of two tablets of levonorgestrel and will be available initially by prescription through Planned Parenthood clinics. Later, according to the privately held company organized to bring Plan B to the U.S. and Canadian markets, the tablets will be available in pharmacies nationwide.

A study (Glasier et al., 1992) at the University of Edinburgh compared Ovral as a morning-after pill with the abortion pill RU-486 (mifepristone). The researchers administered either Ovral or RU-486 to 800 women who requested help after unprotected intercourse. Both treatments successfully prevented pregnancy, but RU-486 caused less nausea and vomiting than did the high-dose birth control pills. In late 2000, RU-486 was approved for use in the United States.

The morning-after insertion of a copper IUD has been used as a postcoital contraceptive. The copper IUD is effective probably because the copper begins to act almost immediately to interfere with implantation, while other inert IUDs could take days or weeks to reach effectiveness. Future protection against pregnancy is an added advantage of IUD insertion, but there is the increased risk of pelvic infection to consider. For a rape victim whose unprotected intercourse may also have exposed her to the risk of sexually transmitted disease, an IUD is not the answer.

There is another alternative for a woman unwilling to wait for a positive diagnosis of pregnancy. It is not a procedure performed the morning after, but it can be done within a day or two of a delayed or missed menstrual period. Called *preemptive endometrial aspiration,* the method is also known as menstrual reg-

ulation, menstrual extraction, minisuction, miniabortion, or even "lunch-hour abortion." A transparent flexible plastic cannula of very small diameter, eliminating the need for cervical dilation, is passed through the cervical os into the uterine cavity, usually without using a local anesthetic. The cannula is attached to a 50-cc syringe that provides minimal but enough suction pressure to evacuate endometrial tissue and blood from the uterine lining. The procedure takes only a few minutes, is relatively painless, and results in a low rate of complications. Such preempting of the uterine cavity will terminate a pregnancy if the woman has conceived and it relieves her from dealing with emotional and ethical considerations of abortion if she finds that necessary. If she is not pregnant, an unnecessary procedure has been performed.

Once there has been a positive diagnosis of pregnancy, the syringe aspiration of the uterus can be successfully used to terminate pregnancy up to 8 weeks of gestation. Now called minisuction or miniabortion, this method is less expensive, takes less time, and is usually less painful than any other method of abortion. If necessary, a paracervical block is used to reduce discomfort when the cannula is inserted through the cervix. The woman is likely to experience only a few menstrual-like cramps, if anything, during the suction. The aspirated material is carefully examined for evidence of the pregnancy, and a repeat pregnancy test and follow-up pelvic examination are performed in 2 weeks. Some practitioners are reluctant to use the syringe method as a very early abortion technique because of the chance that the cannula may miss the implanted conceptus and fail to terminate the pregnancy. They prefer to wait until the seventh or eighth week after the last menstrual period and to use the conventional vacuum suction method to avoid the possible subjection of the woman to two surgical procedures.

The same technique of endometrial suction aspiration can be used diagnostically to obtain a sample of the uterine lining for biopsy. It can be performed on an outpatient basis and can replace, when appropriate, the traditional dilatation and curettage (D and C), which requires general anesthesia and a hospital stay.

The many names for the procedure are an indication of the various uses for which the method is employed. The terms "menstrual extraction" or "regulation" and the technique were originally used by feminist self-help groups in California who developed the procedure to evacuate the menses at the beginning of a period, thus condensing 5 days into 5 minutes. In proving that there were medical techniques that could be performed for women by other *women,* and not necessarily by doctors, the concept of menstrual extraction was of great value. In practice, while there could be situations to justify its occasional use, using regular menstrual extraction for contraception or to rid oneself of the presumed nuisance or inconvenience of menstruation is too risky. Even when performed by the most skilled hands, putting an instrument from the germ-laden atmosphere into the sterile uterus too frequently is asking for trouble. Menstrual extraction is an invasive procedure. It always carries the possibility, although slim, of hemorrhage, perforation, and infection no matter how expertly it is performed.

$\mathscr{A}$BORTION

No currently available method of contraception is infallible 100% of the time. Even oral contraception has a failure rate of 1%, and multiplying that percentage times the number of women in the world who are faithful but fertile users of the pill can result in about a million of them finding themselves pregnant when they do not want to be.

People are not perfect even when they practice birth control conscientiously and consistently. Extenuating circumstances can cause a slipup, even in the most careful person. Statistics indicate that one-third of all couples who use birth control will still have a pregnancy that is unwanted when it occurs. The surveyed population did not include the unmarried woman, for whom an unplanned pregnancy is generally much more significant.

It is well established that legal **abortion** in an accredited facility, performed by a skilled practitioner and done before the 16th week of pregnancy, is safer than pregnancy and delivery. This is in contrast to the status of abortion before the January 22, 1973, decision of the U.S. Supreme Court. Then, kitchen-table abortionists or self-induced abortions using self-destructive methods with broomstraws, coat hangers, and chemicals were the only options and resulted in the death or illness of thousands of American women.

The induced termination of a pregnancy is legal and safe and is a woman's constitutional right based on the fundamental right to privacy. Although in poll after poll the majority of Americans agree that it must be the woman who makes this very personal decision, there is a small but vocal and powerful minority that would like to see that right abolished. Since the legalization of abortion in 1973, there have been constant campaigns that threaten women's decisions governing their bodies and they have been partially successful. For one thing, laws have been enacted that deny equal access to abortion for all women. In June 1977, the Supreme Court ruled that the states need not pay for nontherapeutic abortions for poor women although they pay for childbirth. Congress then voted to bar federal funds for abortions for Medicaid-eligible women unless they furnished "proof" of rape, incest, or life-threatening danger from the pregnancy. But in 1980 the Supreme Court said that both federal and state governments were under no constitutional obligation to pay for even medically necessary abortions sought by poor women on welfare. Then in 1981 Congress eliminated federal funding for abortions resulting from rape or incest. Although 13 states use state revenues to fund medically necessary abortions for poor women and 7 states provide money for abortions when rape or incest is the cause of pregnancy, by current law, pregnancy termination is the one medical procedure *not* funded by federal Medicaid unless it is necessary to save the life of the pregnant woman.

Further significant restrictions on abortion came through provisions of a Missouri law upheld by the Supreme Court in 1989. The decision in *Webster vs.*

Reproductive Health Services barred abortions at a "public facility" even if no public funds were used and the woman paid for the full cost of the procedure. Because even private hospitals associated with medical schools or community hospitals often receive public funding in the form of grants or accept Medicaid payments, public facilities can be broadly interpreted to include virtually all private institutions. The Missouri law also banned public employees, including doctors, nurses, and other health providers, from performing or assisting an abortion not necessary to save a woman's life and mandated medical tests to determine whether a fetus could live outside the uterus. By upholding the restrictions in the Missouri law, the Supreme Court provided the states with new authority to limit the right to abortion, and in the wake of *Webster,* many state legislatures have sought to exercise it by introducing measures that require waiting periods, parental or spousal notification/consent, or the exposure of every woman seeking an abortion to explicit and frightening antiabortion material rather than medical information prior to her "informed consent." It is evident that the states will continue in their attempts to provide for stringent criteria for abortion and that the legal right to abortion is unraveling.

Pro-choice women may have gained a victory in 1973, but there is obviously a strong move to turn back the clock to the days when wealthy women could obtain illegal but safe abortions because they could afford them, while poor women suffered, died, or gave birth to unwanted children. These women watch legislation taking away rights they thought they had won; there is a helpless feeling as events move backward.

The decision to abort is a matter of personal choice, but it is not an easily or casually made decision. Abortion is not considered an everyday kind of occurrence for most women; it may be an unpleasant and frequently painful experience. Few women view an abortion as anything but a difficult and necessary alternative to an unintended pregnancy. It is not a method of contraception. The issue is not that abortion may take the place of sensible contraception but that it is a backup method to contraceptive failure that provides a way out of an untenable situation.

Obtaining an Abortion

According to the Planned Parenthood Federation, between 1992 and 1996, the number of abortions in the United States fell from 1,529,000 to 1,366,000. The CDC estimates that 55% of legal abortions occur within the first 12 weeks. Only 1.5% occur after 20 weeks. Pregnancy termination is the most frequently performed surgical procedure in the United States.

Most legal abortions take place in freestanding nonhospital abortion clinics, which are located all over the country but concentrated mainly in major urban areas. Only a relatively small percentage of abortions (4%) are performed in doctor's offices, and only 20% of general hospitals provide abortion services. Although virtually all other surgery and almost every childbirth occurs in private and public hospitals, many hospitals, with and without religious affiliations, refuse to offer abortions to women who want them. In the few states that still pay for Medicaid abortions, poor women in urban areas are more likely to utilize hospital services if available. When Medicaid excludes abortions or the hospital does not provide them, low-income women have to get their abortions elsewhere or do not obtain them at all. The paucity of hospital abortions presents a major problem for a woman seeking an end to an unwanted pregnancy. The 10th AGI survey, reported by Henshaw and Van Vort (1990) indicated that 93% of the counties in the United States did not have a single facility in which an abortion could be obtained. Women in rural or less populated areas of the country may have to travel to another county, sometimes to another state, to get a health service to which they are constitutionally entitled. Such women, if they are young, may be also the least likely to have the money, time, knowledge, and ability to cope with the difficulties of having to go outside their local area for an abortion. The likely delay in obtaining the abortion adds to the costs as well as the risks of the procedure, which rise for each additional week of pregnancy. For women living in North Dakota, for example, a state with some of the most restrictive laws in the country against abortion and the only state without a Planned Parenthood affiliate, there is only one abortion facility, and no doctor in the state will staff it. The women's health clinic that provides abortion services has to fly doctors in from Minnesota, depending on weather and plane schedules.

Even in metropolitan areas with several abortion providers, choosing the appropriate facility may present problems. The independent abortion clinics vary in their equipment, ambience, attitude, costs, and quality of the services. Abortion can be a highly lucrative, even multimillion dollar business. Abortion mills, concerned more with making a profit than with meeting needs, do exist. Women must be wary of the clinic with a hello-good-bye, in-and-out atmosphere, devoid of respect for a woman's dignity and concerns. The abortion itself must be performed by a licensed qualified gynecologist who has hospital affiliations. There must be appropriate equipment and personnel for the preoperative tests and the procedure, and emergency backup, if necessary. For most women abortion is more than merely a medical procedure, so counseling and information provided by a professionally trained staff with a supportive nonjudgmental attitude must be an integral part of abortion services.

If a local community has a women's crisis line, women's center, or a chapter of the National Organization for Women, a phone call will provide assistance in finding the best abortion facility in a particular area. The nearest Planned Parenthood affiliate, which has a chapter in almost every state, or the national office in New York City can also help to locate a highly rated abortion provider.

Methods of Abortion

The earlier in pregnancy an abortion is performed, the less complex and safer is the procedure. Primarily, the method chosen is determined by the length of the pregnancy that is to be terminated. First trimester abortion refers to pregnancies that are interrupted during the first 12 weeks dated from the first day of the last menstrual period. The main technique of first trimester abortion is through vacuum aspiration, also called vacuum curettage. This is very similar to the previously described menstrual extraction except that the cervix must be dilated to accommodate a larger suction cannula, and more powerful negative pressure is obtained through the use of an electrical vacuum pump. The optimum time and way to terminate a pregnancy is at 8 or fewer weeks of gestation by means of a vacuum aspiration method, either menstrual extraction or suction curettage. After 8 weeks, suction curettage is the appropriate technique.

Before the suction abortion is done, a medical history is taken, and certain routine laboratory tests are performed. Obviously, there must be a positive pregnancy test. Blood tests administered should include a hemoglobin and hematocrit determination to check for anemia, a blood clotting time, an ABO and Rh typing, and a sickle cell anemia test when indicated. Rh-negative women should be given medication to protect against antibody buildup in future pregnancies. A Pap smear, a gonorrhea culture, a VDRL, and a urinalysis are also standard parts of preabortion testing.

The medical procedure begins with a bimanual pelvic examination to determine the size of the uterus and its position in the pelvis. Then, a speculum is inserted to visualize the cervix. The cervix and the vagina are swabbed with an antiseptic solution and the upper portion of the cervix is grasped with a tenaculum to hold it steady during the rest of the procedure. A local anesthetic—usually a 1% lidocaine solution—is injected into either side of the cervix to cause a paracervical block. Some operators use a uterine sound at this point to determine the direction of insertion of the dilators; others eliminate this step and introduce the first of a series of tapered metal dilators. Progressively larger sizes are used until the cervix is dilated enough to permit the entry of the right sized cannula or vacurette. The entire dilating process takes just a few minutes.

Suction cannulas are numbered to correspond to their diameters in millimeters. After 8 weeks, the general rule is to use a size that is 2 mm less than the number of weeks from the last menstrual period. A No. 8 suction curette, for example, would be used for a pregnancy of 10 weeks' duration, and a No. 10 would be used for a 12-week pregnancy. The larger the diameter of the cannula, the stronger the amount of suction.

The cannula is attached to the hose of the electric suction machine. When the machine is turned on, the cannula is gently rotated while moving from the fundus to the cervix of the uterine cavity. In this way, the entire product of conception, including the placenta or chorionic villi, the fetal material, and some of the decidual tissue or remainder of the endometrium, is removed.

During and after evacuation, the uterine muscles contract to prevent hemorrhage and reduce the uterus to its original size. These contractions may cause rather strong cramps for a while, but they usually subside within 10–20 minutes after the abortion. A period of rest and recovery follows, during which the woman usually receives instructions on aftercare and contraception. She may then leave and return to her normal routine, but most women prefer to rest for the remainder of that day and to avoid particularly strenuous activities for a few days. It is usual to experience cramps and bleeding for the first 2 weeks after an abortion, and it is not unusual for spotting to occur for another 2 weeks after that. The next normal menstrual period is likely to start 4–6 weeks after surgery, and most women ovulate within the first 3 weeks. Intercourse is not permitted for a week after abortion, and to avoid getting pregnant again immediately, a method of contraception must be available and used after that. It is possible to conceive even before the first menstruation.

The D and C for Abortion.

Before the introduction of the vacuum aspiration technique, the usual method of pregnancy termination was the D and C, the dilating of the cervix so that a sharp metal curette could be used to scrape the uterine cavity free of the conceptus and remove the parts with a forceps. This procedure needs more cervical dilatation than the suction method, is a far bloodier operation, is more painful and requires general anesthetic and a hospital stay, and often does not evacuate the uterus as completely as the other method. It is, however, a technique with which every doctor trained in OB/GYN has some familiarity. A woman whose physician wants to perform a D and C for a first trimester abortion should find another doctor, even if it means traveling to another community.

Late-Term Abortion—The D and E.

Some abortion facilities will perform a simple suction curettage up to the 14th or 15th week of gestation using a No. 12 cannula and "twilight sleep" for analgesia—an intravenous Valium and Demerol injection. In general, however, a procedure that is an extension of both the conventional D and C and the vacuum aspiration is particularly appropriate for use during the 13th to 16th weeks of pregnancy, although some advocates will perform it through 20 weeks. Called a D and E, *dilatation and evacuation,* the method requires a greater dilatation of the cervix and a cannula of greater diameter. Because the fetus is larger, withdrawal is aided by an instrument called the ovum forceps, which fragments the conceptus. Suction is then used to complete the procedure, and some physicians will administer drugs to minimize blood loss. The term *partial birth abortion* was created recently when the procedure became discussed actively at a religious and political level. There is a medical basis for use of the term. In June 2000, the Supreme Court ruled against a state ban against late-term abortion, arguing that a ban was unconstitutional and that late-term abortion was a medically appropriate method of terminating certain pregnancies. Debate over this procedure is expected to continue, and it remains controversial.

The D and E requires more cervical dilatation than the traditional D and C. Because rapid dilatation of the cervix by the usual metal dilators can not only be very painful and traumatic but can also result in cervical injury or laceration, the cervix may be enlarged gradually by the use of *laminaria tents* or similar synthetic osmotic dilators. Laminaria tents are made from two species of seaweed, *Laminaria digitata* or *Laminaria japonica,* which grow in the North Atlantic and North Pacific oceans. The stems of the plants are dried, cut, and shaped into cylindrical smooth sticks about 6 cm long, and of varying diameter, from 3–10 mm. A string is looped through one end just beyond a plastic disc that prevents the stick from migrating up into the uterine cavity (Figure 13–15). The sticks are sterilized by high-energy gamma irradiation to prevent any possibility of infection.

Laminaria is enormously hygroscopic—it has the ability to absorb and retain water in a moist environment. When a dry laminaria stick is placed in the moist environment of the cervical canal, it gradually swells to three to five times its original diameter, slowly, progressively, and painlessly dilating the cervix. Sufficient dilatation is accomplished within 6 hours. In practice, a woman who will have an abortion with the use of laminaria will require an initial insertion of the stick and is then asked to return the next day for removal and for the abortion. If the laminaria tent were not removed for several days, it would be likely to induce abortion anyway because of the cervical dilatation. The danger of infection becomes so great after 24 hours, however, that the stick should never be permitted to remain in place for that long a period.

Intra-amniotic Instillation

The other technique of abortion after the 13th week is the inducing of a spontaneous abortion by the instillation of a solution into the amniotic cavity around the fetus. One of three solutions may be injected. The most commonly used is a 20%–25% salt solution, hypertonic saline, but prostaglandin or urea may also be the agent.

The method is really *amniocentesis* followed by *amnioinfusion.* A needle is inserted through the abdominal cavity and the uterus into the amniotic sac. If hypertonic saline is to be instilled, about 150–250 ml of amniotic fluid is withdrawn and an equal amount of saline is injected. If prostaglandin is used, a very small amount of amniotic fluid is removed, and 40 mg in 8 ml of PGF_{2a}, the only prostaglandin currently approved by the FDA, is injected. Then the woman is returned to

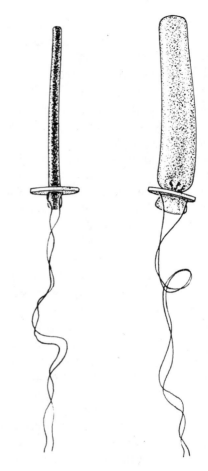

Figure 13–15 Laminaria stick, before insertion and after swelling.

her hospital bed to wait for the onset of labor, which may take anywhere from 12 hours to 2 days. There is no predicting the length of time from intra-amniotic instillation of saline or prostaglandin until labor and expulsion because it varies in different women. So does the amount of discomfort that accompanies the abortion. The process is the same as in childbirth; the uterus contracts, the cervix dilates and effaces, and the fetus is expelled. Fortunate women have a few cramps and it is all over; others may have to experience many hours of painful contractions.

One advantage of prostaglandin is that the time from instillation to delivery is shorter than it is with hypertonic saline. It may not always be effective initially, however, and a second intra-amniotic injection may be required. Other disadvantages of prostaglandin are that it commonly causes diarrhea and vomiting and, because of the more powerful uterine contractions induced, an increased incidence of cervical trauma. Even more traumatically, there is the real risk that the fetus may still show some fleeting signs of life when delivered.

The mortality of the fetus is ensured when hypertonic saline is used, but this method has the greater potential for severe complications. If the solution is inadvertently injected into a uterine blood vessel and gets into the general circulation, the rapid influx of such high salt levels into the bloodstream can result in death.

The intra-amniotic instillation of urea is used in Europe and England but has not been employed to any extent in the United States. Urea is safer, produces fewer side effects or major complications, and is always feticidal. When used alone, however, it frequently fails to induce abortion. Some doctors use urea as an adjunct to prostaglandin, reducing the need for that drug.

Safety of Midtrimester Abortions

Abortion through 16 weeks of pregnancy is statistically safer than continuing the pregnancy and delivering a child. When abortion is delayed beyond the 12th week, however, the relative risk of the procedure increases. The risk of both major and minor complications is affected not only by the delay in obtaining the abortion but also by the choice of abortion method.

Willard Cates and coworkers investigated the morbidity risks of more than 80,000 legal abortions that took place between 1971 and 1975. They determined that the safest procedure at the safest time was suction abortion at 8 weeks or less of gestation. The complication rate increased at 2-week intervals, becoming 91% greater with suction curettage when the abortion was postponed until the 12th week. After 12 weeks of pregnancy, a D and E, the extension of the suction procedure, produced another increase in the complication rate that was higher than that occur-

ring at any time during the first trimester. The risk associated with using D and E as a method of abortion during the midtrimester, however, was never as high as when intra-amniotic instillation of either saline or prostaglandin was used.

The researchers concluded that the relative safety of a D and E for midtrimester abortions should make it the procedure of choice between the 13th and the 15th week, and that specialists should be trained in its use so that this method can be made more widely available in abortion facilities. Those recommendations have been largely realized. D and E has replaced saline instillation as the most common method for terminating pregnancy up to 21 or 22 weeks from the last menstrual period. Beyond 15 weeks of pregnancy, however, a D and E should be done only by experienced personnel who have had appropriate "hands-on" training. There are physicians who lack experience with this method, and some doctors refuse to perform abortions at all between the 13th and the 16th weeks. This is the interval when the uterus is deemed too small and the amniotic fluid too insufficient to perform the instillation procedure. In geographic areas where a D and E is difficult to obtain, a woman who has postponed her abortion beyond the 12th week may have to wait another month before having her pregnancy terminated—and by a method with a higher risk of complications.

In a 1998 comprehensive review article, Gans Epner et al. reported, using 1991 data, that the risk of abortion-related mortality from legal abortions was 0. 8 per 1,000 procedures. The morbidity risk at 8 gestational weeks or less was 0.2 per 100,000 procedures and rose to 5.9 per 100,000 procedures at 16–20 gestational weeks. At 21 gestational weeks or more, mortality rates rose to 16.7 per 100,000 procedures, exceeding the risk of maternal death from childbirth (6.7 per 100,000 deliveries). Abortion-related mortality rates associated with D and E, labor induction, and hysterectomy or hysterotomy (surgical incision of the uterus) all increase at 13 weeks' gestational age or later but are much greater for hysterectomy and hysterotomy (Figure 13–16).

The best available national data on maternal complications resulting from abortion were collected in the

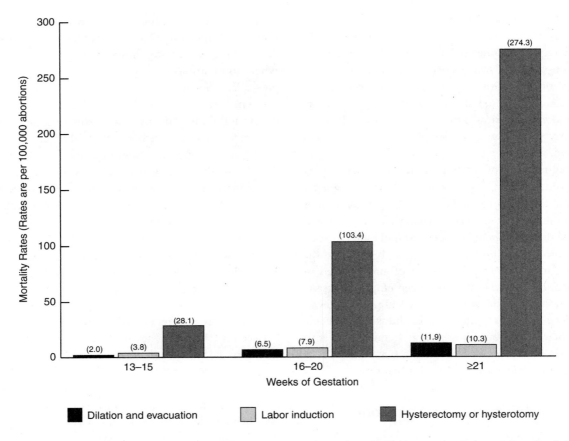

Figure 13–16   Relative risk of major abortion-related morbidity due to length of gestation and choice of method. (From Lawson, 1994)

1970s by the Population Council of New York and the Center for Disease Control in the Joint Program for the Study of Abortion (JPSA) (Gans Epner, 1998). Complications were defined for the purposes of this study as those that result in major unintended surgery, hemorrhage requiring blood transfusion, hospitalization of 11 days or more, or temperature of at least 100.4°F lasting 3 or more days. The JPSA data demonstrated that abortion-related complications are related to both gestational age, as demonstrated previously, and method. Complication rates associated with vacuum aspiration were 2 per 1,000 procedures, 7 per 1,000 procedures for D and E, 21 per 1,000 proce-

dures for saline-induced labor, and 25 per 1,000 procedures for prostaglandin-induced labor.

Although some women procrastinate obtaining an abortion because of ambivalence about the decision or perhaps in a futile hope that the symptoms of pregnancy will just go away, a delay may occur for a variety of reasons for which the woman is not responsible. A woman who normally has very irregular periods or who menstruates during the first month or two of gestation may not even know she is pregnant until after the third month. Or, a woman who starts out wanting her pregnancy may find herself by the third month in the midst of a separation or divorce or some other circumstance that would lead her to decide on termination. Many women may decide on an early abortion, but several months may elapse before they can accumulate the money necessary to pay for it. Health insurance covers pregnancy but infrequently covers ending the pregnancy.

When amniocentesis detects a fetal abnormality, a woman may need to have an abortion very late in the second trimester. It takes that long before all the results of the chromosomal and biochemical tests are in. But it is sensible, because each week of delay increases the relative risk of complications of abortion, that women who do seek an abortion soon after the first trimester have it performed by the D and E procedure.

It has been suggested that while the D and E procedure is safer, cheaper, far less painful, and less emotionally traumatic for women, the instillation procedure is much easier for the physician. The infusion of hypertonic saline or prostaglandin takes 15 minutes, and the doctor goes away, never seeing the woman in labor or the fetus she expels. It is a much "cleaner" way of performing an abortion than is the D and E method, which requires extracting fetal parts with a forceps—a procedure that may be distasteful and disturbing. This could explain the reluctance of many American physicians to perform D and E. But abortion is never pleasant. It can never really be free of emotional challenge either to a woman or her doctor, even in the first 12 weeks when what goes through the suction tube is not identifiable. The physical disadvantages and potential risks to women of the instillation procedure should be of greater importance to physicians than their own discomfort in performing the D and E procedure.

Abortion—The Sooner, The Better

To some degree, abortion is a stressful and problematic experience for all women and hard to deal with even in the first trimester. Abortion after the 12th week becomes an even greater difficulty, physiologically and psychologically. Many physicians do not perform the D and E procedure, and a saline or prostaglandin abortion is a particularly unpleasant, painful, and emotionally upsetting process that should be avoided, if at all possible. If pregnancy termination is the decision, getting it done simply and safely well before the 12th week is the best and wisest choice because there are far fewer complications and little chance of any deleterious effect, either psychological or physical, as a result.

Major studies have been conducted to determine whether prior abortion has any effects on subsequent pregnancies. The findings of investigations in Seattle, Boston, Hawaii, and New York indicated that there was no link between a previously induced abortion and a later complication or unfavorable outcome of pregnancy. The only exception, and the figures were not considered statistically significant, occurred in a Singapore study, in which preliminary results showed a slightly increased incidence of miscarriage after prior D and C but not after suction abortion. Similar conclusions were drawn by Hogue, Cates, and Tietze after their exhaustive 1982 review of the medical literature to assess effects of induced abortion on subsequent reproduction. The researchers found that abortion had no association with infertility, ectopic pregnancy, miscarriage, early delivery, low-birth-weight babies, or greater infant morbidity or mortality. Even multiple abortions produced no increase in adverse pregnancy outcomes, except when D and C procedures with general anesthesia had been performed. Dagg's 1991 review of all the available literature (225 studies) on the psychological consequences of abortion found that negative reactions were rare. Women were more likely to be depressed before the abortion than after it, when the majority had feelings of great relief. Although about a third of the women reported some feelings of regret, sadness, or guilt, 80% rated those feelings as mild. In contrast, the effects of having abortion denied to women produced profoundly negative sequelae. The studies showed that a third of the women denied abortion carry an ongoing anger and resentment for years. Also, the majority of the children (87%) born of such unwanted pregnancies are not given up for adoption, but are raised by their biological mothers, who then continue to harbor negative feelings toward their child.

Of even greater concern, an analysis of studies from Eastern Europe and Scandinavia revealed that those children born to mothers who sought to avoid their birth were much more likely to be troubled and depressed; commit more crimes; drop out of school; and generally have social, interpersonal, and occupational difficulties that lasted into adulthood.

$\mathcal{N}$ONSURGICAL ABORTION— RU-486

An annual 1.6 million legal abortions are performed in the United States and 31 million legal, as well as 22 million illegal, clandestine abortions are performed worldwide. The WHO has estimated that improperly performed, usually illegal, abortions result in the deaths annually of 100,000–200,000 women. Clearly, the development of a safer nonsurgical procedure as an alternative would be a boon. Also, being able to terminate a pregnancy at home, privately, with a self-administered, safe, and effective treatment would be a very attractive option for women. Agents to cause uterine contractions such as prostaglandins and various prostaglandin analogs have been tried in intramuscular and suppository form to induce contractions and subsequent abortion, but without enough success to compensate for the accompanying vomiting and diarrhea, the usual side effects of large doses of prostaglandins. But in the 1980s, a team of French researchers at the pharmaceutical company Roussel-Uclaf developed a synthetic steroid that, although it was not designed for that purpose, turned out to be an antiprogesterone agent, a drug that could cause expulsion of the conceptus from the uterus of a pregnant woman.

The drug was mifepristone and was designated as RU-486, after the manufacturer, Roussel-Uclaf. RU-486 is a progesterone antagonist that binds tightly to progesterone receptors and, by competing with progesterone, successfully blocks its action. Progesterone secreted by the corpus luteum has a number of effects vital to sustaining pregnancy. When the progesterone is blocked by RU-486, it provokes a miscarriage. The endometrium begins to erode and the implanted embryo is expelled along with the endometrial tissue. The drug is taken orally in a single dose of 600 mg, followed 2 days afterward by a prostaglandin analog given orally (misoprostol or Cytotec), by intramuscular injection (sulprostone), or by vaginal suppository (gemeprost). When administered up to the first 9 weeks of pregnancy, RU-486 in combination with the prostaglandin has a 96% success rate in causing a miscarriage. In most instances, the expulsion occurs within 24 hours of receiving prostaglandin. If the abortion is incomplete, the pregnancy must be terminated by surgical abortion. The rate of complications of heavy bleeding and infection with RU-486 are similar to that in surgical abortions, about 1%. Most women experience some uterine pain, but side effects of nausea, vomiting, and diarrhea also may appear after the prostaglandin administration. These are less severe when the second drug is the oral Cytotec.

On the basis of several large multicenter studies in France and England, it is a proven safe and effective abortifacient. However, while available in France, England, and China for many years, it has had great barriers placed against its use in the United States. Antiabortionists have named RU-486 the "death pill" and threatened boycotts against its manufacturers. RU-486 was approved for use in the United States by the FDA in September 2000. The FDA approval enables prescription by physicians who can accurately assess a pregnancy, have read and understood the prescribing information, and who have made backup plans in case of emergency intervention or surgical abortion. Despite its FDA approval, considerable controversy continues regarding the implications of RU-486. In addition to its efficacy as an abortifacient, the drug is able to block corticosteroid as well as progesterone, which may account for its therapeutic ability in certain cancers. When given to women with advanced breast cancer in preliminary trials, 18% had significant tumor regression.

RU–486 has also proven valuable in the treatment of meningioma, an inoperable type of brain tumor, and has dramatically reversed symptoms in Cushing's syndrome, a rare and sometimes malignant adrenal disorder. A multicenter trial of mifepristone in France is assessing its ability to facilitate labor induction in difficult deliveries and reduce the number of cesarean births. Promising research studies have tested the drug's therapeutic effectiveness in glaucoma, ulcers, wound and burn healing, diabetes, and endometriosis. It is known to affect immunity, hypertension, and stress, and there is the suggestion that the drug's ability to block corticosteroids may give it value in the treatment of AIDS (Regelson, Loria, & Kalmi 1990).

THE FUTURE IN BIRTH CONTROL

The question of what can be expected in future alternatives to current methods of contraception can be rather simply answered—not much. Even with the spectacular explosion of knowledge in cellular and molecular biology, no method that really differs substantially from the present techniques of birth control is around the corner, or even around the next decade. The major deterrent to progress in fertility regulation and the reason that contraceptive research is just limping along rather than forging ahead is lack of money.

Support for research on contraceptive development on a worldwide basis has shrunk by nearly 25% in the past 15 years. In the United States, federal allocation of funds for reproductive research, never that great, also has declined. The contraceptive research program at the National Institutes of Health has been budgeted at about the same level, even with inflation, since 1975. The drug industry, which extensively supported the development of oral contraceptives, now has little interest in pouring the kind of time and money it would take into additional contraceptive research. They blame the litigiousness of the American public, citing the costs of insurance, lawsuits, and settlements for contraceptive product liability. The reality is that even with 60 million women in the world on birth control pills, contraceptives are a very small part of the worldwide pharmaceutical market—only about $1 billion. In contrast, there is a $2½ oillion market for cardiovascular drugs. The financial incentive to develop contraceptives is lacking, and without anyone willing to put money into research and development or marketing of contraceptives, nothing much happens. The only companies doing any spending that could lead to new products are Ortho Pharmaceutical Company and Wyeth-Ayerst Laboratories, the rivals for leadership in the $900 million U.S. contraceptive market.

Immunological Methods

Unfortunately, support for contraceptive research has lessened at the very time that major advances are being made in reproductive endocrinology and immunology. Among the newest and most promising possibilities are offered in the area of immunological control of fertility. Recombinant DNA techniques that allow large-scale production by synthetic means of certain antigens have revolutionized vaccine research. Currently, animal tests and preliminary clinical trials are under way to study the safety and efficacy of vaccines that can cause the production of antibodies to human chorionic gonadotropin (HCG). Antibodies to HCG interfere with that hormone's role in implantation and ability to sustain pregnancy. Preliminary investigations seem to indicate that when the antibody level declines, the contraceptive ability is reversed to permit childbearing. Another possibility being considered is to provide passive, rather than active, immunity by giving a woman a dose of antibodies produced by monoclonal antibody techniques.

Other immunological methods under investigation include the production of antibodies to pituitary gonadotropins or to hypothalamic releasing factors, and the development of a way to immunize women against sperm or against their own ova, or against the blastocyst so that implantation is prevented. Any commercial availability of such vaccines to pregnancy is not likely until the first decade of this millennium.

Abortifacients. There are also research efforts to develop a once-a-month pill to induce menstruation whether or not conception has occurred. RU-486, when taken late in the menstrual cycle, leads to menses. Menstruation would preclude the implantation of a fertilized ovum, so the drug has great possibilities as a once-a-month pill with fewer side effects than oral contraceptives. Other lines of investigation involve plants. For thousands of years, a large number of plants have had abortifacient properties attributed to them, and native doctors and herbalists in various countries still prescribe them. The World Health Organization is taking such folk medicine seriously by initiating a study of plants used worldwide in fertility regulation. WHO continues to fund testing in primates for toxicology and effectiveness of the five plants with the greatest apparent potential. For example, one extract that may turn out to be worthwhile is from the Mexican plant zoapatle, the common name for *Montonoa teomentosa* (Gallegos, 1983). Another herb found in the southern part of Nigeria is *Momordica angustisepala,* used by Igbo native doctors to induce abortion in women and confirmed to have abortifacient properties in rodents by Nigerian researchers (Aguwa & Mittal, 1983).

Toward Male Contraceptives

Progress toward the development of a safe and effective pill for males is proceeding but at a slow and careful pace. It may be, as has been suggested, that despite an apparent attitude change and an accompanying more equitable distribution of research funds, the male-dominated scientific community is really reluctant to meddle with the male reproductive tract. More charitably, it may also be that a lesson has been learned in the past 30 years—that hormonal contraceptives have some hazardous side effects. At any rate, no one is rushing into production with the male birth control pill.

Sperm are produced in the seminiferous tubules of the testis under the influence of gonadotropins from the pituitary gland. FSH initiates the proliferation of sperm, and LH, acting on the interstitial cells between the seminiferous tubules, results in the production of androgen necessary for the completion of sperm development. Sperm in the tubules are nonmotile and incapable of fertilizing an egg, but after they are stored in the epididymis of the testis for a while, they acquire maturity and fertilizability. There are two main ways to regulate male fertility with a chemical agent: (1) inhibit sperm production by blocking FSH, LH, or the hypothalamic releasing factors and (2) interfere with sperm maturation in the epididymis. The trouble with using a steroid to suppress gonadotropins in order to interfere with sperm production is that androgen, responsible for sex drive and potency, is also inhibited. A synthetic testosterone derivative called danazol, which has been used as therapy for endometriosis in women, is an orally active antigonadotropin. Danazol, when used daily in combination with testosterone enanthate, an orally active androgen, decreased the sperm count without decreasing the libido. Other androgens, antiandrogens, and combinations of progestins and androgens have been used in clinical trials administered orally, through implants, or by intramuscular injection. Because they either suppress spermatogenesis or interfere with maturation or motility, they have promise as contraceptive agents. The WHO has tested weekly injections of testosterone ethanate for 1 year in 160 men on four continents and reported in 1990 that only one pregnancy occurred—a success rate equivalent to hormonal contraception in women. There were some side effects, including acne, enlarged breasts, and increased libido in a few of the men. As a form of birth control, the method is currently impractical because of the frequency of injections. The clinical trials will continue, using a longer-acting form of androgen and monitoring the men for long-term effects of the increased testosterone levels.

In 1972, Chinese scientists reported the development of a pill for men that is extracted from the seeds and other parts of the cotton plant. Called gossypol, the pill has been tested in China and reportedly has relatively few major side effects while reducing sperm counts below 4 million per milliliter of semen. Dry mouth, dizziness, fatigue, gastrointestinal symptoms, and decreased libido and potency were found in 3%–13% of the men taking gossypol, but fewer than 1% developed a serious side effect of potassium deficiency. The major problem with gossypol, however, may be its possible lack of reversibility. Restoration of full fertility after gossypol ingestion ceases can take 12 months or more, and in 10% of the men, no living sperm were evident in the semen after several years. Research efforts in the United States are being directed toward developing a gossypol analog that would have better reversibility and fewer side effects.

Also used in China is an injection of liquid polyurethane or silicone into the lumen of the vas deferens to form a plug. Chinese researchers claim a contraceptive success rate of 98%–99% and allege complete return of fertility after a simple surgical procedure to remove the plug.

It is unlikely that any form of drug contraceptive for men will be any less free of adverse effects than a similar agent taken by women. While women are justifiably resentful that all the risks associated with pill use have been theirs alone for so many years, most would not feel, unless revenge is their aim, that exposing their husbands or lovers to similar health hazards is a way to solve the problem. The ultimate goal should be the elimination of risk for everyone.

GnRH Analogs for Contraception

Another group of compounds believed to have great potential as birth control agents is the luteinizing hormone-releasing hormone analogs. Since 1971, when GnRH was finally isolated, purified, characterized, and synthesized—an undertaking that required the analysis of hundreds of thousands of sheep and pig hypothalami—more than 1,000 GnRH analogs, structurally different but functionally similar compounds,

have been generated. The chemical modification of the parent GnRH molecule has made it possible to create two kinds of peptide derivatives, the antagonists and the agonists. The GnRH antagonists do what their name implies—they interfere with GnRH activity and are able to block production of FSH and LH, thus inhibiting ovulation or sperm production. The agonists, which require less structural tinkering with GnRH to derive, were expected to be valuable for the fertility-enhancing ability in anovulatory women because they act similarly to GnRH. The profertility applications of the agonists turned out to be disappointing, however, and their effectiveness in inducing ovulation or treating such conditions as amenorrhea or delayed puberty has not been as successful as was anticipated. But in contradiction to their presumed actions, the agonists were shown to have highly active antifertility effects in higher doses. Tests on animals and clinical trials in humans revealed that, paradoxically, some of the compounds were very potent or "super" agonists that could inhibit ovulation or corpus luteum activity and thus provide contraceptive effects. Taken orally, these agonists were inactivated, but it also became apparent that the compounds could exert their pharmacological activity after being administered via other than oral routes—nasally, vaginally, and even rectally. In a study in Sweden, GnRH analogs were administered to 27 women via nasal spray daily for 3–6 months and resulted in the inhibition of ovulation and menstruation with no pregnancies and no apparent side effects, at least in the short term. Upon discontinuation, ovulation and menstruation return (Bergquist, Nilius, & Wide, 1979). A number of other investigations along similar lines have demonstrated that superagonists can clearly inhibit ovulation and thus constitute a promising lead in the search for a new female contraceptive. The most appropriate timing, dosage, and methods of administration and possible adverse long-term effects are all unknown as yet, although GnRH analogs should theoretically be safer and pose fewer problems than synthetic steroid-based oral contraceptives. We are still, however, a long way from "a sniff a day keeps the baby away."

Nevertheless, the promise of superagonists as contraceptives is greater at this point in women than in men. In males, agonists can inhibit or virtually prevent sperm development, but treatment is accompanied by the usual unacceptable side effects of testosterone inhibition and impotence. Men have to take androgen along with the analog to prevent these problems. Compared with the number of clinical trials in women, there has been relatively little testing of GnRH analogs in men, and as yet, the best agonist to use, what dose, and how it should be administered have not been established. It is anticipated that a GnRH analog contraceptive pill for males will take much longer to develop.

So What Else Is New and Improved?

In addition to searching for new methods of birth control, a major focus of contraceptive research is aimed at the improvement of the existing methods. Most of the advances in birth control technologies of the past decade, such as lower-dose oral contraceptives, medicated IUDs, and better ways of barrier contraception, are really improvements on, or rectifying the problems of, known methods. Assuming that the funds for intensified research and testing are available, the candidates most likely to appear first are as follows:

1. Safer oral contraceptives and new ways of delivering hormonal steroids other than oral injection. These include improved long-acting injectables, the intravaginal silastic ring that fits around the cervix, and the silastic two-rod implant under the skin. Also on the horizon is a hormone patch.
2. Progesterone-medicated and copper IUDs that can remain in the uterus for 5–10 years and postpartum IUDs that can be safely inserted without fear of expulsion immediately after delivery.
3. Better barrier contraceptives for women: disposable diaphragms, one-size-fits-all diaphragms, spermicide-infiltrated diaphragms, cervical caps that can remain in place for months without removal, vaginal or cervical spermicide-releasing rings, and female condoms.
4. Improved methods of ovulation detection so that "natural family planning" becomes a more effective means of birth control.

REFERENCES

Aguwa, C. N., & Mittal, G. C. (1983). Abortifacient effects of the roots of *Momordica angustisepala*. *Journal of Ethnopharmacology, 7,* 169–173.

American College of Obstetricians and Gynecologists. (1987, July). Oral contraceptives. ACOG Technical Bulletin No. 106. Washington, DC.

Bahamondes, L., Diaz, J., Marchi, N., et al. (1995). Performance of copper intrauterine devices when inserted after an expulsion. *Human Reproduction, 10,* 2917–2918.

Barkhoff, J. R. (1976). Urticaria secondary to a copper intrauterine device. *International Journal of Dermatology, 15*(8), 594–595.

Beral, V., Hermon, C., Kay, C., Hannaford, P., et al. (1999). Mortality associated with oral contraceptive use: 25 year follow up of cohort of 46,000 women from Royal College of General Practitioners' oral contraction study. *British Medical Journal, 318*(7176), 96–100.

Bernstein, G. S., Clark, V. S., Coulson, A. H., et al. (1986). Use effectiveness of cervical caps. Final Report to NICHD, Contract No. 1-HD-1-2804.

Bernstein, G. S., Kilzer, L. H., Coulson, A. H., et al. (1982). Studies of cervical caps: 1. Vaginal lesions associated with use of the Vimule cap. *Contraception, 26*(5), 444–456.

Bergquist, C., Nilius, S. J., & Wilde, L. (1979). Intranasal gonadotropin-releasing agonist as a contraceptive agent. *Lancet, 2,* 215–217.

Brinton, L. A., Daling, J. R., Liff, J. M., et al. (1995). Oral contraceptives and breast cancer risk among younger women. *Journal of the National Cancer Institute, 87*(13), 827–835.

Cale, A. R., Farouk, M., Prescott, R. J., et al. (1990). Does vasectomy accelerate testicular tumor? Importance of testicular examination before and after vasectomy. *British Medical Journal, 300*(6721), 370.

The Centers for Disease Control and National Institute of Child Health and Human Development. (1986). Cancer and Steroid Hormone Study. Oral contraceptive use and the risk of breast cancer. *New England Journal of Medicine, 315*(7), 405–411.

Collaborative Group on Hormonal Factors in Breast Cancer. (1996). Breast cancer and hormonal contraceptives: Collaborative reanalysis of individual data on 53,297 women with breast cancer and 100,239 women without breast cancer from 54 epidemiological studies. *Lancet, 347*(9017), 1713–1727.

Dagg, P. K. (1991). The psychological sequelae of therapeutic abortion—denied and completed. *American Journal of Psychiatry, 148*(5), 578–585.

Dickey, R. P. (1998). *Managing contraceptive pill patients* (7th ed.). Durant, OK: CIP.

Eschenbach, D. A., Harnish, J. P., & Holmes, K. K. (1977). Pathogenesis of acute pelvic inflammatory disease: A role of contraception and other risk factors. *American Journal of Obstetrics and Gynecology, 128*(8), 838–850.

Forman, D., Vincent, T. J., & Doll, R. (1986). Cancer of the liver and the use of oral contraceptives. *British Medical Journal, 292*(6), 1359–1361.

Gallegos, A. J. (1983). The zoapatle—a traditional remedy from Mexico emerges to modern times. *Contraception, 27*(3), 211–221.

Glasier, A., Thong, K. J., Dewar, et al. (1992). Mefepristone (RU-486) compared with high-dose estrogen and progestogen for emergency post coital contraception. *New England Journal of Medicine, 327*(15), 1041–1044.

Godsland, I. F., Crook, D., & Wynn, V. (1991). Coronary heart disease risk markers in users of low-dose oral contraceptives. *Journal of Reproductive Medicine, 36*(3) (Suppl.) 226–237.

Gollub, E. L., & Sivin, I. (1989). The Prentif cervical cap and Pap smear results: A critical appraisal. *Contraception, 40*(3), 343–349.

Guillebaud, J. (1985). *Contraception: Your questions answered.* London: Pitman Publishing.

Harris, N. V., Weiss, N. S., Francis, A., & Polissar, L. (1983). Breast cancer in relation to patterns of oral contraceptive use. *American Journal of Epidemiology, 116*(4), 643–451.

Harvard Law School, (2000, September 15). Harvard Law School Library receives 1970s-era Dalkon Shield litigation papers. Retrieved from the World Wide Web: http://www.law.harvard.edu/news/librarydalkin.html.

Hasson, H. M. (1978). Copper IUDs. *Journal of Reproductive Medicine, 20*(3), 139–154.

Hatcher, R. A. (Ed.) (1998). *Contraceptive technology* (17th rev. ed.). New York: Ardent Media.

Helmrich, S. P., Rosenberg, L., Kaufman, D. W., et al. (1984). Lack of an elevated risk of malignant melanoma in relation to oral contraceptive use. *Journal of the National Cancer Institute, 72*(3), 617–620.

Hemminki, E., Gissler, M., & Toukomaa, H. (1999). Exposure to female hormone drugs during pregnancy: Effect on malformations and cancer. *British Journal of Cancer, 80*(7), 1092–1097.

Henderson, B. E., Preston-Martin, S., Edmonson, H. A. et al. (1983). Hepatocellular carcinoma and oral contraceptives. *British Journal of Cancer, 48*(3), 437–440.

Henshaw, S. K., & Van Vort, J. (1990). Abortion services in the United States, 1987 and 1988. *Family Planning Perspectives, 22*(3), 102–110.

Hogue, C. J., Cates, W., & Tietze, C. (1982). The effects of induced abortion on subsequent reproduction. *Epidemiologic Reviews, 4*, 66–94.

Holly, E. A., Weiss, N. S., & Liff, J. M. (1983). Cutaneous melanoma in relation to exogenous hormones and reproductive factors. *Journal of the National Cancer Institute, 70*(5), 827–832.

Hooten, T. M., Hillier, S., Johnson, C., et al. (1991). *Escherichia coli* bacteriuria and contraceptive method. *Journal of the American Medical Association, 265*(1), 64–67.

JAMA Women's Health Contraception Information Center. (1997). ParaGard T 380A intrauterine copper contraceptive. Retrieved from the World Wide Web: http://www.ama-assn.org/special/contra/ortho/paragard.htm.

Khaw, K. T., & Peart, W. S. (1982). Blood pressure and contraceptive use. *British Medical Journal, 285*, 403–409.

Kronmal, R. A., Whitney, C. W., & Mumford, S. D. (1991). The intrauterine device and pelvic inflammatory disease: the women's health study reanalyzed. *Journal of Clinical Epidemiology, 44*(2), 109–122.

Laragh, J. H. (1976). Oral contraceptive-induced hypertension—nine years later. *American Journal of Obstetrics and Gynecology, 126*(1), 141–147.

La Vecchia, C., Franceschi, S., Bruzzi, P., Parazzini, F., & Boyle, P. (1990). The relationship between oral contraceptive use, cancer and vascular disease. *Drug Safety, 5*, 436–446.

Lawson, H. W., Frye, A., Atrash, H. K., et al. (1994). Abortion mortality, United States 1972 through 1987. *American Journal of Obstetrics and Gynecology, 171*(5), 1365–1372.

Lee, N. C., Rubin, G. L., Ory, H. W., et al. (1983). Type of intrauterine device and the risk of pelvic inflammatory disease. *Obstetrics and Gynecology, 62*(1), 1–6.

Lee, N. C., Rubin, G. L., & Robucki, R. (1988). The intrauterine device and pelvic inflammatory disease revisited: New results from the Women's Health Study. *Obstetrics and Gynecology, 72*(1), 1–6.

Massey, G. J., Bernstein, G. S., et al. (1984). Vasectomy and health: Results from a large cohort study. *Journal of the American Medical Association, 252,* 1023–1029.

Medina, J. E., Cifuentes, A., Abernathy, J. E., et al. (1980). Comparative evaluation of two methods of natural family planning in Colombia. *American Journal of Obstetrics and Gynecology, 138*(8), 1142–1147.

Mishell, D. R. (1989). Correcting misconceptions about oral contraceptives. *American Journal of Obstetrics and Gynecology, 161*(5), 1385–1389.

Moghissi, K. S. (1976). Accuracy of basal body temperature for ovulation detection. *Fertility and Sterility, 27*(12), 1415–1421.

Neuberger, J., Forman, D., Doll, R., & Williams, R. (1986). Oral contraceptives and hepatocellular carcinoma. *British Medical Journal, 292*(6532), 1355–1357.

Nora, A. H., & Nora, J. J. (1975). A syndrome of multiple congenital anomalies associated with teratogenic exposure. *Archives of Environmental Health, 30*(1), 17–21.

Phillips, J., Hulka, J., Hulka, B., et al. (1981). American Association of Gynecological Laparoscopists. Membership survey. *Journal of Reproductive Medicine, 26*(10), 527–537.

Pike, M. C., Henderson, B. E., Casagrande, J. T., et al. (1981). Oral contraceptive use and early abortion as risk factors for breast cancer in young women. *British Journal of Cancer, 43,* 72–76.

Pike, M. C., Henderson, B. E., Krailo, M. D., et al. (1983). Breast cancer in young women and use of oral contraceptives: Possible modifying effect of formulation and age at use. *Lancet, 2,* 926–929.

Planned Parenthood Federation of America. (1998). Diaphragms and cervical caps. Retrieved from the World Wide Web: http://www.plannedparenthood.org/birth-control/diaphragms.htm.

Population Reports. (1982, July). IUDs: An appropriate choice for many women. Series B, No. 4.

Rabe, T., Feldmann, K., Grunwald, K., & Runnebaum, B. (1995). Liver tumors in women using oral hormonal contraceptives. *Zentralblatt für gynakologie, 117*(3), 153–156.

Regelson, W., Loria, R., & Kalimi, M. (1990). Beyond abortion: RU-486 and the needs of the crisis constituency. *Journal of the American Medical Association, 264*(8), 1026–1027.

Reproductive Health Online. (2000, January 31). Recommendations for contraceptive use. Retrieved from the World Wide Web: http://www.reproline.jhu.edu/.

Rice, F. J., Lanetot, C. A., & Garcia-Devesa, C. (1977, June 22–29). The effectiveness of the sympto-thermal method of natural family planning. Paper presented at the First Assembly of the International Federation for Family Life Promotion, Cali, Columbia.

Richwald, G. A., Greenland, S., Gerber, M. M., et al. (1989). Effectiveness of the cavity-rim cervical cap: Results of a large clinical study. *Obstetrics and Gynecology, 74*(2), 143–148.

Rosenberg, J., Waugh, M. S., & Long, S. (1995). Unintended pregnancies and use, misuse, and discontinuation of oral contraceptives. *Journal of Reproductive Medicine, 5*(40), 355–360.

SafetyAlerts. (2000, September 15). Retrieved from the World Wide Web: http://www.safetyalerts.com.

Schilling, L. H. (1979). An alternative to the use of high-dose estrogens for post-coital contraception. *Journal of American College Health Association, 27*(5), 247–249.

Schlesselman, J. J. (1989). Cancer of the breast and reproductive tract in relation to use of oral contraceptives. *Contraception, 40*(1), 1–38.

Shapiro, H. (1977). *The birth control book* (p. 211). New York: St. Martin's Press.

Shoupe, D., & Mishell, D. R. (1989). Norplant: Subdermal implant system for long-term contraception. *American Journal of Obstetrics Gynecology, 160*(5, Pt. 2), 1286–1292.

Skegg, D., & Spears, G. (1989). Depot medroxyprogesterone (Depo-Provera) and the risk of breast cancer. *British Medical Journal, 299,* 759–762.

Stadel, B. V. (1988). Oral contraceptives and premenopausal breast cancer in nulliparous women. *Contraception, 38*(3), 287–299.

Tietze, C. (1973). Intrauterine devices: Clinical aspects. In E. S. Hafez & T. N. Evans (Eds.), *Human reproduction.* Hagerstown, MD: Harper & Row.

Trussell, J., & Grummer-Strawn, L. (1990). Contraceptive failure of the ovulation method of periodic abstinence. *Family Planning Perspectives, 22*(2), 65–75.

Trussell, J., & Kowal, D. (1998). R. A. Hatcher (Ed.), In The essentials of contraception. *Contraceptive Technology* (17th ed.). New York: Ardent Media.

Vessey, M. P. (1989). Epidemiological studies of oral contraception. *International Journal of Fertility, 34* (Suppl), 64–70.

Vessey, M. P., Lawless, M., McPherson, K., & Yeates, D. (1983). Neoplasia of the cervix uteri and contraception: A possible adverse effect of the pill. *Lancet, 2,* 930–934.

Vessey, M. P., Lawless, M., Yeates, D., & McPherson, K. (1985). Progestogen-only oral contraception: Findings in a large prospective study with special reference to effectiveness. *British Journal of Family Planning 10*(4), 117–121.

Vessey, M. P., Yeates, D., Flavel, R., & McPherson, K. (1981). Pelvic inflammatory disease and the intrauterine device: Findings in a large cohort study. *British Medical Journal, 282*(6267), 855–857.

Wade, M. E., McCarthy, P., Braunstein, G. C., et al. (1981). A randomized prospective study of the use-effectiveness of two methods of natural family planning. *American Journal of Obstetrics and Gynecology, 141*(4), 368–376.

Weir, R. J. (1982). Effect on blood pressure of changing from high to low dose steroid preparations in women with oral contraceptive induced hypertension. *Scottish Medical Journal, 27,* 212–215.

Westhoff, C. L. (1999, January). Breast cancer risk: Perception versus reality. *Contraception, 59* (1 Suppl.), 255–285.

Westrom, L. (1980). Incidence, prevalence, and trends of acute pelvic inflammatory disease and its consequences in industrialized countries. *American Journal of Obstetrics and Gynecology, 17*(5), 509–511.

Yuzpe, A. A. (1979). Post-coital contraception. *International Journal of Gynecology and Obstetrics, 16,* 497–505.

MENOPAUSE

*H*umans are virtually the only species to outlive their reproductive capacities—a true biological difference of great evolutionary interest but unknown significance. In both males and females, the ability to reproduce ceases before the end of a normal life span, but women have a longer post-reproductive period than men. When the average American woman dies at the age of 76, she has not been able to produce a baby for approximately 25 years, or one-third of her life. This female longevity is historically fairly recent; in the past, most women died before or soon after menopause.

Menopause is the final phase of a woman's reproductive ability. It refers to the cessation of the menstrual periods and is considered complete after 1 year of amenorrhea. Although in some women menstruation stops abruptly, menopause is usually a gradual process, with menstrual irregularity making it very difficult to tell precisely when the periods have stopped. *Climacteric* (also known as the perimenopause) is the name given to the gradual changeover, that period of declining ovarian function that terminates in complete menopause. It generally starts in the 40s and is believed to be influenced by the same kinds of factors that affect menarche: race, heredity, climate, nutrition, general health, and socioeconomic status. One-half of all women experience menopause between the ages of 45 and 50, one-fourth before age 45, and one-fourth after age 50. In the United States, the average age of menopause is 51.4. About 8% of women experience premature menopause before age 40. Factors contributing to early menopause include cigarette smoking (Willett et al., 1983), nulliparity (Kato et al., 1998), and medically treated depression (Harlow, Cramer, & Annis, 1995). Menopause is said to be delayed when it occurs after age 55.

CAUSE OF MENOPAUSE

The large number of ovarian follicles with which a woman is born progressively decreases throughout her lifetime. All through childhood, adolescence, and maturity, the follicles are lost by ovulation and atresia. Eventually, the total number is almost exhausted, and the ovarian hormone secretion diminishes. The decreased ovarian estrogen produced by the few follicles that are left is insufficient to inhibit the pituitary gonadotropins, and follicle-stimulating hormone (FSH) and luteinizing hormone (LH) levels greatly increase. In the first years after menopause, the FSH levels in the blood and urine rise 10–20 times above what they were during the reproductive years and stay

high. LH levels also significantly increase. In fact, the major source of human gonadotropins used to induce ovulation in the treatment of infertility is the urine of postmenopausal women. The secretion of FSH and LH continues in the menopause in a pulsatile fashion with a slightly higher frequency and amplitude. None of the other pituitary hormones (prolactin, growth hormone, adrenocorticotropic hormone, thyroid-stimulating hormone) appears to be affected by the loss of reproductive function.

When the level of ovarian estrogens falls below a certain critical amount, the balanced hypothalamic-pituitary-ovarian feedback system is altered. Even though the ovaries may not be totally depleted of follicles, the reduced levels of estrogen secreted no longer cause enough proliferation of the endometrium to result in the usual buildup and breakdown, and the menstrual cycles stop. Menopause is a normal physiological consequence of the progressive loss of follicles that started in a woman before she was born. In a sense, the climacteric starts during embryonic life and continues until death.

DECLINE OF FERTILITY

As menopause approaches, more and more of the menstrual cycles become anovulatory. Cycles in which ovulation does not occur are at first likely to be shorter, and 21-day cycles are not unusual. Any ovulatory symptoms, such as dysmenorrhea, that ordinarily accompany a progestational phase are missing. As ovarian function further decreases, cycles then may become longer because the endometrium is stimulated only by estrogen, and proliferation may take more time. Between the ages of 40 and 45, an estimated 75% of the cycles are ovulatory. After age 46, the percentage drops to 60%. Pregnancy is infrequent between ages 45 and 49, occurring in only 1 of 1,000 births. After age 50, the incidence drops to 1 in 250,000 births. Pregnancy after menopause is extremely rare. It is assumed that such a conception must have resulted from the random ovulation of a surviving follicle and was not associated with a menstrual cycle.

Evidently, there need be little concern about becoming pregnant after menopause has occurred, but for women in their 40s whose periods have ceased, the valid questions are, "How do I know if I reached menopause yet, and when can I stop using a contraceptive?"

The data of Wallace et al. (1979) show that in a woman over 45, the longer the period of amenorrhea, the more likelihood there is that the menopause is permanent. Between age 45 and 49, a 6-month interval without menstruation means a 45% probability of menopause, but in a woman 53 or older, the probability is 70%. That is, after an amenorrhea of 180 days, 55% of women in their late 40s and 30% of women in their early 50s still could expect to have one or more additional episodes of menstruation. Even after 1 year of no menstrual periods, 10.5% of women ages 45–49, 6.4% of women ages 50–52, and 4.5% of women 53 or older could have another cycle, possibly ovulatory. The probability of menopause is greater when the amenorrhea has been preceded by prior irregularity, but if avoidance of pregnancy is important to a woman, it would be prudent to use contraceptives for a *full year* after the last menstrual period.

ℰSTROGEN SECRETION IN POSTMENOPAUSE

While gonadotropin secretion is consistently high, estrogen levels in the postmenopause are subject to very wide variation and may or may not be low. The *kind* of estrogen found in the blood and urine in postmenopause is different from that of premenopause. The major hormone produced by the ovaries during the reproductive years is **estradiol;** the estrogen found in postmenopausal women is **estrone.** Estradiol is much more biologically active than estrone. In some postmenopausal women, estrogen is maintained at a moderate level for the rest of their lives. The extent and rate of its production varies from woman to woman. The following summarizes current knowledge concerning the secretion of estrogens:

1. Estradiol and some estrone are produced by the theca cells surrounding the developing follicles during the reproductive years. The rest of the estrone is derived by the conversion of estradiol and androstenedione by peripheral tissues of the body not located in the ovaries.

2. Androstenedione is a weak androgen. It is produced by the adrenal glands and also by the stromal cells of the ovaries (connective tissue elements containing degenerating theca cells and structures from atretic follicles).

3. After the disappearance of the follicles in the ovaries, the stromal cells, under the influence of high gonadotropin secretion, produce androstenedione, which is converted (aromatized) to estrone by peripheral tissues, principally blood and fat tissue.

4. Even if the ovaries are removed during postmenopause, estrone levels do not decrease significantly, indicating that the adrenal glands produce estrogen by extraovarian conversion of the precursor, androstenedione. The adrenals are the major source of this androgen in the postmenopause, contributing about 85%. If the adrenal glands are removed in a woman who has had her ovaries removed, even then the urinary excretion of estrone does not completely disappear. The origin of this extraovarian and extraadrenal estrogen is unknown.

5. The amount of estrogen in the postmenopausal woman is dependent on the percentage of androstenedione that is converted to estrone. Greater production of estrone and increased rate of conversion have been correlated with increases in age and body weight. Obese women have

more adipose tissue with which to aromatize androstenedione to estrone. This may be why fat women generally have fewer menopausal symptoms than do thin women.

6. There is little evidence for postmenopausal production of estradiol by the ovaries or adrenals. Because many tissues contain alpha and/or beta estrogen receptors, most organ systems are affected by the decline in estrogen levels occurring in menopause. The interesting and challenging questions of menopause treatment for women and physicians stem from what happens when estrogen levels are manipulated.

ESTROGEN REPLACEMENT—IS IT HELPFUL OR HAZARDOUS?

There are approximately 31.2 million women older than age 55 in the United States. In 1990, there were 28.7 million, while in 2020, it is estimated that there will be 45.9 million women over the age of 55. Women who have attained the age of 50 have an average life expectancy of 31 years beyond the menopause. Incredibly, that is only 6 years less than the time they spent having menstrual cycles, assuming menarche started at about the age of 13. Women almost have as much life to live—to look forward to—as they have already lived. To many physicians, the increasing life span in women has only meant an increase in the problems of the postmenopausal period that must be "managed," often by the administration of hormones, although it is characteristically difficult to distinguish many of the effects of aging on the body from the effects of loss of reproductive function. But many women, too, view the "change of life" with dread and anxiety because of the two persistent societal myths of menopause: one, that before menopause a woman is fine, but at age 50 she is over the hill, and two, that the experience of menopause is a very stressful and upsetting event, both physically and psychologically.

Physicians' own expectations for the menopause may be colored by the many grim descriptions that have appeared in the medical world. A prior president of the American Geriatric Society declared that menopause was a "chronic and incapacitating deficiency disease that leaves women with flabby breasts, wrinkled skin, fragile bones, and loss of ability to have or enjoy sex." Public expression of such sentiments certainly would be taboo today, but some doctors still are exposed to these kinds of stereotypical myths during their medical training and practice, leaving them with biases that could influence their perception of women during the menopausal period. Certainly, much of the medical literature views menopause as an illness that should be treated. This is typified by a quote from the second edition of *The Menopause: Comprehensive Management:* "Menopause is an endocrine deficiency state, similar in kind to diabetes and hypothyroidism; hormone replacement is logical therapy" (Edgren, 1988).

But menopause is not a disease like diabetes. It is a normal event, like menarche and menstruation, that occurs in the lives of all women, and not necessarily in the same way. About 15%–20% of women have (besides the obvious cessation of the menstrual periods) no clinical symptoms at all. Evidently in these women, the hormonal and physiological changes that occur are so gradual that they are almost imperceptible. At the other end of the spectrum are another 15%–20% of women who suffer from almost incapacitating physical complaints and a number of psychological disturbances. Their symptoms may include hot flashes, genital atrophy, headache, backache, nervousness and anxiety, depression, memory loss, insomnia, dizziness, breast problems, bloating, nausea, and decreased desire for sex or uncontrollable increased desire. But between these two extremes are the vast majority of women, each experiencing menopause uniquely. A woman in this group may have some of the aforementioned difficulties, such as hot flashes or insomnia, that she can live with but that come and go for years, or she may have symptoms so vague and mild that they can be ignored. Of greater concern is the possibility of increased risk of cardiovascular disease or osteoporosis for women following menopause. Menopause, as well as the treatments for menopause symptoms, may have immediate or delayed consequences.

Our society places high value on youth and beauty. In our youth-oriented culture, the thought of impending menopause can often be the signal of impending old age. Yet, at the beginning of the 21st century, as the baby boom generation approaches retirement and large numbers of women are entering menopause, their positive influence on popular attitudes toward age is evident. The MacArthur Foundation Research Network on Successful Midlife Development reported in February 1999, based on a 10-year study of nearly 8,000 Americans, that people in midlife find it is a good place to be. More than half of the postmenopausal women in this study reported that their major experience at the cessation of their menstrual periods was relief. Utian and Boggs (1999) reported that 51% of the 752 postmenopausal women responding to the North American Menopause Society (NAMS) 1998 survey described being more fulfilled and happier than they were in their 20s. More than half also noted that their menopause had no effect on their sexual relationship.

When the combined efforts of the pharmaceutical industry and a few physicians in the early 1960s promised that women could remain "feminine forever," healthy, young, and sexy by taking estrogen for the presumed miseries of menopause, it is not surprising that the sales of the drug quadrupled in 10 years, as millions of women were encouraged routinely to take it as a cure-all. By the mid-1970s, the decade of **estrogen replacement therapy (ERT)**, there were some urban areas of the country where more than half of the menopausal women were receiving estrogen (Stadel & Weiss, 1975).

The majority of annual prescriptions written for postmenopausal women are for Premarin, the estrogen preparation manufactured by Wyeth-Ayerst. Premarin consists of conjugated equine estrogens, also called natural estrogens.

The treatments available to women and their role in selecting appropriate treatments have changed in the past 30 years. In many ways, this change is welcome in that physicians are increasingly expecting women to actively participate in determining their course of action and to not relinquish that determination to their physicians. However, there is a great deal still unknown about long-term effects of estrogen depletion and even less known about the long-term effects of menopause treatments. Any discussion of treatment options must begin with ERT—estrogen replacement therapy.

Endometrial Cancer

Early in 1975, three published studies aroused suspicion that the miracle drug for the middle-aged woman was probably responsible for a marked increase in uterine cancer. The studies found that the risk of getting endometrial cancer was increased by 5–14 times by taking ERT, and the likelihood was increased with the duration of use and dosage of Premarin. At least 20 more studies subsequently substantiated that the odds of developing endometrial cancer were greater after estrogen use. Cessation of use diminishes the risk, but several reports showed that the risk was increased after only a year of cyclic ERT and remained increased for as long as 10–14 years after discontinuing therapy (Shapiro et al., 1985; Paganini-Hill, Ross, & Henderson, 1989). By the late 1980s, a progestin such as norethindrone, norgestrel, or medroxyprogesterone acetate began to be routinely given along with the estrogen for 1 week to 10 days. Studies had shown that the addition of progestin largely alleviated the endometrial cancer problem. For menopausal women with a uterus, estrogen replacement therapy became **hormone replacement therapy (HRT)**. However, the protection conferred by progestin against uterine cancer is achieved by an increase in progestin-related symptoms—physical, psychological, and with some potentially adverse effects on the concentrations of blood lipids. The addition of progestin also can produce a regular pattern of menstruation-like withdrawal bleeding, a consequence many women find unappealing. Hormone replacement therapy carries with it both benefits and risks. While the addition of progestin is believed to counter the additional risk of uterine cancer, there is concern that some regimens of HRT may increase the risk of endometrial hyperplasia compared with conventional administrations (Lobo, 1999). HRT may cause high blood pressure, and the hypertension disappears when therapy is discontinued. In women with a history of thrombosis, there is an increased risk of venous thromboembolic events with estrogen. In addition, in women taking HRT, breast tenderness and bloating—or PMS-like side effects—may also occur.

Administration of estrogen to postmenopausal women results in a twofold increased risk of gallbladder disease, and many women receiving therapy have subsequently required gallbladder surgery. A previous history of gallstones would thus be a contraindication for estrogen usage.

Uterine fibroids and endometriosis tend to regress in the menopause. While ERT or HRT do not routinely result in the regrowth of fibroids or endometriosis, pain or an increase of uterine size, determined by regular pelvic examinations, would be a reason to stop the therapy.

Breast Cancer

But the greatest concern is the enhanced risk of breast cancer with HRT. Over the past several years, it seems that each new study has contradicted the last study released and added new confusion, leaving women and physicians uncertain. Unopposed estrogen has been known to increase the risk of breast cancer, primarily among women currently or recently on long-term ERT (Collaborative Group on Hormonal Factors in Breast Cancer, 1997; Jacobs, 2000). Because the addition of progestin in HRT counters to a considerable extent the risk of endometrial cancers associated with estrogen-only ERT (or unopposed estrogen), it had been hoped that the same benefit might also be true for breast cancer risk. Studies in the late 1970s and early 1980s suggested that this would not be the case, but these conclusions were countered by other reports questioning the scale and reliability of the studies. Since then, a number of studies have confirmed that the addition of progestin not only fails to reduce risk, but rather adds to the risk of developing breast cancer. Pooled data from epidemiologic studies compiled by the Collaborative Group on Hormonal Factors in Breast Cancer suggested that among current or recent hormone users, the risk of breast cancer was 53% higher for combination therapy and 34% higher for estrogen alone, compared with no hormone use. A report of the Nurses' Health Study found that for each year of use, the risk of breast cancer increased by 9% for combined use and by 3.3% for estrogen alone (Colditz et al., 1998). In his *Menopause Management for the Millennium,* Lobo (1999) draws from his review of the literature to-date that the risk of breast cancer is probably in the range of 20%–30% for women on HRT with moderate doses of estrogen and who are susceptible, noting that it isn't possible to identify which women are susceptible prior to treatment. Studies support a greater link for long-term (more than 10 years) than short-term (less than 5 years) estrogen use. A recent major study published in the *Journal of the American Medical Association* in early 2000 by Schairer et al. made headline news across the country by affirming, through analysis of data from 46,000 women who participated in the Breast Cancer Detection Demonstration Project—the largest study to-date—that combined estrogen-progestin therapies were associated with greater risk for breast cancer than estrogen alone, that such risk is particularly relevant for lean women, and that increased risk is directly related to duration of use and is largely limited to current or recent users. These researchers concluded that risk increases 8% for each year of HRT use and 1% per year for estrogen alone (Schairer et al., 2000). Stated another way, a woman on hormone replacement therapy for a decade doubles her risk of breast cancer.

There is no question that potential risk of breast cancer has made women and physicians alike more cautious about HRT and that these recent studies raise substantial concerns about the wisdom of HRT for most women. It is also true that epidemiologic studies, from which most of these conclusions have been drawn, are not controlled random studies and rely on retrospective reports by large cohorts of women, making them subject to reporting bias. There is a controlled study—the Women's Health Initiative—that has been under way since 1993 from which the earliest reports will be available in 2004. Until that research is concluded, the evidence from studies to-date raises substantial concerns regarding the risk of breast cancer with either unopposed estrogen therapy or combined estrogen-progestin therapy particularly for current and recent long-term users of HRT. These conclusions must be taken very seriously by women in considering whether HRT is an option worth its risks.

Newer Estrogen Therapies and SERMs

Because a number of the "symptoms" of menopause are directly linked to the decline of estrogen, there continues to be great interest in improving hormone replacement therapies to minimize their associated risks and to develop therapies that mimic the positive effects of estrogen without including the negative effects.

Hormone replacement therapies can be adjusted by dosage and by formulations of estrogen and progestin to respond most effectively to a particular woman's situation. Transdermal patches are available as an alternative to oral estrogens. "Designer estrogens" (introduced in Chapter 7) are designed molecules that act like estrogens in some ways and like antiestrogens in other ways. These **selective estrogen receptor modulators (SERMs)** would be ideal if they acted as an estrogen agonist on tissues for which estrogen stimulation in menopause is good (bones, heart, skin, and brain) but as an estrogen antagonist—interfering with the action of estrogen—on tissues for which estrogen stimulation is bad—uterus and breast.

The SERMs that are now available are not yet ideal but are considered promising. As noted in Chapter 7, tamoxifen is a nonsteroid antiestrogen that has some beneficial characteristics for menopausal women, such as some protection against osteoporosis and reduction of LDLs and cholesterol, just as does estrogen. And, just as estrogen does, tamoxifen increases the risk for endometrial cancer. However, because it competes with estrogen binding at estrogen receptor sites in breast tissue, tamoxifen does not increase the risk, and rather actually decreases the risk, for certain breast cancers. Like tamoxifen, raloxifene, marketed as Evista, has a beneficial effect on bone density and blood lipid levels and may reduce the risk for breast cancer. Unlike tamoxifen, raloxifene does not increase the risk for endometrial cancer. Both tamoxifen and raloxifene increase the risk for venous thrombosis and have no beneficial effect on vaginal atrophy and hot flashes.

Finally, certain phytoestrogens—plant-derived substances found in relatively high proportions in soy products—act like weak estrogens. Studies have documented only slight effects of soy-based proteins, for example, on beta estrogen receptors, found in brain tissue and coronary arteries. The current thinking regarding phytoestrogens is that they are worth a try, but their efficacy still needs to be determined.

MENOPAUSAL SYMPTOMS

The change from estradiol to the less potent estrone and the general reduction in estrogen during the premenopausal and the menopausal years can result in varying degrees of what could be distressing symptoms. Ninety percent of women going through the menopause have menstrual irregularities. Mostly the altered bleeding pattern is toward shorter, possibly skipped, cycles with light flow, so heavy bleeding and longer flow should be reported to the physician in case there is some underlying pathology. Other difficulties may be hot flashes, drying of the vaginal tissues that can make intercourse painful, or drying of the lower urinary tract that results in a burning sensation while urinating or predisposes to more frequent urinary tract infections. Alterations in mood and cognitive function and potential susceptibility to dementia may or may not be associated with hormonal changes in the menopause. Health changes that are associated with reduced levels of estrogen are acceleration in the loss of bone tissue and increased susceptibility to heart disease.

Vasomotor Instability (Hot Flashes and Flushes)

A hot flash is the feeling of intense warmth of the upper body; a flush is the visible reddening that may or may not accompany the flash. Hot flashes may occur more often during sleep, thereby provoking a night sweat. Hot flashes are thought to be caused by a disturbance in the temperature-regulating center in the hypothalamus. This special group of neurons in the preoptic anterior hypothalamus is also called the vasomotor center. The area controls body temperature via the autonomic nervous system by causing sweating and by dilation or constriction of all the small blood vessels of the skin. When body temperature increases, impulses from this area are transmitted to skin vessels and sweat glands to cause cooling by vasodilation and sweating. When body temperature is cooled, vasoconstriction occurs, and sweating is abolished.

A hot flash, sometimes preceded by a chill, is a sensation of warmth that may be perceived most intensely on the upper trunk of the body, starting in the lower chest and rising up to the head and neck. Hot flashes are a generalized phenomenon, however, and when skin temperature is measured, the greatest rise occurs over the fingers and toes, although perspiration is most apparent on the upper body. The skin of the face and neck may redden and flush, but in some women only the hands and fingers are flushed. The sensation of heat may be followed by a drenching sweat, particularly at night. Any factor that affects the temperature-regulating mechanism, like lying in bed under a blanket, sitting in a warm room, exercise, eating, or emotional stress can trigger hot flashes. They may occur only once or twice a day, or every half hour; they may last for a few weeks or continue for years. Eventually, they subside, but they can be a distressing and humiliating experience for the woman who has them severely. The stigmatization of menopausal symptoms in our culture can be a major cause of the woman's distress.

The usefulness of estrogen therapy in treating hot flashes is well established—estrogen usually alleviates or eliminates the condition. This does not necessarily mean that lack of estrogen has caused the vasomotor disturbance. Hot flashes do not occur in women born without ovaries or with nonfunctioning ovaries, in girls who were ovariectomized before puberty, or in patients with hypofunctioning pituitary glands. If these females, however, who have never had their own source of estrogen are given estrogen treatment for more than a year and subsequently abruptly withdrawn from treatment, they will then experience hot flashes. This finding has generated a theory that vasomotor instability represents withdrawal symptoms from years of addiction to endogenous estrogen, and some researchers maintain that many of the symptoms attributed to menopause are analogous to those occurring upon withdrawal from drug dependency. The idea that women become estrogen addicts between menarche and menopause may sound odd, but hot flashes definitely appear to be correlated to the withdrawal of estrogen levels. Men can also have hot flashes as a consequence of testosterone withdrawal; 73% of men who have had their testes removed for prostatic cancer will have flashes (Frodin, Alund, & Varenhurst, 1985).

Because of the complexity of the hypothalmic-pituitary-ovarian axis, it is probable that there is more than lack of estrogen involved in the cause of hot flashes. Other researchers have implicated LH, since there is a close association in time between the onset of the hot flash and a surge of LH. But the actual changes in the body's chemistry that precipitate a hot flash are not clearly understood. One theory holds that, since hot flashes are experienced several years before the last menstrual period, the instability of the temperature-regulating system is associated with a middle range of estrogen as it passes from the high range of the reproductive years to the low levels at menopause, and that the effect is mediated through the hypothalamus. Since LH is released during a flash, and LH is stimulated by GnRH, perhaps both LH and GnRH are implicated in triggering a hot flash. The neurons that produce GnRH are in the same area of the hypothalamus as the neurons that control body temperature. Moreover, the same neurotransmitters believed to be involved in the release of GnRH—norepinephrine and dopamine—have also been implicated in temperature regulation. It is possible that when the neurotransmitters cause the release of GnRH, they have overlapping effects that alter the adjacent thermoregulatory neurons, thus causing a hot flash.

During the climacteric, the extent of estrogen deficiency differs among women and has a great deal to do with the extraovarian production of estrone. The amount of circulating estrogen is thus related to the adrenal production and peripheral tissue conversion of androgen (androstenedione), and the latter is directly correlated to body weight.

But not all heavier women are free of hot flashes, and not all thinner women get them, so it is not possible at this time to predict which women entering menopause will experience them, how severe they will be, or when they will end. An estimated 75% of the women who enter menopause in a single year will have hot flashes, and only a small minority will have vasomotor symptoms severe enough to require therapy. The symptoms of heat and sweating are mediated through the autonomic nervous system, and some women have been relieved by a prescription drug called Bellergal, which combines phenobarbital and both sympathetic and parasympathetic nervous system inhibitors. Clonidine, a drug used in treating hypertension, reduces the frequency of hot flashes but is not as effective as estrogen and may have unpleasant side effects of dizziness, nausea, and headache. When hot flashes are bad enough to interfere with daily activities, or chronically disturb sleep, they will respond well to small doses of

estrogen for a short period of 6–12 months or less. Phytoestrogens may be a good option for countering hot flashes for some women. Also, recent trials (Studd et al., 1999) have shown that intranasal applications of estrogen reduced hot flashes for 75% of the women sampled and had far fewer negative side effects than oral administration of estrogen. Tamoxifen and raloxifene are not good options. Tamoxifen tends to precipitate hot flashes; raloxifene provides no benefit for and may also precipitate hot flashes. Generally, while estrogen is clearly the most effective treatment for hot flashes, short-term management of hot flashes may not be worth the risks associated with estrogen replacement, particularly in high doses.

Genital Atrophy

Another symptom of the menopause experienced by some women is the gradual atrophy of the genital organs, generally appearing 10–20 years after menopause. Because the vulvar skin is more sensitive to absence of estrogen than the skin and fat of the rest of the body, the labia majora, minora, and mons pubis shrink in size, and the pubic hair may become scant. Because the strength and elasticity of the muscles and ligaments of the pelvis are also affected, cystocele, rectocele, and prolapse may occur for the first time, especially if there was previous childbirth damage. Most of the problems that women have, however, are a result of the thinning and shrinking of the vaginal and urethral epithelium and wall. The vagina shrinks in both length and width, and the epithelium atrophies. The epithelial cells lose their glycogen, the Döderlein's bacilli disappear, and vaginal secretions are no longer acid. The vagina then becomes much more prone to infections, and pain during intercourse (dyspareunia) may occur. All of these changes can be reversed with low doses of estrogen, but local treatment with estrogen-containing suppositories or creams is also effective, and less estrogen is absorbed into the bloodstream. (Tamoxifen and raloxifene are, again, not good options for genital atrophy.) When atrophy is less severe, symptoms may be alleviated by the use of sterile lubricating gels.

It should be noted that a study of 52 post-menopausal women not taking estrogen replacement therapy confirmed the earlier report of Masters and Johnson concerning the beneficial effect of sexual activity on vaginal atrophy. The women who had intercourse three or more times monthly or who masturbated had less vaginal atrophy than the women who engaged in less frequent sexual activity (here defined as intercourse less than 10 times yearly) or did not masturbate (Leiblum et al., 1983).

Mood and Cognitive Function

Basic research confirms that estrogen has a positive effect on mood and memory, while progestins may attenuate some of these effects (Lobo, 1999). But it is not clear whether estrogen deficiency causes mood changes, loss in cognitive function, or higher risk for Alzheimer's disease. Even less clear is the question of whether ERT is advised to prevent loss in cognitive function or dementias. In a 1998 review article published in the *Journal of the American Medical Association*, Yaffe, Sawaya, Lieberburg, and Grady concluded, based on their review and analysis of articles published between 1966 and 1977, that

> *"There are plausible biological mechanisms by which estrogen might lead to improved cognition, reduced risk for dementia, or improvement in the severity of dementia. Studies conducted in women, however, have substantial methodologic problems and have produced conflicting results. Large placebo-controlled trials are required to address estrogen's role in prevention and treatment of Alzheimer's disease and other dementias. Given the known risks of estrogen therapy, we do not recommend estrogen for the prevention or treatment of Alzheimer's disease or other dementias until adequate trials have been completed." (p. 688).*

Lobo's conclusion, based on his 1999 comprehensive review of published studies, is somewhat different:

> *"The data on estrogen reducing the risk of Alzheimer's disease, however, are remarkably consistent . . . among case-control and cohort studies. This reduced risk also appears to be greater with longer duration of estrogen use. . . . No data exist, however, as to the effect on the risk profile of adding progestin. Although estrogen appears to have a protective effect on the development of Alzheimer's disease . . . the data on the effects of estrogen in the treatment of Alzheimer's disease are inconsistent and somewhat disappointing." (p. 23)*

The best we can conclude at this point is that the jury is still out regarding efficacy of HRT on cognitive function and prevention/treatment of dementia.

Another type of "mood change" associated with menopause is a decrease in libido. Whether this is truly a symptom of menopause or age or culture is unknown. Interestingly enough, though, if it is a result of hormonal changes, it is more likely caused by a decline in testosterone than estrogen. Between her 20s and her 40s, a woman's testosterone levels decrease by about 50%. Estrogen treatments result in an even greater decline in testosterone levels. At this time, any benefits of androgen therapies for menopausal women are fairly speculative.

Osteoporosis

Osteoporosis is literally "holes-in-the-bone," a condition of increased porosity, bone loss, and therefore increased fragility of bone, leading to fractures after little or no trauma to the bone. Osteoporosis is a chronic skeletal disorder associated with aging and is commonly diagnosed after the age of 60, but it can start much earlier, at about age 30 or 35. Although peak bone mass is reached in both sexes at approximately age 30, the rate of bone loss normally after that is statistically greater in women than in men and appears to be associated with menopause. Women in their 30s lose less than 1% of their bone tissue a year, but following menopause, the loss of bone tissue in women averages 3% in the first 5 years and 1%–2% per year after that, particularly in the spinal column. Because women generally have proportionately less bone mass to start with, and generally live longer, which gives them more opportunity to lose bone, their chances of getting osteoporosis are greater. In industrialized Western countries, more than one-third of women older than 65 display some symptoms of osteoporosis.

In its most serious form, osteoporosis results in a predisposition to fractures. When fractures occur in the thinned and weakened vertebra that support most of the weight in the spinal column, the result is a progressive decrease in height and bending of the spine, producing swayback or humpback. Approximately one of four women older than 60 years of age has such spinal compression fractures. Hip and wrist fractures are other dangers. If a woman lives to the age of 90, her risk of hip fracture is approximately 30%. Breaking a limb results in immobilization, which not only aggravates osteoporosis, but in the aged may result in lung collapse, pneumonia, and death.

Osteoporosis is both a natural consequence of aging and a result of estrogen deprivation. Seventy-five percent of postmenopausal women never get the severe form of the disease. It appears that some people are more susceptible than others, that those with a smaller adult bone mass have an increased vulnerability to the development of osteoporosis, although those with a greater adult bone mass seem to be protected. Blacks of both sexes, white men, and obese women have less risk of developing osteoporosis. Other factors involved in bone loss are lack of physical activity, calcium and protein deficiency, and general malnutrition.

Trying to identify which women are at risk for osteoporosis has not always been successful, but there are some factors that appear to be related to a higher risk. Being petite, small boned, and thin; being Caucasian, especially with a Northern European heritage; being Asian; and having a family history of osteoporosis are genetic factors. Other risks for osteoporosis include conditions that have resulted in estrogen deficiency, such as having had ovaries removed before the

age of 40 or having other reasons for prolonged amenorrhea, such as anorexia or bulimia. A dietary calcium deficiency, long periods of immobilization or a general lack of exercise, smoking, and high alcohol or caffeine consumption can also add to the risk. In addition there are some medications taken on a long-term basis such as corticosteroids, excess thyroid hormone, or anticonvulsants that appear to increase the likelihood of getting osteoporosis. But a woman who reaches a good peak bone mass in youth through exercise and calcium intake, who continues to eat well and include calcium-rich foods in her diet, does not smoke, uses alcohol in moderation, and exercises regularly should have less to fear from the decreased estrogen levels at menopause.

Screening tests to measure bone density have not been particularly informative for asymptomatic younger or middle-aged women to determine whether osteoporosis may develop in the future, but they could be used to establish a baseline level of bone mass if there are many risk factors. The preferred test is dual energy x-ray absorptiometry, which calculates the mineral content of the bone at the spine and hip. Computed tomography (CT scan), which exposes the woman to more radiation, can also assess the amount of bone in the spine. Bone mass measurement techniques like these can detect low bone mass in younger women with genetic risk factors and enable them to make changes in diet and exercise that can prevent further bone loss.

Osteoporosis is a painful, crippling, and potentially fatal disease, and its recognition, prevention, measurement, and treatment have provided medical challenges. Numerous studies have indicated that postmenopausal women who take estrogen are less likely to fracture a bone than untreated women. Two retrospective case-controlled studies (Hutchinson, Polansky, & Feinstein, 1979; Weiss et al., 1980) demonstrated that estrogen, taken within 5 years of the menopause in the first study and taken for at least 6 years in the second study, has a protective effect against the incidence of bone fracture, reducing by more than 50%

the likelihood of a postmenopausal woman's breaking her forearm or hip. Evidently estrogen therapy works best during the first 5–10 years after menopause when bone loss is greatest. Another group of epidemiologists (Williams et al., 1982) showed that estrogen use in obese women had little or no effect on bone fracture risk and that the beneficial effect of estrogen on fractures was greatest in thin women, especially in those who smoked cigarettes. A Swedish study of 23,000 women found that women who used estrogen preparations had a 21% reduction in the overall risk of hip fractures, with even greater reductions for women who had started treatment before the age of 60 (Naessen et al., 1990). More recently, researchers found that exercise plus calcium supplements and exercise plus estrogen were both effective in slowing or stopping bone loss in postmenopausal women who were considered, on the basis of their low baseline bone density, to be at risk of fracture. Exercise alone turned out to have little effect, but in a few women accustomed to a high level of exercise (walking briskly for 2 hours per day) the effect of either treatment—calcium or estrogen—was enhanced and bone loss was stopped rather than slowed (Prince et al., 1991). But because of the side effects of the hormone therapy (bleeding, breast tenderness) in the exercise-estrogen group, these authors recommended that exercise and calcium be advised for women with intermediate bone density, reserving estrogen for the women with low baseline bone density.

Besides estrogen, there are other therapies for the treatment of osteoporosis. Calcitonin, a hormone produced by the thyroid gland, lowers blood calcium by stimulating calcium uptake and its incorporation into the bone and inhibits the cells that normally break down bone (osteoclasts). Thus, calcitonin can reduce the rate of bone loss and may even increase bone mass in postmenopausal osteoporotic women. Synthetic calcitonin—salmon, marketed as Miacalcin, is an alternative for women with osteoporosis who are 5–10 years past menopause and who cannot or choose not to take estrogen. Administered as a nasal spray, its primary side effect is nasal irritation. Another alternative

is alendronate sodium, marketed as Fosamax, which is absorbed into bone tissue and inhibits osteoclasts. Fosamax increases bone density in the spine and hip and reduces by 50% the risk of spinal fractures, making its impact comparable to that of estrogen. Fosomax is administered orally daily, upon awakening and 30–60 minutes prior to eating, drinking, or taking medication. To reduce the risk of serious esophageal erosion and digestive upset, a women needs to remain upright after swallowing Fosomax. This is not an appropriate treatment for those with esophageal disorders, advanced kidney disease, or low blood levels of calcium.

The SERMs (see earlier section, this chapter) also provide alternatives to estrogen in treating and preventing osteoporosis. Tamoxifen increases bone mass and, unlike estrogen, reduces the risk for breast cancer. However, like estrogen, tamoxifen increases the risk for uterine cancer and blood clots, and long-term use is not recommended. Raloxifene (Evista) also builds bone mass, is thought to reduce risk for breast cancer, and carries no additional risk of uterine cancer. It does increase risk for blood clots. These are relatively new drugs, and long-term effects when used as treatment for osteoporosis are not known.

Estrogen has been heavily promoted for prophylactic use by menopausal women to prevent or reduce bone loss. But while all women are relatively estrogen deficient in the menopause and estrogen and other therapies have proven benefits, osteoporosis is not an inevitable disease, and only one out of four white women over age 60 develops osteoporosis. The benefit of treatment has to be weighed against the risks.

Although bone health is largely genetically determined, it is also important to build bone health through weight-bearing exercise and a nutritious diet throughout childhood and adolescence. It would seem logical that the more bone mass there is in early adulthood, the less there is to lose in old age. But failure to consume sufficient calcium in later years as well can result in an accelerated and excessive rate of bone loss and set the stage for hip fractures. Increasing calcium intake through diet or supplementation is probably not going to stop bone loss completely, but it will slow the rate of loss and will not do any harm. A number of studies have found that the average intake of calcium in normal women at the time of menopause was well below the recommended daily allowance (RDA).

Long-term low calcium intake, decreased physical activity with increasing age, and some of the aspects of the American diet are believed to be factors that contribute to calcium loss over the years and thereby promote the development of osteoporosis. It has been recommended by a number of investigators that an intake of at least 1 g a day before menopause and 1.5 g daily after the menopause is necessary to maintain the appropriate calcium balance for the prevention of bone loss. Getting that much from the diet alone is difficult, and supplementation with calcium carbonate, calcium gluconate, or calcium lactate pills or powder would be necessary. Some researchers have advised that women should begin such calcium supplementation as early as age 25, and there are a number of over-the-counter pills available. The FDA has, however, warned against the consumption of calcium sources such as bone meal or dolomite (usually found at health food stores) because these products have been found to be contaminated with lead or other substances. There are inexpensive antacid preparations that contain 500 mg calcium carbonate, equivalent to 200 mg elemental calcium, as the sole ingredient. Two to four tablets daily, depending on the diet, would be a palatable way to obtain the recommended total calcium requirement. There are no epidemiological data to indicate that amounts of calcium carbonate in that range have any adverse effects on stomach acid or increase the likelihood of kidney stone formation, but calcium in any form can be constipating. It may be necessary to take a stool softener along with additional calcium.

Coronary Heart Disease

There is a difference in the vulnerability of men and women to coronary heart disease, but the reasons for it are unknown. In the past 30 years in the United States, the ratio of male to female deaths from heart disease at ages 45–50 was 5 to 1, but it was 2 to 1 in Italy, and 1 to 1 in Japan, indicating that the sex difference regarding heart disease is much smaller in less affluent societies. Furthermore, only white women have the sex advantage; it is seen to a much lesser extent in blacks. Even in this country, the ratio of male to female mortality rates steadily declines after age 50, principally as a result of a slower statistical acceleration with age of coronary heart disease death rates for men. Women appear to be protected until menopause, but eventually they almost catch up to the men, and there is a steady increment in their rate of heart disease deaths after the age of 50. Within the first few years of menopause, the risk of cardiovascular disease is not appreciably greater, but it continues to increase with time. Around 60 years of age, the rate of heart attack in a woman equals that of a man 6 to 10 years her junior. Heart disease is the number one killer of women 50–75 years of age, claiming five times as many lives as breast cancer (Huston & Lanka, 1997).

Since the premenopausal state appears to be protective against coronary heart disease, the logical implication is that endogenous estrogen, mediated through the beneficial effects of estrogen on cholesterol levels, is responsible. The assumption that blood serum total cholesterol levels play an important role in the development of cardiovascular disease has come from epidemiological studies indicating that men with high total cholesterol have an increased risk—that for every 1% increase in total cholesterol there is a 2% increase in the risk of heart attack. Virtually all of the studies of the prevention and treatment of heart disease have been done in men, and the male model has shown that the risk of developing coronary heart disease is greater when the blood levels of low-density lipoproteins (LDL = "bad" cholesterol, the major carrier of blood cholesterol that could be deposited in the arteries) are higher and the risk is lessened when levels of high-density lipoproteins (HDL = "good" cholesterol that helps get rid of the cholesterol released from cells) are greater.

There is evidence that unopposed (without progestin) oral estrogen therapy increases HDL levels and decreases LDL levels. The HDL levels do not normally decrease to any appreciable extent in postmenopausal women, so this increase in HDL levels with estrogen replacement therapy is pharmacological. That is, when estrogen is taken orally (not by the transdermal patch form of administration), it improves some of the lipoprotein levels believed to be cardioprotective. Estrogen therapy is estimated to reduce the occurrence of cardiovascular disease by 25%–50% over no treatment, presumably due primarily to its beneficial effect on HDL (Lobo, 1999). Estrogen is also reported to increase cardiac output and decrease blood pressure (Rosano & Panina, 1999). Estrogen's impact on other factors associated with increased risk of heart disease is less certain. These factors include central body fatness, which increases in menopause, and insulin resistance. Also, despite its apparent protective effect on cardiovascular disease, it is as yet unclear whether estrogen helps to prevent strokes in postmenopausal women.

Trying to isolate estrogen as a factor in cardiovascular disease in women is almost impossible because of all the variables that confuse the issue, even if the data are adjusted to take some of them into account. Risk factors for heart disease also include obesity, smoking, use of oral contraceptives, diet, heredity, and general lifestyle. Moreover, women who take estrogen after menopause are more likely to be white, educated, upper middle class, and thinner, therefore having a lower risk of heart disease than women without estrogen replacement therapy anyway (Barrett-Conner, Wingard, & Criqui, 1989). The long-term studies to eliminate this bias have not been done yet.

Taking estrogen in the larger doses found in oral contraceptives decreases HDL levels and increases the incidence of heart attack in premenopausal women, especially if they are cigarette smokers. Also, the increased risk of blood clot formation has clearly been shown to be associated with estrogen administration. Moreover, all of the epidemiological data showing the benefit of estrogen have pertained to the use of estrogen alone, without the added progestin. Unless a woman has had a hysterectomy, however, the use of progestin is necessary to protect against endometrial cancer. It appears that progestins, mainly due to the androgenic properties, counteract the benefits of estrogen on blood lipid levels and also may have a negative effect on the physiology of the blood vessel walls (Lobo, 1990). But some estrogen-only proponents believe that the lifesaving potential of estrogen on heart disease outweighs the risk of getting endometrial cancer, maintaining that uterine cancer is slow growing and is curable at an early stage. Now that recent studies have associated risk of breast cancer with both ERT and HRT, the use of estrogen to protect against heart disease is further challenged.

If estrogen therapy protects postmenopausal women from developing cardiovascular disease, then it would seem that estrogen should be effective in treating heart disease. In fact, as early as the 1970s, it was shown that when men with previous heart attacks were given high-dose conjugated estrogens, the effect was more harm than good and resulted in an increased incidence of heart attacks. In the 1990s, the Heart and Estrogen/Progestin Replacement Study (HERS)—the only large randomized clinical trial on the benefit of HRT in women with cardiovascular disease—found an increased incidence of secondary cardiac events in the first year of HRT treatment.

The relationship between estrogen replacement therapy and cardiovascular disease is still too uncertain for a postmenopausal woman to take estrogen on that basis alone. Moreover, there are other ways to reduce the risk of heart disease besides taking ERT. Exercise, even in moderate amounts, will also increase HDL levels. A group of researchers at the Cooper Institute for Aerobics Research found that previously sedentary women who walked 3 miles a day, 5 days a week, for 6 months, regardless of the pace, had an increase of 6% in HDL levels. The women who walked at the fastest pace (a 12-minute mile) also increased their cardiorespiratory fitness by 16%, about the same as that of women who jog (Duncan, Gordon, & Scott, 1991). Maybe an hour's walk each day to aid the heart is not as easy as taking a daily pill, but it may provide equivalent benefits with absolutely no risk.

A WOMAN'S INFORMED DECISION

Long-term use of estrogen has been advocated for emotional stability, sensuality, a youthful appearance, and a "feeling of well-being." It is for these alleged benefits that estrogen has been most overused and misused. While there are innumerable clinical observations by physicians that indicate that estrogen relieves anxiety, tension, depression, and irritability, there is no evidence from controlled clinical trials that any of these conditions are improved if hot flashes are not present. It could be that the relief of severe hot flashes and the accompanying insomnia has the secondary benefit of alleviating the psychological symptoms that the incapacitating vasomotor symptoms may have caused.

There has been no objective documentation that estrogen therapy contributes to a youthful appearance or a feeling of well-being. Estrogen cannot reverse or retard the aging process. Aging creates menopause, not the other way around. But when youthfulness, attractiveness, and the ability to reproduce are seen as important attributes for women, menopause can be a trying time for even the most stable of individuals. Menopause itself, however, does not turn an emotionally healthy, functional woman into a dysfunctional, depressed neurotic; it is generally agreed that the total behavior patterns and personality of a woman before menopause have a determining effect on her response to menopause. Social and cultural factors are far more likely than hormonal deficiency to affect psychic functions.

Perhaps many women are afraid of menopause and afraid of aging. But with just cause, they are more afraid of cancer. Studies have shown that administration of estrogen increases the risk of developing endometrial cancer, breast cancer, gallbladder disease, and hypertension. Prudent and cautious use of this potentially dangerous drug is necessary.

There are two age-old maxims in medicine. One is that healthy patients are best left untreated, and the other is found in the Hippocratic oath: *primum non nocere,* or "first, do no harm." Estrogens are valuable in treatment but should be reserved for women who have symptoms that are severe and incapacitating or who are identified as being at increased risk for osteoporosis. The decision to take estrogen in the menopause should be individualized, taking into account each woman's special needs. Women must decide whether what estrogen does for their symptoms outweighs what it may do to their health. Women must also be aware that they should not have estrogen therapy if they have any of the following conditions: fibroids of the uterus, endometriosis, previous history of cancer of the endometrium or breast, or any history of blood clot formation. Severe diabetes, elevated blood fat level, or high blood pressure are other contraindications. Indeed, there are a number of drawbacks to estrogen therapy in addition to those already mentioned. These include breast tenderness, weight gain, pelvic pain, vaginal bleeding, leg pain, digestive disorders, and recurrence of allergies. Any women taking estrogen therapy should see her doctor regularly, and if she has any unscheduled vaginal bleeding, she should see her doctor immediately.

Of greatest concern, of course, is the increasing evidence that both estrogen therapy and hormone replacement therapy amplify risk for breast cancer. In their editorial published in January 2000 in the *Journal of the American Medical Association,* Willett, Colditz, and Stampfer conclude, based on the report of Schairer et al., published in the same volume, that hormone replacement therapy increases breast cancer risk, that "Although postmenopausal hormone use has important benefits . . . the commonly held belief that aging routinely requires pharmacological management has unfortunately led to neglect of diet and lifestyle as the primary means to achieve healthy aging. Now is an appropriate time to reassess this emphasis."

If a woman is fully aware of all the ramifications of taking estrogen menopausally and has decided that it is essential, then it is her informed choice.

ℛEFERENCES

Barrett-Conner, E., Wingard, D. L., & Criqui, M. H. (1989). Postmenopausal estrogen use and heart disease risk factors in the 1980s. *Journal of the American Medical Association, 261*(14), 2095–2100.

Colditz, G. A., & Rosner, B., for the Nurses' Health Study Research Group. (1998). Use of estrogen plus progestin is associated with greater increase in breast cancer risk than estrogen alone. *American Journal of Epidemiology, 147* (Suppl.), 645.

Collaborative Group on Hormonal Factors in Breast Cancer. (1997). Breast cancer and hormone replacement therapy: Collaborative reanalysis of data from 51 epidemiologic studies of 52,705 women with breast cancer and 108,411 women without breast cancer. *Lancet, 350*(9084), 1047–1059.

Duncan, J. J., Gordon, N. F., & Scott, C. B. (1991). Women walking for health and fitness. *Journal of the American Medical Association, 266*(3), 3295–3299.

Edgren, R. A. (1988). B. A. Pharmacology of hormonal therapeutic agents. In B. A. Eskin, (Ed.). *The menopause: Comprehensive management* (2nd ed.). New York: Macmillan.

Frodin, T., Alund, G., & Varenhurst, E. (1985). Measurement of skin blood-flow to assess hot flushes after orchiectomy. *Prostate, 7,* 203–209.

Harlow, B. L., Cramer, D. W., & Annis, K. M. (1995). Association of medically treated depression and age at natural menopause. *American Journal of Epidemiology, 141*(12), 1170–1176.

Huston, J., & Lanka, L. (1997). *Perimenopause: Changes in women's health after 35.* Oakland, CA: New Harbinger.

Hutchinson, T. A., Polansky, S. M., & Feinstein, A. R. (1979). Postmenopausal oestrogens protect against fractures of hip and distal radius. *Lancet, 2,* 705–709.

Jacobs, H. S. (2000). Postmenopausal hormone replacement therapy and breast cancer. *Medscape Women's Health, 5*(4). (http://www.medscape.com/medscape/WomensHealth/wh7271.jaco/wh7271.jaco-01.html)

Kato, I., Toniolo, P., Akmedkhanov, A. et al. (1999). Prospective study of factors influencing the onset of natural menopause. *Neurology, 53,* 308–314.

Leiblum, S., Bachmann, G., Kemmann, et al. (1983). Vaginal atrophy in the postmenopausal woman. *Journal of the American Medical Association, 249*(16), 2195–2198.

Lobo, R. (1990). Cardiovascular implications of estrogen replacement therapy. *Obstetrics and Gynecology, 75*(4. Suppl.), 18S–25S.

Lobo, R. (1999). Menopause management for the millennium. Medscape Women's Health. *Women's Health Clinical Management, 1.* (medscape.com/Medscape/WomensHealth/ClinicalMgmt/cm.vol/public/indexcm.vol.html)

Naessen, T., Persson, I., Adami, H-O., et al. (1990). Hormone replacement therapy and the risk for hip fracture: A prospective, population-based cohort study. *Annals of Internal Medicine, 13,* 95–103.

Paganini-Hill, A., Ross, R. K., & Henderson, B. E. (1989). Endometrial cancer and patterns of use of estrogen replacement therapy: A cohort study. *British Journal of Cancer, 59,* 445–447.

Prince, R. L., Smith, M., Dick, I. M., et al. (1991). Prevention of postmenopausal osteoporosis. A comparative study of exercise, calcium supplementation, and hormone-replacement therapy. *New England Journal of Medicine, 325*(17), 1189–1195.

Rosano, G. M., & Panina, G. (1999). Cardiovascular pharmacology of hormone replacement therapy. *Drugs and Aging, 15,* 219–234.

Schairer, C., Lubin, J., Troisi, R., Sturgeon, S., Brinton, L., & Hoover, R. (2000). Menopausal estrogen and estrogen-progestin replacement therapy and breast cancer risk. *Journal of the American Medical Association, 283*(4), 485–491.

Shapiro, S., Kelly, J. P., Rosenberg, L., et al. (1985). Risk of localized and widespread endometrial cancer in relation to recent and discontinued use of conjugated estrogens. *New England Journal of Medicine, 313,* 969–972.

Stadel, B. V., & Weiss, N. (1975). Characteristics of menopausal women: A survey of King and Pierce counties in Washington, 1973–74. *American Journal of Epidemiology, 102,* 209–216.

Steinberg, K. K., Thacker, S. B., Smith, J., et al. (1991). A meta-analysis of the effect of estrogen replacement therapy on the risk of breast cancer. *Journal of the American Medical Association, 265*(15), 1895–1990.

Studd, J., Pornel, B., Marton, I., et al. (1999). Efficacy and acceptability of intranasal 17 beta-oestradiol for menopause symptoms: Randomised dose-response study. *Lancet, 353*(9164), 1574–1578.

Utian, W. H., & Boggs, P. P. (1999). 1998 Menopause survey: Part I. Postmenopausal women's perceptions about menopause and midlife. *Menopause, 6*(2), 122–128.

Wallace, R. B., Sherman, B. M., Bean, J. A., et al. (1979). The probabilities of menopause with increasing duration of amenorrhea in middle-aged women. *American Journal of Obstetrics and Gynecology, 135,* 1021–1024.

Weiss, N. S., Ure, C. L., Ballard, J. H., et al. (1980). Decreased risk of fractures of the hip and lower forearm with postmenopausal use of estrogen. *New England Journal of Medicine, 303,* 1195–1198.

Willett, W., Colditz, G., & Stampfer, M. (2000). Postmenopausal estrogens—opposed, unopposed, or none of the above. *Journal of the American Medical Association, 283*(4), 534–535.

Willett, W., Stampfer, M., Bain, C., et al. (1983). Cigarette smoking, relative weight, and menopause. *American Journal of Epidemiology, 117,* 651–658.

Williams, A. R., Weiss, N. S., Ure, C. L., et al. (1982). Effect of weight, smoking and estrogen use on the risk of hip and forearm fractures in postmenopausal women. *Obstetrics and Gynecology, 60*(6), 695–699.

Yaffe, K., Sawaya, G., Lieberburg, I., & Grady, D. (1999). Estrogen therapy in postmenopausal women: Effects on cognitive function and dementia. *Journal of the American Medical Association, 279*(9), 688–695.

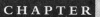

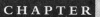

CHAPTER

15

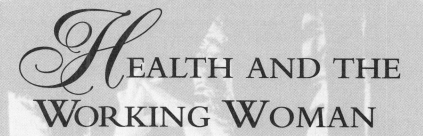

HEALTH AND THE WORKING WOMAN

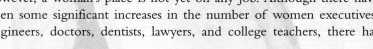

KEY TERMS

Carcinogens	Teratogens
Mutagens	

In the past 40 years, the number of American women working outside the home has grown dramatically. For the first time in U.S. history, and for reasons largely related to both the economic climate and the rise of the women's movement, nearly two-thirds (64%) of adult women older than 16 are employed. And despite depictions on TV and in the movies, they are not all superwomen and supermom professionals, making policy in corporate boardrooms while a nanny cares for the children and a cook makes the meals. More than two-thirds of working women are single, divorced, widowed, single parents, the sole earner in the family, or married to men who make less than $15,000 annually.

A woman's place is clearly on the job more often than in the home; however, a woman's place is not yet on any job. Although there have been some significant increases in the number of women executives, engineers, doctors, dentists, lawyers, and college teachers, there has been little change in the number of women employed in blue-collar jobs. Progress has been made from a decade ago, but very few women are construction workers, electricians, plumbers, or mine workers—the better-paying jobs that are still considered men's work. Only 30% of the professional workforce is female, and the majority of the working women continue to do "women's work"; they are school teachers, librarians, nurses, bank tellers, or clerical workers, and they earn only around 74% of what men make.

As women moved in significant numbers into the job market, from 30 million in 1970 to 60 million in 1997, it began to be evident that the issues of occupational health and safety, formerly believed to concern only men, were highly relevant to working women as well. Like men, women faced the potential hazards of job-related injury and disease, not only as industrial workers, but also in the offices, hospitals, and laboratories where most women work.

In 1970, Congress passed the Occupational Safety and Health Act that established a federal agency, the Occupational Safety and Health Administration (OSHA), and adopted improvement in the workplace environment as a national priority. Along with the Mine Safety and Health Administration (MSHA), the charge to OSHA is the promulgation and enforcement of standards to ensure the greatest protection of workers from job-related injury or disease—a mandate that has embroiled the agency in controversy since its inception because both labor and industry have frequently viewed OSHA's regulatory efforts as less than optimally beneficial. The act also created the National Institute for Occupational Safety and Health (NIOSH), the federal preventive health agency responsible for identifying workplace hazards, developing means of preventing them, and recommending the standards and guidelines to OSHA for the protection of workers.

There are two general types of hazards associated with work: one is traumatic injury, and the other the possibility of illness or death resulting from exposure to toxic agents—chemicals, pathological microorganisms, cotton or coal dust, asbestos, heavy metals, physical agents such as noise, and cumulative or repetitive straining such as back injury.

During the middle 1970s, as more women moved into the workforce, adverse reproductive effects became the focus of greater public, industry, and government interest. The nation's goal of reducing the hazards of the workplace now developed a further dimension—the need to protect the health of women of reproductive age from exposure to substances that could affect reproduction.

But the possibility that adverse effects, such as infertility or birth defects, could be caused or influenced by the working environment resulted in a new kind of dilemma: the potential conflict between the obligation of the employer to provide for occupational health and safety and the rights of women to equal opportunity in employment. New questions of ethics, moral commitment, legality, and constitutionality arose. To what extent could or should another group of individuals—the potential offspring of workers exposed to mutagens or teratogens—be protected? Women had struggled for equal work and equal pay; were their reproductive capacities again to be a barrier? How should a company be able to protect itself against lawsuits brought against it if it could be proved that the next generation was harmed by something in the mother's workplace?

Some companies attempted to solve their problem by developing exclusionary policies that eliminated women of reproductive age from certain jobs. In disregard of the strong probability that any substance toxic enough to threaten a woman's reproductive health is very likely to produce a similar adverse reproductive effect (sterility) in men, they reasoned that because it was economically unfeasible to totally remove the risks, the removal of the women from the job and shifting them to a less hazardous (and lower paying) environment was the only way to protect them and their potential fetuses from hazardous substances. In one highly publicized reaction to such a job restriction policy, five women employees at the American Cyanamid Company chose to have themselves sterilized so that they could return to their former jobs because the money meant more to them than being able to get pregnant. One of the women sterilized was 26 years old, facing divorce, and helping her ill parents with their medical bills.

The fetal protectionist and exclusionary policies were attacked by critics and challenged in the courts. The case that went all the way to the U.S. Supreme Court was that of *Automobile Workers v. Johnson Controls, Inc.,* an automobile lead-battery company. The hazards of lead poisoning have been known for centuries, but it was not until 1975 that OSHA set workplace lead exposure limits for all workers that required companies to remove workers from an environment when their blood levels of lead exceeded 50 micrograms per 100 ml. In 1977, the Milwaukee-based company with plants across the country urged its women employees who were planning to become pregnant to remove themselves voluntarily from lead exposure. How many complied is unknown, but at least six women subsequently gave birth to normal children when their own blood levels, as determined during routine tests, were high (Gunn, 1991). There is no proof that children can be damaged before birth by exposure to lead in utero. There is ample evidence, however, that exposure to lead has a variety of negative reproductive consequences in men, including sterility, impotence, adverse effects on sperm numbers, motility, and morphology—and an increased incidence of spontaneous abortions or stillbirths in their wives. Even the one study linking lead and minor birth defects did not rule out parental exposure as a contributing factor (Bellinger et al., 1987). But of course the company did not ban all married men from areas of the plant with high lead levels. Instead, in 1982 Johnson Controls adopted a policy that prevented all women employees, regardless of age or plans for childbirth, from being exposed to lead unless they could provide medical proof of sterility. One of the first women to be removed from her job was at the Vermont plant and was 50 years old and divorced.

Because a dozen or more other major corporations had similar policies barring all women workers, fertile women, or in some cases, only pregnant women

from exposure to hazardous materials, a ruling in favor of Johnson Controls by the Supreme Court meant that as many as 20 million female workers exposed to toxins on well-paying jobs could potentially be excluded from those jobs. The legal issue was whether the fetal protection policy violated the federal Civil Rights Act of 1964, specifically Title VII, the antidiscrimination statute applicable to employment. The company based its defense on the grounds that the policy was a "business necessity" and claimed that nonfertility was a "bona fide occupational qualification" (usually referred to as a B.F.O.Q.) for a job in a lead-battery factory. In cases alleging deliberate discrimination, the federal civil rights law generally requires the employer to use the B.F.O.Q. defense. Johnson Controls' interpretation of the B.F.O.Q., however, was not accepted by the Supreme Court. In March 1991, the Court declared that the Civil Rights Act prohibited fetal protection policies, that "women should not be forced to choose between having a child and a job," and that women henceforth had the same right to jobs with health risks as did men—a kind of double-edged victory.

The ruling was the end of the fetal protection policies. Because employers could no longer use potential hazards to fetuses as grounds for excluding women from jobs, the Court upheld the rights of women to get the better-paying jobs in traditionally male-dominated industries and allowed women to decide for themselves whether they wanted work that might endanger their reproductive capacities or cause fetal harm.

Obviously, a variety of problems to health and safety are encountered when women work, either at a "man's job" or at a traditionally women's occupation, and they include more than effects on childbearing. As might be expected, however, issues of women's occupational health have focused on the reproductive system. But little is conclusively known and even less is proven concerning the substances or conditions in the working environment that are especially hazardous to reproduction. The severe cutbacks in OSHA's funding and staff resulting from a push toward deregulation in several presidential administrations may also be partially responsible, but OSHA has been slow to issue standards for substances used in industrial plants, offices, laboratories, and homes that have harmful effects on human reproduction. Of the thousands of agents found in the workplace, there are only four—dibromochlorporopane (DBCP, a pesticide), lead, ethylene oxide, and ionizing radiation—that are regulated in part because of their capacity to cause reproductive harm. NIOSH has identified both chemical and physical agents and disease-causing agents. These agents include but are not limited to carbon disulfide (CS_2), lead, cancer treatment drugs (as in the case of health care workers and pharmacists), ionizing radiation, strenuous physical labor, cytomegalovirus (CMV), hepatitis B virus, human immunodeficiency virus (HIV), and so on.

Much of the difficulty in developing standards for regulation or addressing the questions raised by OSHA and representatives of labor and industry results from the paucity of valid scientific data. Until recently, most of the studies by government and privately supported researchers were devoted to other kinds of occupational safety and health hazards to men. Only lately, now that so much of the nation's workforce is female, has the matter of adverse reproductive effects of the workplace become a major occupational health issue.

Over the past 20 years, the research reports have been accumulating. Some studies have been well designed and documented, but others have been based on small samples, provide incomplete information, or are in other ways methodologically flawed. Much more research needs to be done before any definite conclusions on cause-and-effect relationships between jobs and reproductive harm can be drawn.

EFFECTS OF TOXIC AGENTS IN THE WORKPLACE

Some of the chemical and microbiological agents that are known or suspected to be **mutagens, teratogens, or carcinogens** (like DES) that cross the placenta have already been discussed, and many of them can be encountered in the home as well as in the workplace. As previously indicated, there are specific problems associated with attempting to prove a link between exposure to a substance and an adverse reproductive effect such as spontaneous abortion or birth defect. Congenital abnormalities occur at about a 3% rate in the general population; their origin could be genetic, environmental, or through interaction of both. Moreover, the true rate of spontaneous abortion in the general population is unknown and probably underestimated. Many miscarriages may be very early, unrecognized, and unreported; any comparisons of the rate of spontaneous abortion in working women exposed to a particular agent and the rate in nonworking or nonexposed women could be very misleading. Work is certainly not the only factor affecting the outcome of pregnancy.

But even if one keeps in mind the possible shortcomings of the studies and the difficulties in proving the link, there is evidence suggesting that there may be an increased risk of spontaneous abortion for women who work in the following kinds of occupations: research chemists or biologists and women laboratory workers who are exposed to organic solvents like benzene and toluene; hospital workers or laboratory workers who sterilize instruments with ethylene oxide and glutaraldehyde; operating room personnel (anesthesiologists and operating room nurses and technicians) because of exposure to anesthetic agents; women working in the copper smelting industry or with soldering agents. Occupational exposure to heavy metals, pesticides, and herbicides has also been reported to be linked to increased rates of spontaneous abortion in women workers as well as in wives of exposed men.

Finnish researcher Hemminki and his colleagues were the first to suggest (1983) that the occupations of both parents may interact in contributing to an increased risk of spontaneous abortion. They found that the rate of miscarriage was greater for women working in the textile industry when their husbands worked at a large metallurgical factory than it was for women whose husbands worked elsewhere.

In general, there are more data attesting to an increased risk of miscarriage than a greater incidence of birth defects after exposure to workplace toxic agents. Exposure to organic solvents in chemical laboratories has been reported to be related to congenital malformations in the offspring of pregnant workers, and so has employment in the copper smelting industry during pregnancy. There is conflicting evidence, however, for the risks of exposure to anesthetic gases and the rate of birth defects in the children of women hospital workers.

EFFECTS OF PHYSICAL FORCES ON REPRODUCTION

A report by the Council on Scientific Affairs of the American Medical Association (1984a) considered the evidence for adverse reproductive effects as a result of exposure to such physical factors as temperature, atmospheric pressure, vibration and noise, and radiation. They found that neither low nor high atmospheric pressure has been demonstrated to produce teratogenic effects in infants, but that high altitudes were correlated with low birth weights. One report linked increased atmospheric pressure experienced by women scuba divers who dived during pregnancy with increased fetal abnormalities (Bolton, 1980), but the survey sample was small.

Increased temperature or hyperthermia has adverse effects on male fertility and is known to be teratogenic in animals when the temperature has been raised to 43°C (109°F) during embryonic development. In humans, there are data to suggest that fever higher than 104°F that lasts at least 1 day during the third to seventh week of gestation could affect the nervous system of the fetus (Pleet, Graham, & Smith, 1981), but getting body core temperature that high through an ambient working environment is believed to be virtually impossible because no one could tolerate remaining in that hot an atmosphere for long enough.

Of course, ionizing radiation (x-rays) is damaging to all living tissues, including reproductive organs, and the effects are dose related. It is unlikely that today, men and women who are occupationally exposed to ionizing radiation, such as health care workers, are unaware of the potential consequences. They are more likely to take great caution to keep exposures as low as possible. There may be some potential hazards of radiation, however, over which people have no control.

Ionizing radiation is carcinogenic; exposure to low doses increases the risk of cancers like leukemia as much as 20–30 years later. But studies focusing on cancer prevalence in people living near or working at nuclear facilities have had mixed results. Reports from Great Britain indicated increases in leukemia and lymphoma among young people living near the nuclear fuels plant at Sellafield, and the increased incidence appeared to be due to genetic damage to their fathers' sperm (Gardner et al., 1990). Jablon, Hurbec, and Boice (1991) analyzed the incidence of cancer in populations living near 62 nuclear power stations in the United States and found no increased incidence or mortality from cancer. Wing and colleagues (1991) found, however, after an average follow-up time of 26 years, that death from leukemia and all cancers collectively was greater among workers at the Oak Ridge National Laboratory who had been exposed to protracted low doses of radiation. It could be that radiation, even in doses lower than previously believed to be harmful, is carcinogenic if the follow-up on those exposed is long enough.

The adverse effects of ionizing radiation to the reproductive organs are well known, but there is no firm evidence that any differences in fertility, in the rate of spontaneous abortion, or in the frequency of birth defects occur as the result of exposure to other physical forces such as gravity and acceleration, noise, ultrasound, vibration, or ultraviolet and infrared light or laser beams. Neither are there well-documented reports of injuries to reproduction from microwaves or radio frequency waves.

There are epidemiological studies in the scientific literature, however, that suggest that there may be a link between prolonged exposure to low frequency electromagnetic radiation in electromagnetic fields and the risk of cancer, miscarriage, and birth defects. Electromagnetic fields (EMFs) occur wherever electricity flows in an alternating current at 60 cycles per second or 60-hertz. All public power companies supply this kind of alternating current, so EMFs occur from all electrical sources—from overhead power lines and substations as well as household appliances and computers. For example, one widely publicized study found a seasonal increased incidence of miscarriage in a small number of pregnant women who slept under an electric blanket (Wertheimer & Leeper, 1986). Although the study was criticized for not considering that the heat from the blanket, rather than the EMFs, could have caused the problem, some manufacturers of electric blankets have begun to advertise that their blankets are made with reconfigured wiring that reduces EMFs. Pregnant women who usually sleep under electrical blankets and are concerned about EMFs could just turn off the current and add another blanket for the duration of the pregnancy.

The association between exposure to EMFs and cancer is highly controversial, and a cause-and-effect relationship has not been demonstrated. In some studies, children living near power lines appeared to have an increased risk of leukemia and brain tumors (Ahlbom, 1988), and a number of epidemiological studies found an increased risk of the same kinds of cancers in adult electrical workers (linemen, repairmen, and so on) who were occupationally exposed to EMFs (Coleman & Beral, 1988). David Savitz, a researcher at the University of North Carolina, stated that "there currently is not convincing evidence that exposure to EMFs from living near power lines and substations causes cancer." Until further research resolves the issue, however, he urges a policy of "prudent avoidance" (1991).

Because of the growing perception that EMFs emitted from household appliances were connected to leukemia, the National Cancer Institute and the Children's Cancer Group (CCG) collaborated on a large-scale investigation to determine whether exposures to magnetic fields contribute to the development of acute lymphoblastic leukemia (ALL) in children under age 15. ALL comprises 70%–80% of all childhood leukemias in the United States. In a detailed evaluation of the use of electrical appliances and childhood ALL, investigators from NCI and CCG examined whether the use of household electrical appliances by the mother during pregnancy and by the child might be associated with an increased risk of childhood ALL. Electric appliances included in the study were electric blankets, mattress pads, heating pads, water beds, stereo or other sound systems, television and video games connected to a television, video machines located in arcades, computers, microwave ovens, sewing machines, hair dryers, curling irons, ceiling fans, humidifiers, night lights, and electric clocks.

There was no clear conclusion drawn from the data. Although the data showed some association between appliance use and leukemia, there was no consistent pattern of increasing risk with increasing exposures. The scientists speculated that the magnetic fields from electrical appliances are unlikely to increase the risk of childhood ALL (Linet et al., 1997). While EMFs at this point cannot be discounted as a possible cause of cancer, their contribution to cancer, if it exists at all, is likely to be minute when compared with other factors. Smoking cigarettes, for example, increases the risk of cancer about 30 times over normal. Keeping children away from smokers, watching their diets, and monitoring their exposure to sunlight could be better prevention for them against cancer than moving away from overhead power lines.

VDT RISKS TO WOMEN

Almost all secretaries and other clerical workers are women (99.2%), and most of them have had their typewriters or adding machines replaced by video display terminals (VDTs). At least three-quarters of the full-time VDT users are women of reproductive age. Women workers have raised questions about the safety and potential health risks of working at their terminals.

Although most health complaints related to VDTs are focused on head, neck, and back pain; fatigue; eye strain; and stress, some users worried about the reports of an increased number of spontaneous abortions occurring in women exposed to the terminals. In the early 1980s, several locations in the United States and Canada showed statistical oddities or "clusters"—an unusually high incidence of miscarriage—in a group of women office workers. About 16 epidemiological studies were subsequently performed by both private researchers and NIOSH, which produced conflicting results. Most found no effect of VDT use on pregnancy, but two studies did find an increased risk of miscarriage among women who used VDTs more than 15–20 hours per week (McDonald et al., 1988; Goldhaber, Polen, & Hiatt, 1988). The latter researchers, however, acknowledged that there was no biological mechanism to account for the effects and that factors in the workplace (discomfort, stress, monotony of the work) other than the terminals could have accounted for their findings.

A VDT contains a cathode-ray tube to display images on the screen and generates both extremely low frequency (45–60 hertz) and very low frequency (15 kilohertz) electromagnetic fields. Although these low frequency rays were all but ruled out by the studies as having any adverse effect, NIOSH continued to research the possible links between pregnancy problems and VDTs in view of the uncertainty of the effects of even tiny amounts of electromagnetic radiation. In 1991, Teresa Schnorr and her coworkers at NIOSH published the results of a 6-year study described by other epidemiologists as the most carefully done, detailed study to date. The researchers compared two groups of telephone operators from AT&T, among whom are probably the most intensive users of VDTs in the workforce. The operators were similar in age; in number of pregnancies during the period studied; in race, education, and amount of time spent in front of their equipment; and in the number of years employed at the telephone company. They differed only in the presence or absence of a video display terminal at their stations. "Directory-assistance" operators use a VDT,

while "general information" operators do not. In measuring EMFs at VDT workstations and at workstations without VDTs, the researchers found that, in addition to the 45-to-60-hertz EMFs to which all telephone operators were exposed, the women who used VDTs also were exposed abdominally to the 15-kilohertz EMFs. In the 730 women studied, the results were that the rate of spontaneous abortion for all reported pregnancies was 14.9% for the operators exposed to the VDT very low frequency radiation and 15.9% for the operators not exposed. It would appear from this study that there is no added risk of miscarriage due to sitting in front of a VDT. In 1997, the National Institute for Occupational Safety and Health released the results of one of the most extensive investigations ever of reproductive health concerns associated with VDT use. A report (Grajewski, Schnorr, Reefhuis et al., 1997), published in the *American Journal of Industrial Medicine,* concluded that working with video display terminals (VDTs) does not increase a woman's risk of delivering a baby of reduced birth weight or delivering prematurely.

The researchers interviewed 2,430 women employed as telephone operators. During the period covered by the study 707 pregnancies had occurred in which the mothers had been employed at least one day as operators, and in which the pregnancy ended with a live birth. Some 304 of the pregnancies were among operators who had worked with VDTs, and 403 were among women who had not. Some 27 babies of reduced birth weight were delivered by women who had worked with VDTs, or 8.9% of the VDT group, compared with 39 delivered by those who had not worked with VDTs, or 9.7% of that group. No substantial differences were seen between the two groups in the mean birth weight of babies by gestational age. Some 24 preterm infants were born to women who worked with VDTs, or 7.9% of the VDT group, compared with 45 to those who had not worked with VDTs, or 11.2% of that group. NIOSH stated that these new data should provide reassurance to working women, employers, and VDT manufacturers that VDTs do not pose a reproductive risk.

Pregnant women who are chained by their employment to a VDT could take some action to minimize their exposure, just in case. They can work farther away, at least at arm's length (28–30 in.), from the screen, since EMF radiation dissipates rapidly with distance. And because most of the radiation from a VDT comes from the sides of the monitor and from the back where the transformer is located rather than from the front where the person sits, it would be wise to sit well away from a colleague's monitor. Also, IBM, as well as several other computer manufacturers, is now marketing low-radiation monitors in the United States that originally were designed to be sold in Sweden, where there are stringent standards for low frequency emissions from VDTs.

Perhaps the final word on VDTs and pregnancy problems is not in as yet. What has become very evident, however, is that there are other hazards associated with working at the keyboard. Vision problems—eye strain, headaches, blurriness, watering eyes—are one of the most common complaints of VDT workers. People who never wore glasses before may need them for the terminal. Individuals over age 40, who already may be using reading glasses, bifocals, or trifocals, may also need different glasses because they are unable to focus unless they raise their chins or tilt their heads—sure ways to develop neck and back pain. Other musculoskeletal ailments such as tendonitis, bursitis, or carpal tunnel syndrome may be the result of the repetitive motion (also known as cumulative trauma disorder) at the keyboard. The carpal tunnel is the bony and ligamentous passageway through which the nerves pass into the hand. Anything that narrows the tunnel compresses the nerve and causes great pain. Anyone who uses her hands doing the same thing for long hours can get carpal tunnel syndrome, and tedious, repetitive work is often also women's work. Such jobs as working in a meat or poultry packing plant, being a sewing machine operator, a keypunch operator, or a cashier, or sitting at the keyboard of a computer all day, require repetitive motions at a rapid pace. The result can be strain in the tendons of the wrist, painful swelling, and even permanent nerve damage to the hands and wrists.

The answer to many of the problems may be in ergonomics, that is, in making the equipment, job tasks, and environment conform to the person, rather than the other way around. Most of the complaints related to working with a VDT can be ameliorated by paying attention to such factors as being able to adjust the room illumination to eliminate glare; having a chair that supports the body with good alignment of the back; adjusting the height of the chair, the height of the screen, or the angle of the screen; and having the hands in a neutral position over the keyboard with straight, not bent, wrists and the arms parallel to the floor. Some states and cities have passed or considered legislation that would require employers to provide adjustable chairs and tables, special lighting, detachable keyboards; to allow additional rest breaks, offer eye exams; and on request give leaves with no loss in compensation to pregnant VDT operators. San Francisco was the first city to require businesses with more than 15 employees to furnish adjustable chairs, adequate lighting, and regular breaks from the screen.

But even well-designed workstations may not result in a problem-free work environment for office workers. The World Health Organization (WHO) has recognized the "sick building syndrome" as a factor producing symptoms such as headaches, dizziness, or runny noses in office workers. In addition to tobacco smoke, a new energy-efficient, computerized office could have myriad pollutants floating around in the air employees breathe. Indoor pollution can stem from faulty ventilation systems that circulate insufficient fresh air, toxic fumes emitted by chemicals used in a variety of office equipment such as photocopiers and chemical cleaning products, and microorganisms.

WORK DURING PREGNANCY

Another AMA Council on Scientific Affairs report on the "Effects of Pregnancy on Work Performance," released in 1984 generally reaffirmed what many women already know: that in a normal and uncomplicated pregnancy, if a woman wants to, and feels like it, there is no reason why she should not continue to work until her first contraction. As an update to the 1984 report, the CSA issued Report 9 in 1999, which summarized the findings of research published between 1980 and 1998 (American Medical Association, 1999). Although the findings do state that most work during pregnancy does not pose a hazard to the mother or the fetus, there are several associations between work and detrimental fetal outcomes that are cause for concern.

Acknowledging that each individual situation is unique, current research indicates that occupational exposure to certain agents (e.g., lead and mercury) and some occupational infections (e.g., hepatitis, rubella, CMV, herpes) may produce adverse fetal outcomes. Prolonged standing, bending, or shift work presents increased hazards in combination with situations with limited opportunities to rest (AMA, 1999). A recent metanalysis of published research based on 160,988 women in 29 studies also evaluated the association between working conditions and adverse pregnancy outcomes (Mozurkewich, Luke, Avni, & Wolf, 2000). Their analyses of data from many studies from diverse nations and nationalities found a significant association between physically demanding work, prolonged standing, and shift and night work, and adverse outcome of pregnancy. The authors believe that these findings support the need for a better national maternity leave policy for working women with pay, health benefits, and job security.

The AMA's Report 9 concludes that "physicians need to consider the potential benefits and risk of occupational activities and exposures on an individual basis and work with patients and employers to define a healthy working environment for pregnant women. A recommendation that a pregnant woman not perform a particular activity should not be made without serious consideration of the potential health consequences of working versus the hazards of not working. Physicians can encourage employers to accommodate women's increased physical requirements during pregnancy. These include modifications in the work sched-ule to accommodate breaks every few hours, with a longer "meal" break every 4 hours; encouraging adequate hydration; regularly varying work positions with sitting, standing, and walking; and minimizing heavy lifting, especially if associated with bending."

The AMA adopted a set of statements as policy at its 1999 annual meeting, based upon the CSA report; it pledged that as an organization it would do the following:

1. Support the right of employees to work in safe workplaces that do not endanger their reproductive health or that of their unborn children
2. Support workplace policies that minimize the risk of excessive exposure to toxins with known reproductive hazards irrespective of gender or age
3. Encourage physicians to consider the potential benefits and risks of occupational activities and exposures on an individual basis and work with patients and employers to define a healthy working environment for pregnant women
4. Encourage employers to accommodate women's increased physical requirements during pregnancy; recommended accommodations include varied work positions, adequate rest and meal breaks, access to regular hydration, and minimizing heavy lifting
5. Acknowledge that future research done by interdisciplinary study groups composed of obstetricians/gynecologists, occupational medicine specialists, pediatricians, and representatives from industry can best identify adverse reproductive exposures and appropriate accommodations

WOMEN, WORK, AND STRESS

Hans Selye, a Canadian physician and endocrinologist, first developed the concept of physiological stress and stress-related disease. Selye defined stress as the nonspecific response of the body to any demand, or stressor. The key word is *nonspecific:* the stressor can be positive or negative, physical or emotional. It can cause feelings of joy or pleasure; it may result in anxiety or fear—but the body sees little difference and makes no distinction among the stressors. It responds in a non-specific and generalized way—by increased activity of the nervous system and by production of hormones from the hypothalamus, pituitary, and adrenals. These mechanisms make it possible for the body to react to the stressor, cope with it, and adjust the internal environment to make the least damaging and most appropriate response.

The stress response proceeds through three stages. The first one is the alarm reaction, with hormonal and nervous system effects that increase blood pressure and heartbeat, increase energy utilization, and decrease antigen-antibody reactions, thus decreasing resistance to disease. The next stage is the resistance stage. After the initial alarm, the body responses return to normal and there is no further reaction to the given stressor while the body repairs the damage. Most stressors are mild or of short enough duration to elicit only the alarm and resistance stages. But if the stressor continues and is severe enough, the body is no longer able to cope and goes into the exhaustion stage. The hormonal and nervous system responses again reappear and can lead to tissue damage and disease. In experimental animals, even death can result.

By Selye's definition, any stimulus that produces the stress response is a stressor and can be a variety of agents—physical, chemical, or internalized as an emotion. It follows, therefore, that stressors are continually encountered and are a part of living, associated with all life experiences and activities. It is not only impossible to avoid them, but undesirable to try to avoid them. The stress response is essential to keeping us alert and motivated enough to respond to life's challenges. Ideally, according to Selye, the level of stress in our lives should be *eustress*, an amount that is positive and leads to productivity. It is the *distress*, the continual and unrelieved tensions and frustrations—the kinds of emotions that result in internal fruitless wheel spinning—that can lead to illness. One significant aspect of stress-related disease, however, is how an individual perceives and

interprets the stressing agent. Something that is devastatingly stressful for one person could be seen as unimportant to another or even pleasurable to a third. Another important determinant is the way in which one deals with the stressor. Some people will use physical releases and exercise off their stresses; others may chainsmoke or use alcohol or other drugs for release of tensions and compound the damage. Because human behavior in response to stressors is so variable, it is impossible to know for certain the extent to which stress alone is actually involved in human illness.

"Stress," however, is accepted as a known risk factor for coronary heart disease and has been implicated in the development and course of a number of other so-called male diseases, such as gastric ulcers, hypertension, and colitis. Certain occupations, too, have long been acknowledged as carrying a higher level of stress and pressure. The coronary-prone male executive was epitomized by the Type A personality type described by cardiologists Rosenman and Friedman in 1974—the hard-driving, fast-talking, ambitious, competitive workaholic. As women began to enter the workforce and take on male jobs, many in executive ranks, there were predictions that they would take on the Type A behaviors and begin to suffer the same stress-related diseases as males: more heart attacks, ulcers, and high blood pressure.

Whether the increased participation of women in male-dominated professions is going to result in their acquiring more male diseases and decrease their longevity advantage remains to be seen. As yet there is little evidence to warrant the assumption. For reasons that are not clearly understood, but probably are related to diet and exercise, the incidence of cardiovascular disease in both sexes is decreasing. Women still continue to live longer than men, and the gap is increasing, not narrowing. Moreover, research thus far suggests that when workers of either sex suffer apparent stress-related cardiovascular problems, it is not the executives at the top who get heart attacks, but the people in the middle and lower levels of the job hierarchy who are more subject to health problems. It appears that lack of decision-making capacity on the job can be directly correlated with the incidence of heart disease. Studies by the Metropolitan Life Insurance Company (1979) that followed successful and prominent men and women listed in *Who's Who* found that high-level executive men outlived other middle-class men by 29% and that executive women outlived all other women as well as working men. It is evidently not the pressures of work alone that are unhealthy; rich, successful, powerful men and women who are in control of their lives can take a lot of work-related stress and thrive. Presumably, then, the frustrations and insecurities of middle-management positions, the associate and assistant executive jobs that more women are beginning to occupy, are more likely to result in stress-related illness. The really high-risk jobs for coronary heart disease may be at job classification levels where the psychological demands are great but the worker control is lowest—the positions where most women workers are concentrated.

But to put concerns about working women and health into appropriate perspective, it should be recognized that consistently, according to the National Center for Health Statistics, all women who work in any job classification enjoy better health than all nonworking women. They also appear to be healthier overall than working men. Although women workers tend to have more health problems of a mild nature and shorter duration, men workers have more chronic illness, more work injuries, and more life-threatening diseases (Verbrugge, 1982). Another more recent study also showing that working women are healthier was conducted by epidemiologists Donna Kritz-Silverstein, Deborah Wingard, and Elizabeth Barrett-Conner at the University of California, San Diego. They followed 242 middle-aged white women in an upper-middle-class suburb north of San Diego for 15 years to assess their relative risks of heart disease and diabetes. Of the women, 129 worked outside the home and 113 stayed at home. The researchers found that the working women had significantly lower cholesterol and blood-sugar levels as well as favorable levels of other biological variables, which resulted in their being healthier in general and having less risk of heart

disease and diabetes. Moreover, 80% of the employed women worked as professionals, managers, or administrators, again substantiating that being in an executive-level position does not result in stress-related cardiovascular problems (Kritz-Silverstein, Wingard, & Barrett-Conner, 1992).

The Framingham Heart Study, in which 6,000 residents of the Massachusetts city have been observed since 1950, followed a subgroup of 387 working women and 350 nonworking housewives for the development of heart disease. The report by Haynes and Feinleib (1980) confirmed that there was no increase in the risk of heart attack for working women generally as compared with housewives who had never worked outside the home. There was, however, a higher rate of coronary heart disease in one group of women who were clerical workers—secretaries, typists, clerks, and bookkeepers—when compared with other working women and homemakers. But even in that group, analysis revealed that there was no greater incidence of heart disease in single women clerical workers; the rates were boosted by the increased incidence that occurred particularly in women who were mothers and married to blue-collar workers. The researchers discovered that the clerical workers, compared with other working women, were likely to have nonsupportive employers, little or no job mobility, and a tendency to suppress anger and bottle up their resentments. These results lend substantiation to the theory that a routine, dead-end job with few satisfactions besides the paycheck carries a greater risk.

Lois Verbrugge's (1984) analysis of data from the National Interview Study, however found that clerical women in the United States have the best overall health profile, with low rates of injury and of chronic illnesses which might restrict or limit their activities, and average health services use. She suggested that in the Framingham clerical workers, it was the combination of an unsatisfying work situation *plus* child-rearing duties *plus* financial pressures that resulted in the greater incidence of heart disease. Wolfe and Haveman's study (1983) of more than 2,300 working women further substantiated that the added burdens of child care and housework can be detrimental to the health of working mothers, who had greater problems with illness than working women without children. The mothers reported that they generally devoted about the same amount of time to the children and the house after getting a job as before, which might provide a clue to their additional ills.

Clearly, it would appear that working, in itself, is no more stressful for women than it is for men. It is more likely that it is the "pluses," when a woman is powerless to deal with them, that could be unhealthy. Stress factors for a working woman are not difficult to identify. They are built into a job when a woman is stuck in a low-paying, low-status position, when she is subjected to sexual harassment on the job, or when she trains a man for a job and then finds him promoted before she is. Work-related stress is intensified when a woman performs the same duties as a male employee or occupies a position of comparable worth and then finds out that the man makes more money than she does. Pressure can come from outside as well as on the job. For a working mother with preschool children, stress is when a child is sick, the sitter is sick, or the car is sick. For a woman with school-age children, it is stressful when she cannot leave work early enough to get to a parent-teacher conference before the teacher leaves; for the teacher, it occurs when she has the same problem with her own child's teacher. When a woman has to be a full-time worker and a full-time homemaker, when she has simultaneous responsibilities and conflicting role expectations, continual high levels of stress may result. Many women experience at least some of these "pluses"; a few may even be subjected to all of them. There would be less concern for the effects of job stress on the working woman's health if more ways of reducing those burdens were available—through job sharing, flexible time scheduling, better and more accessible day care facilities, and shared parental responsibilities—and if there were greater efforts toward eliminating the inequities, discrimination, and resultant frustration that working women experience in some jobs.

VIOLENCE IN THE WORKPLACE

Since the 1980s, there has been a growing awareness of violence in the workplace, including such actions as assault; nonfatal injuries; homicide; aggressive acts such as hitting, kicking, pushing, biting, and scratching; sexual attacks; or any other physical or verbal attacks directed toward the worker. Although females comprise 45% of the workforce, they experience approximately 55% of work-related assaults and 58% of assault-related injuries that result in lost work time, a majority of these occurring in the domestic services and home health care industry (Hewitt & Levin, 1997).

Efforts to reduce violence in the workplace include such actions as implementing environmental controls (adequate lighting, open visibility of cash registers, and so on); mandatory training in the management of assaultive behavior, and implementation of policies and procedures to reduce violent behavior in the workplace. Much effort is being directed toward places of employment providing postincident trauma counseling and for places of employment to assume responsibility for providing a safe and healthful workplace.

REFERENCES

Ahlbom, A. (1988). A review of the epidemiologic literature on magnetic fields and cancer. *Scandinavian Journal of Work and Environmental Health, 14,* 337–343.

American Medical Association. (1999). Report 9 of the Council on Scientific Affairs (A-99). Effects of Work on Pregnancy. Chicago.

Bellinger, D., Leviton, A., Waternaus, C., et al. (1987). Longitudinal analyses of prenatal and postnatal lead exposure and early cognitive development. *New England Journal of Medicine, 316,* 1037–1043.

Bolton, M. E. (1980). Scuba diving and fetal well-being: A survey of 208 women. *Undersea Biomedical Research, 7,* 183–189.

Coleman, M., & Beral, V. (1988). A review of epidemiological studies of the health effects of living near or working with electricity generation and transmission equipment. *Internal Journal of Epidemiology, 17,* 1–13.

Council on Scientific Affairs. (1984a). Effects of physical forces on the reproductive cycle. *Journal of the American Medical Association, 251*(2), 247–249.

Council on Scientific Affairs. (1984b). Effects of pregnancy on work performance. *Journal of the American Medical Association, 251*(15), 1995–1997.

Gardner, M. J., Snee, M. P., Hal, A. J., et al. (1990). Results of case-control study of leukaemia and lymphoma among young people near Sellafield nuclear plant in West Cumbria. *British Medical Journal, 300,* 423–429.

Goldhaber, M. K., Polen, M. R., & Hiatt, R. A. (1988). The risk of miscarriage and birth defects among women who use visual display terminals during pregnancy. *American Journal of Industrial Medicine, 13,* 695–706.

Grajewski, B., Schnorr, T. M., Reefhuis, J., Roeleveld, N., Salvan, A., et al. (1997). Work with video display terminals and the risk of reduced birthweight and preterm birth. *American Journal of Industrial Medicine, 32*(6), 681–688.

Gunn, E. (1991, March 17). Hazardous duty. *The Milwaukee Journal.*

Haynes, S. G., & Feinleib, M. (1980). Women, work and coronary heart disease: Prospective findings from the Framingham heart study. *American Journal of Public Health, 70*(2), 133–141.

Hemminki, K., Kyyronen, P., Nieme, M. L., et al. (1983). Spontaneous abortions in an industrialized community in Finland. *American Journal of Public Health, 73*(1), 32–37.

Hewitt, J. B., & Levin, P. F. (1997). Violence in the workplace. *Annual Review of Nursing Research, 15,* 81–99.

Jablon, S., Hurbec, Z., & Boice, J. D., Jr. (1991). Cancer in populations living near nuclear facilities. *Journal of the American Medical Association, 265*(11), 1403–1408.

Kritz-Silverstein, D., Wingard, D. L., & Barrett-Conner, E. (1992). Employment status and heart disease risk factors in middle-aged women: The Rancho Bernardo study. *American Journal of Public Health, 82*(2), 215–219.

Linet, M. S., Hatch, E. E., Kleinerman, R. A., Robison, L. L., Kaune, W. T., et al. (1997). Residential exposure to magnetic fields and acute lymphoblastic leukemia in children. *New England Journal of Medicine, 337*(1), 1–43.

McDonald, A. D., McDonald, J. C., Armstrong, B., et al. (1988). Work with visual display units in pregnancy. *British Journal of Industrial Medicine, 45,* 509–515.

Metropolitan Life Insurance Company. (1979). Longevity of prominent women. *Statistical Bulletin of the Metropolitan Life Insurance Company, 60*(1), 2–9.

Mozurkewich, E. L., Luke, B., Avni, M., & Wolf, F. M. (2000). Working conditions and adverse pregnancy outcome: A meta-analysis. *Obstetrics and Gynecology Review, 95*(4), 623–635.

Pleet, H., Graham, J. M., & Smith, D. W. (1981). Central nervous system and facial defects associated with maternal hyperthermia in four to fourteen weeks gestation. *Pediatrics, 67,* 785–789.

Rosenman, R. H., & Friedman, M. (1974). *Type A behavior and your heart.* New York: Alfred A. Knopf.

Savitz, D. (1991). Questions and answers. Power lines and cancer risk. *Journal of the American Medical Association, 265*(11), 1428.

Schnorr, T. M., Grajewski, B. A., Hornung, R. W., et al. (1991). Video display terminals and the risk of spontaneous abortion. *New England Journal of Medicine, 324*(11), 727–733.

Verbrugge, L. M. (1982). Sex differentials in health. *Public Health Reports, 97,* 417–437.

Verbrugge, L. M. (1984). Physical health of clerical workers in the U.S., Framingham, and Detroit. *Women and Health, 9*(1), 17–41.

Wertheimer, N., & Leeper, E. (1986). Possible effects of electric blankets and heated waterbeds on fetal development. *Bioelectromagnetics, 7,* 13–22.

Wing, S., Shy, C. M., Wood, J. L., et al. (1991). Mortality among workers at Oak Ridge National Laboratory: Evidence of radiation effects in follow-up through 1984. *Journal of the American Medical Association, 265*(11), 1397–1402.

Wolfe, B., & Haveman, G. E. (1983). Time allocation, market work, and changes in female health. *American Economic Review, 73*(2), 134–139.

CHAPTER

16

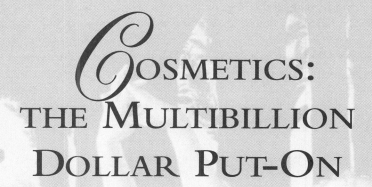

Cosmetics: the Multibillion Dollar Put-On

*P*eople probably have more awareness of their skin than of any other organ system of the body. Not that skin is the largest organ; in terms of surface area, the lungs, the circulatory system, and the digestive tract are bigger. But skin is so very obvious. There it is, covering the entire body, and unlike other organs, it is completely visible. The skin functions as the only barrier between the outside environment and the body inside. It protects against thermal, chemical, and physical injury. Relatively waterproof, the skin allows the body to exist in dry air without shriveling like a raisin and permits one to soak in a tub for hours without appreciably swelling. And, because it is so abundantly supplied with nerve endings, the skin acts as one enormous sense organ, constantly receiving information from its surface for transmission to the brain.

Along with its other functions, and perhaps of greater importance to most people, skin also defines the individual. It provides humans with an identity. The "real me" inside, with all the flaws or attributes of character, remains hidden and internal; what the world sees first of me is the skin covering the contours of face and body. All people are literally sisters and brothers under the skin; without it, everyone would look very much the same.

Skin and its derivatives, hair and nails—the body's facade, are obviously the major media of sexual attraction. Enhancing their appeal has been part of every culture for thousands of years. Eons ago, some enterprising prehistoric human probably first used oils extracted from plants to soften the skin or to smooth the hair. Perhaps, recognizing something powerful and splendid about the vivid colors of nature, primitive men and women mixed red clay or copper ore with water, daubed it on the face, and invented the first makeup. The face and body became the canvas for visible symbols, for dramatizing cultural ideas. Paint pots and implements to grind and apply eye shadow and liner have been unearthed in Egypt and dated to 10,000 years ago. Archeologists digging in Sumerian tombs have found 5,000-year-old lipsticks. Throughout the ages various substances have been applied to the skin to clean, perfume, or color it, camouflage or disguise it, frighten off enemies, ward off evil spirits, protect it from the weather, make it look younger, and generally, to make a statement about self: look at me, this is who I want to show! There is nothing new about cosmetics; they have been in use for thousands of years.

What is new is the emergence of the cosmetics *industry*, which packages, promotes, and sells. Before the 20th century there was very little marketing of cosmetic products. Preparations were mostly made up in the home from "recipes" that used ingredients purchased from the pharmacist. In 1849, 39 manufacturers produced a total of $355 worth of cosmetics that cost only $164 to make (Corson, 1972). Today, the cosmetics industry has multibillion dollar annual sales depending on exactly which items are included in the thousands of formulations on the market. The dollar figure varies, according to whether sales of shampoos, deodorants, toothpaste, or mouthwash are contained in the totals. It is probably valid to include all such products in one mass group. All of them affect the buyers in the same way: to make ourselves better, to make ourselves more appealing. With the largest advertising budget of any commercial enterprise in America, the cosmetics industry, through the media of TV, magazines, and newspapers, offers health, success, fulfillment, new attractiveness, and a whole new lifestyle if only people will buy, buy, buy the products.

The primary focus of cosmetics advertising is directed at women, the greatest consumers of the products. Major cosmetic sales are in beauty aids. Women who believe they do not use cosmetics, that is, facial makeup or nail polish, still buy shampoos, hair conditioners, and toilet soaps. Even the most widely used cosmetic product, toothpaste, is sold as a beauty enhancer. The promotion of toothpaste may be based on sex appeal or plaque removal, depending on whether the sales pitch is to be sex or cavities. And while skin-care products designed strictly for men are viewed by the industry as an additional opportunity for revenue, the major profit is derived from cosmetics purchased by women.

We live in a beauty culture, a world fostered by a cosmetics industry in which stereotyped models of feminine attractiveness—the beautiful people—set the standards. Every year a new image of fashion and beauty is packaged and promoted like the products themselves, by advertising "hype," and to achieve the image, one apparently must only buy the product. Looking different and somehow also looking alike, the models are tall, slim, with marvelous teeth and gorgeous hair, ever widening the gap between fantasy and reality. Real-life women are urged by the fashion magazines and the TV commercials to *get the look,* variously described as clean, natural, glowing, sun warmed, polished, rain-wet, glossy, sheer, silky, satiny, or sensational. They are promised that if they use a certain product they can get rid of the frizzies, the greasies, split ends, and unsightly dandruff. They are persuaded to curl, straighten, color, perm, and 30-minute deep-condition their hair. They are told that they must exfoliate, clarify, moisturize, and replenish their skins, and if only they will apply this lotion or that cream, its special, unique, secret, and rare ingredients will prevent, smooth out, or eliminate the effects of aging.

Perhaps there are those who are able to perceive the whole cosmetics scene as the massive put on it is and remain unaffected by the industry's massive put-down of women's real bodies and faces, which it literally does. But in a society where women are generally overvalued for their personal appearance and undervalued for their contributions and competence, most women are to a certain extent vulnerable to the messages. What teenage girl does not harbor a secret desire to be the subject of a "makeover," believing that the answer to looking better is out there somewhere; and the media tells us where; in a tube, a bottle, a box. Few women are immune. Even feminist author Susan Brownmiller, who admittedly has an anti-makeup bias, acknowledges that she dyes her own prematurely gray hair, although she considers it a "shameful concession to the wrong values." A job has been done on all of us.

All women—wealthy, poor, teenage, mature, women who work, those who stay home, the feminist woman, and the self-described nonfeminist—buy cosmetic products. Cosmetic use is hardly debatable; cosmetics have been used for countless millennia, and we will undoubtedly continue to use them. Virtually all of the studies by psychologists and social scientists have reaffirmed what most people instinctively know—physical attractiveness is better than unattractiveness. Looking good makes you feel good about yourself and improves your self-esteem. Good looks can make you liked, get you viewed as a better and more intelligent person, get you hired, get you promoted, and get you elected to office. Regardless of what this implies about the superficialities of human judgment and our interactions with each other, there are valid psychological and tangible benefits to be derived from trying to enhance our appearance. Wearing makeup does not have to be a guilty concession; it can still be a choice, and as informed consumers women should at least have the knowledge to choose products that are not overpriced or unsafe to use. Knowing about skin, hair, nails, and the composition of cosmetics can provide the information to understand what products can reasonably be expected to do. It should then be easier to look the way one wants to without accumulating a bathroom full of useless and expensive and possibly even dangerous mistakes.

SKIN STRUCTURE

Skin consists of two principal layers, each of which has its own subdivisions. The top cellular layer that faces the outside is the **epidermis.** Epidermis, relatively thin except on the palms of the hands and soles of the feet, also gives rise to specialized skin derivatives, the hair, glands, and nails. The surface of the skin is marked by numerous tiny ridges and furrows and many minute orifices, the openings (pores) of the sweat glands and hair follicles. The underlying and supporting **dermis,** much thicker than the epidermis, is also called the true skin, which is probably why a skin doctor is never called an "epidermatologist." The dermis contains the blood vessels to nourish the epidermis. The two layers of skin are intimately held together by tiny elevations, or papillae, of dermis that project into corresponding depressions of the epidermis. Continued strong friction or heat can cause an accumulation of fluid and the separation of the epidermis from the dermis, or a blister.

Below the dermal layer is the *subcutaneous layer* or *superficial fascia,* which anchors the skin to the underlying muscle. The subcutaneous layer is loosely constructed and contains fat that varies in amount in different parts of the body. In some areas, the fat forms a continuous layer; in hefty individuals, the layer reaches more than an inch in thickness. The fat serves as a reserve energy supply and further insulates the body and cushions it from injury. The characteristic more rounded body contours found in women result from a different distribution and, usually, a greater percentage of subcutaneous fat (Figure 16–1).

Epidermis

The epidermis is the skin's frontier. Its function is to protect against the invasion of microorganisms, against fluid loss or gain, mechanical injury, or any of the other onslaughts of an ever-changing environment. Most of this barrier is provided by 10 or 12 rows of dead cells at the surface of the epidermis called the *stratum corneum,* or horny layer. The lifeless cells of the horny layer are continually being scraped, rubbed, or worn off. As they are sloughed off, they must be replaced from below by the rapidly dividing cells in

the *stratum germinitivum,* or basal layer. Actually, the entire living body is wrapped in a husk of dead cells that contains a tough insoluble semitransparent protein called *keratin,* from a Greek word for "horn." The flat, scalelike surface cells of the stratum corneum contain soft keratin with less sulfur content than the hard keratin of the hair and the fingernails and toenails.

Where the epidermis is thickest, it is stratified into five layers. Figure 16–2 illustrates the epidermis and the layers within it. Rapid cell reproduction occurs in the basal layer. The new cells are pushed upward into the spiny or prickle-cell layer, so called because the cells appear to have little spiny projections between them which represent cellular attachments. After the cells get into this layer, they stop reproducing and start producing keratin. Above the spiny layer, cells begin to accumulate granules of keratohyalin, a precursor to

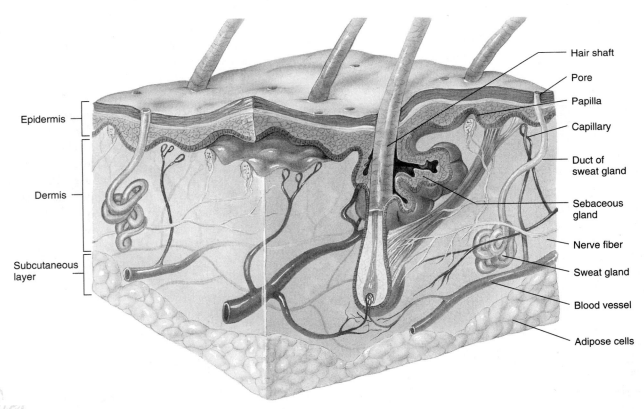

Epidermis

Dermis

Subcutaneous layer

Hair shaft

Pore

Papilla

Capillary

Duct of sweat gland

Sebaceous gland

Nerve fiber

Sweat gland

Blood vessel

Adipose cells

Figure 16–1 Three-dimensional diagram of the skin in cross section.

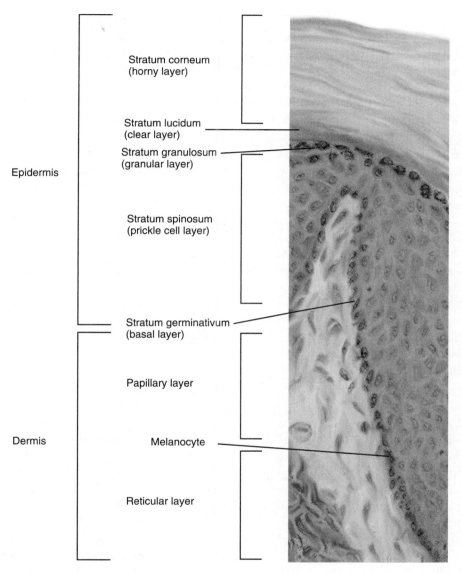

Figure 16–2   Diagram through thick skin showing all five layers. The melanocytes produce pigment to protect the cells from the damaging rays of the sun.

keratin, and are then called the granular layer. Beyond the granular layer, the cell boundaries and nuclei seemingly disappear. The cells look glassy and closely packed, forming the clear or lucid layer that contains a semifluid substance derived from keratohyalin. By the time the cells reach the top of the epidermis, they are flat, scaly, and lifeless, and they are retained in the horny layer until they are shed off as little dead flakes. The rate of growth in epidermis is such that it completely replaces itself from the bottom up every 15–30 days, depending on the area of the body. All five layers are not evident when the epidermis is thin. In those locations, the basal layer gradually and imperceptibly passes into the horny layer.

Hair.

Humans may look naked and hairless compared to other mammals, but we have about the same number of hair follicles as our primate relatives, the gorillas, chimpanzees, and orangutans. Most of our hair follicles, however, give rise only to tiny colorless *vellus* hairs, or "down." Hairs are actually present almost everywhere on the body and are missing only on the palms, soles, nipples, the skin around the nails, and at the various body openings. Children have as many hairs or hair rudiments as adults, but until puberty their only coarse *terminal* hairs are on the scalp, eyebrows, and eyelashes. With maturity and the production of sex hormones, the hair follicles enlarge and become more active. Terminal hairs replace the vellus hairs in the pubic area and under the arms. In men, similar terminal hairs appear on the chest, face, shoulders, legs, and arms. Women have the same number of hairs on their bodies as men, even on their faces, but many of them are small and not as noticeable.

All hair follicles are formed before birth and arise early in the third month of fetal life. A tubular hair follicle begins as a downgrowth from the epidermis into the underlying dermis. The epidermal hair bud becomes bulb shaped at its base and develops a concavity that is invaginated by a mass of connective tissue, blood vessels, and nerves called the dermal papilla. The epidermal cells that lie directly over the papilla are known as the germinal matrix. The germinal matrix cells are analagous to the basal cells of the epidermis in that the product of their repeated cell divisions, in this case a hair, also consists of cells that become cornified and die.

Nourished by the blood vessels in the dermal papillae, the matrix cells proliferate. As they push up toward the surface of the skin, they grow farther and farther from their source of nutrients; become progressively keratinized; and differentiate into an outer cuticle of scaly dead cells, a middle keratinized *cortex* with variable amounts of pigment, and in some hairs, a central medulla. The cuticle and cortex are composed of hard keratin, similar to that of nails or the feathers and scales of birds and reptiles. Medullary keratin is softer and the same as that in the horny layer of the epidermis. The medulla is poorly developed and frequently absent. It is not present in the short and fine vellus hairs, is missing from some of the hairs on the scalp, and is rarely found in blond hairs. The *shaft* of a hair is that part that extends beyond the surface of the skin. The *root,* enclosed within a tubelike follicle, expands at its base into the bulb, the only part of the hair with living, germinating cells (see Figure 16–3).

Shed hairs that still contain some live cells can be analyzed in the same manner as other body tissues. It is also not difficult to determine microscopically if hair has been subjected to bleaching or dyeing. It is further possible to detect traces of minerals such as lead, arsenic, cadmium, or mercury in hair, but such chemical analysis, although much favored in the plots of mystery novels, does not necessarily mean that the elements have been ingested in toxic amounts. Anything in contact with the hair—water, hair sprays, shampoos, dyes, permanent wave solutions—may deposit or remove minerals from the hair.

Glands.

Sweat glands.   Sudoriferous or **sweat glands** are epidermal derivatives located in the dermis and are widely distributed over the entire body surface except on the nail beds of the fingers and toes, the margins of the lips, and on certain parts of the external genitalia. Sweat glands empty their secretion onto the surface of the skin by way of a tiny opening. The watery sweat, or perspiration, is a mixture of certain solids (mostly salts) in solution. It has a cooling effect on the body and also helps to eliminate wastes.

Sebaceous glands.   One or more **sebaceous glands** are always associated with a hair follicle, having differentiated during the development of the follicle by budding off from the epidermal downgrowth. There appears to be a kind of inverse relationship between the size of the sebaceous glands and the size of the hair; that is, follicles that contain the smallest, finest hairs have the largest glands. The sebaceous gland drains its fatty secretion, *sebum,* into the follicle to oil

(A)

(B)

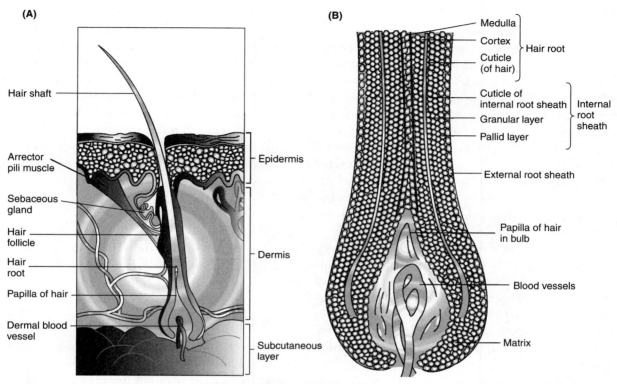

Figure 16–3   (A) Diagram of a hair within its follicle. (B) The follicle expands at its base to form the bulb that contains the dermal papilla. The cells of the germinal matrix lying directly over the papilla give rise to the hair. Pigment cells or melanocytes in the germinal matrix are responsible for hair color.

the hair and pour out over the skin surface. In some locations on the body, the glands develop independently of hair follicles and open by their own duct directly onto the skin.

The hair follicle openings on the surface of the skin are commonly called "pores," although sweat gland openings are also pores. The diameters of the follicle openings are generally related to the size of the sebaceous glands they contain. People who have oily skin have larger glands and hence more conspicuous or enlarged pores. Pores are not doors, and they cannot be opened or closed by heat, by cold, or by any other method. Astringents are solutions that irritate the facial skin to cause a slight swelling and may temporarily make the pore openings appear smaller. Any slight inflammation of the skin, such as a mild sunburn, can

cause a similar edema and "shrink" the pores. Of course, pores can be made less obvious by covering them with makeup.

Except in the eyelashes, hair follicles and hairs are located on a slant rather than at a right angle to the skin surface. The sebaceous glands and a small bundle of smooth muscle fibers, the *arrector pili,* are usually found on the slanting side. The arrector pili muscles are controlled through the autonomic nervous system. When the outside temperature is lowered, or some hair-raising event has occurred, the muscles contract to pull on the follicles and make the hairs erect—literally, to make them stand on end. At the same time, little mounds of skin on the surface are produced by the muscular contraction. We call them goose bumps or goose pimples.

Nails. Fingernails and toenails also develop during fetal life from downgrowths of the epidermis into the dermis underneath. The **nail** itself is a cornified curved plate of hard keratin that rests on a thickened surface of epidermis called the nail bed. The exposed part of the nail is the body, pink because the blood in the capillaries of the dermis shows through the nail translucence. The hidden part of the nail is the root, from which it grows. The root is covered by a curved fold of skin, the cuticle, and a half-moon-shaped whitish area, the lunule, appears on the part of the body closest to the cuticle. Why the lunule is opaque and does not let the capillaries show is not clearly understood.

The half-moon is most visible in the thumbnail, becomes progressively less apparent in the other fingers, and is generally completely hidden by the nail fold on the little finger. The white spots that occasionally appear on the nails are caused by air bubbles between the keratinized cells. They are probably caused by an interruption of keratinization during growth of the nail.

Nails grow an average of 0.5 mm per week, more rapidly in the fingernails than in the toenails and faster in the summer than in the winter. The rate of growth is greatest in the longest finger, least in the little, and intermediate between the two in the other fingers.

Hangnails are the result of cracks or splits of the skin alongside the nails. They may stem from excessive skin dryness from frequent washing of the hands but are more usually caused by a nervous picking at the skin.

The cause of brittle and splitting nails is unknown, but it is suspected that exposure to environmental agents (detergents, solvents, nail polish remover) may be a factor. Eating large amounts of gelatin (collagen) is supposed to be helpful, but there is no real evidence that it works. Gelatin not only has little nutrient value, but it lacks the amino acids necessary for keratin formation. Unless a person is protein deficient (highly unusual for Americans), eating protein will not affect the nails. One of the more common reasons for weak and brittle nails that break easily is dryness, especially in winter. Frequent applications of petroleum jelly or hand cream to the nails and cuticles will help. Also, nails absorb water and swell when immersed for long periods. As they dry out they shrink and weaken, so wearing protective gloves when working with water, cleansers, detergents, or any other chemicals is a good idea. Nail polish can actually help strengthen weak nails, but nail polish remover is very drying, so manicures should be stretched as long as possible—10 days to 2 weeks—to avoid overexposure to the remover.

THE SKIN—COMMON SENSE AND NONSENSE

Skin Color

The fairer the skin, the more the skin color is modified by blood in the capillaries of the dermis and in the larger arteries and veins just under it. The translucent epidermis allows the blood vessels to show through, resulting in a pinkish tone. On the face and neck where the epidermis is thin and the blood vessels are close to the surface, dilation of the vessels during anger or embarrassment will cause the skin to blush. Fear or anxiety may cause a constriction of the blood vessels, and the skin blanches and turns pale as it takes on the color of the underlying connective tissue. Naturally rosy cheeks, or a high color in some people does not mean they are healthier but merely that genetically they have thin skins with many blood-filled capillaries close to the surface and showing through.

The major reason for skin color differences is owing to the activity of pigment-producing cells called **melanocytes.** Sandwiched in among the dividing keratin-producing cells in the basal layer of the epidermis, the melanocytes synthesize a yellow, brown, or black pigment called melanin. Melanin is produced by oxidation of an amino acid, tyrosine, with the aid of a copper-containing enzyme, tyrosinase, and bound to proteins inside the melanocyte to form granules called melanosomes. Melanosomes are then transferred to the other epidermal cells by the threadlike extensions or dendrites of the melanocytes.

The purpose of the melanin is to protect the skin from the harmful effects of ultraviolet rays of the sun. The pigment absorbs the damaging ultraviolet radiation that could, in excessive doses, cause sunburn and skin cancer. The more pigment produced, the darker the skin and the greater the protective power. The actual number of melanocytes is the same in everyone, no matter what the skin tone. Black, white, and Asian skins all contain similar numbers of melanocytes, about 1,000–2,000 per square millimeter, depending on the body area. Racial differences in color and individual differences in skin hue are determined genetically and are the result of greater melanin production by the melanocytes and wider dispersal of the pigment.

When fair skin receives a heavy exposure to sunlight, the melanin that is present oxidizes and darkens. This is followed by an increased production of melanin by the melanocytes and a thickening of the epidermis to reflect more of the radiation. Over a period of several days, the skin becomes tanned or darker. Skins that are darker to begin with tan more readily. Well-tanned or naturally very dark skins are protected to an extent against the harmful effects of sunlight, but even black skins can become sunburned and are not immune to overexposure.

Suntans: Are They Worth It?

Every year millions of fair-skinned people spend millions of hours trying to acquire a tan. A golden, glowing tan is highly prized and admired. It makes the teeth appear whiter, the eyes brighter, and the complexion smoother and more even. Troubled skins are likely to improve, perhaps because the sun's drying effect reduces the number of microorganisms on the skin, perhaps because of the increased blood flow to the skin. Even getting the tan can be a relaxing and pleasant experience if it takes place on a vacation beach rather than in the backyard. For some, a tanned skin is a sign of affluence, indicating leisure and the ability to afford a trip to a resort area. But while tanning may be beneficial to the psyche, in the long run it is harmful to both appearance and health. The notion that a suntan is healthy and beautiful is fallacious. All it means is that the skin has responded to ultraviolet radiation by stepping up its protective mechanism, a process that ultimately can not only irreparably affect the appearance of the skin but also set the stage for the development of skin cancer.

Even without trying to get an annual "terrific tan," there is a visible difference in the appearance of the skin on the face, head, neck, arms, and hands that always has been exposed to the sun when compared with the skin on the abdomen, which rarely sees the light of day. Skin that has always been protected by clothing is still "baby skin"—softer, smoother, and finer textured. If this is the normal difference between covered and uncovered skin, imagine what will happen to the skins of sun worshippers after years of ritual tanning. The thickened epidermis and the increased production of melanin is not enough to prevent the damaging rays from penetrating down to the dermis of the skin. The cumulative effect of the sun causes irreversible damage to the resiliency of the connective tissue fibers in the dermis. Getting a gorgeous tan in one's 20s could result in a premature wrinkled, leathery looking skin in one's 40s.

The risk of permanent effects of tanning is greatly increased when the tanning process is started with a sunburn, as it is by almost everyone. Few people have the patience to wait for the tan to come slowly, taking the sun in small doses of 10–15 minutes a day, increasing by 5 minutes daily, using an effective sunscreen all the while, and sunning only in the early morning or late afternoon. They want a tan quickly and are willing to endure soreness, wakeful nights, and peeling to get the final bronzing. It is believed, however, that once the skin is burned initially, even moderately, the ultraviolet rays are able to penetrate into the dermis despite the tanning of the outer layers. Once the elasticity of the fibrous tissue has been damaged, the result is premature wrinkling of the skin, and nothing can reverse it. Some investigators are even convinced that any skin tanning means skin damage.

Skin Cancer. The relationship between ultraviolet radiation and **skin cancer** is well established. The most common forms are basal cell cancer, which rarely metastasizes, and squamous cell cancer, which occurs less frequently but is more likely to spread. A third type, melanoma, is highly dangerous but much less common. Its cause is not as clearly correlated to over-exposure to sunlight, but melanomas occur more frequently in people with fair complexions.

Eighty to 90% of basal and squamous cell cancers occur on the parts of the body that are exposed to the sun. The incidence of skin malignancies in this country has increased, and it is no coincidence that this has accompanied the increase in the number of tennis players, joggers, golfers, swimmers, and sunbathers and the time spent in outdoor sports and activities. More cases of the disease occur in southern areas of the country where there is more sun and greater exposure, and people with fair skin are particularly vulnerable. Naturally dark-skinned individuals are not immune to skin cancer, however, although the risk is less.

Obviously, there are other factors besides ultraviolet radiation that are involved in skin cancer. The disease sometimes occurs on areas of the body not exposed to the sun, and there are inveterate sunbathers who never get skin cancer. As with all cancers, there are probably genetic or environmental factors that combine with the damaging effects of the ultraviolet rays. There is no way of predicting whether frequent bouts with sunburn during youth will result in skin cancer in the later years, but there is evidence that even several short exposures to a very hot sun are capable of causing a malignancy.

Sunscreens. **Sunscreen preparations** are designed either to reflect the rays of the sun or to absorb them, mimicking the body's own defenses against radiation. Zinc oxide ointments or any other preparation that contains an opaque substance, such as titanium dioxide

or kaolin, are very effective sunblocks; that is, they reflect the damaging rays. Most people dislike sunblocks because they minimize tanning and are not cosmetically pleasant to use, but they are necessary for those who cannot tolerate any exposure to the sun. The most effective solar radiation absorbing agents are those containing para-amino benzoic acid (PABA) or derivatives, such as glyceryl PABA or octyl dimethyl PABA; but occasional allergic reactions occur when using PABA, chemically related to benzocaine. Of somewhat lesser effectiveness are preparations containing benzophenone or cinnamate compounds derived from cinnamon oil. These products are able to reduce the intensity of the ultraviolet rays by absorbing them, thus permitting a longer period of exposure, but no product, despite its claim, is able to provide "tanning without burning." If sunbathing takes place in intensive sunlight for an extended period, sunburn will occur in the same way that a burn can occur right through a deep tan.

It is important to read the label before buying any suntan oil or lotion. A product that contains vegetable fats, such as sesame seed oil, olive oil, or cocoa butter, may have some limited sunscreening properties but will primarily only lubricate the skin. Baby oil has a mineral oil base and is virtually useless as a sunscreen.

To help consumers figure out which sunscreen to use, the Food and Drug Administration (FDA) adopted a rating method called the "sun protection factor" or SPF of 2–45 that can be found on most brands of lotions or oils. The numbers in the system refer to the amount of additional exposure to the sun that can be tolerated if the product is used. For example, an SPF of 8 means that if the product is applied and not washed or perspired off, one could remain in the sun eight times as long as without the product. A person with a very fair and sensitive skin who burns after 30 minutes of exposure to the sun could apply that product and theoretically stay out for 4 hours without burning but probably should not count on it. Individuals who burn easily and never tan should use a product with an SPF factor of 12 or more. For average skin that burns moderately and tans gradually, the FDA recommends using a product with an SPF of 6 for the first exposure to the sun. Sunblocks with an SPF above 15, even going up to 25, 30, or 45, offer little additional protection. As long as the sunscreen is reapplied often enough throughout the day, and especially after swimming, the lower SPF products are sufficient. An SPF 20 delivers protection to the fairest of skins for 10 hours—probably enough sunbathing for even the most avid sun worshipper. An SPF beyond 20 would offer no advantage because there are not enough hours of sunlight, even on a summer's day, to warrant it.

The kind of sunscreen preparation used may be important as well. Sunlight contains two kinds of solar rays, ultraviolet A (UVA) and ultraviolet B (UVB). A study by Hanson and Simon (1998) found that the appearance of prematurely aged skin—wrinkles, sagging, leathery looking—can be caused by ultraviolet A (UVA) radiation, a type generally not blocked by many of the preparations on the market that protect against UVB. Zinc oxide blocks UVA, and some sunscreens contain it in a more transparent form, so it is important to read the label. If sunbathing is desired, an SPF of at least 15 is recommended by dermatologists. A better and more protective recommendation for those exposed to the sun is to wear long sleeves and a hat.

Increased consumer awareness of the role of ultraviolet light in causing premature aging as well as most skin cancers has generated the introduction of a number of tanning products by major cosmetics manufacturers. Called tan accelerators, the products, which generally contain moisturizers and tyrosine, are intended to speed up the skin's production of melanin and thus shorten the time to the "golden glow." Most are to be applied on several consecutive days before exposure to the sun as well as during exposure. While the idea is beguiling, most people report that the tan accelerators, despite claims by the manufacturers, do not seem to work.

Another route to a fake tan is through self-tanning creams and lotions, supposed to provide skin darkening without sun exposure. These products contain a colorless chemical called dihydroxyacetone (DHA),

considered safe by the FDA as a skin dye. DHA reacts with the cornified outer layers of the epidermis to produce a brown color, which gradually fades off as the stratum corneum is replaced from underneath. Because the degree of darkening depends on the thickness of the skin layers, the result may be uneven and, in the opinion of many, artificial looking. These products do not contain sunscreens. Users who go out in the sun may look tanned but are still at risk for sunburn and skin damage.

Although the products just described may yield disappointing results, they are safe to use. But oral suntanning pills, which are sold by tanning salons and through magazine and newspaper advertisements, could pose a serious health risk for users. The tablets contain canthaxanthin, a synthetic food-coloring agent. Because canthaxanthin is highly fat soluble, it is deposited in skin and is used in animal feed to produce a yellow color in chicken skin. At best, canthaxanthin turns the skin yellow-orange. It has never been evaluated for safety as an oral tanning agent, is not harmless, and evidently could have toxic or even lethal effects when used for that purpose. A 1991 report (Bluhm, Branch, Johnston, & Stein) told of a fatal outcome as a result of ingesting canthaxantin. A previously healthy young woman who had taken a course of "tanning pills" obtained from a tanning salon subsequently died of aplastic anemia, a severe depression of the bone marrow. Why anyone would think an orange cast to the skin looks like a tan is puzzling, but the same effect could be obtained safely by eating enormous quantities of carrots! It takes a lot of carrots, which contain the yellow-orange pigment betacarotene, to turn the skin orange, but at least carrots are healthy.

Photosensitization. Some individuals will get a very severe sunburn or have a severe skin reaction characterized by itching, burning, inflammation, and skin rash even if their exposure to the sun is minimal to moderate. Such increased sensitivity to the sun is possible when certain drugs have been ingested; certain chemicals in soaps or perfumes have been applied to the skin; or if there is already the presence of a skin disorder, such as lupus erythematosus or herpes simplex, that becomes aggravated by exposure. The photoallergic response can result from a wide range of substances. Antibiotic drugs, such as the sulfonamides and their derivatives (oral diabetic drugs, thiazide diuretics) and the tetracyclines, are known to be particular offenders in some people. So are some tranquilizers and antihistamines, quinine, barbiturates, aspirin, and foods containing riboflavin. Anyone taking a drug known to be implicated in photosensitivity reactions (check the *Physician's Desk Reference* or other sources of information on drug action) must *beware of the sun*. A photosensitivity reaction can leave a permanent pigmentation of the skin (Figure 16–4).

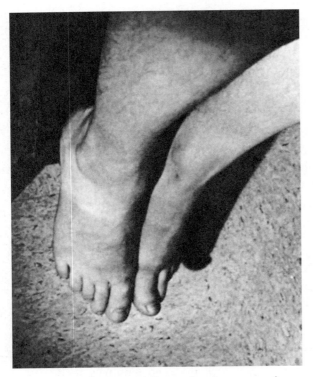

Figure 16–4 Photosensitivity reaction that occurred as a result of exposure to sunlight while taking a tetracycline antibiotics, demeclocycline hydrochloride, as a treatment for acne. Skin darkening persisted for more than a year.

As in All Things, Moderation. Basking in the sunshine is great, and so are water sports, tennis, and any other outdoor athletic activities, as long as unprotected exposure does not take place during the period of the day when the maximum amount of ultraviolet radiation reaches the earth's surface. There is no reason to doubt that the admonition to get plenty of fresh air and sunshine is good advice for a healthy existence, as long as it is done wisely. One known beneficial effect of exposure to sunlight on the skin is that ultraviolet rays do stimulate production of vitamin D by the activation of 7-dehydrocholesterol. But since vitamin D can also be obtained from the diet, and many foods are fortified with it, a normal adult can get all that is needed through proper nutrition. Sun is good, but there is no benefit to going out of one's way to get a suntan, and there is every evidence of detriment. Exposing the skin unnecessarily to get it darker results in accelerated aging and the possibility of skin cancer. The most recent absurdity is the indoor tanning parlors. Regrettably, indoor tanning continues to be a popular activity and theoretically poses the same solar risks, but inside a booth. Because patrons of tanning facilities will also later be outdoors receiving sun exposure, however, it may be difficult to separate the effects of the indoor from the outdoor tanning. In a review of studies of tanning lamp exposure and melanoma, it was noted that there may be a lag time before longer-term effects of this relatively new kind of exposure can be documented (Swerdlow & Weinstock, 1998).

Wrinkled Skin

The dermis of skin is a loose interweaving network of connective tissue proteins called collagen, elastic, and reticular fibers. The collagen and elastic fibers are responsible for the ability of the skin to stretch and contract to accommodate body movement or for changes in size or shape of the body. Generally, although there is great individual variation, skin tends to lose its resiliency with age. For example, if the loose skin on the top of the hand of a young man or woman is pinched up between the fingers, it will instantly return to normal when released. In an 85-year-old, the skin will remain wrinkled up anywhere from 5–15 seconds after release (Figures 16–5 to 16–9).

Facial skin normally wrinkles at right angles to the lines of pull of the facial muscles underneath. After years of facial expression, the lines become accentuated and exaggerated. Because there are more abundant elastic fibers in the dermis of the face and scalp than elsewhere, their natural degeneration with time,

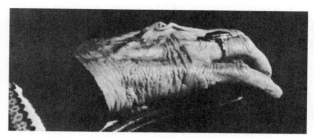

Figure 16–7 The older woman's skin remains wrinkled 10 seconds after release. The elastic and collagen fibers in the dermis have lost much of their resiliency with age.

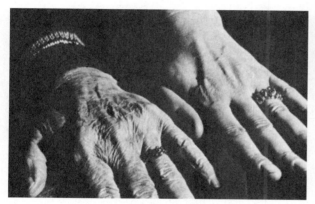

Figure 16–5 Hand of a woman of 85 (left) and hand of a woman of 35 (right). Although there is great individual variability, skin elasticity tends to be very different in these two age groups.

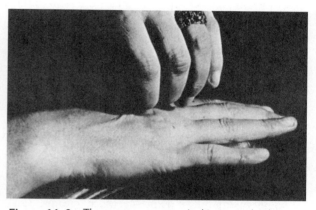

Figure 16–8 The younger woman's skin is pinched up between the fingers.

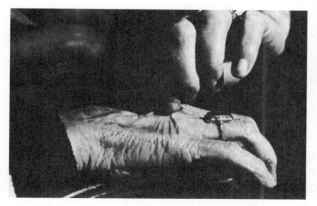

Figure 16–6 The skin on the hand of the older woman is pinched up and stretched between the fingers.

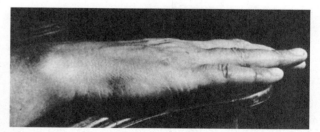

Figure 16–9 Young skin is elastic and instantly returns to normal after being released.

accompanied by the decrease in water content of the skin and the pull of gravity, results in the appearance of permanent wrinkles on the face. Skin aging depends to a great extent on heredity, and a good way to retain an unwrinkled skin after 40 is to be born to parents who also have smooth skin at that age. Of course, one could also try going through life without smiling, frowning, laughing, or talking—a stony-faced alternative to normal communication.

Facial lines and wrinkles are a natural consequence of aging, and they result from the normal deterioration of the bundles of collagen and elastic fibers in the dermis. The process can be accelerated by overly enthusiastic sunning. Smoking will also hasten the formation of facial wrinkles. But there is no way of preventing the eventual appearance of wrinkles—no cosmetic product that "creams" the skin rather than washes it, no matter how faithfully used, and no regimen of facial exercises, massage, masks, or saunas. Facial exercises merely tone the facial muscles and have no effect on the skin above them. Vigorous facial massage could actually help to break down the fibrous connective tissue and create new lines in a hurry. There are some cosmetic aids that can form an oily film that make tiny lines appear less apparent, but nothing except plastic surgery can cure or remove wrinkles.

Some of the most outrageous claims are implied by some of the most expensive face creams. One "extra-rich nourisher" sells at $55 for 2 oz and contains a "unique kind of collagen." Its uniqueness is questionable because it is actually the insoluble protein from the collagen fibers of animal connective tissue, which has been made soluble chemically. The collagen is present presumably to "sink into skin" and "attack the reason for fine dry lines." Note that there is no direct promise that the collagen will penetrate the dermis to rejuvenate or repair the worn-out connective tissue fibers, but the name of the product and the wording of the claim tend to leave that erroneous impression. The other ingredients in this costly cream provide quite valid ways of dealing with fine dry lines because they form a barrier to water evaporation and thus to skin dryness; but the same effect can be accomplished for much less money.

One substance that *may* have some effect on aging of the skin as a result of sun damage is tretinoin, a vitamin A derivative. Exactly how tretinoin works is not clearly understood, but it apparently stimulates epidermal cell division and increases their turnover rate, increases blood flow, decreases melanin synthesis, and causes an increase in collagen bundles in the dermis. The results are a thinner and more compact stratum corneum, a thicker underlying epidermal layer, an evening out of blotchiness and pigmentation, possibly an appearance of translucence and a rosy glow, and a smoothing out of fine wrinkles. Tretinoin has been known to cause regression of premalignant lesions and has been found to significantly improve or remove stretch marks. Not everyone is able to use tretinoin, however. Some skins are too sensitive and become chapped, red, and irritated. Even if the product is tolerated, a person using it should not expect immediate results. It could take 3–6 months of daily use before any changes are apparent, and if use is discontinued, the benefits gradually diminish and disappear.

Alpha-hydroxy acid (AHA), which is also known as glycolic acid, is a component of a number of nonprescription, age-defying creams and lotions. Its effectiveness on fine wrinkles varies with the original condition of the skin and the concentration of AHA. Dermatologists can order and obtain AHA in concentrations of 15%–20% from some manufacturers. At that strength, AHA acts similarly to tretinoin—it increases skin cell turnover, increases collagen production, and usually causes redness and swelling. Over-the-counter preparations cannot, by FDA safety regulations, contain more than 10% AHA and are usually 8% in strength. If the concentration is not listed on the label, it is likely to be quite low. AHA is not regulated by the FDA because it is legally a cosmetic, not a drug, since manufacturers make no claims of effectiveness. The results of a clinical trial of the efficacy of 8% AHA, which was used by 74 women whose ages ranged from 40–70 years for a period of 22 weeks, were that the product was "modestly useful" in improving fine wrinkles and creating a more even skin tone (Stiller et al., 1996). Evidently not all dermatologists are convinced, however. In an article in the *Archives of Dermatology* titled "Snake Oil for the 21st Century," AHA was included, at least in the author's opinion, in a list of questionable skin products promoted and sold by dermatologists (Bigby, 1998).

Probably the latest advancement in wrinkle treatment used by plastic surgeons is the injection of botulinum toxin type A (Botox) into frown lines, forehead lines, "crow's feet" around the eyes, and vertical lip lines. *Clostridium botulinum* is a microorganism that produces a lethal toxin in improperly canned foods. The toxin made within the clostridial cell is a neurotoxin; that is, it acts at the junction between a nerve cell and a muscle cell to prevent the transmission of impulses from nerve to muscle. As a result, botulinum toxin causes muscular paralysis and weakness. The bacteria produce eight different types of toxins, each with a different potency. Very low dose Botox, or type A toxin, has been used therapeutically for a variety of medical reasons, including eyelid twitching, for the past 20 years, but injection for cosmetic purposes into muscles of the head and neck became popular in the past decade as an alternative to surgical treatment. Botox injection temporarily relaxes (partially paralyzes) the muscles responsible for facial lines, wrinkles, and furrows, and injections may have to be repeated. The treatment is allegedly safe with no significant complications other than bruising (Kane, 1999; Fagien, 1999; Binder, Blitzer, & Brin 1998).

Dry Skin, Oily Skin

The ideal in women's facial skin is a smooth, umblemished complexion in which the little orifices from the sweat glands and the sebaceous glands exiting through the hair follicles are not enlarged (large pores); that does not look dry, flaky, or chapped; or does not appear greasy from too much oil on the surface. Women with such skins are fortunate to have inherited the combination of genes to produce it. Many women do have dry skins, not only on the face but all over their bodies, and have either chronic or seasonal problems with itching and flaking skin. Other women have varying degrees of oiliness or possibly a combination of some areas that are dry and others that are oily. Oily skins are perceived as unsightly, but unless the condition precipitates a skin disorder, they are far less of a problem than dry skin.

Dry skin occurs when the water loss from the top layer of the epidermis occurs more rapidly than it can be replaced from the underlying tissues. The keratin in the epidermis must contain at least 10% water for the skin to be soft, pliant, and supple. If the percentage of moisture falls below this level, the cornified layer dries out, becomes brittle, and flakes off. The skin feels tight and dry, and in the extreme, the skin on the hands, for example, can crack and bleed. Water is constantly being supplied upward to the keratin from underneath. The skin retains its hydration because there is a barrier layer in the epidermis to prevent rapid movement of water; without it, moisture would evaporate off too quickly. Besides the barrier layer, two other factors prevent rapid water loss and promote water retention. One is the presence of hydrophilic (water-loving) substances in the horny layer that bind the water these cells need. These water-soluble and water-attracting substances could be removed from the skin by washing or by perspiration, but they are protected from loss by a thin film of water-insoluble sebum. Sebum, the fatty secretion of the sebaceous glands, is a complex mixture of lipids containing fatty acids (mostly palmitic and oleic acids), neutral fats or triglycerides, wax esters, cholesterol esters, and squalene, a precursor to cholesterol. This "skin fat," in combination with sweat, forms a coating on the surface and functions to help slow down the too rapid evaporation of water. Sebum also coats the projecting edges of the dead keratinized cells, smoothes them down, and thus reduces the surface area for evaporation. Creams, lotions, and "moisturizers" for dry skin attempt to duplicate and enhance the functions of sebum.

Sebaceous glands are largest and most numerous on the skin of the forehead, around the nose and mouth, and over the cheekbones, attaining a density of 800 per square centimeter compared with 100 glands per square centimeter in other locations. Their number and activity are under both hereditary and hormonal control. The production of sebum is greater in teenagers, the increase resulting primarily from the secretion of androgen but affected by estrogens and progesterone as well. The luster of youthful skin, that shiny, glossy glow so prized and promised by the cosmetic ads, is essentially caused by the same sort of sebaceous gland activity that is labeled a "too oily" skin when a woman is past adolescence. There are vast individual differences in sebum production, and these differences cause the differentiation between dry, normal, and oily complexions. Obviously, when the amount of sebum produced is neither too scanty nor too excessive, and when the rate of water loss from the surface of the skin is balanced by the rate at which water moves from the dermis into the top layers, the skin appears neither dry nor oily, but normal.

Any skin type, even naturally oily, can become dehydrated when water evaporation exceeds the capability for replacement. Environmental and hormonal factors play a role in inducing dessication of the horny layer. Water loss is greater when the temperature is elevated, the humidity is low, and the wind velocity is increased. Warm weather alone is not necessarily drying, even in lowered humidity, because sweat on the skin surface keeps it moist. A warm, dry, windy day, however, may cause a problem for those whose skins are naturally drier. Dry-skinned people can really suffer in the winter months, when the combination of cold, dry outside air and overheated, low-humidity indoor air is likely to result in the "winter itch," a dry skin condition. The daily bath or shower will also add to the difficulty in the winter because washing the skin removes the oily sebum film. Ordinarily, this defatting of the skin surface is only temporary because the increased activity of the sebaceous glands soon renews the barrier effect of the sebum. The replacement is less rapid, however, in people who through heredity or age normally produce less sebum. Fewer, cooler, and quicker baths in the winter time would probably benefit everyone's skin. The use of emollients to replace the surface skin lipid layer and to retard evaporation will also be helpful.

Once the skin has become dry, brittle, and cracked, it will take more than the application of a lotion or cream to restore it. The most direct way to heal chapped and roughened skin, common on the hands and face during the winter months, is to rehydrate it. Moisture can only be replaced with moisture, not with fats, which have no effect on returning hard, dry keratin to softness and pliability. Merely attempting to replace the lost oils on the skin is not enough. An oily barrier must be applied to prevent further evaporation after the skin is hydrated.

Hand lotions and creams are emulsions of water and oils; the water provides moisture to the skin and the oils are supposed to form a barrier to keep it there. But when the skin has become very dry and is painfully chapped, lotions and creams in themselves cannot add enough moisture or provide enough of a retardant to further water loss. Rather than relying on the products alone, restoring moisture can better be accomplished by soaking the hands in water, drying them, and then slathering on a thick layer of petroleum jelly (Vaseline). The skin will pick up the moisture during immersion, and the petroleum jelly barrier will retain it.

The same method of petroleum jelly occlusion is used commercially to combat chapped lips, since various lip balms are basically petrolatum plus solidifying waxes. The straight Vaseline treatment after soaking is appropriate for the hands because one can always go to bed with cotton gloves on. Using petroleum jelly on the face is less appealing; it messes up the sheet and is too greasy to wear under makeup. All night creams and most daytime moisturizers, however, contain mineral oil, which is liquid petroleum jelly. They also contain other ingredients in a more elegant formulation to provide similar benefits with greater aesthetic qualities. The ability of any moisturizing cream or lotion to aid a flaky and chapped skin is enhanced when the skin is moistened before application. This means that putting the preparation on when the skin is still wet is going to make the barrier work more effectively.

Does everyone's skin need the protection of a moisturizer? Cosmetics manufacturers, whose business is selling products to make a profit, tend to advocate the use of moisturizers in some form as beneficial for all women. In areas where the year-round climate is hot and dry or in the northern parts of the country where the inside of most houses during the winter months is similar to a desert atmosphere, it may be that a barrier film is needed even by women with a normal skin-oil to skin-moisture ratio, but moisturizers are of no benefit to those with oily skins. They may further aggravate the skin in those who are troubled with acne.

Skin dryness or oiliness is, after all, highly subjective and variable. It may change, even in the same individual, under different conditions—with the environment, with the amount of skin cleansing, with the kind of makeup used, and to a certain extent, even with the emotional state. Unless the dryness or oiliness is very unsightly or is related to a skin disorder, it is probably overrated as a problem. Dry skin does not cause wrinkles. Heredity, aging, and exposure to ultraviolet light causes wrinkling, and no amount of creaming or moisturizing is going to prevent it. Wrinkles can be more apparent when the top layers of the skin are dehydrated and lifted up rather than lying flat to refract light evenly. Scanning electron microscopy photographs of the horny layers taken before and after the use of moisturizing lotions seem to indicate that the primary action of such products appears to be the lubricating and flattening down of the uplifted or flaking layers of cornified cells. The effect results from the oils and additives in the product and not from the moisture or water component (Garber, 1978). If the skin feels tight and looks dry, any emollient preparation, even something as mundane as Vaseline or plain mineral oil or pure solid vegetable shortening, will put a fatty film on the skin surface and accomplish the same purpose. In 1995, the FDA approved topical tretinoin for improving the appearance of sun-damaged skin. Tretinoin sloughs off dead skin and regenerates collagen ("Tretinoin (Renova) Approved for Treatment of Wrinkles," 1996).

Commercial products may contain a more pleasant combination of ingredients that makes using them more agreeable than applying shortening or baby oil to the face. Moisturizing lotions also contain, in addition to oil and water, substances called *humectants.* Humectants, such as glycerine, sorbitol, urea, propylene glycol, polypropylene glycol, or in "organic" products, honey, are highly hygroscopic and are capable of attracting moisture. Advertisements imply that such agents have the ability to draw the water out of the air and bring it to the skin surface. It is very unlikely that humectants actually transfer water from the atmosphere to the skin. They are, in fact, nondirectional. If humectants were used alone or in high enough proportions they would be just as likely to pull the water out of the skin. The only way that a high concentration of glycerine (or glycerol, which is the same substance) can be useful for dry skin is under conditions of very high atmospheric humidity of 90% or more. Of course, if the humidity is very high, dry skin would not be a problem. The main purpose of humectants in moisturizing lotions is to bind with the water in the emulsion and therefore keep the preparation itself from drying out or shrinking through evaporation. Humectants also smooth and soften the skin surface and make the application of the lotion easier.

Skin Mythology

The public gets a lot of advice concerning facial skin care, and much of it is utter nonsense. Women are constantly being told by beauty "experts" to let the skin breathe, to let the skin rest, to nourish it, to let it thirstily soak up the oils it craves, to flush out its pores, to pat or massage it, and to coddle it with applications of all kinds of substances. During the past few years when anything "natural" or "organic" has been very popular, recipes for do-it-yourself cleansers, toners, masks, and various remedies have been appearing in magazines and newspapers. There was a time when the expression "ending up with egg on your face" meant discomfiture or embarrassment. Now it means that a mixture of egg, honey, oatmeal, and so forth has been applied to deep-clean, tone, prevent blotches, moisturize, or in other ways provide innumerable benefits.

The homemade preparations composed of vegetable oils, herbs, fruit juices, and cereals are certainly cheaper than cosmetics. They can have similar emollient or drying properties and provide the same effect as many commercial products. They can also be equally allergenic, sensitizing, irritating, or acne producing on some skins as the chemicals in commercial cosmetics, and there is no particular benefit in buying cosmetics that contain "organic" substances. Moreover, the notion that the skin requires a little nourishing snack in the form of mayonnaise or a little drink of apple cider vinegar in preference to other emollients or astringents is patently absurd. Human epidermis does not "eat," need to be nourished, or in any way fed from the outside. Neither does it "drink," soak up oils, "breathe," or need to breathe. Skin gets all the nourishment and oxygen it needs delivered to it from the underlying blood vessels in the dermis. Little if any gaseous exchange occurs from the environment. Skin can be nourished only from the inside. Eating the eggs, oatmeal, strawberries, avocados, cucumbers, or whatever, is a better way to get a healthy and good-looking skin than by mashing the foods up in a "berry-butter-beautifier" or "protein mask."

Letting the skin breathe may refer to nonocclusion of the openings from the sweat glands and the hair follicles. Certain cosmetics are said to clog the pores. Virtually all facial makeups, powders, and moisturizing creams and lotions are occlusive to an extent, but even heavy facial makeup is unable to block perspiration, as anyone who has sat up close to the actors during a stage performance can verify. Cosmetics that contain large amounts of oil may be occluding to hair follicle openings, but thorough face washing with soap unclogs the clogged pores, and this is sufficient for most women. Some skins do have a lower tolerance for occlusive oily makeups and respond with "acne cosmetica," a condition to be described later. But not everyone gets clogged pores or pimples from wearing makeup. At night, however, common sense indicates that makeup should always be completely removed.

Skin Care

Essential to keeping skin healthy and good looking is keeping it clean. Cleansing the skin removes the flakes or dead cells, dust or soot particles, dried perspiration, accumulated skin oils and remnants of cosmetics, and skin bacteria that act on organic materials to cause odors. Water alone does a good job of rinsing away dirt if enough of it is used for a long enough period of time in conjunction with a brush or a harsh cloth. To more easily remove the impurities that are embedded with skin fat in all the little skin folds and follicle openings, however, a cleansing agent should be used. The most efficient agents are those that surround or dissolve dirt particles so that water can rinse them away and not merely redistribute them.

The cosmetics industry implies that different methods of cleansing are necessary for different kinds of epidermis. Some manufacturers, with an eye toward the current interest in computer technology, have begun to use computerized skin analysis to determine the exact preparations to be purchased by every skin type. A vast array of substances for facial cleansing are on the market—morning cleansers for dry skin, evening cleansers for oily skin, creamy cleansers containing milk, scrub creams, facial baths, and various extraordinarily priced "cleansing bars."

Although many cosmetic "experts" would probably disagree, most dermatologists concur that the best method for washing any face is using soap and water. Toilet soaps are a mixture of the sodium salts of various fatty acids—mostly stearic, palmitic, and oleic—and are essentially the same fat and lye compound that has been used to remove dirt for thousands of years. Today's soaps, however, contain extra ingredients that are supposed to confer special qualities. Superfatted soaps such as Dove, for example, contain 3%–5% more fat, and transparent soaps, such as Neutrogena, contain glycerine. Many soaps claim to have deodorant effects. Because the antibacterial hexachlorophene can no longer be used in soap, most of the deodorizing effect of deodorant soaps is the same as that of any soap—the removal of dirt and body oil. Acne soaps contain sulfur and tar, which are drying agents and may be irritating to some skins. Castile soap contains coconut or olive oil, and soaps that float are inflated with air. Ivory soap smells like soap; it contains less perfume or oil than some other brands and could be less sensitizing to some skins. Some soaps are completely made of synthetic detergents and are "nonsoap" soaps, but they are neither better nor worse than any others.

All soaps get the skin clean. Choosing one over another is a matter of personal preference. As pointed out by *Consumer Reports,* all modern soaps have been adjusted to an appropriate pH, and none is harshly alkaline. Oily skinned individuals are able to tolerate more frequent washing, whereas people with dry skins will probably want to wash no more than twice a day. Those with very dry skins may prefer a soap containing more creams or oils—the superfatted variety. Spending a lot of money on exotic beauty soaps does not guarantee that they have any particular qualities beyond cleansing power. Soap is soap.

Lasers for Skin Treatment

Over the past few decades, the use of lasers for a variety of skin treatments has assumed an increasingly important role for cosmetic surgeons and dermatologists. Lasers are frequently used to minimize wrinkles; permanently remove unwanted body hair; ameliorate postoperative scarring; and eliminate birthmarks, spider veins, colored tattoos, and the little brown benign skin lesions resembling a freckle. Compared with surgery, laser treatment may offer advantages when patients are properly selected and the physician is well experienced, but it is not without risk of bleeding, infection, and serious complications (Alster & Bettencourt, 1998; Grossman, Majidian, & Grossman, 1998).

Laser beams have varying wavelengths, which determine how deeply the beam penetrates into the skin. The CO_2 laser is used in resurfacing of the face to reduce or eliminate fine wrinkles and thus can replace dermabrasion or chemical peel. Pulsed-dye lasers coagulate blood proteins within the vessels, causing their disintegration and subsequent absorption and are used for spider veins. Larger vessels generally require the use of argon lasers. Neodymium-YAG lasers are used to remove colors in tattoos. Lasers are high-energy machines—the procedures can cause swelling and pain. Unfortunately, scarring or pigmentation changes also are possible.

Facial Makeup

There are many women who inherit the kind of facial skin and coloring that really needs no covering or enhancement. Through genetics, and with no particular effort on their part, they have smooth, unblemished, velvety skin that is the epitome of a beautiful complexion. Such skin is often remarkably indifferent to the way it is treated. Flawless skin is, after all, most similar in quality and texture to baby and children's skin, and no special regimen of creaming, cleansing, or any other kind of coddling with high-priced products is used on youngsters. For such lucky women, perhaps a little mascara and a lip gloss would be as much makeup as they would ever use.

Other women whose facial skin has small imperfections, whose pigmentation is not as even, whose skin texture is not as fine, may choose not to meet the world with a bare face. They may use a number of cosmetics—foundation, blusher, eye makeup, lipstick—as the most practical solution to being born with skin that is less than perfect. Although there is a prevalent belief that there is value in going without makeup, using no makeup is not necessarily better for *normal* skins. Some women, however, have unusually sensitive skins that cannot tolerate cosmetics without reacting adversely. Some women are prone to acne eruptions long after the usual adolescent acne should have disappeared and would do better to avoid very oily makeups that will aggravate their conditions. Women who tend to have dry skin will probably choose oil-based cosmetics but may want to avoid pancake or matte finish makeups. Even though they contain more emollients, they also contain more chalk and talc that absorb oils and draw moisture out of the skin.

Probably the best way to find a number of products for personal use, given that each woman has her own requirements, is to remain highly skeptical about the advertised claims and experiment around, trying to spend as little as possible. When it comes to buying cosmetics, the old axiom "you get what you pay for" is not necessarily true. In most instances, what you get, whether you spend a little or a lot, is essentially the same combination of ingredients.

"Hypoallergenic" Products. Consumers may be surprised to learn that the cosmetic labels that claim that a cosmetic or an entire line of products is "hypoallergenic," that is, less likely to cause an allergic or adverse skin reaction, are meaningless. There are no scientific studies showing that products that make such claims actually contain ingredients that have a lower potential for causing sensitivity or irritation than any other similar products not claiming hypoallergenicity. All cosmetics contain allergens for some people; to completely avoid reactions to cosmetics would require abolishing the use of all of them.

The FDA has been unsuccessfully trying since 1974 to issue a regulation that would require manufacturers to withdraw cosmetics labeled "hypoallergenic" from the market, unless testing on human subjects indicated that a product so labeled caused significantly fewer adverse reactions than competing products not making such claims. The FDA's efforts were challenged legally by Almay and Clinique, two of the largest manufacturers of alleged hypoallergenic cosmetics. When the FDA's proposal was upheld in U.S. District Court, the two firms appealed the decision. In late 1977, a federal court ruled that the FDA's regulation was invalid because it had not demonstrated that the word "hypoallergenic" was perceived by consumers in the way described in the regulation and that the agency's definition of the term was hence unreasonable.

Manufacturers may now continue, as they have in the past, to advertise and label their products as hypoallergenic without having to provide any substantiation. A cosmetic marketed as hypoallergenic may indeed contain fewer sensitizing ingredients, but its content may be the same as that of any other similar product, a fact easily ascertained by reading the labels. An FDA regulation that did not suffer the same legal fate as the hypoallergenic proposal (although this was not due to lack of effort on the part of the industry) requires that the ingredients used in cosmetics be listed on the product label in order of predominance in

amount. Women who know they are allergic to certain chemicals can be afforded some protection by looking for the presence of the offending ingredient in the product. Unfortunately, "trade secrets," "fragrance," and "flavor" are categories presently exempt from the required labeling. Each of these broad classifications may in themselves contain dozens of chemicals that are capable of provoking an adverse reaction. The FDA is considering a change in the regulation to include certain flavor or fragrance ingredients.

Federal Regulation of Cosmetics

The majority of cosmetic products are probably safe for use by the majority of people. Their harmlessness is only an optimistic assumption, however, because there is actually no proof of their safety. Moreover, there is not much chance of getting that verification. Of course, cosmetics manufacturers have reputations to protect and stand to lose a great deal if the safety of their products becomes suspect. Most firms do test their products before putting them on the market, but there is no law that requires that they certify them for safety before sale, no necessity for them to report the results of their tests to the FDA, and no mandate that they inform the FDA of consumer complaints of adverse reactions to their products. Under current legislation, there is no way of knowing how many cosmetics manufacturers exist, what they are making, what the products they sell contain, or whether or not they are hazardous. An estimated 8,000 chemical ingredients are used in formulating cosmetics, and only for about 75—the color additives—is there any necessity for documenting safety and effectiveness.

The privileged status of cosmetics, exempt from the regulations governing all other substances under the purview of the FDA, has its basis in the Food, Drug, and Cosmetic Act. Passed by Congress in 1938, the law defines cosmetics as articles "rubbed, poured, sprinkled, or sprayed on, introduced into, or otherwise applied to the human body for cleansing, beautifying, promoting attractiveness, or altering the appearance without affecting the body's structure or function."

This means that some cosmetic products, such as deodorants or antidandruff shampoos, because they do affect body structure or function, are legally drugs and have to meet tests for safety and efficacy before marketing. But many cosmetics that by definition are excluded from regulation contain ingredients that not only can cause adverse skin reactions but also can be absorbed, ingested, or inhaled to result in the same kind of systemic health problems as those caused by the chemicals in drugs and food additives. There have been reports of microorganism contamination of eye makeup and hand lotion, skin photosensitizing chemicals in bar soap, asbestos in talcum powder, formaldehyde in nail hardeners, highly skin-sensitizing feminine deodorant sprays, and carcinogens in hair dyes. No one really knows, for example, to what extent cosmetic ingredients may be absorbed through the skin, what happens to the molecules once they get into the bloodstream, or what their long-term effects may be. The safety of beauty products is a largely ignored major issue in women's (and men's) health. The apparent disinterest in cosmetic safety regulation may stem from the general assumption that there already are existing rules, codes, and ordinances controlling the sale of cosmetics. The government, after all, seemingly extends its regulatory presence into the marketing of all commodities. Under current laws, however, the only way in which an unsafe cosmetic product can be removed from the marketplace is for the FDA to prove to a court that the cosmetic is misbranded or adulterated. Unlike drugs, food, drug and cosmetic color additives, and medical devices, cosmetics do not have to be pretested for safety before being sold. Millions of consumers, therefore, have become the ex post facto experimental subjects for the possible and potential hazards of cosmetics.

Every few years another Congressional report points out major weaknesses in the FDA's ability to regulate the cosmetics industry. The industry maintains it can regulate itself, but a Government Accounting Office study released in 1990 found, among other shortcomings, that 884 chemicals used by the cosmetics industry are on a federal toxic substances list, that companies rarely disclose safety test results to the FDA, and that only a tiny percent of the 5,000 cosmetic distributors file consumer injury reports. Consumer groups have argued that the government should have the same control over cosmetics that it has over the other items regulated by the FDA and that the 1938 statute needs to be rewritten to close loopholes and give the FDA more clout. Perhaps some needed changes will be forthcoming, but in a governmental atmosphere of deregulation, cosmetics safety reform legislation, although introduced in the Senate, has not as yet been enacted. Were a bill to pass, it likely would require premarketing certification for safety of all cosmetics and mandate that manufacturers report all complaints of adverse reactions that they receive.

In a move toward greater consumer protection, the FDA extended its regulatory authority over cosmetics by labeling requirements. All cosmetics manufacturers must now list ingredients on the product labels. Moreover, if a cosmetic manufacturer has not substantiated the safety of a product, the label must carry the following message: "Warning—the safety of this product has not been determined." While the regulations are of benefit to consumers, they are not as far reaching as would be expected. Cosmetics used in beauty shops (hair dyes, permanent wave solution, and so on) need not carry warning labels. Furthermore, because the FDA has no authority under law to examine the data on which the manufacturers' claims of safety are based, the effectiveness of the regulation is obviously weakened.

Generally, when companies have tested new formulations of their products for safety and effectiveness, they have used animals as subjects. While many people accept the use of animals in medical research, it is somewhat more difficult to justify animals used for tests of cosmetics, a vanity item. Clearly, in any scientific research—medical or cosmetic—there is no valid reason for cruelty or mutilation of research animals. In awareness of growing consumer concern and the possibility of animal rights legislation, several of the largest cosmetics manufacturers have announced an end to animal testing. Others have scaled down the use of animal tests, while Procter & Gamble has offered a half-million dollar program of research grants to develop alternatives to animal testing (Donato, 1989). Such alternatives could include computer modeling instead of animal tests or the use of cultured cells from the dermis as a skin substitute (Erickson, 1990). It should be noted that "humane" cosmetics, or "cruelty-free" products are offered by the Body Shop, established in 1976 by Anita Roddick as a tiny alternative cosmetics company in England. Currently the Body Shop has stores in major cities worldwide.

Read the Labels!

While the ingredient listing on the labels in itself does not provide the kind of regulatory control over cosmetic formulation that is necessary, it is a step forward and is significant for several reasons. First, consumers have the right to know what is in the products that they buy. People are then able to avoid suspect chemicals that have been implicated as carcinogenic, have produced adverse allergic skin or systemic reactions in them, are known to be photosensitizing, or that can aggravate an existing skin condition such as acne. Second, the listing can result in comparison shopping and promote truth in advertising. For years there have been rumors that a lipstick that costs $17.50 may contain the same 15¢ worth of ingredients as a lipstick selling for 79¢, but the expensive one has the prettier tube and the more prestigious brand name and is sold in a department store instead of a drug or discount store. Now it is possible to actually compare the value of competing cosmetic products and to personally decide whether the costly one is worth the price difference.

Cosmetic companies maintain that the evaluation of a product's worth has little to do with the listing of ingredients. They claim that the quality and purity of the ingredients may vary among the expensive and cheaper brands and that these criteria cannot be listed on the label. The validity of such arguments, similar to those used to justify the inordinate price differences between generic and brand-name drugs, is difficult to evaluate. It may be that some products contain commercial-grade chemicals and others pure grade. It may also be true that different grades of chemicals may mean that varying amounts of degradation products or impurities are present. There is no assurance, however, that expensive products use a better grade of chemical. The only information that is available is the identity of the ingredients; whether being expensive and creatively advertised makes an individual product better or purer is controversial.

Two skin lotions, for example, are contrasted in the chart that follows. They both purport to perform essentially the same function. The more costly product is termed a "clarifying" lotion, which serves to remove the top layers of dead skin cells and leave skin looking "its cleanest, freshest, healthiest." The cheaper preparation is a "texture" lotion, meant to "remove dirt" as well as "stimulate and refresh skin for a smooth, glowing complexion." Because the ingredients are listed in order of predominance, the consumer can judge whether the difference between the two products warrants the fourfold difference in price.

Lotion A ($16.50 for 13.5 oz)	Lotion B ($6.50 for 16 oz)
SD alcohol 40	water
water	SD alcohol 40
witch hazel	witch hazel
glycerine	propylene glycol
acetone	sodium borate
sodium borate	isopropyl alcohol
menthol	methylparaben
caramel	fragrance
D&C red #33	D&C red #33
	FD&C blue #1

What Do the Labels Mean?. The preceding example demonstrates that it is possible to compare ingredients to see how one product stacks up to another more expensive or cheaper brand without understanding much about the purpose or the action of the chemicals. It is going to be increasingly difficult for a manufacturer to continue to make exaggerated claims about what a product with a "miracle" or "European" formula can accomplish when all the "secrets" must, by law, be listed on the label. According to the FDA regulation, the materials in the formula must be presented in the descending order of their predominance and by established and uniform names so that the consumer is not confused or misled by the use of different terms for the same substance. The terminology was developed by the Ingredient Nomenclature Committee of the Cosmetic, Toiletry, and Fragrance Association (CTFA) and is published in the *Cosmetic Ingredient Dictionary.*

The names may be uniform and consistent, but their intelligibility to anyone without a degree in organic chemistry would appear to be doubtful. When confronted by 10 tiny lines of long and technical terms on the bottle, one's normal response might be the presumption that such a complex combination of chemicals must surely be worth every bit of the price! It is important to remember, however, that the formula listing is qualitative only and that the concentration of the ingredients is lacking. If water is the first ingredient listed, the product is mostly water, and the components near the bottom of the list are not going to be present in greater concentrations than just a few percent. Those small amounts are not likely to contribute much to the effectiveness of the product and are there mostly as stabilizers or preservatives. Moreover, after a little persistence, there is no reason to feel completely intimidated by the chemical jargon. Once a person becomes accustomed to being a label reader, the terms may begin to take on familiarity. Perhaps one may never feel comfortable with "diisopropanolaminecarbomer 041" (a preservative and emulsifying agent), but after seeing the ubiquitous "glycerine" or "paraben" on bottle after bottle, it may be no more strange than the sugar, BHA, and BHT on the breakfast cereal box.

Consider, for example, the ingredients listed previously for the two lotions. The first three are water, SD alcohol 40, and witch hazel. The alcohol is one of a group of ethyl alcohols that have been denatured, that is, adulterated to prevent them from being drinkable in accordance with government regulations. Witch hazel is an extract made from the bark and leaves of a small tree. It has astringent, or puckering, action on the skin, as does the sodium borate. Astringents are mildly irritating and make the skin feel tingly. Menthol has a slight anesthetic effect and provides a cool feeling as it evaporates. Glycerine and propylene glycol are humectants; their purpose is to prevent the liquid from evaporating too quickly. Acetone and isopropyl alcohol are fat solvents, similar in function to the SD alcohol. Methylparaben is a widely used antibacterial preservative. Caramel, as most people know, is burnt sugar and is present as a coloring agent. So are the D&C and the FD&C colors. D&C means that the color may be used in drugs and cosmetics only and not in foods; and "F" preceding the D&C means that the color has been certified for use in foods as well.

D&C red #33 belongs to a group known as azo dyes, which are known to cause allergic reactions in some individuals. FD&C blue #1 is a food coloring that has been banned from use as a food additive in Europe and the United Kingdom. Both colors are members of the family of dyes known as coal-tar colors. The safety of any coal-tar color additives in foods is highly suspect. All have been implicated as carcinogenic in animals and allergenic in humans. There is controversy concerning their safety in cosmetics. The potential hazard when small quantities are absorbed through the skin or ingested in lipstick is unknown. Many people do have adverse skin reactions to coal-tar colors in cosmetic products.

It might also be observed that the purpose of both of these lotions, degreasing the skin and removing or exfoliating the top layers of dead surface cells, can be accomplished just as easily by washing with soap and a terry washcloth and drying with a towel. If more "clarifying" is desired, a complexion brush, a polyester fiber sponge, or a natural sponge could be used.

For someone who has experienced an allergic reaction—a skin rash, edema, itchy eyes, puffy lips—and needs to avoid other products that contain the suspected ingredient, it would be worthwhile to invest in Ruth Winter's *A Consumer's Dictionary of Cosmetic*

Ingredients. This excellent handbook, available in paperback, describes the origin, function, and safety of specific cosmetic components in nontechnical, easily understandable language. It is an indispensable and enlightening reference for anyone interested in separating out the realities of cosmetic function from the advertised claims. But since carrying a dictionary to the cosmetic counter is not really feasible, and since most people want to know what is in a product before they buy it, it is also possible to remember a few fundamentals about cosmetic ingredients.

Foundations. Cosmetics contain various combinations of oils, fatty acids, alcohols, preservatives, humectants, colors, fragrances, and chemicals that stabilize, emulsify, foam, reduce surface tension, and generally aid in keeping the other ingredients together or enable them to go on the skin better. In a typical foundation or makeup base, the mineral oil, lanolin oil, lecithin, and spermaceti are all emollients; so are apricot oil, sesame oil, grape seed oil, wheat germ oil, or any other vegetable oils, no matter how exotic they may sound. Stearic acid, palmitic acid, oleic acid, and myristic acid are all naturally occurring fatty acids. In their alcohol or salt derivatives, they are used as emulsifiers or stabilizers. TEA stearate, for example, is triethanolamine stearate, an emulsifier. Talc and kaolin are chalk and clay, respectively, and they are color and covering agents. Propylene glycol, glycerine, and sorbitan or sorbitol are humectants and skin softeners. Mica, titanium oxide, iron oxides, ultramarine blue, and all the coal-tar colors provide the various shades for the foundation. Methyl, butyl, or propyl parabens are antibacterial, antifungal preservatives.

Lipsticks. All lipsticks are combinations of oil and wax with red pigments to stain the lips and a perfume that is present more to eliminate the fatty taste that may be present in the ingredients than to provide odor. Typical organic pigments could be eosin red (D&C red #21), orange-red (D&C orange #5), and blue-red (D&C red #27), or inorganic pigments, such as bromo-acid (tetrabromo fluorescein) and derivatives of fluorescein. Lip gloss and lip shine are composed of the same ingredients but contain more lanolin and mineral oils. Frosted lipsticks may contain guanine crystals or bismuth oxychloride for the pearlized look.

Eye makeup. Only inorganic pigments are permitted in eye shadows, mascara, and eyeliners since coal-tar colors are prohibited from use in the eye area. The pigments are dispersed in a wax, gum, or resin along with perfume, oils, and preservatives, such as propylparaben, imidazolidinyl urea, or p-hydroxybenzoate. The major colors are iron and chromium oxide pigments; aluminum powder for silver; the ultramarines; and carmine, a crimson pigment derived from the dried bodies of female cochineal insects.

There is substantial evidence that mascara is subject to potentially dangerous bacterial contamination. Serious eye infections and even loss of vision have resulted after an accidental scratch of the cornea with the applicator from a contaminated tube of mascara. Mascara should never be used longer than 3–4 months and should be thrown away after that to avoid the danger of contamination. An old brush should never be inserted into a refill mascara container without cleaning and sterilizing it first. No eye makeup should ever be shared with another person, and one should never try on eye shadow from the tester well or pot at the cosmetic counter. If the corneal epithelium is scratched while applying mascara, the scratch should be treated immediately and both the eye and the mascara should be cultured to detect the presence of specific organisms. *Staphylococcus* or *Fusarium* species have been associated with mild infections, but *Pseudomonas* has been implicated in corneal ulcers and resultant blindness (Centers for Disease Control, 1990).

Less serious adverse effects of eye area cosmetics include sensations of stinging and burning experienced immediately or a short time after application of the makeup or clinical manifestations of response, such as puffy lids or eyes that are bloodshot and teary. Sometimes these symptoms are not the result of ingredients in the makeup but occur because of a physical irritant, such as a flake of mascara or eye shadow or a lash extender inadvertently falling into the eye. Allergic reactions can often be initiated by the practice of drawing eyeliner across the upper and lower inner, instead of exterior, lids. Another consequence of inner eyeliner application is the permanent disposition of black pigment with possible burning and tearing as a result. No long-term adverse effect is known, but neither is there any known treatment for the condition (Pascher, 1982).

Deodorants and antiperspirants. An average adult produces from 1–3 pints of perspiration a day, depending on physical activity, temperature, and humidity. Most of this water is produced by approximately 2 million *eccrine sweat glands* distributed over the body. They open directly into the skin surface and primarily function to regulate the body temperature. Heat and nervous tension cause copious secretion of sweat, and evaporation on the body surface provides cooling. Sweat is a salt-containing dilute acid solution that is colorless and virtually odorless.

The other type of sweat glands are the *apocrine glands* that develop with puberty and are found in relatively small numbers, either singly or in clusters, under the arms, in the anogenital region, on the abdomen, and around the nipples. The mammary glands and the wax-producing glands are modified apocrine sweat glands (Figure 16–10).

Apocrine glands are much larger than eccrine glands and are usually associated with a hair follicle, although a few open directly onto the skin surface. The apocrine gland secretion is a milky fluid that contains more solids and does become malodorous when it undergoes decomposition by skin bacteria. The underarm, abdomen, and anogenital areas of the body are, therefore, a greater potential source of unpleasant body odor. Fresh perspiration on clean skin has little odor. Even with daily washing, however, odor can develop when apocrine sweat is no longer fresh and remains on the skin. Some form of odor control is used by an estimated 90% of women and 80% of men. Deodorants prevent odor by covering it or by destroying or inhibiting the growth of bacteria on the skin

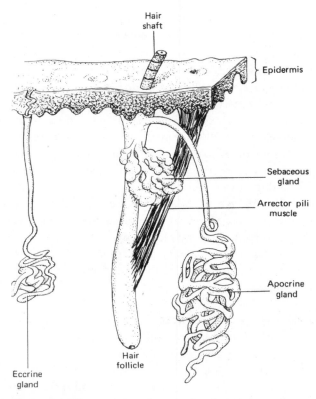

Figure 16–10 Diagram of sweat glands and their relationship to a hair follicle. The secretion of the apocrine glands, which open into hair follicles, is responsible for body odor on unwashed skin. Eccrine glands help regulate body temperature.

surface. Antiperspirants reduce the volume of perspiration in a localized area. Perfumes mask odors, and powders absorb moisture.

Deodorants may contain propylene glycol, salts of stearic acid, or other antibacterial agents. Not all deodorants have antiperspirant activity; if they do, they must be so labeled. No antiperspirant can stop wetness, and it would not be desirable if it did, for that would completely block the gland ducts. All antiperspirants in this country are aluminum salts. Exactly how they work is unclear. The aluminum is evidently absorbed on the top layers of keratin and the sweat gland openings. It may mechanically narrow the orifice by astringent action, increase the duct's permeability to water and thus resorb the sweat, or perhaps simply attract water during the crystallization of the hydrated form, alum. The most effective antiperspirant is a 10% solution of aluminum chloride, which can be purchased at the pharmacy very cheaply. Its disadvantage is its high acidity in contact with skin and its tendency to destroy clothing. Almost all commercial antiperspirants compromise with a 20% solution of aluminum chlorhydrate, sometimes complexed with zirconium salts. This is not as effective, but neither is this solution as irritating to skin or to fabric.

According to most surveys, the one category of cosmetics most likely to cause adverse reactions was the deodorant/antiperspirant group. All such products carry a warning concerning application to broken skin and indicate that use must be discontinued if a rash develops.

Artificial Nail Products ("Acrylics"). The cosmetic ideal is for long, perfectly shaped, perfectly polished fingernails; therefore, women unable to grow their own may use artificial nails. Fake nails may be made of plastic that is bonded to the nail plate with acrylic glue or may be acrylic polymers, which are "sculptured" and shaped onto the surface of the nail plate to form the nail. Natural nails also are sometimes repaired with silk or linen wrap and acrylic glue. Any of these practices is not without risk and could be damaging to the natural fingernails for several reasons. Because the artificial nails are longer, they are subject to a greater "fulcrum" effect at their base. That is, a nail could catch on something and, because it is bonded to the real nail, pull the nail away from the underlying nail bed. Also, because moisture is trapped underneath the nonporous false nail, the nail bed can easily become subject to bacterial or fungus infections. Some people have severe reactions to the glue and get dermatitis, even on their eyelids when they touch their eyes (Guin, 1998). A particularly dangerous form of adhesive, liquid methyl methacrylate (MMA), was prohibited by the FDA in the 1970s because the chemical could result in severe damage, even deformity, of the fingernails, which in many instances would not grow back. In Florida, however, where a number of manicurists were fined and lost their licenses, the restricted glue evidently was still being used at less-expensive nail salons because it was cheaper. Authorities in Florida believe MMA continues to be used in some salons nationwide because it can be easily obtained from dental and beauty suppliers for other uses (*The New York Times,* 1998).

Nail glue also has caused other problems unrelated to false fingernails. The plastic bottles containing nail adhesive closely resemble bottles containing eyedrops, and a number of people have accidentally dropped nail glue into their eyes. People who are frequent users of eyedrops or who may have difficulty reading the tiny print on the bottles, such as contact lens wearers or glaucoma patients, should be particularly cautious.

ACNE—THE MOST COMMON SKIN DISORDER

The occurrence of **acne** is so frequent that the disease has been called the bread and butter of dermatologists. It is said to be responsible for more office visits than any other skin problem. But even this may not accurately reflect the true prevalence of the condition. Many people do not go to see a doctor at all but self-medicate with one of the hundreds of available over-the-counter preparations. At least 75% of the population suffers from acne at one time or another, predominantly during the adolescent years. Some authorities maintain that no one passes from puberty to adulthood without some manifestation of a blemish, bump, or blotch.

While the majority of acne cases occur during adolescence, the disorder sometimes appears to hold off until postadolescence. Some men and women get acne in their late 20s or 30s when they never had a pimple as a teenager; some are troubled with "teenage acne" all of their reproductive lives, and many women are troubled with distressing eruptions of premenstrual acne.

What Does Not Cause Acne?

Clearing up acne when it occurs is often not too difficult; clearing up the confusion about its onset and prevention is a different matter. Acne is not precipitated by diet or by eating chocolate, hamburgers and fries, soft drinks, or any other greasy or sweet food. Plewig and Kligman (1975) reported a study in which acne patients ate a special candy bar each day that contained 10 times the usual quantity of chocolate, with no particular effect on the acne. There is also no unequivocal evidence that high fat intake results in an oilier skin. Many people are convinced, however, and know through experience that for them, eating certain foods appears to result in a flare-up. The sensible recourse is to avoid those particular items. Some individuals may have food allergies that cause or aggravate acnelike eruptions. Long-term ingestion of iodides and bromides present in some drugs or vitamins can also make existing acne worse or reinitiate it in a former sufferer, but the amount in iodide-containing foods (shellfish, peanuts, cabbage, spinach) or iodized salt is believed to be too minimal to worry about.

Despite common misconceptions, acne is nobody's fault. It has nothing to do with infrequent washing, and obsessive cleanliness is not going to help. Neither does acne result from constipation, lack of sleep, or too little or too much sexual activity. In those who are acne prone, there may be some externally applied or internally ingested substances that are acnegenic, that is, have a greater ability to induce acne. In adults, one such factor may be "acne cosmetica," which will be discussed later.

What Causes Acne?

The disease is a disorder of the sebaceous glands associated with hair follicles—the pilosebaceous unit. The gland-containing follicles that are especially prone to acne lesions are most numerous on the face and the upper trunk, and those that have exceptionally large sebaceous glands and tiny rudimentary hairs. It is the production of sebum from these glands that "fuels the acne flame," as described by Plewig and Kligman.

Sebum is normally synthesized by the sebaceous glands in response to circulating hormones, and the glands are especially sensitive to androgens. Androgen cannot be said to cause acne, however. Even with the advent of improved techniques for assay in blood or urine, no consistent hormonal excess, deficiency, or imbalance has ever been determined to exist between acne sufferers and those who do not have acne. Investigators have never found any chemical difference between the sebum produced by an individual with acne and the sebum of a person who does not have acne, or even between the sebum in one part of the body of an acne victim compared with the sebum in another part. Some people get acne; others do not, and the reason is essentially unknown. One generally accepted theory is that there is a gene-determined susceptibility and an end-organ response, the end-organ being the pilosebaceous unit. At puberty when the hormone levels rise, the end-organs respond. Why, at some point in life, the end-organs stop responding is not clear. The same follicles of the face, neck, and back that may erupt in acne during adolescence cease for no apparent reason to be influenced by the identical hormonal stimuli sometime during the third decade of life. In most people, acne then spontaneously disappears.

There are other perplexing factors associated with this common skin condition. Some acnes produce scars; other acnes, equally severe, cause little or no scarring. Although it is accepted that large sebaceous glands and excessive sebum production are related to acne, some people have very oily skins and little acne, whereas others have a lot of acne but produce little oil. Still others have a lot of oil and acne. Another mystery is that when women get acne later in life well beyond adolescence, the acne usually is limited to the chin.

The causes of acne are still imperfectly understood; the mechanics of its occurrence are better known.

What Happens in Acne?

Acne is always associated with the pilosebaceous unit composed of a hair follicle and sebaceous gland. In the susceptible individual, the problem is believed to arise with a *hyperkeratinization,* or abnormal piling up of cells of the follicle lining and the wall of the gland. The dead cells accumulate in the follicle ducts and prevent the sebum from exiting onto the skin surface, and the clogged duct begins to distend as the oils continue to pour into the canal. Several kinds of bacteria and fungi normally present in the follicle and on the surface of the skin find the sebum an excellent growth medium, and the follicle canal soon bulges with sebum, dead cells, and microorganisms. The result is a blocked pore occluded with excess sebum. It is called a whitehead or comedo (plural, comedones). A closed comedo may progress to become an open comedo, or blackhead. The accumulating material gradually causes the pore opening to dilate, allowing the impacted mass of horny cells to protrude from the orifice. Blackheads are not caused by neglect or dirt. The black in a blackhead is the result of the dark pigment melanin, which has moved up to the surface with the cells.

A closed comedo may also rupture to form an inflamed pus-filled pimple, technically called a papulopustule, which actually represents a blowout of the follicle wall. As the oils from the gland continue to clog up the follicle lining, microorganisms called *Propionibacterium acnes* that inhabit the depths of the follicle metabolize the sebum through enzymatic action to form fatty acids and glycerol. These free fatty acids not only stimulate further proliferation of the keratinized cells blocking the follicle but also act as an irritant to the follicle walls. Eventually the walls rupture, releasing toxic oils and bacteria into the surrounding tissues (Figure 16–11).

Treatment of Acne

Acne can be mild, moderate, or severe and is usually divided into four major grades. Grade 1 acne is the kind with just whiteheads and blackheads and never leaves scars. Grade 2 acne has visible pimples, but if further inflammation does not occur, scarring rarely results. Grade 3 includes the large inflammatory lesions, and grade 4 is the most severe form of cystic

acne. Because in acne the follicle opening is plugged with sebum and cellular and bacterial debris, much of the therapy for mild and moderate acne is based on methods to induce the ducts to remain open and to stimulate blood flow to heal the lesions. The mainstay of such treatments are the topical applications of chemicals called "exfoliants." These chemicals irritate the top layers of the skin to cause an inflammatory response that results in reddening, then thickening, and finally the scaling off or peeling of the horny layer of the epidermis. While the skin looks dry and scaly, there is actually no measurable decrease in the amount of sebum production.

Various exfoliants are used in the treatment of acne, and some of them are available without prescription. Benzoyl peroxide in a 5% or 10% concentration is the strongest of the over-the-counter agents. It can be found under such trade names as Benoxyl, Loroxide, Oxy-5, Persadox, Panoxyl, Persagel, Besnagel, Topex, Dry and Clear, and Desquam-X. Salicylic acid is also a traditional exfoliant, but according to dermatologists, its concentration must be at least 5% for effectiveness. Most commercial preparations contain less than that amount and would not be expected to be of as much value.

A very potent irritating and peeling agent is retinoic acid (tretinoin) available by prescription only. The drug produces a strong inflammatory response, and reactions can be very intense but very effective. In a kind of double-whammy assault on severe acne, some dermatologists prescribe both benzoyl peroxide and retinoic acid, one in the morning and the other in the evening. Not all skins can tolerate the increased irritation, however.

Newer agents, some with retinoidlike activity, are often equally effective and produce less skin irritation. They may be used alone or in combination with tretinoin and include adapalene; azelaic acid; tazarotene; and Velac, a gel containing both tretinoin and the antibiotic clindamycin. There are also reformulations of tretinoin designed to retain potent activity but reduce irritation.

Some of the very familiar and widely advertised topical acne remedies contain sulfur and resorcinol,

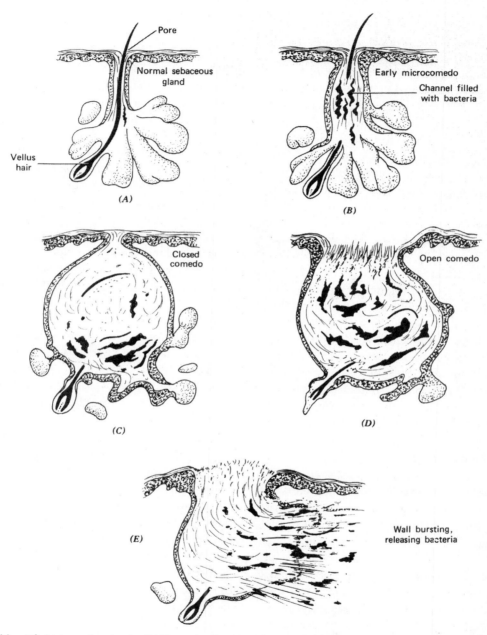

Figure 16–11   Life history of a pimple. (A) The type of pilosebaceous unit especially prone to acne: the hair follicle has a tiny vellus hair and large sebaceous glands. (B) Early development of the comedo: the follicle duct has become distended with keratinized cells, and a few bacteria-filled channels are evident. (C) Whitehead or a closed comedo: the pore opening is occluded with sebum; the dense keratin forms an impaction of concentric layers that dilates the follicle; there are numerous and larger spaces containing bacteria and fungi. (D) Blackhead or open comedo: the impacted mass moves up to dilate the pore opening, and the comedo is filled with keratin, bacteria, fungi, hairs, and oils. (E) The blowout, or pus pimple: the epithelial lining of the follicle wall ruptures and releases bacteria and toxins to cause inflammation of the surrounding tissue.

two agents traditionally prescribed for topical application by dermatologists for generations. Today, doctors generally agree that sulfur and resorcinol are virtually without value in the treatment of acne. Still, there are a lot of people who are attached to Acnomel or Clearasil, despite evidence of their ineffectiveness. There are many over-the-counter remedies that clear up mild acne, although doctors cannot explain how they work.

Medicated cosmetics are useless both in the treatment and in the prevention of acne. They have no exfoliant activity, and any antibacterial agents in the formulation serve only to preserve the cosmetic from deteriorating. Bacteria involved in pustule formation are deep in the follicle and not on the skin surface. Reaching them requires the use of a topically applied or orally ingested antibiotic.

When acne is severe, antibiotics are prescribed in addition to the effective exfoliants. Many dermatologists are enthusiastic advocates of antibiotic therapy, but while the drugs are undeniably helpful for some acne victims, they can be both a blessing and a disaster. Vaginitis, colitis and other gastrointestinal symptoms, and photosensitivity reactions are not uncommon.

The breakthrough in treatment for the physical and psychological destruction of severe cystic acne came in September 1982, when the FDA approved Accutane (Hoffman-La Roche Laboratories), or isotretinoin, also known as 13-*cis*-retinoic acid, for the treatment of acne that is unresponsive to conventional therapy, including systemic antibiotics. Accutane has been called a real miracle drug; it is not only highly effective in the treatment of severe acne, but it also appears to cure it. In most acne sufferers treated with the drug, prolonged remissions occur that continue years after discontinuance of drug therapy. Accutane has a profound effect on reducing the sebum production in the sebaceous glands, which tends to explain its initial effectiveness. But although the sebum levels tend to return to normal after the drug is stopped, the benefits continue—a result that is not clearly understood.

Almost all individuals treated with Accutane experience dryness, chapping, and itching of the skin. Forty percent get some form of conjunctivitis, and

temporary contact lens problems could result. Other symptoms during treatment, although they rapidly disappear after discontinuation, can include mild musculoskeletal complaints, skin rash or hair thinning, nonspecific urogenital or gastrointestinal symptoms, fatigue, headache, or an increased skin sensitization to sunburn. The powerful drug may also be linked to depression. After isolated reports of some patients who became depressed while taking Accutane and even reports of a few suicides, the FDA required that Hoffman-La Roche change its label. The manufacturer, who said there was no proof that Accutane caused the problems, that cystic acne sufferers often experienced depression, that 4 million Americans had taken Accutane, and that the possible side effect was exceedingly rare, complied with the directive. Letters were sent to doctors informing them of the new label, which now states, "Accutane may cause depression, psychosis and rarely, suicidal ideation, suicide attempts and suicide." Hoffman-La Roche suggested that physicians should carefully observe patients who are on the drug for signs of depression (*The New York Times*, 1998). *Accutane is a known teratogen and should never be taken during pregnancy.* Effective contraception should be used for at least a month prior to beginning therapy, and a pregnancy test should be done 2 weeks before starting Accutane. It is a good idea to begin therapy in the middle of a normal menstrual period; it is imperative to continue to have pregnancy tests monthly and to use two forms of contraception (e.g., diaphragm and condom, condom with spermicide) or abstinence during treatment and for at least a month after cessation of treatment. Because it is not known whether the drug is excreted in breast milk, it should not be taken by nursing mothers. Because isotretinoin is a vitamin A derivative, vitamin supplements containing additional vitamin A should be avoided during treatment.

In clinical studies of patients receiving Accutane, about 25% developed abnormal blood lipid levels that included an elevation of triglycerides, a reduction in the high-density lipoprotein (HDL) levels, and a small increase in blood cholesterol levels. All of these changes went back to normal when the treatment was stopped, but individuals who have high blood lipid levels to begin with should be monitored during treatment.

The effects of severe acne on the individual are so devastating that most are happy to accept the possibility of side effects and the current expense of treatment in order to be cured. As more is learned about the mechanisms of action of isotretinoin and the optimal dosage schedules, it is probable that the drug can be used for less severe acne as well. Oral retinoids are believed to have great potential in a broad spectrum of skin diseases. They have been tested clinically in psoriasis and are being evaluated in the prevention and treatment of skin cancer.

The wide variety of treatments available for acne means that some combination of agents is bound to be effective in controlling the disorder in everyone. In most instances, however, quick improvement should not be expected. Generally, it takes about 6 weeks to 3 months before any marked effect of therapy is obvious.

Mild acne can probably be kept in check without consulting a physician, particularly if the nonprescription remedies are chosen wisely.

Grown-up Acne—Premenstrual Variety

There are estimates that one-third of all women experience premenstrual facial breakouts, and if very mild manifestations are included, some have placed the incidence as high as 60%. The general assumption is that in some unknown manner, progesterone is responsible for premenstrual acne, but there is no clear explanation for the increase in skin eruptions a week or so before menstruation. Some investigators claim that excessive sebum is produced in the postovulatory phase of the cycle, but others maintain that sebum production remains constant throughout. It has been observed that during the luteal phase, the follicle openings appeared to become smaller in diameter. This narrowing of the ducts, presumably the effect of progesterone, may aid to block the orifices and lays the groundwork for the acne flare-ups just before the menses. It is recognized that the amount and type of

progestin in oral contraceptives are important in the effect of the pills on acne.

Opinions vary as to how or whether premenstrual blemishes can be prevented. The acne appears in women who have premenstrual weight gain and also in those who do not retain water. Some doctors prescribe salt restriction and diuretics; others believe that the elimination of water has no prophylactic effect. Hormonal therapy might help, but it seems more reasonable to treat the premenstrual acne in the same manner as any other acne—that is, by topical applications of effective exfoliants—rather than to initiate pill taking, which may not be effective for the acne anyway.

Acne Cosmetica. There is evidence that women in whom acne has persisted since adolescence, or women who have bouts with premenstrual acne, may aggravate the condition by the use of certain cosmetics that contain ingredients that have the ability to induce the formation of comedones, that is, are comedogenic. The term "acne cosmetica" was coined in a 1972 paper by Kligman and Mills. The investigators described the occurrence of a mild but persistent form of acne in women that was associated with the long-term use of heavy and oily creams, lotions, and moisturizers. Acne cosmetica seems to be prevalent in women who are known to be acne prone, but it also has afflicted women who went through their teen years without so much as a single pimple. The two workers tested samples of the leading brands of facial creams by the rabbit-ear assay method (the sensitive external ear canal of the rabbit easily responds to comedogenic chemicals after short periods of topical application) and determined that about half of the popular creams contained substances that would produce comedones in the rabbit ear canal. Fulton and Black (1983) expanded the tests to include a large range of foundation makeups, acne preparations, and some of the various surfactants, emulsifiers, preservatives, and miscellaneous substances used as ingredients in cosmetics.

It was determined that cosmetic ingredients with a high potential for causing acne were fatty acids, fatty acid esters, and fatty acid alcohols such as isopropyl myristate, isopropyl isostearate, sodium lauryl sulfate, butyl stearate, and hexadecyl alcohol. Substances found to have negligible or no comedogenic ability were candelilla wax, titanium dioxide, glycerin, caster oil, iron oxide pigments, propyl gallate, methyl paraben, propylene glycol, and mineral oil. Mineral oils, in fact, would probably cause the least problems compared with vegetable oils, especially olive oil and cocoa butter in high concentrations. Russell (2000) notes that although cosmetics may get more than their share of blame for causing acne, patients should use oil-free, noncomedogenic cosmetics and avoid oils from hair products and suntan lotions.

It should be emphasized that the rabbit-ear assay method is probably ultrasensitive compared with the human face. The tested substances were applied to the rabbit daily and not washed off with soap and water. Even the most powerful acnegens in the rabbit are likely to be only weakly acnegenic in the human. Women who are not acne prone could get acne cosmetica only by providing what Fulton has called 24-hour acnegenic coverage—starting the day with a comedogenic foundation, removing it at night with a comedogenic cleansing cream, and then faithfully applying a comedogenic night moisturizer before going to bed. Following this kind of regimen for a couple of months would invite acne-form eruptions, and it makes little difference how expensive the cosmetics are. This program of cosmetic use, it might be noted, is frequently advised for dry-skin care and forms the basis of various beauty plans heavily promoted by cosmetics companies, particularly for older women.

Women who have persistent postadolescent acne, who have oily skins, or who have a tendency to premenstrual flare-ups, would probably respond more easily to comedogenic cosmetics. Because the more lipid or lipidlike the ingredients in the product, the more potent is its comedogenicity, such women should avoid all oily heavy cosmetics. It would probably be better for a woman with acne to avoid *all* cosmetics, but this advice, while logical, is unrealistic. A woman with a flawless complexion can more easily go without cosmetics; one with a troubled skin may have a greater desire for cover-up. If wearing makeup is seen as a necessity, the only answer is to try to wend one's way through the morass of "oil-free," "oil-controlled," "pore-minimizer," "oily-skin," and "water-base" foundations to find those that are free of offending oils and also free of comedogenic potential. Unfortunately, cosmetics are usually the exception to "what you see is what you get." A product may actually contain a lot of oil but still claim to be for oily skins or be water based. A simple test can determine whether a makeup is actually free from oil. If a few drops of the foundation are placed on 100% cotton bond paper and left for 24 hours, an oily halo will form around any makeup containing oil. The test is not foolproof; some oils may evaporate so quickly that the halo will not be apparent.

As yet there is no company that has developed an entire group of noncomedogenic cosmetics. When selecting makeup, women with acne-prone skin should read the labels to check the ingredients and be certain to stay away from cosmetics containing isopropyl myristate or isopropyl isosterate if these substances are near the top of the list.

The industry has apparently not found the production of oil-free, noncomedogenic cosmetics to be that lucrative. There are fewer such cosmetics to choose from and the range of colors is much less. Women accustomed to the spreadability of other foundation creams will probably find oil-free makeup more difficult to apply because it is quick drying. Obviously, no moisturizer, even one presumably formulated for oily skin, should be used under the oil-free foundation.

HAIR: FOLLICLE FACTS AND FALLACIES

Except in certain areas, the hair on human bodies has little functional value. Around the body openings—the nose, ears, anogenital areas—the hair is protective to a certain extent, mostly acting as a filter against foreign particles, and the hair on the brows and lashes helps to safeguard the eyes from sweat and specks that may obscure or interfere with vision. It is believed, however, that the only reason hair on the face, the head, and under the arms has survived in the human race is probably for decorative purposes. Scalp hair in particular is a body ornament. There is certainly enough evidence from anthropology, archeology, history, folklore, and the works of poets, painters, and sculptors to attest to the fact that humans have always had a great emotional investment in the appearance of their hair.

It has been suggested that today we appear to have a greater interest than ever before in the keratin growing out of our scalp follicles. Some have even said that the preoccupation approaches that of an obsession with hair. Whether contemporary men and women have more concern with their hair than did their ancestors is uncertain, but it is undeniable that this part of the human body does have important cosmetic significance in our culture. Perhaps our fascination with hair is inordinate, but there has never before been such an opportunity to indulge our interest. Until recently, people had not been exposed to mass media advertising that promotes the sale of an astonishing number of hair-care products. When we are confronted by such a baffling array of things to do to and for our hair, it only reinforces our uneasy presentiment that something needs to be done. There are options for everyone—for those whose hair is too straight, too curly, too fine, too coarse, too oily, too dry, too dark, too light. Much expense and time can be saved by knowing about the physical and chemical structure of hair and the composition and action of hair-care products. We may find ourselves in less of a love-hate relationship with our hair when some of the myths concerning its growth, color, texture, and care are debunked. It should be remembered, however, that there are variations in hair characteristics between one person and another. There are even differences between the hair on different parts of the head in the same person. Therefore, the method or substance that "works" on one head will not necessarily produce the same effect on someone else's hair.

Hair Growth

Many people are convinced that cutting hair makes it grow faster, perhaps because, in the opinion of one beautician, "it takes the weight off the ends." Hair growth, however, is cyclic. It does not grow continuously, but only during certain definite periods. During the growing phase of the cycle, the cells at the roots of the hair follicle proliferate rapidly and the hair grows longer. When a hair reaches its limit in length—characteristically short for the body hairs, longer for the scalp in both sexes and beard hairs in men—it stops growing and rests for a while, being retained in its follicle. During the resting phase, the base of the hair becomes a solid, completely keratinized, club-shaped mass, and it sends out little rootlets that fasten it to the remains of the follicle. After a resting period, a new bulb forms at the base of the follicle below the old clubbed hair. The new hair forms and pushes upward, loosening the old hair from its attachment and causing it to be shoved out and shed. Periods of growth and periods of rest for hair follicles are about equal, except for the hair on the face and the scalp. Each follicle, however, has its own individual rhythmic cycle. In any given area on the body, some of the hairs are actively growing, some are resting, and some are being shed. Unlike some other mammals, humans do not molt seasonally to replace the summer coat with a winter growth, but hairdressers have pointed out that people appear to lose more hair in the autumn of the year. Apparently about the time the leaves on the trees are being shed, so are the hairs on the head, but there are no quantitative published studies to substantiate the observation.

Obviously, because hair grows from the bottom up, cutting or shaving it cannot affect its rate of growth or its texture. All hairs on the scalp are growing at different times, however, so cutting the ends periodically will even off the longer hairs and the stragglers, and the hair will probably look better. It takes about 7 weeks to grow an inch of hair on the head. Hair on the legs, which grows about 0.05 inches weekly, does not become coarser or grow faster after shaving. It does, however, become more stubbly, because the soft and tapered ends of the hairs have been bluntly cut off. If those hairs were permitted to be shed and replaced, their successors would again feel soft. Because shaving, once started, is more or less continuous, hair on the legs always feels prickly.

The life span of an eyelash is about 4–5 months, and only 30 days of that time are spent in active growing. The lash is in the resting phase for the remainder of the period before being shed. Hair on the head has a much longer period of growth (anywhere from 2–6 years), rests for only 3 months or so, and is then shed. If uninterrupted by cutting, scalp hair can attain very long lengths in some people, a feature that is genetically determined. Of the 100,000 hair follicles on the average scalp, 90% are actively growing and 10% are resting at any given time. The normal 50–100 hairs that are shed daily to end up on the comb, the brush, or in the shower drain have, therefore, been on the scalp an average of 4 years. If a hair is pulled out during its growing period, the root will be tapering and cylindrical. If a resting hair is plucked, it will have a rounded club-shaped root (Figure 16–12).

A certain amount of thinning of the hair on the head in both sexes is a normal consequence of aging because there is a progressive increase in the number of follicles that are in the resting phase as one grows older. While hair evidently grows faster between the ages of 16 and 46, there is an accompanying gradual decrease in the density of the hair, most noticeably on the forehead. Actual baldness, however, is about six times more prevalent in men than in women and is a genetic trait that is sex influenced; that is, the genetic factors become evident only when male hormone is present in the body. Hair loss that is mournfully excessive at an early age, beginning in some men even before their 20s, is rarely caused by any medical problem and is more likely the result of their having the gene for male-pattern baldness. Whether it happens early or late in life, men who become bald will probably find little consolation in the fact that androgens,

responsible for hair growth, male secondary sex characteristics, libido, and potency are also responsible for hair loss when the genetic predisposition is present. Eunuchs (male castrates) rarely become bald. Why the same hormones that cause activity of follicles should later result in their inactivity is unknown.

Lowered estrogen levels after menopause may result in unwelcome changes in hair distribution in some women—more on the face and less on the head. Facial hair may be made less obvious by bleaching or removed by tweezing or electrolysis, but for many women little can be done for thinning of the hair on the head except to disguise the thinness with styling. Women may have increased hair loss with age, but they do not become bald. Less estrogen after menopause is not the only reason that some women experience hair thinning. High fever, severe infection, or the flu can sometimes cause a transitory hair loss, but thinning also may be a sign of a medical condition such as faulty thyroid gland production, kidney disease, or autoimmune disease. There are nearly 300 prescription and over-the-counter medications that have been linked to hair loss in some women. They include drugs for hypertension, certain antidepressants, and amphetamines.

The only treatment known to help a small percentage of men with male-pattern baldness and women with thinning hair is minoxidil. When minoxidil is applied to the scalp twice a day, about a quarter of the men (especially if they are under age 26) and about 19% of women experience moderate regrowth. About a third of the users get fuzz and the rest get nothing. The drug must be applied for several months before the user knows whether it works. It costs $20–$30 a month and must be used continuously. Once use ceases, regrown hair falls out within a few months. Another such drug is finasteride. It is approved only for men because it is a major cause of birth defects. Women are advised in the television ads to not even touch it.

Hair Structure

The hair shaft consists of the cuticle, the cortex, and the medulla and is almost completely composed of the

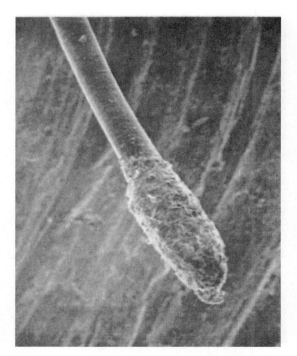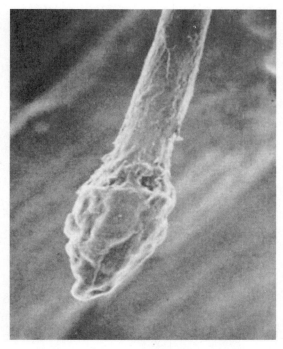

Figure 16–12   A scanning electron micrograph of the roots of two hairs. The hair on the left was pulled out during the growth phase. Note the narrow tapering end. In contrast, the clubbed root on the right is from a hair plucked during the resting stage.

protein, keratin. Between 90% and 99% of the dry weight of hair is keratin, making hairs the most durable parts of the body. Hair is tough; it survived on Egyptian mummies for thousands of years. Durable as it is, however, hair can be damaged by weathering and by various cosmetic manipulations. For 2–6 years, a hair on the head is washed, combed, brushed, exposed to ultraviolet light and extreme temperatures, and may undergo various chemical treatments from dipping in a chlorinated pool to processing with dyes and permanent wave solutions. Small wonder it may not always look good. Obviously, the gentler one treats the hair, the better it is likely to appear.

The cuticle, for example, is made up of a very thin and heavily keratinized single layer of cells. Cuticle cells look like overlapping shingles on a roof, except that their free edges point upward. Covered by a layer of lipid from the sebaceous glands, the cells move over each other to function as a flexible protective armor plate for the hair shaft. Cuticle cells that lie flat against the cortex reflect light evenly off the surface oil film and are responsible for the quality of hair called shininess. Disrupting the cuticle to make it swell and uplift in order to tint or wave the hair, or treating the hair in a less than gentle manner—backcombing it, blow-drying it, sunning it—will result in an uneven diffraction of light. The hair no longer appears shiny and looks dull. Various conditioners can glue the cuticle scales back down and coat them with oils so that the hair again appears glossy (Figure 16–13).

Split ends are merely a separation of the cell layers at the ends of the hair shaft. The longer the hair, the longer it has been there to be exposed to the elements, the daily combing and brushing, and perhaps the

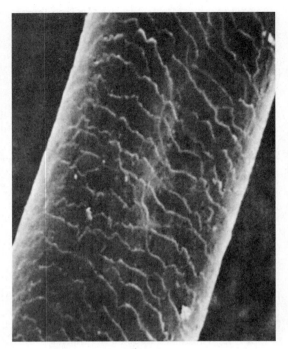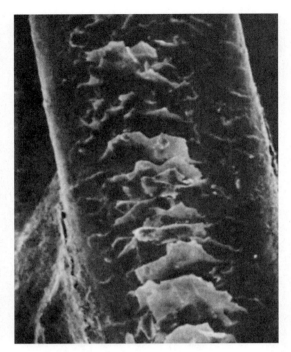

Figure 16–13 As seen with the scanning electron microscope, the cuticle cells of the unprocessed hair on the left are lying flat against the cortex. This hair will look shinier than the hair on the right, which has been both bleached and permed. Note the disrupted and uplifted cuticle cells.

nontender treatments used to improve its color or curl. It is inevitable that even without any chemical processing, long hair will begin to separate at the ends. The cure for split ends is to cut them off. There are conditioning products that can temporarily hold the layers together, but split ends will always reappear unless they are removed (Figure 16–14).

The cortex is the main bulk of the hair shaft, and it consists of long and intertwined molecules of keratin. Most studies of keratin have been made on wool fibers (because of their economic value) and feathers, and the exact structure of human hair keratin is not known. It is believed to be a keratin complex composed of a sulfur-rich nonfibrous protein matrix that lies between fibrous protein chains low in sulfur content. The fibrous parts of the keratin complex are made up of long protein molecules aligned in a characteristic alpha helix (spiral stair-

case) configuration. The molecular arrangement, which could be compared to lengths of rope tied and wound around each other, is generally accepted to be as follows: three alpha helices are wound around each other to form a protofibril; 11 protofibrils are twisted and coiled to make up a microfibril; and the microfibrils are aligned together into the macrofibrils within the matrix of the cortical cells. A hair may be visualized as a number of supercoils imposed on primary coils—a kind of overly twisted rope (Figure 16–15).

Several kinds of chemical bonds hold the keratin complex together. The most common linkage is the *hydrogen bond,* important in stabilizing and forming the coiled chain. Some of the hydrogen bonds are easily broken by wetting the hair, and this forms the basis for setting hair while it is wet. If the wet hair is stretched—over rollers, for example—the bonds reform into a new

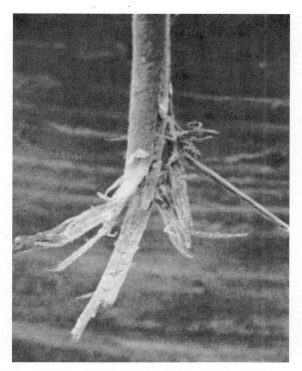

Figure 16–14 Split ends. This is the same overly processed hair shown in Figure 16–13.

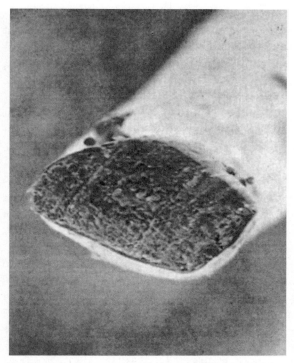

Figure 16–15 The molecular structure of the cortex is almost suggested by this scanning electron micrograph of the cut end of a hair. The keratin complex is made up of a number of macrofibrils or twisted coils set in a matrix of high sulfur proteins that links them together.

and temporary curl position when the hair subsequently dries. Hair sprays are aqueous solutions of shellac or the resin polyvinylpyrrolidone (PVP), which stiffens the hair to hold the reshape in shape. Heat will also break hydrogen bonds so that they may be realigned. Electric rollers and curling irons can set in a curl, but the result is generally not as lasting as one formed through wetting and setting. Blow-drying works on the same principle. The hairstyle is directed into place by stretching the hair over a brush while drying it with hot air. But because wet hair in the presence of heat is highly susceptible to mechanical damage, the brush or comb that stretches the hair during a blow-drying should be used slowly and gently.

Permanent Waves The curl formed by wetting and setting is only temporary and lasts until it "falls" or the hair is dampened. A permanent realignment of the protein chains to form a permanent wave can be accomplished by breaking the *disulfide bond*. This sulfur to sulfur link is responsible for the strength, great stability, and cohesiveness of keratin. Water cannot disrupt the disulfide bond, and strongly alkaline thioglycolate compounds, substances with a characteristic strong and unpleasant odor, are used to rupture the bond. Thioglycolates are the essential ingredients in permanent-wave solutions.

When getting a "perm," the hair is washed and set while wet on the perm rollers—the smaller the roller, the tighter the curl. Then the rolled hair is soaked with the waving lotion that swells and raises the cuticle so that the keratin of the cortex can be made softer and more malleable, and its chemical bonds can be broken. After a certain period, the alkaline hydrolysis is stopped, and the bonds are reformed in the new position with the "neutralizer," usually an acidifying agent combined with an oxidizing agent such as sodium or potassium bromate or persulfate, or most commonly, hydrogen peroxide. The neutralizer counteracts the swelling and restores the disulfide links.

Permanents applied correctly and with the right timing do not necessarily cause hair damage—at least no more damage than other cosmetic manipulations. But more expensive permanents do not guarantee better results. The solutions in the $25 or the $100 permanent may be very similar. What one may be paying for in the more costly process is the skill and experience of the operator. Most of the problems with frizzy hair, split ends, dryness, and breakage occur as a result of an inexperienced hairdresser. Too much wave lotion left on too long or inadequately neutralized can cause a disastrous effect that is irreversible, and cutting off the perm after it grows out is the only recourse. Home permanents are usually weaker solutions than the ones used in salons, but overprocessing is also possible at home.

Failure of permanents to "take" may be caused by a hair texture that is more resistant to waving and that may require more skill in application, another reason to select an experienced hairdresser. Failure of the wave is not caused by pregnancy or menstruation and is very unlikely to be associated with the taking of any medication. One woman said her hairdresser maintained that her perm did not take because she lacked a medulla in her blond hair, which is nonsense. The medulla, frequently absent from hair, is of little importance to the hair when it is present.

A permanent, applied correctly, will generally look best on unpermed hair. Unless the hair has been permitted to grow out completely and the old permanent has been cut off, there will be unavoidable structural modifications to hair after the repeated chemical processing of permanents.

Hair Relaxers

Hair relaxers are products used to straighten naturally curly hair. They get the curl out in a way similar to how permanents get the curl in—by the use of strongly alkaline chemicals to swell and disrupt the overlapping hair cuticle layers so that penetration of the cortex to change its configuration can take place. Conventional lye relaxers contain sodium hydroxide, generally work quickly, and are frequently used in professional salons. No-lye versions are two-part relaxers that generally can be purchased in retail stores. They contain a somewhat milder alkali such as calcium hydroxide and an acid carbonate as the activator, act on the hair more slowly, and thus minimize the chances of overprocessing. The no-lye relaxers may not produce hair that is as straight hair as that produced by the lye relaxers, but they have equal potential for causing overstressed hair. Consistent use of relaxers could result in scalp irritation or lusterless hair with decreased manageability and shine. Internal damage to the hair shafts caused by relaxers can decrease elastic properties and result in hair breakage or even loss. The commercially available products provide instructions about measuring, mixing, and the time required for each step, and these instructions should always be followed. Moreover, like other cosmetic products that contain caustic chemicals, child-proof packaging is not standard for hair relaxers, and accidental ingestion can be a significant health risk for children.

For those who want a reprieve from the use of caustic hair relaxer agents for very curly hair, there are other forms of hairstyling that have been handed down through generations. Experienced hair braiders twist, braid, and weave in hair extensions. The joining together of strands of hair forms locks, also known as dreadlocks. Over time, the strands become entwined, meshing, spiraling, coiling, and locking together like a cylinder. None of these braided, twisted, or coiled styles is free of maintenance, and each requires once-a-week shampooing, conditioning, and for dreadlocks, scalp massage with a light natural oil (Kinard, 1997). Getting hair braiding, especially if enhanced with hair extensions, is time consuming and costly when done professionally because the process could take up to 10 hours for very long and thin braids. With care, however, the braids will stay looking good for 4–12 weeks ("Hair Today, Hair Tomorrow," 1998). Braids and other popular hairstyling techniques, if pulled too tightly, may cause "traction alopecia," which is hair loss as a result of excessive pressure on the hair follicles and is sometimes accompanied by pigmentation (McMichael, 1995).

Hair Color

The pigment in hair is provided by the activity of melanocytes in the germinal matrix, the cells that proliferate to give rise to the hair. The pigment is deposited mainly in the cortex of the hair shaft. The color of the hair and its depth depend on the size, number, and kind of pigment granules, or melanosomes, and on the presence or absence of air bubbles in the cortex. The black-brown pigment melanin is the predominant color in deep black, brown-black, ash brown, ash blond, and platinum blond hair. Golden blond, red, or auburn hair contains greater quantities of the yellow-brown pigment, phaeomelanin. White hair is caused by a progressive reduction in the activity of the melanocytes and the eventual cessation of pigment production. White hairs mixed in with partially pigmented and fully colored hairs results in the appearance of graying. Actual gray hairs are very rare.

The eventual loss of pigment in hair is determined genetically, occurs in some people quite early in life, and is more obvious in brunettes. Graying is irreversible, and any reports of repigmentation as a result of taking various vitamins or eating a particular diet have not been substantiated, although malnutrition, protein deprivation, or illness can cause changes in the hair that include temporary loss of pigmentation. Stress has not been proved to accelerate graying, and neither can a trauma turn hair white overnight. The only possibility that could provide a basis for all the eyewitness reports to such a happening is that a stressful experience might result in the quick loss of a number of thinner normally pigmented hairs that were in the resting stage. The thicker coarser unpigmented hairs that were present all the time would then suddenly become exposed, giving the appearance of a rapid color change. Then when the new hairs grow in, they too would be unpigmented, providing more "evidence" of the overnight phenomenon.

Coloring the Hair. Reportedly, nearly 60% of American women color their hair, but a substantial number of men are also displeased with their natural color or do not think that gray is that good looking.

People who want to change the color of their hair can do it several different ways. A temporary rinse contains a water-soluble color that merely coats the outside of the hair and does not actually dye it or change the hair structure. The ability of the product to color the hair is, therefore, limited. It can provide highlights, lessen the appearance of graying, or intensify and darken the natural shade, but the effect is removed with the next shampoo, although the color may adhere more strongly when the hair has previously been bleached or has been otherwise processed. The coating is water resistant, but it can be affected by rain or even perspiration, and sometimes it will rub off on the pillow or clothing. These disadvantages make the rinses hardly worth the time or money for most people.

A semipermanent tint contains dyes or stains that barely penetrate the hair shaft but that adhere strongly enough to the cuticle to provide a color coating that lasts through four to six shampoos. Such a product may come in many shades, but there is no possibility of lightening the hair by using it. It can only diminish graying and produce a color several tones darker than the original. Loving Care is a widely sold product of this type. It alters hair structure somewhat, but only minimally.

Permanent dyes are coloring agents that provide a deeper and more lasting color effect. Three kinds of dyes are used: an oxidation procedure that utilizes hydrogen peroxide; vegetable hair colorings; or metallic salts. The most commonly used type that can lighten hair to a different shade and that remains until new growth appears is the oxidation dye.

The oxidation-dye procedure may be a single process in which two components, an alkaline dye and a peroxide system, are mixed, applied to the hair for 30 minutes, and then rinsed off. Usually referred to as a "tint" by the hairdresser, it remains until the "roots," actually the new growth, appear and a "touch-up" must be performed. In the touch-up, the previously dyed strands are exposed for a lesser time than in the original procedure. Obviously, the older portions of the hair shaft can become progressively altered. Single process dyeing can produce an extremely dark shade or a color several shades lighter than the natural one.

The double-process method permits any possible color desired—even going to platinum blond hair from black hair—but is hardest on the hair structure. The hair is drastically bleached or "stripped" to remove most of the color in the cortex by a strong persulfate powder and peroxide mixture. After stripping, the hair is redyed with a "toner" to the desired shade. New growth has to be stripped and toned at intervals to maintain the color. Frosting or streaking is double processing of either random tufts of hair all over the head or of selected clusters of hair strands. The hair to be processed is pulled through a special cap with holes and wrapped with foil during the bleaching. This is a time-consuming and expensive procedure but does expose less of the total hair on the head to the chemical manipulations. It also needs to be repeated far less frequently.

Hair Dyes and Cancer. The oxidation or aniline dyes, also inelegantly known as coal-tar dyes, are the only permanent hair coloring agents that penetrate through the cuticle to the hair cortex. The molecules of the other nonpermanent dyes are too large to move through the cuticle barrier, and they remain on the hair surface. Oxidation dyes are able to enter the hair shaft only because they contain amine bases, such as paraphenylenediamine (PPD) and paraaminophenol and their derivatives. These components of the dyes are small molecules crucial to penetration of the hair cuticle. Although they are not in themselves dyes, they are dye intermediates. Once introduced into the shaft, they undergo a coupling reaction with an oxidizing agent, hydrogen peroxide. This transforms the amine bases into large dye molecules too big to get washed out of the cortex, and the color is therefore locked in.

At the end of the dyeing process, the excess chemicals are rinsed off when the hair is shampooed.

For a long time, paraphenylenediamine has been recognized as a strong skin sensitizer able to cause severe allergic reactions or even blindness should it accidentally get into the eyes. This substance or the other dye intermediates that are used are, however, essential to the dyeing process, and there are no substitutes. Although Congress had banned the use of coal-tar dyes in the 1938 Food, Drug, and Cosmetic Act, coal-tar *hair* dyes were exempted from the ban provided that their manufacturers include a warning statement on the bottle labels. All permanent hair-dye labels tell the consumer that adverse reactions are possible and warn that a "patch test" should be made on the skin for 24 hours before the product is used to dye the hair. Whether many people actually perform such a test at home after they buy the dye at the drugstore or supermarket is speculative. Certainly, the precaution is infrequently observed at the hairdresser's.

Allergic responses to the dyes are only part of the problem. Reports that indicated their carcinogenicity have also appeared in the medical literature since the early 1950s. It was only after the results of several animal studies were announced in 1977, however, that the FDA began to consider taking action against these long-used products that had been immune from federal regulation for 40 years.

In the studies, conducted under the sponsorship of the National Cancer Institute, rats and mice were fed doses of 4-methoxy-*m*-phenylenediamine, or 4MMPD, also called 2,4 diaminoanisole or 2,4 DDA, and its sulfate, 4-methoxy-*m*-phenylenediamine sulfate, or 4MMPD-sulfate. These chemicals, coal-tar dye ingredients more likely to be found in the cool or drab tints—black, brown, or ash blond tones—had been suspected of being carcinogenic. According to the results of the rodent-feeding study, 4MMPD and 4MMPD-sulfate caused a significantly increased incidence of several kinds of cancer.

Because of these findings, the FDA, prohibited by current law from outright banning the chemicals, proposed that a warning label for the dyes containing the suspect ingredients be placed on the bottles and also proposed that a large poster be displayed in each beauty shop that would urge customers to check the bottle labels for the ingredients. The mandated label was to state, "Warning: Contains an ingredient that can penetrate your skin and has been determined to cause cancer in laboratory animals."

The cosmetics industry reacted to these proposals with predictable resistance and distributed a pamphlet to all beauty salons ridiculing the animal studies. The circular, an attempt to mollify the public's concern about the safety of the hair dyes, pointed out that humans put dye on their hair and do not ingest it and that the doses that caused cancer in rodents were the equivalent "to a person drinking more than 25 bottles of hair dye every day for a lifetime." But while people are not drinking hair dyes, evidently the chemicals are able to be absorbed through the skin of the scalp in varying amounts. It has been calculated that about 4–6 mg of dye are absorbed into the body during the coloring process (Kiese & Rauscher, 1968). While some have questioned the validity of extrapolating animal results to humans, such animal bioassays are one of the scientifically established ways of screening chemicals for carcinogenicity. Neither is the effect of the substance presumed to be related to the high dose. It is not true that virtually any substance will be carcinogenic if the exposure to it is high enough. If a substance is noncarcinogenic, it does not cause cancer at the maximum dose tolerated by the animal. Large numbers of industrial chemicals, pesticides, and food additives have been fed to animals in large doses and have not been implicated in cancer formation.

Screening studies proceed on the assumption that if the maximum tolerated dose causes cancerous tumors in a small number of test animals, a very small amount will cause some cancer in large numbers of animals or people. There is not complete agreement, however, that substances that cause cancer in animals will also cause cancer in humans, and considerable criticism has been directed at the hair-dye animal studies.

Also at the heart of the hair-dye controversy are the conflicting results from other cancer-risk studies. Cancers that have been reported as occurring in test animals when paraphenylenediamine was injected were not found to occur when the chemical was topically applied to the skin.

As for hair dye and cancer in humans, epidemiological studies as yet have not confirmed any association or increased risk of any kind of cancer among users of hair dyes or the hairdressers who apply the dye.

The two top manufacturers of hair coloring products have eliminated the suspect 4MMPD and 4MMPD-sulfate from their dye formulations. Because there are more than 30 such dye intermediates and their derivatives used in oxidation hair dyes, the substitution of similar chemicals for the questionable ingredients may or may not have lessened the possibility of risk. Although the use of hair dye does not appear to carry risk of cancer overall, it cannot be assumed, in view of the conflicting evidence, that it is completely harmless.

Other Permanent Dyes. Metallic dyes for coloring the hair have been used for centuries. The name of one commercial preparation, Grecian Formula, implies there is a time-honored quality in its ingredients. The dyes, salts of various metals such as lead, silver, and copper, are advertised for use on gray hair as "color restorers," as if they had some magical power that could make hair without pigment resume its natural pigmented shade. When a small amount of formula containing lead acetate, for example, is combed through the hair daily, the salt reacts with the sulfur of hair keratin to form lead sulfide, which coats the cuticle of the hair. Gradual color change from gray to yellow to brown to black are obtained with time. The result is a flat-looking unnatural color that becomes worse with time, is incompatible with oxidation dyes or with permanent waves or straightening, and is very difficult to remove. Moreover, lead colors are toxic. While they may be safe on intact skin, their use is highly questionable if any abrasions exist on the scalp.

Another coloring agent that has been known for centuries is henna, an extract or powder made from the dried leaves and twigs of several varieties of a Middle Eastern bush, *Lawsonia alba, Lawsonia inermis,* or *Lawsonia spinosa.* The chemical substance responsible for the dyeing ability of henna is 2-hydroxyl-1, 4-naphtho-quinone, which is also prepared synthetically and is called lawsone.

Henna has been widely promoted as a completely nontoxic, nonallergenic "organic" dye that produces body, shine, highlights, and completely natural colors, as opposed to those artificial chemical dyes with all their additives. But unless the hair is black, dark brown, or no lighter than medium brown to begin with, the use of 100% henna powder can produce downright startling, highly unnatural results. Even if one finds the shade satisfying, continued use of henna appears to alter the hair keratin, and the hair becomes stiff, dry, and brittle.

Shampoos

Shampoos are meant to clean the hair by removing dirt, sebum, cosmetics, and dead scalp cells that have accumulated on the hair shafts since the last time the hair was washed. Cleaning the hair is not the only function of a shampoo, however, because there are a number of other functions that most people want and expect from the cleansing agent such as leaving the hair shiny, fragrant, healthy looking, and manageable, among others. Moreover, since everyone's hair is different—curly, straight, long, short, oily, dry, dyed, bleached, or permed, some qualities produced by using a particular shampoo may be more desirable to one person than to another. My "soft and manageable" may be your "limp and lank," or what is fluffy body for my hair could be dry and wiry for yours. The only way for a consumer to differentiate among all the claims and options is to try to ignore them and to forget the promises and the gimmicks. After realistically assessing the condition of one's own hair, the best way to pick a shampoo from the dazzling number available is to start with a cheap one and keep trying until a preferred product is found.

Only a few shampoo formulas still contain soap, which performs well in softened water but leaves a dulling deposit in hard water. Most of today's shampoos contain synthetic detergents or *surfactants,* substances that can enhance the washing ability of water by making the water "wetter," by emulsifying the dirt particles and by surrounding the dirt and oil with an electrical charge so that they may be easily rinsed off rather than being returned to the hair or the scalp. The surfactant may be either *anionic,* or negatively charged; *cationic,* or positively charged; *amphoteric,* or both negatively and positively charged; or *nonionic,* possessing no electrical charge. Johnson's Baby Shampoo, one of the largest sellers in the country, contains an amphoteric surfactant that makes it milder—it does not sting the eyes. Its mildness makes it a less effective cleanser, however, so adults would have to use more of it more often. Most adult shampoos contain primarily anionic surfactants.

A typical liquid shampoo is likely to contain lots of water—about 60%–80%—and about 10%–25% surfactant (usually sodium lauryl sulfate); 5%–15% foam builders; and 0.1%–2% sequestering agents, substances that keep the other ingredients from precipitating out to cloud the shampoo. Other additives are varying amounts of thickening agents to give the shampoo a proper consistency so it will not run down into the eyes, and conditioning and finishing agents to control the hair and put the luster back on it. Surfactants are degreasing substances that tend to remove the luster. Small amounts of preservatives and sometimes a substantial amount of perfume (herbal, lemon, strawberry, new-mown hay, fruit salad, whatever) to add to the shampoo's appeal or to cover up the odor of the other ingredients complete the formulation. Manufacturers attempt to build product differentiation into shampoos in a number of different ways, but few of them appear to be relevant to the actual quality of the product. All shampoos are essentially the same.

Some of the antidandruff shampoos contain various antiseptics, which are hardly necessary because it has never been shown that dandruff is an infection or associated with microorganisms. Simple dandruff, the shedding of the top cornified layers of the scalp skin, is experienced by everyone to some degree and appears several days to a week after shampooing. Any shampoo will control dandruff if the hair is washed frequently enough. The medicated shampoos may delay the return of dandruff symptoms for a longer period of time, however, and for this reason may be preferred by people who do not want to wash their hair more often than once a week. Seborrheic dermatitis is a skin condition characterized by inflammation, severe itching, and flaking and is the only kind of dandruff that could actually require the use of a special shampoo. Some skin diseases such as psoriasis produce dandrufflike symptoms but will not respond to antidandruff shampoos.

The shampoos formulated to control dandruff may contain potentially toxic compounds such as zinc pyridinethione (ZnPT) or selenium sulfide. Both are considered to be safe for use in shampoos. The ZnPT is not readily absorbed through the skin, whereas the selenium, which does have considerable absorption potential, presumably has only intermittent and limited contact with the scalp.

Apparently the only difference between a shampoo for dry hair and a shampoo for oily hair is the amount of surfactant—there is less of it in the dry hair formulation. In a survey, *Consumer Reports* found that many people who characterized themselves as having dry hair preferred a shampoo for oily hair and that an equal number of those who said they had oily hair preferred the formulations for dry hair. They concluded that the "dry" and "oily" designations were just another advertising gimmick.

"Low pH," "acid balance," and "nonalkaline" are also qualities with little meaning or advantage other than the enhancement of product appeal. The pH is a measure of the alkalinity or acidity of a substance on a scale of 1–14; anything that is neither acid nor alkaline will be neutral with a pH of 7. The pH of the skin, as a result of its film of sebum and perspiration, ranges from 4.5 to 6 or 7, depending on the area of the body. Most shampoos have pH values between 5 and 8.

Unless the pH of a shampoo were as alkaline as 10 or over (Ivory soap has a pH of 9), it is certainly not going to have any lasting effect on hair or the scalp. Because the total application period of a shampoo is only a few minutes and it is rinsed off with tap water (which could be acid or alkaline, depending on how the water is treated in a particular area of the country), there is even less reason to be concerned about the shampoo's pH.

Shampoos may also contain protein, conditioners, balsam, egg, beer, or other kinds of gums or mucilages to coat the hair shafts—hair may then appear thicker or shinier, have body, and "bounce." An individual may or may not find that these additives make the product better; it is largely a matter of personal preference. One trouble with trying to make a shampoo perform all kinds of additional cosmetic functions is that its major features—cleaning ability and rinseability—tend to become lessened with each addition. If a conditioner is necessary, it is probably better to choose a shampoo without all the extras, and then use a separate conditioning agent after shampooing (Figure 16–16).

Hair Conditioners

The function of hair conditioners is to reduce static electricity that causes the individual hairs to repel one another and also to restore a shiny appearance, improve the texture, and increase the manageability of processed hair. The primary active ingredients in conditioners are cationic surfactants for controlling the hair and increasing the tensile strength, providone (PVP) and protein to coat the hair and add thickness for body, and a variety of oils to provide sheen and lubrication.

The cationic surfactant is a *quaternary ammonium compound*. One of the frequently used quaternaries is benzalkonium chloride. Any kind of hair treatment even combing, can cause a negative electrostatic charge on the hair, and the cationic agent neutralizes that charge by adhering to the hair fiber. In that way, it eliminates flyaway hair and adds to the hair's tensile strength to give it more body and set-holding ability. PVP is a plastic resin and, in a similar fashion to other gums and resins in conditioners, forms a film on the

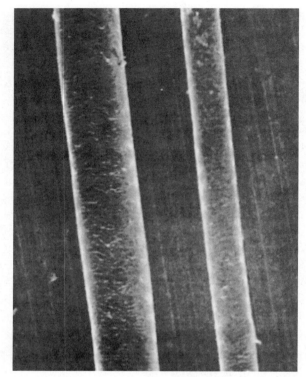

Figure 16–16 Thick and thin hairs. Hair that is thin in diameter may not necessarily be "thin" in numbers of hairs on the head. Hairs with thin shafts that are also in sparse supply would probably benefit from preparations that adhere to the hairs and "thicken" them.

hair shaft to give it more substance. Both quaternary compounds and PVP stick themselves onto the hair shaft (the chemists' term is adsorption) and are not substantively incorporated into the hair itself.

The "protein" in the protein conditioners is not really protein at all. Label reading will show that the protein preparations contain "hydrolyzed animal protein," actually a number of amino acid building blocks or subunits of protein that are obtained when animal collagen or elastin—the source of the protein—is chemically treated to break it down. The amino acids supposedly penetrate the hair shaft to incorporate themselves into the keratin protein of the hair to repair damage and restore the protein chains—a remarkable

accomplishment, if it were possible. There is no evidence that the hair is chemically changed by the addition of protein conditioners. Processed hair tends, however, to adsorb more protein onto the shaft than virgin hair.

The addition of nucleic acids to conditioners is another biochemical marvel. The hair preparation manufacturers are evidently hoping that by now everyone has heard of DNA and RNA but does not remember much about how they work. One label reads, "Contains proper amounts of the nucleoprotein team, DNA and RNA, which assists in the initiation of reconstruction and insures maintenance reconstruction of the hair. The nucleoproteins . . . are in a ratio of three RNA to each DNA and are actually genetically coded for the reconstruction of keratin protein." Autolyzed yeast is the sole protein source in the list of ingredients, so the conditioner appears to be using yeast DNA and RNA to synthesize human protein. This is enormously impressive. Even if the yeast nucleic acids could conceivably have any reconstructing ability, they would make yeast protein, and few people would want *that* growing out their hair follicles. To make human keratin, the conditioner appears to be carrying out a successful gene transfer experiment, a procedure usually performed only in laboratories equipped to do DNA recombination. Or perhaps we are to believe that the yeast is cloning hairs? Either way, this information should certainly be shared with molecular biologists, who are obviously unaware that an astounding breakthrough in genetic engineering is occurring each time the conditioners are used.

It should not be inferred that conditioners—actually, reconditioners—are not useful. They glue the cuticle scales back down against the cortex, they tend to fill in any missing cuticle, and they serve to hold the split ends together for a while. The public, however, should not be "scientifically" deluded into believing they have any other effect. Besides, not everyone needs a separate conditioner after shampooing, and its use will not necessarily make all hair look better. Depending on the hairstyle and type, it may be desirable for the hair to have a certain amount of "flyaway," and conditioning could make hair too soft or even too controlled. There is evidence to indicate that cationic surfactants are the best conditioners after hair processing and that PVP adds more material onto the hair shaft than hydrolyzed protein. Most conditioners take the shotgun approach anyway and contain a little of everything.

Setting lotions that are applied after shampooing and partial drying contain cationic surfactant additives. Variously known as *styling lotion, gel, spray,* or *mousse,* the products contain as a primary ingredient a quaternary compound to coat the hair and hold it in a relatively stiff "wet look" until the hair is brushed out.

Some have suggested that protein conditioners are a wasteful and unnecessary use of protein in a protein-starved world. While there may be some justification in the argument, in this country the protein that is used is second class; it comes from animal by-products and is lacking appropriate nutrients for complete human nutrition. The use of so-called protein in hair preparations, along with all the other vitamins, minerals, and assorted biochemicals that are added to shampoos and conditioners, makes the products more expensive. Unless it is discovered that all those extras really do a better job than preparations without the additives, there is no point in buying them.

The aware cosmetic consumer has probably concluded by now that most formulas for hair-care products are very much the same. If one finds, after wading through all the miracle claims, that a particular product does have benefit and aesthetic appeal, so be it—it is a good product.

ℛEFERENCES

Alster, T. S., & Bettencourt, M. S. (1998). Review of cutaneous lasers and their applications. *Southern Medical Journal, 91*(9), 806–814.

Bigby, M. (1998). Snake oil for the 21st century. *Archives of Dermatology, 134*(12), 1512–1514.

Binder, W. J., Blitzer, A., & Brin, M. F. (1998). Treatment of hyperfunctional lines of the face with botulinum toxin A. *Dermatologic Surgery, 24*(11), 1198–1205.

Bluhm, R., Branch R., Johnston, P., & Stein, R. (1991). Aplastic anemia associated with canthaxanthin ingested for "tanning" purposes. *Journal of the American Medical Association, 264*(9), 1141–1142.

Centers for Disease Control. (1990). *Pseudomonas aeruginosa* corneal infection related to mascara applicator trauma—Georgia. *Journal of the American Medical Association, 236*(912), 1616.

Corson, R. (1972). *Fashions in makeup.* New York: Universe Books.

Donato, M. (1989, July 12). Beauty and the beasts. *Chicago Tribune.*

Erickson, D. (1990). Skin stand-ins. Dermal substitutes promise to reduce animal testing. *Scientific American, 263*(3), 168.

Fagien, S. (1999). Botox for the treatment of dynamic and hyperkinetic facial lines and furrows: Adjunctive use in facial aesthetic surgery. *Plastic and Reconstructive Surgery, 103*(2), 701–713.

Fulton, J. D., & Black, E. (1983). *Dr. Fulton's Step-by-Step Program for Clearing Acne.* New York: Harper & Row.

Garber, C. A. (1978). Characterizing moisturized skin by scanning electron microscopy. *Cosmetics and Toiletries, 93*(4), 74–78.

Grossman, A. R., Majidian, A. M., & Grossman, P. H. (1998). Thermal injuries as a result of CO_2 laser resurfacing. *Plastic and Reconstructive Surgery, 102*(4), 1247–1252.

Guin, J. D. (1998). Eyelid dermatitis from methacrylates used for nail enhancement. *Contact Dermatitis, 39*(6), 312–313.

Hair today, hair tomorrow. (1998). *Ebony, 53*(7), 70–73.

Hanson, K. M., & Simon, J. D. (1998). Epidermal transurocanic acid and the UVA-induced photoaging of the skin. *Proceedings of the National Academy of Sciences of the United States of America, 95*(18), 10576–10578.

Kane, M. A. (1999). Nonsurgical treatment of platysmal bands with injection of botulinum toxin A. *Plastic and Reconstructive Surgery, 103*(2), 656–663.

Kiese, M., & Rauscher, E. (1968). The absorption of p-toluenediamine through human skin in hair dyeing. *Toxicology and Applied Pharmacology, 13,* 325–331.

Kinard, T. (1997). *No lye! The African American women's guide to natural hair care.* New York: St Martin's Griffin.

Kligman, A., & Mills, O. (1972). Acne cosmetica. *Archives of Dermatology, 106,* 843–850.

McMichael, A. (1995). Caring for hair problems in blacks. *Modern Medicine, 63*(10), 22.

The New York Times. (1998, February 26). Special edition, women's health.

Pascher, F. (1982). Adverse reactions to eye area cosmetics and their management. *Journal of the Society of Cosmetic Chemists, 33,* 249–258.

Plewig, G., & Kligman, A. M. (1975). *Acne Morphogenesis and Treatment.* New York: Springer-Verlag.

Russell, J. (2000). Topical therapy for acne. *American Family Physician,* 357–365.

Stiller, M. J., Bartolone, J., Stern, R., et al. (1996). Topical 8% glycolic acid and 8% l-lactic acid creams for the treatment of photodamaged skin. *Archives of Dermatology, 132*(6), 631–636.

Swerdlow, A. J., & Weinstock, M. A. (1998). Do tanning lamps cause melanoma? An epidemiologic assessment. *Journal of the American Academy of Dermatologists, 38*(1), 89–98.

Tretinoin (Renova) approved for treatment of wrinkles. (1996). *Medical Sciences Bulletin, 18*(6), 2.

Our Health in Our Hands

KEY TERMS

Calorie   Kilocalorie

Iatrogenic disease

*H*ealth, according to the old saying, is the one thing that money can't buy. Illness can happen to anybody; being rich has never been a guarantee against getting sick. Somewhere along the way, however, we seem to have forgotten that health is not for sale. For the past 30 years the American public has evidently been convinced that health *could* be bought for everybody, if only enough money were spent, if only enough were invested in health care—the diagnosis and treatment of disease.

The spiraling costs of health care have leveled off somewhat in the 1990s and now account for more than $3,925 per person and more than 14% of the nation's total production of goods and services. The ever-growing share of government dollars spent on doctors, medical schools, health workers, hospitals, and technology leaves that much less for housing, education, creating new jobs, or cleaning up the air and water. The health care industry has raised our taxes and our prices as the costs of health care insurance are passed along to the consumer by the employers. Health insurance in 1998 represented 6.6% of total employee compensation.

Although the bills from the expensive health care industry continue to strain the national economy, the expenditures might be justified if all Americans, regardless of their economic status, were not only receiving quality health care but also living longer and healthier lives as a result. But increasing the spending has not produced better quality care. On the contrary, there is evidence that duplication, waste, inefficiency, and downright fraud exist within the system. Moreover, there are large segments of the population that have limited access to quality care. Even more dismaying, there has been little improvement in overall public health, despite the high costs of medical care. There has been a 10% decline in mortality from heart and blood vessel disease in the past 30 years, but deaths from cancer, chronic respiratory diseases, and cirrhosis of the liver continue to rise. In fact, in the late 1960s a health authority suggested that if the amount spent on health were either doubled or halved, it would have no significant effect on longevity. At that time only $40 billion was spent. Now that the amount has increased 17 times, that observation has sadly proved to be more accurate than expected.

Americans rely on doctors to keep them well, paying dearly for the expectation, but the most highly sophisticated medical treatment can do little for those diseases that cause most of the health problems. The major causes of death in both men and women are cardiovascular diseases (heart attack, stroke, high blood pressure, arteriosclerosis) and cancer. Their incidence, it is now being recognized, is at least partly related to certain risk factors that can be controlled by individuals themselves. These killer diseases might be partially or perhaps even totally preventable if people would take the responsibility for preventing them. Some health analysts have even called certain ailments "diseases of choice," implying that we can choose to be sick or we can choose to be well—it is up to us. There is mounting evidence that correlates lack of exercise and overweight to cardiovascular disease, a high fat diet with cancer, alcohol abuse with cancer and cirrhosis of the liver, and smoking with virtually all health problems. Doctors can treat disease once it has struck, but they cannot be responsible for our health. Our health may be influenced more by what we do to and for ourselves than by how much professional medical care we get.

Better health can never be bought by buying more doctors, more hospital beds, or more computerized brain and body scanners that cost millions of dollars each (Figure 17–1). A better way of spending some of our health care taxes and insurance premiums might be in educating people toward the prevention of illness and the preservation of health. It has been suggested that if people were to modify their behavior to incorporate good health habits into their lives—no smoking, drinking, or harmful drugs, maintenance of a normal weight, getting plenty of exercise and plenty of rest—there would be a reduction in the number of premature deaths, an overall improvement in health, and a containment of the exorbitant costs of health care. John Knowles, late president of the Rockefeller Foundation and a foremost proponent of the personal responsibility for health, stated that the next major advances in the health of the American people will be determined by what individuals are willing to do for themselves and for society at large. It has been said that many cancer deaths could be prevented by changes in people's eating, drinking, and smoking habits.

Not all Americans, however, are in a position to choose a different lifestyle, and the accusation that they can is sociologically naive. Perhaps the decision not to smoke or drink is a choice available to anyone, but a major part of the individual assumption of responsibility for health is obviously profoundly limited when individual living conditions include unemployment, poverty, homelessness, and deprivation. The poor, needy, aged, and uneducated and disadvantaged people of this country—about 35 million of them—suffer more illness than the advantaged, but certainly they have neither chosen their lot nor their diseases. Moreover, their health care needs are not always met. The United States, which spends more on health per person than any other nation and is envied by the

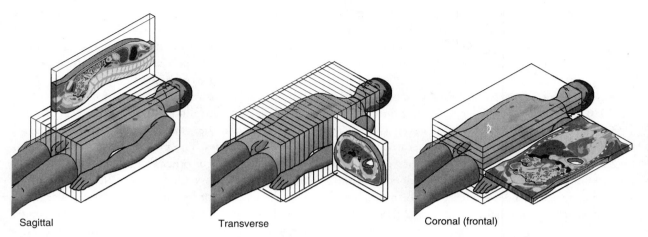

Sagittal   Transverse   Coronal (frontal)

Figure 17–1   A CT (computerized tomography) scanner provides multiple perspectives on cross-sectional views of the body.

world for the quality of its medical training, care, and technology, is the only industrialized country in the world that does not ensure health care for everyone. More than 44 million Americans are without health insurance. Many of them work at low-paying jobs and make enough income to disqualify themselves from government health care programs but cannot afford health insurance. And while Medicaid and Medicare are supposed to take care of those people who cannot pay and qualify for assistance, these programs provide uneven and inadequate coverage in many parts of the country. It is a myth that Medicare and Medicaid offer the needy and elderly health care equivalent to that received by the middle and upper classes.

It must also be remembered that although bad health habits can contribute to the incidence of some diseases, they are not the sole determinants of all illnesses. Our genetic constitutions are an important factor in our health—we do not choose our genes. Illness and mortality in many instances can be reflections of hazardous environmental conditions—of polluted air and water, of toxic substances or carcinogens in the food we eat, and of occupational dangers. There are many people who suffer from illness caused by factors beyond their control. They get sick and they die, but personal responsibility has played a minor role.

The benefits of taking charge of one's own health are not an illusion—they are real and measurable. Self-care can have an enormous impact on the prevention of illness, on life expectancy, on personal quality of life, on everybody's insurance premiums and taxes. The only danger lies in trying to shift the entire burden for health maintenance to the individual. We cannot do it completely by ourselves. We have to be assisted in our quest for health by improved and quality health care and by the elimination of the economic, social, and environmental conditions that contribute to disease. Taking good care of ourselves can play a great part in preserving the nation's health and in helping to control costs, but the individual's responsibility for health is an accompaniment, not an alternative, to the responsibilities of society and government for the improvement and maintenance of the public health.

Government public health priorities for the decade of the 1990s were outlined by a 1990 report released by the Department of Health and Human Services. The report, called *Healthy People 2000,* listed 298 specific objectives to be achieved during the rest of the decade. The objectives, collaboratively drafted and developed by the Public Health Service, 300 medical organizations, and state health departments, were aimed at increasing the healthy life span, reducing the substantial disparities in the quality of health among different Americans, and providing access to preventive health services to all people. Such praiseworthy public health national goals for the year 2000 would perhaps be more impressive had there not been a similar 1980 goals report listing 226 objectives for the year 1990, only half of which were achieved (National Center for Health Statistics, 1990). Government initiatives for health promotion and disease prevention are needed but evidently are difficult to implement in the absence of major changes in our system of health care. Perhaps the population has to wait until 2010?

GETTING HEALTHY, STAYING HEALTHY

Along with the rising costs of health care, there has been a rising dissatisfaction with the care delivered by the traditional medical establishment. Increasing numbers of people are searching for nontraditional methods of healing, some of which are considered nonscientific or even absurd when judged by the usual standards. It is not surprising that the public is disillusioned and disappointed by orthodox medicine. There is evidence not only of the limitations of a health care system based on sickness rather than on health but also of its adverse effects. Recent knowledge concerning the prevalence of **iatrogenic disease** (disease that is doctor induced), of unnecessary surgery, and of excessive and even irrational prescribing of drugs has hardly been reassuring. Faith in the system has been shaken, and a lot of people are ready for a different approach to health and illness, one that stresses that health is more than the absence of disease or infirmity—it is also the feeling of "ease" rather than "dis-ease." Proponents of this view are holistic. They believe that health care should consider all the dimensions of an individual's life—the physical, emotional, intellectual, spiritual, and interpersonal—to find the cause for disease. Total health, then, is seen as a balance of all factors, a wholeness of body, mind, and spirit that allows the attainment of an individual's total potential for well-being. This kind of medical care is more interested in wellness and prevention than in treatment of illness and concerned as much with the improvement of quality of life as with being free of disease.

There are also hundreds of therapies that are included under the general umbrella of alternative medical techniques. The practitioners range from traditional physicians or other established professionals to Indian shamans, psychic healers, New Age proponents, or teachers of healing philosophies. Their forms of healing may have their basis in known and accepted methods of preserving health, that is, through changing or modifying unhealthy lifestyles. Other modes of treatment may be mystical or experimental. Adherents of holistic health generally keep an open mind to alternative ways of relieving physical or emotional pain. Herbal healing, homeopathy, hypnotism, acupressure and acupuncture, rolfing, reflexology, meditation, and even laying on of hands are unscientific by traditional standards, but they sometimes are successful in producing cures or pain relief when orthodox treatment has failed. Recognizing that the belief in the treatment and the practitioner of a therapy is frequently of greater importance than the content of the therapy, the sole test of the usefulness of a technique is usually pragmatic—if it works, use it.

Obviously, some of these modes of healing are of limited usefulness and downright dangerous in serious illness, injuries, or infections. Waiting to see whether nutritional therapy works when chemotherapy has a proven track record is a foolhardy course to pursue. A better test of the safety and effectiveness of a nontraditional technique is whether or not it can actively harm an individual. The decision to use an alternative method involves making the same kind of *informed* choice one uses for the usual forms of medical care. Herbal remedies, for example, may be more natural than the drugs prescribed by a physician, but they may be, nonetheless, drugs. They should be subject to the same kind of scrutiny. A nutritional regime that promises a cure for disease, instant permanent weight loss, or that "cleanses out the body" may be harmless or a waste of time; it could also be of dubious safety. Many women have learned not to be passive recipients of current medical care, but passive acceptance of the claims of the alternative and unorthodox therapies without investigation and knowledge is hardly progress. When exploring some of the unconventional pathways to good health, it would be wise to retain some of the cynicism and informed skepticism with which the standard surgery and drugs of the doctors are being viewed.

Of all the described ways to wellness, of all the methods and techniques used to attain a healthy life, the bottom line is still good nutrition, good exercise, good relaxation. These are the three inseparable elements of health. The rest of this chapter takes a physiological look at nutrition and physical activity with a view toward providing information that can result in better nutrition and more exercise.

Nutrients

The human body is a marvel of engineering and, with just a few minor exceptions, excellently designed to carry out all of its specific functions. Similar to all machines, the body, too, needs fuel in the form of energy to propel it throughout its daily living—to keep the heart beating and the blood circulating, to inhale and exhale the air, to contract the muscles for movement, to power cell division and the synthesis of new tissue that means growth, to do all of the work of the life processes that keep the body alive and active. Humans get their energy from the carbohydrates, proteins, and fats in their diet. The energy value of the food is expressed in terms of a unit called the **kilocalorie** or **Calorie** (with a capital *C*). A Calorie is the amount of heat that is required to raise the temperature of a kilogram of water (1,000 g) from 14.5 degrees Celsius to 15.5 degrees Celsius. The calorie (with a small *c*) is really 0.001 Calories, but it is used so often in association with food that it is usually understood to mean the kilocalorie. When oxidized or burned inside the cells of the body, 1 g of carbohydrate provides 4 calories, 1 g of protein also provides 4 calories, and 1 g of fat yields 9 calories. The process by which food is combined with oxygen for the release of energy takes place in all the cells of the body and is called *cellular respiration*. The energy is not released as heat, which would be destructive and useless to the cells. Instead, it is captured to form a high-energy molecule called *adenosine triphosphate* or ATP. Then, when the cell needs energy to power its physiological work, it can get it from the ATP. Cellular respiration, without which no living cell could survive, results in the production of energy as ATP and of carbon dioxide and water. The entire process looks like this:

Food molecule + oxygen →

ATP + carbon dioxide + water

Actually, the carbohydrates, proteins, and fats in the foods eaten are not in a form utilizable by cells; their molecules are too large to pass into the cells. Before they can be a source of energy, the three foodstuffs must be broken down into their smaller building block molecules. The chemical conversion of carbohydrates into simple sugar, proteins into amino acids, and fats into fatty acids and glycerol is called digestion, and it takes place within the digestive tract.

Figure 17–2 is a diagram of the digestive system. Food taken in at the mouth is acted on within the tract by digestive enzymes produced both by the digestive tube itself and by glands located outside the tube and emptying into it. When digestion is complete, the simple sugars, amino acids, and fatty acids and glycerol are absorbed by the cells lining the small intestine. All of the sugars and amino acids and a small quantity of the end products of fat digestion get into the bloodstream and are carried to the liver first before they are transported to the rest of the body. The majority of the fatty acids and glycerol molecules bypass the liver. They are absorbed into the lymphatic system but also get into the bloodstream eventually via a large vein near the heart. All undigested substances left over after absorption are expelled from the body as waste or feces.

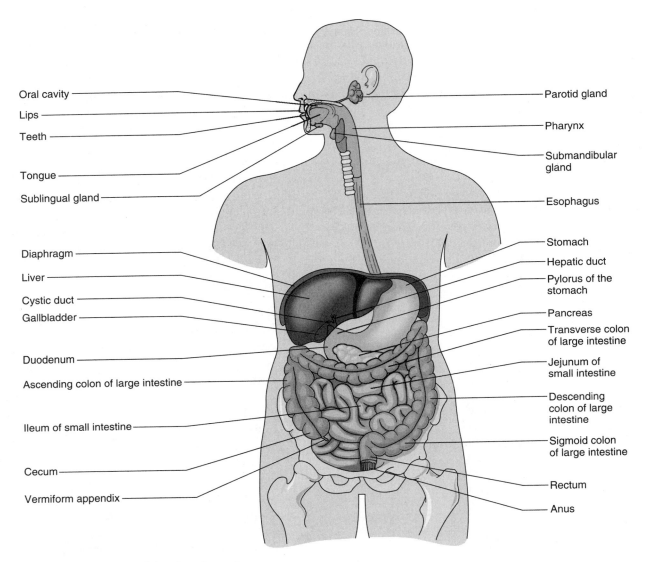

Figure 17–2 Diagram of the digestive system.

While carbohydrates, proteins, and fats provide the energy in food, other required components of the diet are minerals, vitamins, and water. These substances do not contribute energy but are no less vital for survival. All of these chemical substances on which humans and other animals rely for the continuation of life processes are called *nutrients.*

Carbohydrates

In the typical American diet, 50%–60% of the energy is provided by carbohydrates, compounds made up only of carbon, hydrogen, and oxygen. Because carbohydrates are found abundantly in plants, they may provide as much as 90% of the energy in the diet (with adverse effects on health) in developing countries where protein is unobtainable or too expensive.

In the process called photosynthesis, green plants use the energy from the sun to combine carbon dioxide and water to form *glucose,* the predominant building block of carbohydrate. All the more complex carbohydrates are variations and multiples of glucose. The plant cell converts the glucose to larger carbohydrates and also to fats, proteins, and vitamins, utilizing the minerals and nitrogen obtained from the soil. The main sources of carbohydrates in the diet are tuber and root vegetables, legumes (beans and peas), cereal grains, and fruits.

There are three groups of carbohydrates, divided on the basis of size and complexity of their molecules. Glucose is the best known and most prevalent *monosaccharide,* or simple sugar, and is the main sugar of carbohydrate metabolism and energy production in the body. "Blood sugar" is glucose. Other monosaccharides are fructose or fruit sugar and galactose, a component of milk sugar.

Disaccharides are formed from two monosaccharides linked together. *Sucrose,* or table sugar, which comes mainly from the juices of sugar cane, sugar beets, or maple trees, is composed of glucose and fructose. Honey is about 50% fructose and 50% glucose plus a trace of vitamins and minerals usually considered inconsequential. *Lactose* is another disaccharide and is made up of glucose and galactose. *Maltose,* which rarely occurs in foods but is an intermediate product of carbohydrate digestion in the body, has two glucose units.

Polysaccharides are very long chains made of hundreds, thousands, or even millions of glucose units. The most common polysaccharides are plant starch, or *amylose* and *amylopectin; cellulose;* and animal starch, or *glycogen.* Cellulose forms a large part of the diet, but it cannot be utilized for energy because humans lack the enzyme for breaking it down to glucose. Although cellulose cannot be digested, it does add to the mechanics of the digestive system by contributing fiber and bulk. A moderate amount of cellulose and other indigestible materials or roughage is necessary for normal bowel activity and is obtained from whole-grain cereals and raw fruits and vegetables. An increased incidence of diverticulitis (inflammation of small pockets in the wall of the colon), cancer of the colon, and heart disease has been correlated to a low fiber intake in the diet.

Few of the food nutrients that provide energy, except when they are highly refined as in table sugar or salad oil, are ever "pure." Even flour, which is primarily starch, has a 6%–10% protein content. Dry peas and beans contain 20% protein, and soybeans are different from other legumes in that they contain even more protein and fat and less starch.

Fats and Lipids

Because fats provide more than twice the calories per gram than both carbohydrates and proteins (9 calories/g in fats versus 4 calories/g in the latter two), foods containing fats will be higher in calories and energy content. More than 33% of a typical American diet is fat, much of it coming from animal sources.

The term *fat* is usually used synonymously with "triglycerides," "true fat," "neutral fat," or "visible fat," and it refers to body fat or adipose tissue as well as to food fats, such as butter, margarine, lard, and vegetable shortening and oils. *Lipid* is a broader term; it includes the phospholipids, the sterols such as cholesterol, and all the other substances that contain fatty acids and are insoluble in water. Triglycerides are used for cellular energy in animals and plants. The other lipids form parts of cellular membranes, are involved in the transport of triglycerides in the bloodstream, or are important in the synthesis of other important compounds. Cholesterol, for example, is the precursor for the synthesis of sex hormones, bile salts, the adrenal cortical hormones, and vitamin D.

Triglycerides. Containing only carbon, hydrogen, and oxygen atoms, a triglyceride molecule consists of three molecules of fatty acids linked to one molecule of an alcohol called glycerol, commonly known as "glycerine." The fatty acids can either be all the same kind or all different. Palmitic, oleic, and stearic are the most common fatty acids found in nature. They are found frequently in food fats and are the common fatty acids in human body fat. Palmitic and stearic are examples of *saturated* fatty acids. A saturated fatty acid contains all the hydrogen it is capable of containing, attached to the carbon atoms. In *unsaturated* fatty acids, such as linoleic, linolenic, and arachidonic, the place on a carbon atom that would ordinarily be attached to a hydrogen is unoccupied. The carbon atoms are then joined by double instead of single bonds; like this: (—C=C—). When a fat contains fatty acids with two or more double bonds between carbon atoms it is said to be *polyunsaturated*. The consistency of fat at room temperature is determined by the degree of saturation with the hydrogen atoms. Animal fats are composed largely of saturated fatty acids and are solid, but fats from plant sources are found in a liquid state as oils because they contain unsaturated fatty acids. Margarine, Fluffo, Crisco, and Spry are vegetable oils that have been partially saturated and converted to a solid form by hydrogenation, the addition of hydrogen atoms. Cocoa butter (chocolate fat) and tropical oils such as palm kernel, palm, and coconut oil are exceptions to the unsaturated quality of vegetable fats.

Linoleic and linolenic acids are called the *essential* fatty acids because they cannot be synthesized by the body and must be obtained in the diet. The essential fatty acids are necessary precursors to the biosynthesis of prostaglandin by human tissue.

In addition to providing the source of certain necessary fatty acids, fat in the diet is also required as a carrier for the fat-soluble vitamins in the food. Without dietary fat, there would be great difficulty in absorbing vitamins A, D, E, and K from the intestine.

The fat stored in the body, found within the adipose cells of adipose tissue, is desirable and advantageous as long as not too much is accumulated. Moderate fat deposits provide roundness and shape to the body in both males and females and is a reserve source of energy. Fat insulates the body, conserves against heat loss, and also supports and cushions the body organs. But the body's requirements for fat as a nutrient can be met by 15–25 g of food fats eaten daily. The typical diet contains 10 times that amount—about 110–260 g—or more than a quarter of a pound of fat. Much of the excess body fat in overweight individuals does not come from dietary fat, however. When the food energy ingested in the form of fat, protein, or carbohydrate exceeds the amount of energy needed for body activities, it is converted to body fat and stored in the adipose tissue.

Lipids Other Than Triglycerides.

Phospholipids. Phospholipids are similar to triglycerides, but one of the fatty acids in the molecule has been replaced by a phosphate-containing substance. In the phospholipid *lecithin,* found in egg yolk and soybeans, the substance is choline, a nitrogenous base. Some of the claims for the value of high lecithin intake have bordered on the miraculous. It has been said to lower blood cholesterol levels; dissolve gallstones; prevent heart disease; and when combined with seaweed, vitamin B_6, and cider vinegar in a low-calorie diet, emulsify and "burn up" fat to cause spot-reduction from special places. There is little or no evidence that extra ingestion of lecithin provides any of these benefits. When lecithin is digested in the body, it breaks down into glycerol, fatty acids, phosphate, and choline. The body cells are able to synthesize both choline and lecithin on their own.

Probably the most important function of phospholipids in the body is that they form part of the structure of all cells, mainly in the membrane elements.

Cholesterol. Cholesterol is a member of a third class of lipids called sterols. It is found in the fatty portions of all foods of animal origin and is, therefore, present in the diet of most people. Much of the cholesterol of the body is converted by the liver to cholic acid and combined with other substances to form bile salts, which are necessary for the digestion and absorption of fats. Cholesterol is also essential for the synthesis of hormones by the adrenal glands, the ovaries, and the testes. Along with phospholipids, cholesterol forms a part of the structural components of all body cells.

After 6 months of age, dietary consumption of cholesterol is unnecessary because the body will make what it needs from other substances, and normal adults produce about 200 mg of cholesterol daily. Most of this endogenous cholesterol is manufactured by the liver, but it is also synthesized by all the other cells of the body. When foods high in cholesterol are eaten, the production of endogenous cholesterol is somewhat but not completely cut back. Thus, the habitual ingestion of high cholesterol-containing foods in most people causes a rise in blood cholesterol levels. Common foods that contain large amounts of cholesterol are those high in saturated fats, such as butter, whole milk, and cheeses made from whole milk, and meats that are heavily marbled with fat. Egg yolks, organ meats such as liver and kidney, and shrimp also contain appreciable amounts of cholesterol.

There is a great deal of evidence to link high blood levels of cholesterol with atherosclerosis, considered to be the leading cause of coronary heart disease and stroke. Atherosclerosis is a condition in which fatty plaques of lipids, mostly cholesterol, are deposited on and in an artery wall. The cholesterol deposits slowly build up, become fibrous and calcified, and eventually cause narrowing and hardening (arteriosclerosis) of the artery. The artery can become so narrow that it becomes closed, cutting off the supply of blood to a vital area supplied by the diseased vessel, or part of the plaque can break off and become a thrombus or clot that blocks the vessel, which may also lead to a heart attack or a stroke.

It should be emphasized that the relationship of a high intake of saturated fats and cholesterol to high blood cholesterol levels and the incidence of heart disease and stroke is no longer controversial. It is known that a low-fat diet and exercise lower blood cholesterol. Changing the nutritional lifestyle to incorporate a low-fat, low-cholesterol diet along with regular exercise is not only prudent but potentially lifesaving.

When polyunsaturated vegetable fats such as soybean, safflower, and sunflower oils are consumed, they lower cholesterol by enhancing its excretion. But because these oils indiscriminately decrease the "good" high-density lipoprotein (HDL) cholesterol along with the "bad" low-density lipoprotein (LDL) cholesterol, the monosaturated oils such as canola, olive, or walnut, which reduce only the LDL cholesterol, may be preferable. In addition, certain unsaturated fats called omega-3 fatty acids, found in canola and olive oils and in large amounts in deep-sea fish, appear to be protective against heart disease. Diets that are high in any kind of fat, however, have been associated not only with heart disease but also with cancers of the bladder, breast, colon, ovary, and pancreas.

Fat is not an evil food, however, that should be eliminated from the diet or make people feel guilty when they sometimes eat food with a high fat content. Although most nutritionists recommend that no more than 25%–30% of the *total* daily calories should come from fat, this does not mean that food containing more than 30% in fat calories should never be consumed. Doing that would mean completely removing from the diet any margarine, oil, almost all meats and dairy products, almost any kind of nuts, ice cream, virtually all desserts—for most people taking all the pleasure out of eating and requiring a sort of asceticism. It is true that all of these foods contain well over 30% of fat calories—some are 70%–80%—but the issue really is how much and how frequently such foods should be eaten. As long as the total diet balances out to 30% or less of fat calories on a daily basis or even over time, the diet will be nutritious, enjoyable, and protective of health. One can occasionally eat very small amounts of high-fat foods, treating them like appetizers or condiments, and combine them with frequent eating of far greater amounts of low-fat foods such as grains, pasta, fruits, and vegetables. No one is advocating a monklike subsistence, but remember the old saying: don't live to eat, instead eat to live.

Figuring out the fat content of the food consumed (which is often conveniently indicated on the nutrition label) requires knowing the number of calories and the grams of fat in a serving. Because there are

9 calories in each gram of fat, simply multiply the number of grams of fat in the serving by 9 and divide that number by the total number of calories. For example, a 3½ oz serving of chicken with skin has 239 calories and 14 g of fat. Multiply $14 \times 9 = 126$, divide by the number of calories (239) to equal 0.53, or 53% from fat. Of course, that assumes the chicken was broiled, roasted, or microwaved, not fried in fat. Removing the skin of the chicken before eating it also will decrease the fat content. Or one could look at a serving (tablespoon) of peanut butter with 95 calories and 8 g of fat. Eight times 9 is 72 divided by 95 equals 76% of the calories in peanut butter from fat. Try this formula on some of the snack foods or packaged deli meats in the supermarket that claim to be "low fat" or "lite" for some surprises.

The Monsanto Company, the same people who gave us Nutrasweet (aspartame, a sugar substitute used in 161 soft drinks and 3,000 other products) has tried to duplicate Nutrasweet's phenomenal success with another food substitute—a fake fat. Introduced in 1990 after approval from the FDA and called Simplesse, the fat substitute technically is "microparticulated protein." The substance is made from egg white and whey, the watery part of milk, whipped and cooked into a fatlike consistency that feels like fat in the mouth but with less than half the calories of animal fat. Simplesse cannot be used in foods that are fried or baked, so it may never be as ubiquitous as Nutrasweet, but it is used in ice cream, dips, and salad dressings. Olestra, a product of Proctor & Gamble, is a synthetic fat that cannot be digested and therefore provides no calories. It is currently used in many snack items. Fake fat and fake sugar sound promising, but there is little evidence that such substitutes actually help people lose weight or cut down on their intake of fat or sugar. Apparently, many people feel so virtuous about eating the substitutes that they may allow themselves greater portions of fatty or sugary foods at other mealtimes. According to the nutrition experts, another problem with the newer low- and no-fat, no-cholesterol cakes, cookies, and frozen desserts is that they lack the nutrients and fiber of the fruits, grains, and vegetables people actually should be consuming. But for those really trying to reduce the fat in their diets, low-fat or fat-free foods may be distinctly beneficial, especially if they eat more fresh fruit or a vegetable salad when it has a no-fat dressing on it. Research has shown that two-thirds of American adults currently eat the low- or no-fat products ("Just What Is a Balanced Diet Anyway?" 1992). But it is important to check the labels, especially of the fat-free pastries, because zero fat does not mean zero calories. Although the fat is reduced or absent, the sugar is still there.

It is worth noting that not all experts agree with the National Research Council's recommendation that everyone should reduce their dietary fat to 30%. Some think the reduction is too great and others believe it to be insufficient. To a number of authorities, a diet with 20% of the calories from fat or even less, one that is low in saturates and cholesterol and high in fiber, would be better protection against coronary heart disease and cancer. The issue currently remains controversial and was not clarified by a study from the University of California–San Francisco School of Medicine (Browner, Westenhouse, & Tice, 1991) that estimated that if all Americans indeed reduced their fat intake to 30%, the effects on mortality from coronary heart disease and cancer would be far from spectacular. The researchers reported that, based on their mathematical extrapolations, about 40,000 of the 2.3 million deaths that would otherwise occur annually in adults would be deferred by only 3–4 months, mostly in people 65 and older. Does this study mean, as one bewildered student asked, that the population can continue to gorge on high-fat goodies with no risk to health? Not a chance. A more likely explanation is that there are still unknown factors in the proven relationship between blood fats and heart disease and dietary fats and cancer, that there is no one pathway that can absolutely guarantee a longer life span, and that the quality of life in good health is as important as the quantity. The control of dietary fat and cholesterol need not become an obsession or subject to food fads like the oat bran craziness of the past decade. Instead, it can be recognized that limiting the fat content of the diet is one legitimate and well-documented way of pursuing a healthy lifestyle.

Proteins

Most of the body is composed of water, but the solid part is three-quarters protein. Without exception, every cell contains protein fundamental to cell function and structure. The 20-odd amino acids that are the structural units of proteins contain carbon, hydrogen, oxygen, and nitrogen plus small quantities of other atoms such as sulfur and phosphorus. The proteins in food provide the amino acids necessary to build new tissue or maintain and repair the tissues already built.

Actually, the basis of all life is the protein synthesis going on within the cells. The energy-supplying role of food protein is secondary; its major importance is the support of normal growth and repair of the body's cells, tissues, and organs.

When proteins are eaten, they are digested down to amino acids, absorbed from the small intestine, and taken to all the cells of the body to be utilized in making the types of proteins needed. Protein synthesis can take place only when all of the 20 amino acids are present in an adequate supply. As long as there is enough nitrogen available (via protein food intake), the cells of the body are capable of manufacturing most of the amino acids normally present in animal proteins. Nine of the amino acids, however, cannot be synthesized in human tissues because the enzymes necessary to their formation are lacking. (Actually, our DNA lacks the genes required to direct the manufacture of those particular enzymes.) Those nine amino acids are called *essential* because they must be obtained from the diet. They include isoleucine, leucine, lysine, methionine, phenylalanine, threonine, tryptophan, valine, and histidine.★

The other amino acids are just as essential in the cellular formation of protein, but they are not essential from the diet. Almost all foods eaten contain some protein, but not all of them have the same quantity and kinds of amino acids. Only animal proteins, such as meat, poultry, fish, eggs, and dairy products, have all the amino acids, including the essential ones in the amounts and proportions appropriate for protein synthesis. For these reasons they are called *complete* or *high quality proteins.* Other foods, such as gelatin made from animal collagen and elastin, or soybeans, are rich in protein but do not contain all the essential amino acids. Most plant proteins are deficient in several of the essential amino acids, usually threonine, tryptophan, or lysine. Protein foods from vegetables and grains that lack essential amino acids are called incomplete sources of protein because they have a lower biological value than animal protein. Some plant foods have a lower percentage of protein and may be more difficult to digest because the cellulose in the plant wall resists the action of digestive enzymes. The protein present in the plant cells will probably pass right on through the tract as part of the bulk. Dried beans, for example, have to be softened by long periods of cooking to improve their digestibility.

As the prices of meat and fish and even cheese become increasingly astronomical, it is necessary to appreciate the fact that protein synthesis in the body can be supported without ingesting much animal protein or even any at all, although pure vegetarianism can result in inadequate nutrition unless foods are selected very carefully and wisely. A money-saving and nutritious way of eating mixes low-cost incomplete proteins from plant sources with complete protein from animals. Asian cooking, for example, uses only a little meat or fish along with a lot of rice and vegetables. Another way of obtaining quality complete protein is by combining two vegetable proteins so that they supplement each other. Legumes lack some essential amino acids; cereal grains lack others. Peanut butter on whole wheat bread, however, or beans and rice together provide good nutrition. But because the body has no mechanism for storing amino acids in the way that it accumulates fats or carbohydrates for future use, it is important to try to mix complementary protein foods at the same meal. In this way, all 20 amino acids necessary in the manufacture of protein will be present in the body cells at the same time. If it is not always feasible at a given

---

The mnemonic device Pvt. T. M. Hill stands for the first letters of the essential amino acids.

meal to combine complementary proteins, as long as a variety of incomplete and complete amino acid–containing foods are consumed during any given day, there is no problem.

VEGETARIANISM

Large numbers of Americans, for various reasons, have decided to eliminate animal flesh from their diets. Their motives are diverse. They may believe there are harmful constituents—hormones, antibiotics, pesticide residues—in meat, poultry, and fish. They may practice a religion or special lifestyle that requires the exclusion of animal products. They may want to reduce the saturated fat content of their diet. They may want to make a personal contribution to the alleviation of the world protein shortage. Every year 60 million people worldwide die of starvation, and hungry people could be fed with the grain and soybeans now eaten by livestock. It does, after all, take 21 lb of grain fed to a steer to make 1 lb of beef protein. Those who give up red meat may have environmental concerns. Not only do beef and dairy farming add to pollution, but millions of acres of forest and the countless species they support have been destroyed to provide crop-growing or grazing land for the $57 billion-a-year cattle industry. Or the nonflesh eaters simply may be unable to afford meat, fish, or fowl; a diet based on plant foods can cost one-quarter that of one centered on meat.

There need not be any nutritional disadvantage to practicing vegetarianism as long as the diet is carefully selected. Depending on the foods included, a vegetarian diet may even be superior to the typical American diet, loaded with extra calories and saturated fats. The lacto-ovo-vegetarian diet, one that includes milk, eggs, and other dairy products, will provide sufficient calories, a good quality balance of essential amino acids, and adequate vitamins and minerals. It is nutritionally safe and appropriate for all age groups, including children. Some "vegetarians" eliminate only red meat and permit fish and chicken or turkey, claiming that they feel better or even smell better when beef or pork has not been eaten. Any benefits derived from the exclusion of red meat with its higher fat content would likely be long term rather than immediate. It is doubtful whether the body, after digestion of animal protein to amino acids, is able to distinguish the source of those amino acids.

A pure vegetarian or "vegan" will not eat animal products in any form and chooses his/her diet from cereals, legumes, nuts, fruits, seeds, and vegetables. Vegans may have a little more difficulty maintaining adequate nutrition, but with knowledge and appropriate food selection, it is still possible to stay well nourished. The vegan must make certain to get enough calories for energy needs. A pure vegetarian diet usually contains so much bulk that it is hard to eat enough to meet caloric requirements. It is also important to include protein-rich legumes in the diet and to combine them at the same meal with cereal grains. Furthermore, the diet must be supplemented with vitamin B_{12} and calcium because B_{12} is found only in foods of animal origin, and the major source of calcium is milk. Ingestion of soybean milk fortified with vitamin B_{12} and significantly increasing the intake of the calcium-containing green leafy vegetables will provide adequate amounts of these two nutrients. Eating nuts and seeds is also important. These foods are a source of protein and vitamins and contain the fat necessary for absorption of fat-soluble vitamins from the intestine. As a safety measure, it would probably be sensible for vegans to consider vitamin supplementation in tablet form.

A purely vegetarian diet that even vegans might find difficult to pursue is one that would eliminate even nuts and seeds because of their fat content, reduce fat to no more than 10% of the total calories, allow only nonfat milk and nonfat yogurt, and remove all stimulants, including coffee. In a small experimental study by Ornish (1990), however, such a diet was found actually to reverse some of the coronary artery blockage in 18 of the 22 people with heart disease who followed the diet for a year. Members of the experimental group, who also exercised at least 30 minutes three times a week and practiced meditation and other stress-control techniques, were compared with a control group of 19 people with heart disease who followed a diet with 30% of their calories from fat—the kind recommended by the American Heart Association and many nutritionists. The heart patients in the control group not only had no improvement in their coronary arteries, but their condition worsened over the year. Only the people who reduced the fat, calories, and stress in their lives and exercised had measurable improvement in their arteries.

This kind of diet—extremely low in fat—compared with the typical American diet with 30%–40% of its calories derived from fat, admittedly would be a drastic regimen to follow for most people without heart disease. But as nutritionist Jean Mayer, the late president of Tufts University, pointed out, such an extremely low-fat diet was the normal human diet for millions of years and is still eaten by some societies. Our American way of eating is only 100 years old.

Ornish's diet is a well-balanced, albeit very conservative vegetarian diet. But vegetarians who eat *only* cereal grains or *only* fruits and nuts, associating this kind of restriction with some sort of purification or spiritual reawakening, are extremists who are playing with fire, nutritionally. The body will always put a higher priority on energy than on maintaining and repairing the body proteins. A low-calorie diet that is also low in protein, inevitable on this kind of limited regimen, is very dangerous to health. The carbohydrates and fats in the diet are insufficient to supply the energy needs, so the body is forced to use proteins pulled out of the structural components of the cells for energy. Normal protein synthesis necessary for building and replacement of tissues then suffers, and the body literally wastes away.

The risks to health of a severely inadequate diet depend on the previous nutritional status and the length of time during which strict adherence to the diet takes place. An individual who has gone through infancy and childhood in a well-nourished state may not immediately suffer the consequences of nutritional deprivation. There are hundreds of millions of people in the world, however, even some in this country, who are energy deficient and protein deficient and never by choice. They exist in a state of semistarvation, subject to disease and early mortality because they simply cannot get enough food to lead healthy and active lives. To invite a similar condition through a self-inflicted dietary regime is irrational.

How Much Protein Is Enough?

Many people are convinced of the virtues of a high-protein diet. Increased consumption of protein is said to improve health, sex life, energy, and athletic performance and to be beneficial for losing weight. Weight lifters and body builders eat a lot of animal protein and take protein supplements. Quick-weight-loss diets of the "eat-all-you-want, calories-don't-count" variety extol the advantages of high-protein, low-carbohydrate eating. "To stay in shape," claims one cookbook with better recipes than nutritional advice, "don't count calories, count protein grams . . . if you start filling yourself with prote instead of just cals, you'll look and feel better and have more *real* energy than you've ever had in your whole life."

The widespread misconception illustrated here is that "prote" is a major energy source for the body. Carbohydrates and fats are the primary providers of "real" energy, however, and calories obviously do count. As pointed out before, amino acids, unlike carbohydrates and lipids, cannot be stored in the body to any extent. Once the quantities of amino acids needed for protein synthesis have been taken up by the cells and utilized, any *additional* amino acids are converted and oxidized for energy. If the total energy intake in calories is too great, the excess amino acids will simply be converted to fat and retained in the adipose tissues.

Very high consumption of protein during dieting is based on a mistaken interpretation of the fact that it takes somewhat more energy to digest and metabolize pure protein when it is eaten than to digest and metabolize carbohydrate and fat. Protein in pure form, however, does not occur in protein foods; it is usually accompanied by fats and carbohydrates. The energy requirement to utilize protein, therefore, is not likely to be much of a factor in weight reduction. Moreover, a gram of protein contains as many calories as a gram of carbohydrate. There is no advantage to replacing carbohydrate with protein to lose weight; a balanced diet with restriction of total calories is more important.

During periods of rapid growth, such as in infancy and childhood, an increase in dietary protein is necessary for tissue building. Greater amounts of complete protein must be supplied to ensure optimum growth and development. For similar reasons, more protein is also needed by a pregnant woman to synthesize new tissue and by a lactating woman for milk formation. Other circumstances under which more protein is required occur during convalescence from a debilitating illness. Recovery from surgery, for example, increases the need for protein in the diet in order to repair and heal the injured tissues. After hemorrhage, more protein would obviously be necessary to replace blood tissue. For an athlete, however, a small extra amount of protein might be utilized during athletic training as the muscles get larger, but exercise or athletic performance does not increase the requirement for protein. The additional energy needed can be met by generally increasing food intake.

Under ordinary conditions, the adult body is in a state of protein balance. The rate of protein synthesis equals the rate of normal breakdown of body protein. Healthy adult men and nonpregnant, nonlactating healthy adult women need to eat enough protein to maintain that equilibrium. The recommended daily dietary allowance for adults is somewhere between 40 g and 70 g of protein, depending on the size of the individual. The value is approximately 0.4 g protein per pound of body weight. A 125-lb woman should, therefore, eat about 50 g of protein per day.

One ounce of meat, which also contains fat and water, yields an average of 7 g of protein. An ounce of cheddar cheese also contains 7 g, and a cup of skim milk will provide 9 g. Getting the daily required amount of protein (which already includes a liberal safety margin) is no problem, and it is obvious that most people in this and other developed countries probably already consume more protein than they need. There is every reason to ensure that there is enough protein in the diet, but there is no evidence that a superabundant high-protein diet of 200 g per day confers any special advantage. Whether that much is worthless and wasted, or actually fattening, depends on the total caloric intake.

VITAMINS

Life could not be sustained on chemically pure protein, carbohydrate, fat, and water only. Animals and humans need to eat *foods* because foods contain additional factors necessary for survival. These accessory food substances—the vitamins and minerals—do not contribute energy, but they are nonetheless essential. They must be ingested at relatively frequent intervals throughout the life span of an individual. Because they are required in such small quantities, sometimes only in trace amounts, they are frequently referred to as micronutrients.

Vitamins are organic compounds other than amino acids, fatty acids, glycerol, or monosaccharides that are essential for normal metabolic processes. They must be components of the diet because they cannot be manufactured within body cells, or at least cannot be synthesized in the necessary amounts. The term for these food factors was coined by a Polish biochemist who was working with a substance that prevented a disease called beriberi in chickens. Because the active compound was an amine and it was necessary to the life (vita) of the chickens, he called it a "vitamine," although presumably he could just as easily have named it "aminevite." When other such factors were subsequently discovered, it was evident that they were not chemically related and hardly any of them were amines. The final "e" was dropped, and the chemicals became called vitamins. As each one was identified, it was assigned a letter name.

Today there are 13 or 14 vitamins recognized as essential to the human diet. The higher figure includes choline, which is a vitamin for various animals, although its need for humans has not been proved. Table 17–1 summarizes the 13 vitamins, their richest sources, their biological role, and the associated deficiency diseases.

Vitamin needs. Vitamin needs are expressed by means of the Dietary Reference Intakes (DRIs). The DRIs consist of four parameters, including the 1989 Recommended Dietary Allowances (RDAs), Tolerable Upper Intakes, Estimated Average Requirements, and Adequate Intakes (National Academy of Sciences, 1997).

The DRIs represent the latest attempts to identify the quantity of any given nutrient that is needed to promote optimal health and prevent chronic disease. The DRI has been established for the major nutrients involved in bone health—calcium, phosphorous, magnesium, vitamin D, and fluoride—and for the eight B vitamins and choline. For the remaining nutrients and energy, the 1989 RDAs will continue to be used until the DRIs are established.

The Estimated Average Requirement is defined as the amount of a nutrient that will maintain a specific biochemical or physiological function in half the people of a given age and sex group.

Adequate Intakes. For some nutrients, there is insufficient scientific evidence to identify a specific requirement. In these cases, an Adequate Intake is offered instead. Adequate Intake is defined as the average amount of a nutrient that appears sufficient to maintain a specified criterion. The RDAs for vitamins include a generous margin of safety to cover possible wide variations of individual needs and to provide for the possible losses of vitamins that occur with the preparation and storage of food.

Tolerable Upper Intakes. Because some nutrients can be hazardous, even deadly, in large amounts, Tolerable Upper Intake Levels have been established for some nutrients. These levels represent the maximum amount of a nutrient that appears safe for most healthy people and beyond which there is an increased risk of adverse health effects.

Should people take vitamin pills as insurance against an unbalanced diet? The only answer is—maybe. No one appears to have the definitive word. Certainly, pharmaceutical companies that manufacture vitamins would have us believe that we need supplementation to lead healthy, active lives, full of vim and vitality, and they advertise accordingly. Most nutritionists, however, maintain that taking extra vitamin pills in the presence of an adequate diet is an unnecessary expense. Furthermore, there are no scientific data to indicate the necessity for supplementation when people are eating reasonably well.

It is not too difficult to determine whether there are aspects of individual eating patterns or lifestyle that may increase the risk of inadequate vitamin intake. There are the meat and potatoes people—those who never learned to like anything green. They have stringent food preferences that limit the variety of foods ingested. Other individuals may be voluntarily restricting their diets in order to lose weight and are thereby unbalancing their nutrients. Some may be involuntarily restricting their normal diets because the cost of meat and fresh fruits and vegetables has become more than they can afford. Heavy smokers sometimes show reduced blood levels of vitamin D, and heavy drinkers are more likely to have poor eating habits. Other kinds of drugs, either over the counter (antacids, laxatives) or medically prescribed, can cause vitamin depletion by interacting with the nutrients in foods. Some of the chemotherapeutic drugs used in the treatment of cancer, certain antibiotics, and various anticoagulants can act as antivitamins or interfere with vitamin absorption, effects that could be ignored by the prescribing physicians.

Obviously, swallowing vitamin pills should never be a substitute for the optimal nutrition obtained through the wise selection of a variety of good foods. But under certain circumstances, something only individuals themselves can know, vitamin pills may be a feasible way of defending against a probable deficiency. The most sensible way to take vitamin pills, if one chooses to buy them, is to figure out which vitamins (and minerals) are potentially lacking in the diet and to supplement only the ones needed as inexpensively as possible. Because vitamins exert their effects in only small quantities, pills that contain enormous amounts

TABLE 17–1 Vitamins

Name	Rich Sources	Function	Deficiency	Potential Toxicity When Large Amounts Are Consumed
Water-soluble vitamins				
Thiamine (B$_1$)	Pork; whole grains, enriched cereal grains; legumes (lost when cereals are milled and refined)	Component of coenzyme; energy release	Beriberi; impairment of cardiovascular, nervous, and gastrointestinal systems	None; excreted in urine
Niacin (nicotinic acid)	Lean meats, liver; peanuts; yeast; cereal bran and germ	Component of two coenzyme systems; energy release	Pellagra; "4 Ds": dermatitis, diarrhea, depression, death	None; may cause harmless symptoms of flushing of skin, dizziness, and nausea
Riboflavin (B$_2$)	Milk; eggs; liver; kidney; heart; green leafy vegetables (lost in dehydrated vegetables)	Component of various enzymes involved in energy release	Dermatitis; light sensitivity of eyes to light; sores at corners of mouth	None
Pantothenic acid (B$_3$)	Liver; kidney; egg yolk; wheat bran; fresh vegetables (esp. broccoli and sweet potatoes); molasses	Component of coenzyme A; energy release	Fatigue; GI distress; personality changes; numbness and tingling of hands and feet; muscle cramps	None
Biotin	Milk; liver; kidney; egg yolk; yeast; also synthesized by bacteria in intestine	Coenzyme carrier of carbon dioxide	Scaly skin; seborrheic dermatitis in infants	None

Vitamin	Sources	Function	Deficiency	Toxicity
Folic acid (folacin; pteroylglutamic acid)	Green leafy vegetables; liver; kidney; lima beans; asparagus; whole grains; nuts; legumes; yeast	Blood-cell formation	Anemia	Generally none; reports of folate hypersensitivity, possible neurotoxicity at 15 mg daily
Cobalamin (B_{12}; cyanocobalamin)	Only foods of animal origin; beef, liver, kidney; milk; eggs; oysters; shrimp; pork; chicken	Essential for function of all cells	Anemia; nerve fiber degeneration	None
Pyridoxine (B_6)	Yeast; wheat and corn (20% lost in processing grain); egg yolk; liver; kidney; muscle meats	Components of coenzymes for protein synthesis; central nervous system metabolism	Anemia	None until doses of 600 mg; neurotoxicity, depression at megadoses
Ascorbic acid (C)	Citrus fruits; tomatoes; green vegetables	Collagen formation; capillary integrity; synthesis of adrenal cortical hormones; aids in iron absorption from intestine	Scurvy: bleeding gums; easy bruising; swollen joints; impaired wound healing	Inconclusive; reports of kidney stones, diarrhea, nausea at megadoses over 2–5 g; interference with absorption of B_{12} and trace minerals

(continues)

TABLE 17-1 (continued)

Name	Rich Sources	Function	Deficiency	Potential Toxicity When Large Amounts Are Consumed
Fat-soluble vitamins				
A (A alcohol = retinol; A aldehyde = retinal; A acid = retinoic acid)	Whole milk; liver; kidney; cream, butter; egg yolk; yellow and green vegetables; fruits	Night vision; growth; reproduction; health of epithelial cells; cell membrane maintenance	Night blindness; skin lesions	Very toxic in high doses of 20–30 × requirement; effects reverse on discontinuation
D (ergocalciferol = D_2; cholecalciferol = D_3)	Fatty fish; eggs; liver; butter, fortified milk; cod-liver oil; also through exposure to ultraviolet light	Normal bone formation; promotes absorption and retention of calcium and phosphorus	Rickets in children; osteomalacia in adults	Highly toxic in large doses; possibly fatal in children
E (alpha-to-copherol)	Wheat germ oils; other vegetable oils; beef liver; milk; eggs; butter; leafy vegetables	May function as antioxidant in tissues; possible role in prevention of cell degeneration	None known in humans; sterility; muscular dystrophy; red cell fragility in animals	Reportedly nontoxic up to 1 g/day; effects of long-term megadoses unknown
K (naphthoquinones)	Synthesized by intestinal bacteria; also lettuce, spinach, kale, cauliflower	Essential for blood clotting	Increased clotting time	None

in excess of the RDA are more costly and a waste of money. In some instances, an excessive intake can have adverse effects.

Reasonable quantities of the water-soluble vitamins are safe to take. If unneeded by the body, they are merely going to be excreted to provide the sewage system with vitamin supplementation. (Someone once said that the greatest source of vitamins is middle-class urine.) Excessive amounts of water-soluble vitamins have been found to be harmful, and the overconsumption of fat-soluble vitamins can be toxic. Vitamins A and D are stored in the body for long periods of time, are metabolized very slowly, and are excreted with great difficulty by way of the bile. It is virtually impossible, however, to get too much A or D from the diet, and the only way for toxic effects to occur is by taking these vitamins in tablet or capsule form. Daily ingestion of more than 25,000 International Units (I.U.s) of A (30,000–100,000 I.U.) will cause toxicity, with neurological symptoms of irritability and headache, liver problems that can lead to cirrhosis, and dermatological problems such as brittle nails and dry, rough skin. Excessive vitamin A can also be teratogenic to fetuses.

Carotene, a plant pigment found in carrots, sweet potatoes, apricots, peaches, and other yellow and orange fruits and vegetables, is the provitamin for A, which is converted to vitamin A in the body cells after ingestion. Plants contain a number of carotenoid pigments; but the alpha, beta, and gamma carotenes as well as cryptoxanthine, the yellow pigment in corn, are those important in human nutrition. Beta-carotene, along with vitamins C and E, is an antioxidant nutrient. Antioxidants like these and antioxidant enzymes are compounds that deactivate the millions of harmful free radicals in the body formed as a side effect when the body cells use oxygen. Free radicals are unstable molecules that can damage tissue, and a number of studies have suggested that a higher intake of antioxidants is related to a lower incidence of such diseases as cancer, heart disease, rheumatoid arthritis, or cataracts and also can slow the aging process. This is why fruits and vegetables containing beta-carotene, vitamin C, and vitamin E should be eaten daily. A

National Academy of Sciences recommendation is that five servings of vegetables and fruit should be consumed daily. If that sounds like a lot of fruit and vegetables, a half a cup of small or diced fruit or of vegetables is considered a serving. So is a small apple, banana, or orange.

The reason it is better to get vitamins from foods rather than relying on supplements is that the foods also provide additional nutrients, some of which may also protect against disease. Moreover, the epidemiological research that linked the antioxidant vitamins with disease protection was based on high fruit and vegetable intake in the populations studied and not on people taking vitamin pills. Unlike vitamin A, beta-carotene in supplemental form is nontoxic because the body can regulate its conversion to vitamin A. Whether supplement pills of beta-carotene, C, and E beyond dietary intake would retard aging or prevent disease is as yet unknown.

Like vitamin A, excessive vitamin D—more than 50,000–75,000 I.U. per day—will cause toxic symptoms and possibly the development of kidney and bone disease. Even consumption of far lesser amounts could increase intestinal uptake and decrease intestinal excretion of calcium. The results may be unwanted calcium deposits in soft tissues (kidney, heart, lung, arteries).

Natural versus Synthetic Vitamins

In almost any drugstore, there are several kinds of vitamin preparations on the shelf. If the pharmacy is part of a large chain, the "name" brand will be more expensive than the "house" brand. In health food stores, the vitamins are presumably "natural" and are even more costly. Vitamins labeled natural have presumably been extracted from a food rather than formulated synthetically in the laboratory. Many people, believing that natural vitamins are superior and provide special benefits, appear to be quite willing to pay a high price for the products so labeled.

All of the compounds presently considered vitamins have been isolated. Their chemical formulas are known and, with the exception of vitamin B_{12}, they can all be synthesized in the laboratory. In manufacturing synthetic vitamins, the same chemicals found in nature are used. The same chemical reactions that take place in the cells are duplicated. In every way, the synthetics are identical in structure and biological activity to the vitamins occurring naturally in foods, and no form of chemical analysis or biological assay can tell them apart. Not only are there no known advantages to "natural" vitamins, but there is some question about how natural they are. In the *Journal of Nutritional Education,* pharmacologist Adolph Kamil described a visit to two manufacturers of natural vitamins in California. These companies make most of the preparations sold under the famous natural brand names in health food stores and drugstores across the country. He discovered that while "Rose Hips Vitamin C Tablets" contained some naturally extracted C, there was also a lot of additional synthetic ascorbic acid or C in the preparation. The reason for the addition was that natural rose hips contain only 2% vitamin C. If no synthetic were added, he was informed, "the tablet would have to be as big as a golf ball." Because the labels on the finished bottles neglected to mention the additional source of vitamin C, the consumer presumes that the product is entirely extracted from rose hips.

In a similar fashion, the natural B vitamins were composed of large amounts of synthetic B compounds combined with small amounts that had come from yeast and other natural sources. Of all the manufactured vitamins, only vitamin E was actually completely derived from vegetable oils. It also was sold as inexpensively as the synthetic variety. As Kamil pointed out, however, the wheat germ, soy, and corn from which the E was extracted *was not* organically grown, that is, without the usual chemical fertilizers and pesticides. Moreover, the vitamin was concentrated using the usual chemical solvents and procedures, and even the gelatin capsule in which it was enclosed contained a chemical preservative to keep it from getting rancid. All in all, the result was hardly a natural or organic vitamin E.

Vitamins, whether extracted from food sources or chemically synthesized, are the same in every way except price. Anyone who wants the benefits of natural vitamins should spend the extra money to get them the most natural way—from the nutritious foods that contain them.

High-Dose Vitamin Therapy

Knowing that illness can result from the absence or insufficiency of a particular vitamin tends to promote the idea that if a little of that substance is good, a lot is going to be better. It is tempting to believe that something as easily available and relatively inexpensive as vitamin pills can have miracle powers to provide superhealth. There are many claims for the preventive and curative effects of massive doses of the various vitamins. Although there are many proponents of such megavitamin therapy, there is no really convincing evidence to confirm the advantages of excessive consumption. It should also be emphasized that when huge amounts of a vitamin are taken to alleviate a disease that is not the result of a nutritional deficiency, the vitamin is likely to be acting as a pharmacological agent or drug, and not in the usual manner as a vitamin. Self-prescribed long-term supplementation can be vitamin abuse, not use.

Intake of vitamin A in excess of nutritional requirements has been claimed to improve vision, prevent infection, and protect against cancer. Greater than the RDA for vitamin D, especially when taken in codfish liver oil—the "natural" way—has been said to have all kinds of benefits. There is no scientific substantiation for the claims that large doses of A and D in the absence of deficiency are beneficial in any way. As previously indicated, the abuse of A and D is actually dangerous.

Vitamin E has been advocated for almost everything—leg cramps, asthma, coronary heart disease, sterility, impotence, ulcers, burns, wound healing, high cholesterol, menopausal symptoms, prevention of cataracts, and aging—to mention only a few of them. Although hundreds of studies on vitamin E have been conducted and some have shown promising results on the prevention of cataract formation, enhancement of the immune system, reduction of the risks of cancer and heart disease, and alleviation of some of the symptoms of Parkinson's disease and other disorders, there is currently insufficient basis for any definite answers. More research and evaluation is needed before the benefits of large doses of E can be confirmed. The RDA for vitamin E is 10 mg of alpha-tocopherol, the most potent form. This is equivalent to 30 I.U.s. Most research has failed to find any toxic effects for doses 10 times the RDA, but most of the soft gel tablets available in health food stores and that people are taking are 400 I.U. each, or 13.3 times the RDA.

After Nobel Prize laureate Linus Pauling wrote the book *Vitamin C and the Common Cold,* millions of people began to take ascorbic acid in the recommended 1–5 g daily so they could prevent the most common of human ailments. An imposing 15 g daily was advised for treatment of a cold. There was not enough data to confirm or deny the benefit of high intake of C to prevent colds, although there are some indications that increased ingestion of C may reduce the severity, if not the incidence, of colds. Pauling also pursued the idea of vitamin C being effective against cancer through enhancement of natural resistance to the disease, and in collaboration with other proponents, conducted studies that reported a beneficial effect on cancer patients. At a symposium sponsored by the National Cancer Institute to assess the biological functions of vitamin C and its relation to cancer, one of the researchers summarized current epidemiological data on the role of ascorbic acid in cancer prevention. Of 46 epidemiological studies, 33 have reported significant protective effects on cancer from vitamin C. Evidence exists for reduction of risk for cancers of the esophagus, larynx, oral cavity, pancreas, stomach, rectum, lung, breast, and uterine cervix. Again, these studies were based on consumption of vitamin C in food, not as supplements, so other components in fruit or other unknown factors may confer additional protection. The conference participants also reviewed the antioxidant functions of vitamin C, its relation to the immune system, its inhibiting effects on tumor growth, both *in vitro* and *in vivo,* and its ability

to reduce the toxic effects of radiation in experimental animals (Henson, Block, & Levine, 1991). The case for vitamin C in the prevention of cancer, however, appears stronger than for the treatment of cancer, which is still very controversial.

Vitamin C ingestion has been generally viewed as nontoxic, but massive consumption may not be harmless in some individuals. Although the data have been disputed, Herbert and Jacob (1974) showed that large doses of C can destroy vitamin B_{12} when the two are ingested in foods together, thus potentially interfering with the absorption and metabolism of B_{12}. A rebound scurvy effect can develop when megavitamin doses of C are withdrawn (Siegel, Barker, & Kunstadter, 1982), and Cochrane (1965) reported that babies born to mothers who took more than 400 mg of C during pregnancy later developed scurvy although they were fed a normal diet. The feeding of large doses of C to laboratory animals has caused diarrhea, very acid urine, and bladder and kidney stones; and gastrointestinal symptoms have occurred in some people on greater than 1-g doses. In general, it would be wise to be cautious in taking really substantial amounts of vitamin C until more information is available. Moreover, anyone having a complete physical examination should be aware that fecal excretion of vitamin C interferes with the fecal occult blood test for colon cancer and should abstain from C ingestion for several days before the exam.

Some vitamin preparations that contain 10–15 times the RDA for the B-complex vitamins are called "stress-formula," under the assumption that such high potency in these vitamins will relieve emotional distress and depression. Since the B vitamins are necessary for the metabolic function of all cells, they are, of course, essential for the proper function of nerve cells. It is not surprising that a deficiency of any one of them—thiamine, riboflavin, niacin, pantothenic acid, folic acid, biotin, B_6, and B_{12}—would produce mental symptoms. There is no evidence to indicate that during periods of emotional stress and in the absence of deficiency, taking amounts of B vitamins in excess of the RDA is of any benefit. The idea may have originated in studies that reported that the occasional depression that occurs in women on oral contraceptives was linked to an absolute vitamin B_6 deficiency. When the vitamin was administered, the symptoms of depression were relieved (Adams et al., 1973). It is also known that a riboflavin deficiency is more frequent during periods of physiological stress (after surgery, trauma, illness) and during pregnancy and rapid growth periods in children. There are many who believe, however, that psychological stress also increases the need for the B vitamins, but there is little corroboration for the supposition.

Orthomolecular psychiatry is a controversial method of treatment that advocates megavitamin therapy for such emotional disorders as schizophrenia, hyperactivity of children, childhood autism, and various kinds of neuroses and psychoses. Orthomolecular psychiatrists may still use the traditional forms of treatment but also add very high doses of water-soluble vitamins and, frequently, special diets. The usefulness of megavitamin therapy in the treatment of psychiatric disorders has been challenged by the American Psychiatric Association, and the methods and claims of its practitioners have not been well accepted by most psychiatrists.

The true believers in a megavitamin dosage hailed the practice as an exciting breakthrough. The critics denounced it as faddist with the possibility of adverse effects. Megavitamin therapy may be beneficial, but, unfortunately, one can never be completely certain currently that taking doses of nutrients at 20–100 times their usual daily level does not have some potential for harm. Generally speaking, an excess or "mega"-anything taken into the body frequently turns out ultimately to have undesirable effects.

Vitaminlike Compounds

For a substance to be classified as a vitamin, there are certain criteria to be met. For one thing, the compound must have an established biological role; that is, it has to be a proved essential dietary requirement, the absence of which would lead to a visible deficiency. Second, true vitamins are not able to be synthesized in the body's cells in adequate amounts to meet physio-

logical needs. Finally, the established vitamins are present in foods in very small quantities and exert their metabolic effects at very low levels. While these requirements may seem somewhat arbitrary, they do define, on the basis of current knowledge, the concept of what constitutes a vitamin.

Choline is a substance frequently listed with the B vitamins, although it can be synthesized in the body from the amino acid glycine. While it is known to be a vitamin for many young animals, its need by humans has never been established. Choline in animals is necessary to prevent the accumulation of fat in their livers, but although fat infiltration of the liver is common in chronic alcoholism or in protein-calorie deficiency, feeding choline has never been successful in curing this disorder in humans. Choline, however, does have many important functions in the body. It is a component of cell membranes and of myelin, the insulating covering around the nerve fibers. It is a part of the lipoproteins involved in the transport of fat-soluble substances and is necessary for the synthesis of acetylcholine, which functions in the transmission of nerve impulses.

The sugarlike inositol and para-aminobenzoic acid (PABA), also sometimes included in the B vitamins, are important growth factors for lower animals or microorganisms, but there is no evidence that they are vitamins for humans.

Bioflavonoids are a group of compounds that include hesperidin, rutin, flavonones, flavones, and flavonols. They are widely distributed in plant foods, found particularly in citrus and other fruits, berries, such vegetables as cabbages, brussels sprouts, and onions, and in tea, vinegar, and red wine. It is estimated that the average daily intake of flavonoids amounts to about a gram from a normal mixed diet. There is evidence that some bioflavonoids have an antibacterial and antiviral activity. There has also been research to indicate that many of the flavones appear to have a tumor-inhibiting effect. The substances also have a vitamin C–like activity, and large doses have been used therapeutically in patients with increased capillary fragility or permeability. While a bioflavonoid deficiency has been produced in animals, it has never been demonstrated for humans.

Minerals in Human Nutrition

Of all the 92 naturally occurring chemical elements in nature, more than 50 are found in human body tissues. Fewer than half of these are known to be essential to human body function. Those minerals known to be required in the diet at levels of 100 mg daily or more include calcium, phosphorus, sodium, potassium, chlorine, magnesium, and sulfur. Pertinent information concerning their source and function is listed in Table 17–2. The remaining mineral nutrients are called *trace elements* because they are needed in daily amounts of only a few milligrams. They are listed in Table 17–3.

There are a number of minerals found in minute quantities in the body. They include tin, nickel, silicon, and vanadium. These are elements that *may* be essential and vital in human metabolic processes, but no human requirements have been established for them as yet.

With the possible exception of iron in women who have heavy or prolonged menstrual periods, deficiencies of the trace minerals are rare in developed countries. In the opinion of some researchers, however, the current popularity of high-fiber diets could result in various mineral deficiencies, most notably calcium. Evidently, increasing the fiber content of the diet may impair the absorption of iron, copper, and calcium from the intestine. There has also been a suggestion that a chemical reaction between phytic acid in fiber and some minerals, such as calcium, causes trace mineral inactivation.

Taking huge doses of trace mineral supplements in the belief that they enhance energy or protect against disease is risky, despite the advice of the salespersons in health food stores. For example, zinc supplementation is known to cause copper deficiency and anemia. Broun, Griest, Tricot, and Hoffman (1990) described cases of a life-threatening form of anemia and bone marrow depression caused by ingestion of excess zinc. The authors concluded that daily consumption of 100–150 mg of elemental zinc will result in copper excretion, a negative copper balance, and the likelihood of anemia.

Dietary Guides

People are born knowing how, but not what, to eat. There is no inherent instinct that makes us choose a properly balanced diet. In fact, there appears to be every evidence that left to their own devices, people will probably select diets that are inadequate to meet the body's requirements for essential nutrients. Perhaps the human body utilizes proteins, carbohydrates, fats, vitamins, and minerals, but individuals eat *food,* not nutrients. And food is not just an adequate diet. Food means Mom, home, and the family—love and emotional identity. Food is not just for hunger; it means comfort when one is upset and a reward when one is being indulgent. Food is getting Chinese carryout, having a pizza delivered, a dinner party, or splurging in a restaurant. There can be any number of social and psychological considerations that affect eating and food choices, and getting good nutrition at the same time is not automatic. People have to be educated to select the foods consistent with optimal health. One practical approach to nutrition education is the use of the Food Guide Pyramid (Figure 17–3).

The Food Guide Pyramid helps consumers by recommending the type and quantity of foods to eat from five major food groups. The suggested amounts per day are 6–11 servings of bread, cereals, and other grains; 3–5 servings of vegetables; 2–4 servings of fruits; 2–3 servings of meat, fish, poultry, and alternatives; 2 servings per day of milk, cheese, or yogurt. It is also recommended that consumers use fats, oils, and sweets sparingly because they provide food energy while contributing few nutrients. Miscellaneous food not high in calories such as spices, herbs, coffee, tea,

TABLE 17–2 Essential Minerals Needed in Amounts of 100 mg/Day or More

Element	RDA (adults)	Rich Sources	Functions in Body
Calcium	800 mg	Milk, cheese; leafy vegetables, legumes, nuts; whole grain cereals; bones from sardines and other canned fish	Normal bone and teeth structure, muscular contraction, blood coagulation, nerve membrane stability
Phosphorus	800 mg	Protein-rich foods	Normal bone and teeth structure, production and transfer of high energy phosphates, absorption and transportation of other nutrients, regulation of acid-base balance
Sodium	5 g (five times more than actual physiological need)	All food, table salt	Osmotic pressure of body fluids, muscle function, permeability of all cells
Potassium	4 g	All foods	Muscular activity, especially heart, and proper nerve function
Chlorine	Same as sodium	All foods, table salt	Osmotic pressure regulation, water balance, acid balance
Magnesium	350 mg	Most foods, especially vegetables; milk, meat, cocoa, nuts, soybeans	Enzyme activity, energy release, nerve and muscle function
Sulfur	0.6–1.6 g	All proteins, particularly those rich in cystine and methionine	Component of vitamins, hormones, enzyme systems, important in detoxification mechanisms

TABLE 17–3 Essential Trace Elements

Element	RDA (adults)	Rich Sources	Functions in Body
Iron	10 mg (males), 15 mg (females)	Organ meats (liver, heart, kidney, spleen), egg yolk, fish, oysters, whole wheat, beans, figs, dates, molasses, green vegetables	Oxygen transport, cellular respiration
Copper	2.5 mg	Liver, kidney, shellfish, nuts, raisins, dried legumes	Enzyme component, hemoglobin formation
Cobalt	Unknown	Animal protein sources	Part of Vitamin B$_{12}$
Zinc	15 mg	Meat, especially liver, eggs, seafoods, milk, grain	Enzyme component, part of insulin molecule
Manganese	300–350 mg(?)	Bananas, whole grains, leafy vegetables	Normal bone structure, normal function of reproductive and nervous systems
Iodine	100–140 micrograms	Fish, iodized table salt	Necessary for normal thyroid function
Molybdenum	Unknown	Beef kidney, legumes, some cereals	Enzyme component
Selenium	Unknown, probably 50–100 micrograms is adequate	Seafood, meat, grains raised in selenium-rich soil	Enzyme component, similar to vitamin E in function
Chromium	Unknown, probably 20–50 micrograms is adequate	Meat, corn oil	Normal glucose metabolism
Fluorine	1–2 mg	Fluoridated water, milk	Resistance to dental caries

and diet soft drinks can be used freely. The guide is depicted in the form of a pyramid to indicate that the grains, at the base, deserve most emphasis in the diet, while items at the tip, consisting of fats, oils, and sweets, are meant to be used sparingly.

Today's eating habits have changed considerably. There are new categories: "health foods," "junk foods," "fast foods," and engineered or synthetic foods. Surveys have indicated that Americans now spend one-third of their food budgets at restaurants, mostly of the fast-food chain variety. The country has seen a veritable explosion of carryout or eat-it-there quickie and relatively inexpensive places. Preparing meals from scratch takes more time, time that a working man or woman may not have, and convenience foods have become a major dietary inclusion for many people. The food companies, scrambling over each other to cash in on the convenience food dollar, have produced

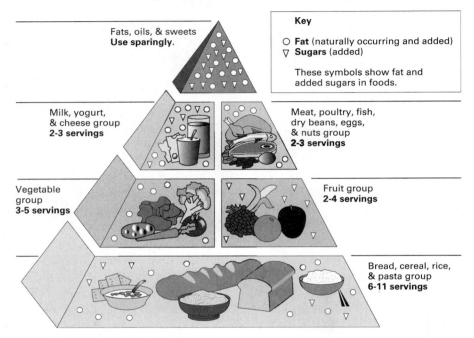

The Food Guide Pyramid
A guide to daily food choices

Fats, oils, & sweets
Use sparingly.

Key

○ **Fat** (naturally occurring and added)
▽ **Sugars** (added)

These symbols show fat and
added sugars in foods.

Milk, yogurt,
& cheese group
2-3 servings

Meat, poultry, fish,
dry beans, eggs,
& nuts group
2-3 servings

Vegetable
group
3-5 servings

Fruit group
2-4 servings

Bread, cereal, rice,
& pasta group
6-11 servings

Figure 17–3   Food Guide Pyramid. (Courtesy of USDA and DHHS, 1992. The Food Guide Pyramid: A guide to daily food choices. Leaflet No. 572, Washington, D.C.)

a number of products for the supermarket shelves and freezers to compete with the fast-food chains. How do these new foods fit into the Food Guide Pyramid?

A typical contemporary diet may be balanced, but a new form of malnutrition—overnutrition, rather than undernutrition, is now a danger. For example, a Big Mac covers several food groups: meat, dairy, vegetable, and bread and is thus properly "balanced." But although that Big Mac (or a Double Whopper or any other fast-food equivalent) is apparently nutritionally sound, it provides more than 1,100 calories, more than 14 teaspoons of fat (mostly saturated), and more sodium than anyone needs when it is eaten with large fries and a chocolate shake.

The grouping of foods is an effective and easy way of learning about a nutritious diet. Because it is gener-

ally taught at the elementary school level, it can impress upon children the necessity of eating a variety of foods and getting fresh fruits and vegetables daily. If people past grade school continue to consume smaller amounts of dairy and protein two times per day and increased amounts of cereals, fruits, and vegetables more times daily, they are certain to be choosing an adequate diet. Many adult Americans, however, would welcome and use a more complex and sophisticated approach to selecting their meals. There has been an increasing awareness that it is not so much that "you are what you eat" but that what you eat may largely determine what you are (or whether you are) 20 or 30 years from now. The payoff of today's good nutrition could be the prevention of the killer diseases that accompany aging.

*Ē*ATING RIGHT IN THE NEW MILLENNIUM

It is generally acknowledged that the nation's eating habits—its convenience foods, its snacks, and its sweets—are gnawing away at its health. We conquered malnutrition caused by deficiencies—hardly anyone gets rickets, pellagra, and beriberi anymore. We have replaced these diseases with the malnutrition caused by oversufficiency. But although consumers have a vested interest in nutritional education, every time the government has attempted to provide some guidelines to sensible eating, it has generated huge controversies.

The first effort came in the form of a report prepared by the Senate Select Committee on Nutrition and Human Needs. First released in 1977 and revised in early 1978, the report, called *Dietary Goals for the United States,* was both praised and vehemently attacked. The dietary goals were an unprecedented attempt to change the high-fat, cholesterol, sugar, and salt consumption of the American public. Essentially the goals recommended the following:

1. Reduce the overall fat consumption from the current 40%–45% in the diet to about 30% of the caloric intake.
2. Reduce the amount of saturated fat so that it amounts to only about 10% of the total energy intake; then balance that with polyunsaturated and monounsaturated fats, which should then account for about 10% of energy intake each.
3. Reduce the amount of cholesterol ingested to about 300 mg daily.
4. Reduce salt intake so that it amounts to only 5 g or 1 teaspoon per day.
5. Increase the consumption of complex carbohydrates and naturally occurring sugars from about 28% intake to about 48% of energy intake. Reduce the consumption of refined and processed sugars down to about only 10% of total intake.
6. To avoid overweight, decrease energy intake and increase energy expenditure.

The dietary goals were basically the same recommendations made for a "prudent diet" by the American Heart Association in 1973. The goals, however, were emphatically denounced by many scientists and several special interest groups. The National Livestock and Meat Board objected because of the implied recommendation to reduce consumption of meat and increase consumption of poultry and fish. The egg producers protested reducing egg ingestion. The sugar interests said there was no scientific basis for lowering sugar intake. The National Canners Association was displeased that there was the suggestion that more fresh or frozen vegetables should be used. The American Medical Association's statement (1977) contended that there was insufficient evidence that diet was related to disease and that dietary advice should not be prescribed to the general population but is best dispensed by physicians to their individual patients.

In 1980, the United States Department of Health and Human Services and the United States Department of Agriculture, with an eye toward the vehement controversy engendered by the goals, jointly issued essentially the same message but framed it in words carefully chosen to offend fewer lobbies. The *Seven Dietary Guidelines* said the following:

1. Avoid too much fat, saturated fat, and cholesterol.
2. Eat a variety of foods.
3. Maintain ideal weight.
4. Eat foods with adequate starch and fiber.
5. Avoid too much sugar.
6. Avoid too much sodium.
7. If you drink alcohol, do so in moderation.

Another report, issued in 1982 by the National Academy of Sciences' National Research Council, did little to allay the controversy and created additional disagreement. Called *Interim Dietary Guidelines on Diet, Nutrition, and Cancer,* this statement again called for reduction of fat intake by 25% to reduce breast and prostate cancer and added the avoidance of salt-cured, salt-pickled, and smoked foods to reduce the incidence of esophageal and stomach cancer. There was also the recommendation to add more fruits, vegetables, and whole grains to the diet, especially those containing vitamin C and vitamin A, with a particular admonition to include cruciferous vegetables—cabbage, cauliflower, broccoli, and brussels sprouts, which have been identified as possible defenses against cancer. Alcohol was to be used in moderation, especially in smokers, because the combination of smoking and alcohol is associated with a greater incidence of certain cancers.

To continue the chronology of efforts to get the public to change its eating habits to reduce the incidence of disease, the *Dietary Guidelines* were reissued in 1985, 1990, and 1995. The advice was essentially unchanged; the differences in the wording reflected an evolution based upon the nutrition research accumulated during the 1980s and 1990s. The advice on weight, for example, went from "Maintain ideal weight" in 1980 to "Maintain desirable weight" in 1985 to "Maintain healthy weight" in 1990 to "Balance the food you eat with exercise" in 1995. Other revisions included the change from "Eat foods with adequate starch and fiber" to "Choose a diet with plenty of vegetables, fruits, and grain products," which emphasizes which foods to eat rather than their content. Regarding fat in the diet, the advice to "Avoid too much" that was in the previous guidelines changed in 1990 to "Choose a diet low in fat, saturated fat, and cholesterol," and the recommendations on sugar, salt, and sodium also went from "Avoid too much . . ." to "Choose a diet (sugars, salt, and sodium) only in moderation." The guidelines on alcohol and on eating a variety of foods remained unchanged.

It is undeniable that actual *proof* that high dietary fat causes heart attacks and breast and colon cancer, that high salt consumption causes hypertension, and that high sugar consumption causes diabetes and heart disease is lacking. There also are no guarantees that the fiber and vitamins in fruits and vegetables will lower the risk of cancer. There are only epidemiological studies that suggest *correlations* between diet and those diseases. Heredity, age, and in some instances, gender, are acknowledged to be risk factors of higher priority. But there is no way in which we can change our genes, age, or sex—we are stuck with our characteristics. Following the guidelines is a prudent and not terribly drastic way to lower one of the risk factors—an overly rich diet. Perhaps there are only correlative data pointing to the value of the recommended ways of eating, but there have never been *any* data to suggest that reducing fat, cholesterol, sugar, and salt and increasing fruits and vegetables and whole grains are in any way correlated to a disease process. Eating to achieve the goals or guidelines is not an improper diet; it will result in a wholesome and nutritious diet. The recommendations constitute no threat to health and, from all indications, are likely to promote health.

When the messages on what to eat get mixed, however, and when the questions of how and in what manner nutrition affects health and disease are mired in controversy, all of us can become more vulnerable to the advice of the self-styled "authorities" who proclaim that they know the true way to superhealth and energy. Who, after all, does not want to be brimming with vim and vigor and glowing with vitality? A mishmash of misinformation is easily accessible through some magazine articles and popular books, from promoters of various food supplements, and by word of mouth. Many of the articles are likely to contain a nugget of fact buried in a mound of hypotheses. Because there is much about nutrition that still remains to be determined, it is impossible to categorically prove or disprove all the claims. Fortunately, most of the food mythology is harmless. Because special foods or food supplements may be bought in special stores, nutrition misinformation may have its greatest effect on the pocketbook. There is always the potential of harm, however, when people take seriously such notions as "pasteurizing milk destroys its enzymes" or that "fasting and enemas cleanse the body of noxious poisons." And when all health problems are self-diagnosed as being caused by nutritional inadequacy and self-treated by nutritional or "metabolic" therapy, real danger to health exists.

Several physician "experts" have written best-selling books on weight reduction that contain unsubstantiated nutritional advice of highly dubious value, illustrating that some doctors are equally guilty of spreading nutritional nonsense. It is not usually recognized that doctors frequently know as little or less about nutritional matters than their patients. The amount of nutritional education physicians get during their professional training is very sparse, and few ever receive a formal nutrition course in medical school. Eminent nutritionist Jean Mayer, the late president of Tufts University, had charged that the nutrition teaching in most medical curricula was, and still is, "miserable." Although the need to upgrade the education of physicians in nutrition has been recognized, and about 100 of the 134 medical schools in the United States and Canada now offer "some sort of course," according to the Association of Medical Colleges, relatively few schools have a mandatory course incorporated into a doctor's undergraduate or graduate education.

With a little effort, excellent information about health, nutrition, and food safety can be obtained by subscription or at the library from a number of monthly publications put out by consumer advocacy groups or universities, registered dietitians, or other sources. These newsletters include the *Nutrition Action Health Letter,* published by the Center for Science in the Public Interest; the *Tufts University Diet and Nutrition Letter;* the *Mayo Clinic Nutrition Letter;* the *University of California, Berkeley Wellness Letter; Nutrition and Health,* from Columbia University; and *Environmental Nutrition,* published by a group of RDs, Environmental Nutrition, Inc. They provide up-to-date, in-depth articles on all aspects of nutrition. But even if one were to subscribe to every one of these publications, it would be clear that at this time, no one has all the answers on nutritional issues. Even with the scientific studies or clinical research currently under way, it is unlikely that any new pill, mineral supplement, special food, or dietary regime that is going to guarantee good health and long life will be discovered. One must always be wary of claims for the exaggerated virtues of a particular food, foods, or other nutrients. Promises of a quick cure for illness through diet or supplements should be viewed with skepticism, especially if the dietary supplements are sold by the promiser.

ARE HEALTH FOODS HEALTHIER?

Depending on whom one asks, health foods could be considered all, some, or none of the following: (1) minimally processed foods that contain no chemical additives; (2) wheat germ, protein supplements, sunflower and pumpkin seeds, various kinds of sprouts, and other brown, bland, and uninteresting foods; (3) plant foods that are organically grown in soils fertilized only with manure or compost and without the addition of pesticides; (4) foods bought in a health food store and costing more money.

Because the terms "natural," "organic," and "health" are used so frequently and for so many products, it is not surprising that they have become almost impossible to define in any kind of meaningful way. Even a tobacco company proclaims that its cigarettes use only "natural flavorings." When those words are used in relation to foods, however, most people usually think of the back-to-nature foods—simpler, whole, unrefined, unfabricated. Such foods have always been available, but it is only recently that one finds that higher prices must be paid for the privilege of buying them. As many food companies have discovered, there are big bucks in the health food industry.

There is apparently little chance that food can be grown in any large-scale quantities without retaining some traces of lingering pesticides. Although no reports of illness have directly been attributed to pesticide residues on foods, the possibility of harm exists. Without insecticides and rodenticides, however, crop losses would be inevitable, and the diseases carried by insects and rodents would become health hazards. Since most of our foods contain various residues, a certain amount of pesticide contamination is impossible to avoid. In one study, 55 products purchased at a health food store contained a greater incidence of pesticide traces than similar products not called "health" or "natural" (Barrett & Knight, 1976). Obviously, the level, or toxic threshold, for a potentially hazardous substance is very important. The federal government is responsible for making certain that pesticides as well as other environmental contaminants in food do not exceed established tolerance levels for safety. The public relies on agencies such as the Agriculture Department, the Environmental Protection Agency, and the FDA for protection. That these agencies could be doing a better job of checking food safety often has been charged by consumer groups, and reports of contamination by drugs, pesticides, bacteria, or general bacteria in meat, poultry, or fish are frequent. Accusations of additional gaps in the government inspection of foods for antibiotics, lead, and food dyes also have been discouraging. But the consumer might take comfort in the fact that at least consumer advocate groups are watching the watchdogs.

Not all of the chemicals intentionally added to foods are harmful, and some are of definite benefit to the consumer. We may have been educated to know the value of whole grain products, for example, and recognize that we should eat whole wheat bread and bran muffins. An overwhelming majority of the population still prefers to eat white bread, pancakes, and English muffins. White flour is, therefore, enriched with thiamin, niacin, riboflavin, and iron to partially restore some of the nutrients lost in the milling of whole wheat. Milk is fortified with vitamin D, margarine with vitamin A, and salt with iodine. There are even some substances, such as benzoic acid, that are naturally found in certain foods at levels greater than that permitted as additives. But although there is little evidence, as some popular writers have alleged, that we are slowly being poisoned by our food supply, not all food additives have been systematically and thoroughly tested. It is possible that some are capable of posing a real threat to health.

Two chemicals that are suspect are BHA and BHT. Butylated hydroxyanisole and butylated hydroxytoluene are antioxidants. They are added to fat-containing foods to extend their shelf life and prevent them from becoming rancid. BHA and BHT are added to cereal packaging, gum, vegetable oil, shortening, snack foods, and most oil-containing products. Improved manufacturing techniques have largely eliminated any

necessity for the addition of these antioxidants, and they provide no benefit. Studies in which animals have ingested large quantities of BHA and BHT have produced inconclusive results, but many believe that these two chemicals have not been adequately tested for carcinogenicity or other potentially adverse effects.

On the other hand, and in one more example of the inconsistencies and controversies in nutritional research, mutagenic substances for bacteria are generally assumed to be more or less carcinogenic in humans. Antioxidants such as propyl gallate and BHA have been shown to effectively inhibit mutagen formation.

Another questionable additive that may ultimately be banned is sodium nitrite. Nitrites are added to cured or smoked meats, poultry, and pickled fish to prevent botulism (a lethal form of food poisoning) and in the case of meat, to add an appealing red color and distinctive cured taste. It has been known since the late 1960s that the added nitrites combine with protein derivatives called amines to form nitrosamines, proven carcinogens (especially stomach cancer) in laboratory animals. Not only nitrosamines, but the nitrites themselves are evidently capable of causing cancer in laboratory rats. The presence of salt in these foods may be a promoting or enhancing factor for the formation of carcinogens. The government appears to be aiming toward a gradual phaseout of the use of nitrites while giving the meat industry time to develop alternative methods of preservation. Foods containing nitrites are estimated to account for about 7% of the food supply. The public could probably get along without the color or even the taste imparted by nitrites, but in the absence of other ways to prevent botulism, an outright ban on the additive would effectively remove such common foods as hot dogs, ham, bacon, and luncheon meats from the diet. There are many who believe the loss would not be that great. Because these foods have a high saturated fat content, are an expensive source of protein, and contain an additive of uncertain safety, they should be avoided and eaten only occasionally.

In final analysis, it is worth looking for foods without certain additives, but these need not necessarily be purchased in a health food store or carry a premium price. The food industry has recognized that the words "all natural, no preservatives or additives" are golden, and many foods now carry that designation. It is still important to read the label to make certain that unwanted substances are not in the ingredients. The supermarket, moreover, has a whole line of health foods—whole wheat flour, buckwheat groats, wheat germ and bran, dried fruits, polyunsaturated oils without antioxidants—and the cost may not be as high. The produce department is full of health foods, and so is the dairy section. If one wants specialty or more exotic items, they are likely to be found only in the specialty health food shops, but the regular stores have always had the staples that are equally as nutritious and less expensive.

JUNK FOOD

Like health food, junk food may have several definitions. To the nutrition experts, food that is excessively high in fat and sugar content relative to the amount of other nutrients, is nutritional trash, "empty calories" that will fatten instead of nourish. To the food industry, however, which spends millions of advertising dollars to entice the public to eat the high-calorie, low-nutrient, sugar-rich items, the foods are not junk at all. They are high-quality snack foods—soda pop, candy, cookies, pastries, various kinds of chips and curls, and the "nutritious" sugar-coated breakfast cereals. These products are so heavily promoted that it is almost impossible for an average TV watcher to remain unsusceptible to their mouth-watering "crunchy" or "creamy-smooth" goodness. Even those who make every effort to consume nourishing food—those nutritious low-fat, plenty of fruits and vegetables, whole grain kinds of meals—cannot be blamed for the occasional lapse from virtuous eating. Almost everyone sometimes indulges in the munchies. If gastronomic heaven means Twinkies, Mallomars, or a bag of Cheetos, Neetos, Fritos, or Doritos every once in a while, it is not a very large sin. Satisfying a junk-food yen is of

little significance if overall nutrition is good, and no one can expect to be totally wholesome all the time. The real problem with junk occurs when it becomes the main course, when the stuff from the vending machine or the candy stand substitutes for lunch or dinner and crowds the other nutrients out of the diet.

Another deceptive but magic word that has meant millions of dollars to the food industry is *light,* or *lite,* with the promise of fewer calories and, depending on the food, less fat, sugar, or salt. Currently, potato chips, ice cream, soft drinks, beer, and almost every other possible kind of snack is marketed as *original* and as *light,* with the implication that the light way is the right way to satisfy one's craving for high-calorie foods with less guilt. Curiously, the consumer always has to pay more for less—"light" items almost invariably are more expensive.

Although "light" junk foods may look better to calorie- and fat-conscious eaters, they still should be consumed only rarely. For example, Milky Way II is the "light" version of the Milky Way chocolate bar, one of the best-selling candies in the country. The original Milky Way has 280 calories and 11 g of fat; the reduced version has 190 calories and 8 g of fat—the same amount of fat in a glass of whole milk. Removing some of the fat and sugar in candy bars, cookies and cupcakes, or other "junky" foods does not turn them into nutritious foods, especially since the reduction is probably accomplished with synthetic additives.

Partial Junk Foods

Soft drinks, candy, and other sugary goodies, a bagged snack that crunches and curls—these are the acknowledged high-ranking junk foods. There are some foods, however, that have some redeeming nutrient value even though they are high in calories and high in fat; that is, they could be viewed as less "junky." Popular fast-food items, for example, could not be called completely nonnutritious, but as previously indicated they may contain an awesome number of calories. Most of those calories are in the form of fat, and much of it is saturated. Unless one is actively trying to plug up the coronary arteries or to become fat, fast-food meals should be limited to the occasional lunch or dinner, and other meals that day should contain fruits, vegetables, and the whole grain foods.

Sugar—The Hidden Assassin?

Sugar, the refined white granulated sweetener that comes in 5-lb bags or 1-lb boxes from the store, is the leading empty nutrient. Sugar tastes good and provides calories, which is all that can be said for it. It is not that sugar calories are different from other calories; it is only that it is so easy to get so many of them. Being easily dissolved and concentrated in solution, large amounts of sugar can be obtained from relatively small quantities of food. Sugar-rich foods thus provide a very poor nutrient return for the amount of caloric investment. When a high percentage of ingested calories is in the form of sugar, it becomes almost impossible to get all the necessary nutrients and still take in few enough calories to maintain a reasonable weight.

It would appear to be easy to avoid excessive sugar consumption. Just take the sugar bowl off the table and stop eating and drinking soda pop, candy, cookies, sugared bakery goods, and the like. Unfortunately, people have much less control over the amount of sugar ingested than they think. According to a *Consumer Reports* study, before 1930 only 30% of the sugar used in this country was purchased by industry while 64% went home with the consumer in the bag or box from the corner grocery. Today, in a complete reversal of the manner of consumption, only 24% of the sugar is bought by people at the store. Sixty-five percent of the sugar is now sold to the food industry, which places an amazingly high concentration of it in processed foods. Much of the sugar consumed is unwittingly obtained in such foods as ketchup, salad dressing, canned and dehydrated soups, frozen TV dinners, canned and frozen vegetables, yogurt, or breakfast cereals. Tests performed on dry breakfast cereals have indicated that they contain an average sugar content of 25%, ranging from a low of 1%–3% in Shredded Wheat, Cheerios,

and Puffed Rice up to an astounding 58%–68% in such presweetened varieties as King Vitaman, Sugar Smacks, and Super Orange Crisp (Shannon, 1974). Even a Hershey Bar has only 51% sugar content. Consider the nutrient value in an ounce of breakfast cereal that is more than two-thirds sugar; one could obtain equivalent results by pouring sugar in the bowl and sprinkling the cereal on top!

Ira Shannon and his associates analyzed more than a thousand food and drink items for sucrose (sugar) concentration and came to the depressing conclusion that nearly everything has sugar added to it. There is even sugar in salt. Sugar has become the leading food additive. Although estimates vary, it can safely be assumed that every man, woman, and child in the United States is ingesting about 130 lb of sugar annually, much of it inadvertently obtained in processed foods. How detrimental all this sugar consumption is to health is inconclusive, but there is a rapidly growing body of medical literature that correlates excessive sugar intake with a number of health problems.

There is little argument, for example, against the evidence that the sweet tooth is the decayed tooth. There may be other factors such as genetic susceptibility that contribute to cavities, but the causal relationship between the amount and frequency of sugar consumption and dental caries is well established. Tooth decay is not a minor problem in a country that spends $34 billion annually on dental bills. Cutting down on cavities means cutting down on all sugar and sugar-containing foods, especially on sticky or slowly dissolving sweets between meals. Brushing and flossing after every meal, or at least rinsing with warm water after eating any carbohydrate, will help. Some authorities maintain that while sugar restriction is necessary, fluoridation of the water supply is of paramount importance. Currently, half of the children aged 5–17 have no cavities at all as a result of fluoridation of their water supply, even though they are probably eating as much or more sugar than ever before. About 60% of the water supply in the United States is fluoridated. Many areas have naturally fluoridated water; if not, the mineral generally is added by local governments. Fluoride in the water is incorporated into the tooth enamel and hardens it, making the teeth resistant to decay. Fluoridation, therefore, is especially important in children before the age of 6, when the permanent teeth erupt, but it helps reduce cavities in adults as well.

With the possible exception of the Sugar Association, almost everyone would agree that sugar should not be a major component of the daily diet. Obviously, the known high-sugar junk foods—soft drinks, candy, cookies, and rich pastries—should be indulged in only very rarely. Trying to reduce the less visible sources of sugar is more difficult, however, and requires some diligent label reading. The list of ingredients on any canned, packaged, or frozen food must reveal the contents in descending order by weight. Unfortunately, the percentage of sugar need not be given, but if sucrose, dextrose, maltose, any kind of "ose," any kind of syrup, or the words "natural sweeteners" appear high on the list or more than once, the product should be avoided.

It should also be recognized that sugar is sugar. Calling it "brown," "turbinado," or "natural" does not offer any advantage. Brown sugar is made by spraying molasses syrup into refined sugar crystals, and the turbinado sugar so prominently displayed in health food stores is partially refined sugar. The few additional nutrients are in such minute quantities as to be negligible. Honey, like sucrose, is composed of the simple sugars, glucose and fructose, plus a minuscule amount of potassium, calcium, and phosphorus—not enough to be significant in the daily recommended allowance.

The term *sugar-free* means that sweeteners other than sugar are used in the product and does not necessarily mean it is low in calories. Carbohydrates such as sorbitol, fructose, honey, or corn syrup are often used in "sugar-free" foods and all have the same number of calories per gram as sugar. Only when artificial sweeteners such as saccharin or aspartame are used as sweeteners instead of sugar will the product have fewer calories. *Read the labels.*

THE CASE FOR SALT REDUCTION

The average American's daily intake of salt is 2–4 teaspoons (10–20 g). This is considerably above the Recommended Dietary Allowance of 3–8 g or 1,100–3,300 mg of sodium, and there is no reason to presume that this huge amount of intake is desirable or good for health. To the contrary, a great deal of evidence indicates that it is dangerous to health. High-salt intake is linked to hypertension or high blood pressure, an affliction affecting an estimated 60–75 million Americans and especially prevalent in African-Americans. Untreated, the condition can lead to stroke, heart disease, and kidney failure. A number of studies have shown that hypertension can be experimentally induced in animals fed a high-salt diet. Moreover, in parts of Japan, where the mean daily salt intake is 26 g, 40% of the people are hypertensive and have a higher death rate from stroke. Conversely, there is a low incidence of hypertension among several groups of primitive people in which the salt intake is very low. A mainstay in the treatment of hypertension, along with the administration of antihypertensive drugs, has long been the reduction and restriction of salt. Still, the relationship between salt consumption and hypertension is highly controversial. There are a number of other factors involved in high blood pressure, and recent research has challenged salt's role. Some studies have suggested that inadequate intake of other dietary minerals, particularly calcium, may be equally important as sodium. It could also be that only a small percentage of people with normal blood pressure are sensitive to salt. But although there is no direct proof that high salt ingestion causes high blood pressure, it is reasonable and prudent to assume that extremes of intake may relate to hypertension. Cutting back on sodium and salt intake and eating low and no-fat calcium-rich dairy products may prevent the development of high blood pressure in those with a genetic predisposition to the disease and, by possibly reducing blood pressure, also prevent development in nonhypertensive Americans.

The taste for a lot of salt is acquired, and we have all been conditioned to it. Up until 1977, all baby foods contained added amounts, primarily to suit the mother's taste since infants have no special like for it. It is certainly possible to become unconditioned, however, by reducing salt intake. In many people, once that takes place, most foods begin to taste too salty. Unfortunately, cutting back on salts is not that easy because salt or sodium are so ubiquitous. About one-third of the ingested salt is present in food before cooking. About 40% of daily intake comes from processed foods. The rest is added with the salt shaker. More may be ingested via drinking water in some areas, and certain medications contain considerable amounts of salt. The first way to cut down is obvious—to follow the advice of the old adage and hide the salt cellar. Cook with little or no salt, and add none at the table. Another way is to purchase foods with no added salt. Many companies have recognized the marketing potential of low-salt products, and more than 40 potato chip producers are currently promoting salt-free "natural" chips. One can also reduce the use of condiments and obviously salted processed foods, but it is undeniably more difficult to limit sodium consumption when almost everything canned, bottled, packaged, or baked contains sodium bicarbonate, monosodium glutamate, sodium benzoate, sodium nitrate, sodium citrate, sodium saccharin, sodium aluminum phosphate, and so on. Many of these sodium-containing additives are in foods for reasons other than flavor and are necessary. They are curing agents, preservatives, stabilizers, or leavening agents, and they cannot be summarily removed unless an equivalent non-sodium-containing replacement in terms of taste, safety, and quality is found. It would be easier to watch salt intake if all foods were labeled, not only with the ingredients, but with a range of sodium content as well. The 1994 food labeling regulations affecting virtually all foods sold in grocery stores should make it easier to watch sodium intake. It would also help to have the government mandate, or at least strongly urge, that manufacturers restrict unnecessary salt addition and seek ways to reduce or replace sodium in their products.

OVERWEIGHT AND OBESITY

Another bonus of conforming to healthy dietary recommendations is that it is more difficult to become overweight. The low-fat, low-sugar, and high-fiber foods of the guide make it easier to maintain a proper weight. The standard American diet—eating on the run, calorie-rich convenience foods, and snacks—can, in contrast, make staying slender a constant struggle. We find ourselves in a double bind when it comes to food and eating. The marketing messages say *buy and eat this remarkable abundance of good-tasting high-calorie food;* the media messages on movie and TV screens and on the pages of any magazine say *thin is sexier, thin is beautiful, the best-looking body is the tall and incredibly slender body.* The media-promoted ideal, however, is psychologically destructive; it leads people to dislike their bodies and encourages them to embark on faddish, unbalanced, nonnutritious diets. We could all benefit from both marketing and media messages that say *no one has to be thin for beauty's sake, but maintaining a normal weight for size, height, and age is healthier.*

To standardize definitions of overweight and obesity, the National Institutes of Health released *Clinical Guidelines on the Identification, Evaluation and Treatment of Overweight and Obesity in Adults* in 1998. Body size is expressed in terms of the body mass index, which equals one's weight (kg) divided by height in meters squared (m). Overweight has been defined as a BMI greater than or equal to 25 kg/m2. Individuals with a BMI of 30 or greater are considered obese. Waist circumference has been found to be an independent predictor of risk factors and morbidity. Men with a waist circumference of more than 102 cm (greater than 40 in.) and women with a waist circumference of more than 88 cm (greater than 35 in.) are considered to be at high risk. Reams of data are cited to support definitions. Studies (Rexrode et al., 1997; Kuczmarski, Carrol, Flegal, & Troiano, 1997) have indicated that the lowest risk of dying was among women with a BMI of 22–23.4 and men with a BMI of 23.5–24.9. Men and women with a BMI of 30 or greater have been shown to have about 50%–100% higher mortality than those with a BMI of 25 or less. The risk was 10%–25% greater for those less severely overweight—with BMIs of 25–30.

A number of health problems are associated with true obesity. Excessive fatness is correlated to hypertension, coronary heart disease, thrombophlebitis, diabetes mellitus, respiratory and gastrointestinal (liver and gallbladder) disorders, pregnancy difficulties in women, and certain kinds of cancer. Obese people are likely to have an increased incidence of osteoarthritis in weight-bearing joints, have a greater number of accidents, and are at significantly greater risk when undergoing surgery. In addition to all the risks to physical health, fat people are likely to have greater emotional distress. They are stigmatized as foodaholics, gluttons who lack willpower, and they suffer not only social but even job discrimination in a society that is repulsed by fatness. Such ordinary activities as taking public transportation, food shopping, buying clothing, or eating in a restaurant without being stared at are severely limited for them.

It is evident that most American adults are above average in weight. Even the leanest Americans, as measured by the skinfold test, have more subcutaneous fat than people in other more active and healthy societies.

A 1996 nationwide telephone survey of 107,804 men and women found that more than two-thirds of American adults were either attempting to lose weight or trying to keep weight off. A primary factor in their lack of success was that significant numbers of the dieters were not following the recommendation of combining calorie restriction with at least 2½ hours of weekly exercise. Among those who were trying to lose weight, only about 20% were combining diet and exercise. Despite a preoccupation with dieting and an annual expenditure of billions of dollars on dietary foods, aids, "fat farms," "fat" doctors, exercise machines, and innumerable other ways and devices to lose weight, many are losers only in the war against excessive weight. In the past decade, the number of obese Americans increased to 33%. Overall, 31% of men and 35% of women are obese (Figure 17–4).

What Causes Obesity?

The most recent edition of the U.S. Dietary Goals addresses the problem when it tersely states, "To avoid overweight, consume only as much energy (calories) as expended; if overweight, decrease energy intake and increase energy expenditure." The cause and the treatment appear to be very straightforward. Overweight, which leads to obesity, results when more calories are on the energy intake side of the equation than on the energy output side. The answer to reducing overweight is simple: eat less and exercise more. It takes 3,500 calories to make a pound of fat. Even just a couple of hundred extra calories a day above the amount expended—a glass of beer and a handful of peanuts or potato chips, a doughnut and coffee, or two glasses of Coke or Pepsi—will put on about an ounce a day. In 6 months there will be a gain of almost 12 lb.

For many people, weight gain is just that simple. They owe their overweight to good food and a sedentary life—taking the elevator instead of climbing stairs, driving instead of walking, watching sports instead of participating in them. Unfortunately, while overeating may be at the root of a weight problem, the total picture of obesity is neither clear-cut nor simple. There is no one etiology; there is not even one single kind of obesity common to all fat people. Excessive fatness is a disorder that is associated with a multitude of reasons that include anatomical, neurological, behavioral, psychological, genetic, and social factors. The bases for getting fat and staying fat may be highly complex and different in different people, but current thinking places the major emphases on several areas: early overnutrition, inherited metabolic differences, lack of physical activity, and a combination of social factors that include home, family, education, economic status, and all the other environmental experiences that could contribute to the development and maintenance of overweight.

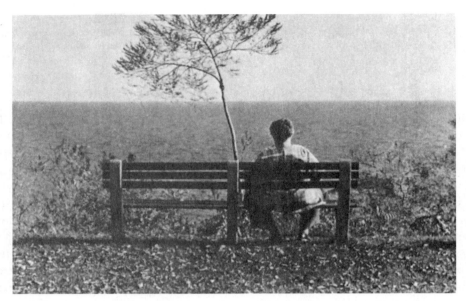

Figure 17–4   Thirty-five percent of female Americans are designated as obese, a medical term defined as more than 20% over desirable weight.

Parental obesity, which also may have genetic and environmental origins, also is believed to be one of the most important factors in predisposing a child to become obese. But not all fat babies become fat adults, and there are inherent risks in instituting nutrient restriction and weight control measures in infancy. Early nutrition plays a lifelong role in health, and parents should be moderate and cautious in attempts to regulate calorie intake in babies or children because it can interfere with optimal growth.

Some people seem to be able to maintain a stable and ideal weight no matter how much they eat; others gain weight if they even look at food, or at least it appears that way. Moreover, many of the obese do not consume any more calories than the nonobese, and some actually eat less. That observation has led to the idea that there may be some difference in metabolic efficiency that exists between the fat and nonfat, and there has been active research investigation into the possibilities. For example, the role that brown adipose tissue might play has attracted a lot of attention. White fat, the kind distributed all over the body, is mainly a storage site; brown fat is a site of heat production or thermoregulation and acts as a kind of chemical furnace in hibernating species, in other animals exposed to cold, and in newborn animals and human infants, where it is believed to be important in the maintenance of body temperature. In human babies, brown fat is found at the nape of the neck and in between the shoulder blades but constitutes only about 1% of the total body weight. In adults, there is some evidence that brown fat still exists, but just where it is located and what function it has are controversial. The connection of brown fat with human obesity is based on studies with genetically obese rats who were shown to have a defect in their brown adipose tissue that reduced their ability to burn up calories in response to exposure to mild cold, thus contributing to their obesity. It has been speculated that a similar ineffectiveness or a lesser quantity of brown fat may be a factor in human obesity. The brown adipose tissue theory may be a lead toward solving some of the unknowns of obesity, but any practical applications of the hypothesis have a long way to go.

TABLE 17–4   Body Mass Index (BMI)

Height (in feet and inches)						Weight (in pounds)								
4'10"	91	96	100	105	110	115	119	124	129	134	138	143	167	191
4'11"	94	99	104	109	114	119	124	128	133	138	143	148	173	198
5'	97	102	107	112	118	123	128	133	138	143	148	153	179	204
5'1"	100	106	111	116	122	127	132	137	143	148	153	158	185	211
5'2"	104	109	115	120	126	131	136	142	147	153	158	164	191	218
5'3"	107	113	118	124	130	135	141	146	152	158	163	169	197	225
5'4"	110	116	122	128	134	140	145	151	157	163	169	174	204	232
5'5"	114	120	126	132	138	144	150	156	162	168	174	180	210	240
5'6"	118	124	130	136	142	148	155	161	167	173	179	186	216	247
5'7"	121	127	134	140	146	153	159	166	172	178	185	191	223	255
5'8"	125	131	138	144	151	158	164	171	177	184	190	197	230	262
5'9"	128	135	142	149	155	162	169	176	182	189	196	203	236	270
5'10"	132	139	146	153	160	167	174	181	188	195	202	207	243	278
5'11"	136	143	150	157	165	172	179	186	193	200	208	215	250	286
6'	140	147	154	162	169	177	184	191	199	206	213	221	258	294
6'1"	144	151	159	166	174	182	189	197	204	212	219	227	265	302
6'2"	148	155	163	171	179	186	194	202	210	218	225	233	272	311
6'3"	152	160	168	176	184	192	200	208	216	224	232	240	279	319
6'4"	156	164	172	180	189	197	205	213	221	230	238	246	287	328
BMI	**19**	**20**	**21**	**22**	**23**	**24**	**25**	**26**	**27**	**28**	**29**	**30**	**35**	**40**

Further evidence for the genetic basis of obesity was provided by two different investigations, each using identical twins as subjects. One of the studies suggested that some people may have an inherited ability to turn excess food directly into fat (Bouchard et al., 1990). The research involved 12 pairs of lean, male, identical twins who were isolated for 4 months and fed an extra 1,000 calories daily over what they had been eating prior to entering the study—a total of 84,000 extra calories over the study period. To no one's surprise, all of the pairs gained weight (from 9½

lb to 29 lb), and the twins in each pair gained almost exactly the same amount of weight and on the same places in the body. But when the researchers looked for reasons why some of the twin pairs appeared to be so much better at gaining weight than the others, they discovered some differences in the way in which the subjects' bodies used the excess calories. The twin pairs that gained the most weight added it mostly as fat deposited on the trunk and in the abdominal area. In the men who gained the least amount of weight, however, 40% of the extra calories were added as body tissues (muscle mass) and much less was deposited as trunk and abdominal fat. The body uses up about nine times more calories (energy) in the process of turning food into muscle protein rather than into fat, so evidently some of the twin pairs were able to use up more of the additional calories in this way and gain less weight—a metabolic ability that the investigators suggest is genetic in origin. The heavy gainers, who were metabolically more efficient at turning the excess calories directly into fat, may have an inherent tendency toward obesity. People who are this efficient at storing energy as fat would have greater difficulty losing weight, even on a low-calorie diet, unless they increased their energy expenditure through exercise.

The study to determine whether similar results would occur in pairs of women twins, that is, whether some women also could be protected from excessive weight gain by metabolic genetic differences, has not been done as yet. Women generally have less muscle mass than men to begin with, tend to diet more than men, and tend to regain weight more easily.

The other twin study (Stunkard et al., 1990) looked at the body weights (corrected for height) of 93 pairs of identical twins who had been reared apart, 154 pairs of identical twins reared together, 218 pairs of fraternal twins reared apart, and 208 fraternal twins reared together. The researchers found that identical twins, whether reared together or apart, had nearly identical body weights. Much more variance occurred in fraternal twins, whether reared apart or together, leading the investigators to conclude that, although environmental factors are significant in obesity, genetic differences play a major role in determining body weight.

These studies should not be interpreted to mean that genetics has to doom people to obesity. Perhaps those with a predisposition to plumpness cannot make themselves thin, anymore than short people can make themselves tall, but extreme obesity is not a given. Very few wealthy people are obese, and it is unlikely that they all have inherited the metabolic propensity for turning excess calories into muscle. Among the rich, there are evidently cultural pressures for thinness, which lead them to various stringent measures of exercise and dieting to avoid excessive weight gain.

Getting Rid of Excess Weight

Putting weight on is so easy; taking and keeping off unwanted pounds can be frustratingly unsuccessful. There are any number of "cures" for overweight—more than 17,000 have been published to date. It would be easy to subscribe to a diet-book-of-the-month club. Each promises a new, revolutionary, quick, painless way of weight loss. Many of them are "doctor's" diets, leading nutritionists to wonder how all the doctors who write diet books get to become instant experts on dieting. They cannot become experts in brain surgery or any other specialty without training, so why is nutrition counseling fair game?

Almost any diet that restricts calories works, at least initially, but there is a difference between weight loss and fat loss. For some of the self-help diets that are low in carbohydrates, high in protein, and relatively low in salt, the most dramatic loss for the first few days or weeks of the regimen is in body water. Although dieters usually do not stay on a diet from the latest best-selling book long enough to create problems for themselves, any unbalanced diet, especially one that lacks sufficient carbohydrates for body function, is potentially a hazard to health. There are risks of fatigue, nausea, and headaches, especially in the early days of the diet. More seriously, there may be calcium depletion, increased serum cholesterol, kidney failure in those predisposed to kidney disease, and gout in those predisposed to that difficulty.

According to Marketdata Enterprises, a research firm that tracks the $35 billion diet industry, at any given time half of the adult women and nearly a third of the adult men in the United States are on diets. They turn to the self-help books or they may join group programs. Dieters try total fasts, over-the-counter liquid diets, and medically supervised liquid diets. People get hypnotized, have acupuncture, and have subcutaneous fat sucked out of their bodies, and the seriously obese may undergo surgical procedures that include wired jaws and stapled stomachs.

One diet that was touted as being the end to all other diets swept the country about 25 years ago. It was called the Last Chance Liquid Protein diet, and it was enormously popular, probably because dieters did not have to face any solid food at all. After a substantial number of deaths occurred among people who had been on it for a number of months, it became evident that this diet was indeed the "last," and its popularity fizzled out. The currently marketed over-the-counter and prescription liquid diets, which provide 400–800 calories daily through a high-protein powder to be mixed with milk or water, are undoubtedly safer than the liquid diets of the 1970s, but they still are not without risks. Any diet containing fewer than 800 calories daily will cause rapid weight loss but if prolonged will also result in breakdown of lean (muscle) rather than fat tissue, cause nitrogen loss from the body, and is hazardous.

The nonprescription liquid diets contain sugar, a protein blend, fiber, and the artificial sweetener, aspartame, and are to be mixed with water. Two of the shakes and one "sensible" meal daily constitute the diet plan. Like the majority of the products in the hugely successful weight-loss industry, such liquid diet powders purchased at the supermarket or drug store are untested, unregulated, and heavily promoted by sometimes deceptive advertising. The medically supervised liquid diets derive more of their calories from protein and fewer from carbohydrates and are actually liquid fasts—the dieter gets no food until after 12–16 weeks. The prescription Optifast and Medifast programs have become highly lucrative for hospital clinics and physicians and have been criticized as the "patient's diets which make doctors fat" (Wolfe, 1989).

Although liquid meal replacements are appealing to the nation's dieters because they provide quick weight loss, are easy to take, and remove the necessity for decision making about food choices, they do nothing for long-term eating habits. Most people on liquid diets invariably go back to their old ways of eating. This is the big problem with any diet that does not consist of moderate eating from a variety of foods. The very notion of going on the diet builds in the idea of going off the diet once the weight loss has occurred. Usually, the weight is quickly regained once the individual goes back to the original eating habits. The up-and-down, gain-and-loss pattern has been called the yo-yo syndrome or the "rhythm pattern of girth control." Getting thin and staying thin requires a complete reeducation of eating and exercise habits. Those calorie-laden fattening goodies that added weight in the first place are always going to be available; permanent weight loss has to mean a permanent lifetime change in behavior. Besides, yo-yo dieting may not be innocuous and has been found to have negative health consequences. Data based on 32 years of follow-up from the 5,127 people in the Framingham Heart Study showed that both men and women whose body weight fluctuated often or greatly had a higher risk of dying from heart disease than those whose weight remained stable. The researchers also found that the greatest up-and-down weight cycling occurred in young women, who were the most likely to be dieting (Lissner et al., 1991).

Many people, however, believe that permanent change is too difficult. They would prefer to follow a yellow brick road to weight reduction—maybe the Wizard can come up with something, perhaps a chemical drug to get rid of fat.

There is strong evidence that appropriate medications can enhance weight loss efforts when combined with calorie restriction, physical activity, and behavior therapy. Unfortunately, some serious side effects have been observed. For example, a commonly prescribed pair of weight loss drugs (fenfluramine and dexfenfluramine) were associated with valvular heart disease. As a result, they were withdrawn from the marketplace. Sibutramine and orlistat remain as therapeutic options. Sibutramine's effect is mediated via neurotransmitters, whereas orlistat functions to block dietary fat absorption. Although it received FDA approval in 1998, orlistat is associated with significant gastrointestinal side effects that may limit its popularity.

The candies to raise blood sugar before a meal, the bulk producers to give a full feeding, the "starch blockers" that have no effect at all on the absorption of starch calories, the antihistamines such as phenyl-propanolamine (PPA), advertised as the most potent nonprescription appetite suppressants, are all over-the-counter aids that have never been proven to be effective unless a restricted food intake accompanies their use. More dollars than pounds are lost when these preparations are used. Besides, phenylpropanolamine is not an innocuous drug. It has side effects similar to amphetamines; reportedly has caused high blood pressure, heart irregularities, and kidney problems; and is potentially toxic to the central nervous system. Anyone with hypertension, cardiovascular disease, or thyroid or kidney problems should not use these ineffectual appetite suppressants, but there are surveys that suggest that one in three high school and college women are popping these over-the-counter diet pills, some ingesting double or triple the manufacturer's recommended dosage. After a review for safety and effectiveness of 113 ingredients found in over-the-counter weight control products, the FDA in 1992 ruled that 111 of them had to be eliminated. The two ingredients in the weight-control products that were allowed to remain, although future action was anticipated, were PPA and benzocaine, a substance supposed to numb the taste buds. The consumer advocacy group Center for Science in the Public Interest (CSPI) wants phenylpropanolamine banned.

Although experience tells us there is no such thing, the search for a calorie-free lunch continues. Dozens of new artificial sweeteners are in development, and additional "all-natural" fat substitutes are making their way onto the market. As previously indicated, there actually is no scientific evidence that food substitutes really are effective in weight loss, but if people use them to cut fat and sugar content in the diet, they could be valuable. It may not be true for everyone, but there is some evidence that for many people the real secret to losing weight and keeping it off could be simply to eat a nutritious diet and exercise regularly. That is, reduce the fat in the diet to 20% of total calories; substitute low-fat for high-fat items; eat a lot of grains, fruits, and vegetables; and exercise 1 hour daily. With that kind of plan, one can virtually forget about the calories since so few of them come from fat.

For the extremely obese adult who remains seriously overweight despite very restricted diets, there are several drastic surgical treatments that have been endorsed by a panel of experts from the National Institutes of Health. Candidates for surgical treatment would be individuals whose obesity is associated with potentially serious health problems. The stomach stapling (vertical-banded gastroplasty) and stomach bypass surgeries are used to diminish the capacity and the outlet of the stomach, thus restricting the ability to consume foods. The complication rate is a rather appalling 10% and includes postoperative wound infection, bleeding, ulcers, and long-term gastrointestinal complaints such as distressing diarrhea and excessive gas. Patients typically lose 100 or more pounds in the first year or two after surgery and then begin to gain weight again, so the procedures serve more as obesity control than cure.

The gastrointestinal tract does more than digest and absorb food. It secretes hormones and may have other, as-yet-undiscovered functions. Thus, surgical intervention for obesity can still be considered experimental. It should be restricted to individuals for whom obesity is a proven health hazard, who are 100 or more pounds overweight, and for whom all other methods have failed.

One other treatment of last resort is wiring the jaws shut. The patient has to carry around a wire cutter in case of impending nausea because of the danger of vomiting and choking on the vomit. Because liquids through a straw are all that can be consumed, the method should produce weight loss. But chocolate shakes and high-calorie liquids from a blender can also be sipped through a straw, so even this combination of what appears to be a medieval torture and a very boring diet may not be successful.

Liposuction is not a treatment for obesity. It is a procedure performed by plastic surgeons to remove fat in one specific spot in people who still have good skin elasticity (less than 40–45 years of age) and are no more than 10–20 lb overweight. Called suction-assisted lipectomy, the operation uses a long, hollow tube or cannula that is inserted under the skin in a fatty area through a small, inch-long incision. The cannula is attached to a pump operating at about 1 atmosphere of pressure. As the surgeon repeatedly pokes the cannula into the fat, the pump sucks it out, leaving Swiss cheese-like patterns in the fat tissue. At the conclusion of the procedure, the cannula is withdrawn, and the skin is pushed down to collapse the holes in the fat. The operation is performed under general anesthesia and can be used in several areas in which fat accumulates, such as the inner and outer thighs, buttocks, behind the knees, under the arms, the breasts, and the abdomen. The cost, which is nonreimbursable as cosmetic surgery by insurance companies, can vary depending on the surgical site and the surgeon. Complications, beyond those associated with general anesthesia, can include burning and tearing sensations; skin pigmentation; persistent edema; and, when overzealous surgeons remove too much fat, depressions in the skin at the operative area. Nevertheless, many patients are evidently delighted with the results, and half of the abdominal suctions reportedly performed by one surgeon are on the "potbellies" in men.

The measure of success for any weight-reduction program is whether the lost pounds stay off. The unbalanced crash diets and drug therapies have not been successful in that regard, and surgery is certainly not the answer except for a few highly motivated individuals for whom all other methods have been tried. So what does work? The only method that seems to be beneficial and is, therefore, getting a great deal of attention currently, although long-term effectiveness is still unknown, is some form of behavior modification. Actually, applying principles of behavioral psychology to eating is not new. Group support programs such as Weight Watchers have been using reward and reinforcement techniques for more than 40 years. The difference may be the current emphasis on self-management and self-control. Basically, the idea behind behavior modification for weight loss assumes that because eating is learned behavior, weight reduction can be promoted by changing the basic eating and activity patterns that lead to overeating and underactivity. One of the main ingredients of the program involves learning to set realistic goals and appreciating that small weight losses over a long period of time are desirable. The prime component is always the emphasis on permanent changes in lifestyle. Self-help is the key to behavioral change, and the focus is on the environmental or situational control of eating. The individual is educated to new adaptive behaviors by "shaping," practicing a series of small attainable changes that ultimately bring one to the final achieved goal.

A number of books have been written as guides to the use of behavioral modification techniques in weight control. Several suggestions to aid in making the appropriate changes in habits are common to all of them. They include the following:

1. Keep a food diary to create awareness of what is eaten, the time it is consumed, the location where eating takes place, and the mood or feelings during the eating period.
2. Sit down at the table while eating; do not stand, watch TV, listen to the radio, or read.
3. Eat slowly. Chew each mouthful until it disappears, put down the fork in between mouthfuls if it helps, savor the food—never bolt it down. Eating too rapidly does not give the stomach a chance to sense the presence of food and signal the brain that it is becoming full.
4. Do not put the meal on a large plate so that it looks small and becomes lost; use a small plate and then put small quantities of food on the fork or spoon. Get in the habit of leaving a little food; an adult no longer has to belong to the "clean plate club." Clear the table immediately after eating, put the food away, and leave the room.
5. Never shop for food on an empty stomach.

WEIGHT LOSS THROUGH EXERCISE

We probably would all agree that a sugared doughnut is low-nutrient junk food while 8 oz of plain yogurt is worthwhile and nutritious. Nevertheless, they both contain the same number of calories. If the calories in either a doughnut or a cup of yogurt are above an individual's energy needs, the body is going to store them as fat. It makes no difference where the extra calories come from. Overeating on yogurt, whole wheat bread, or apples and oranges instead of beer and pretzels may be a more nutritious way of gaining weight, but in the absence of an increased energy expenditure, the end result will still be an additional inch of pinch. As discussed previously, if the daily intake is a few hundred calories more than the output, the gain will amount to nearly 2 lb a month.

Consider the average American female, for example, who, at 145 lb and medium build, is carrying around 20 more pounds than she should or wants to have. Suppose also that her weight has remained stable for several years and that she is neither gaining nor losing weight. It can, therefore, be assumed that in a typical day, she balances the number of calories she expends by the number of calories ingested. Ms. Average Female has several ways in which she could shed those 20 lb. Knowing that there are 3,500 calories in a pound of fat, she can reduce her intake by 500 calories a day and maintain her present level of activity. In 7 days she will have lost 1 lb ($500 \times 7 = 3,500$ calories = 1 lb). At that rate it will take 20 weeks to lose 20 lb.

With a few simple mathematical calculations, however, she can figure out how to lose the extra weight by increasing her energy expenditure. Moving the body through 1 mile of distance will use up about 100 calories. A slow amble, a brisk walk, a jog, or an actual run expends an equal amount of energy; surprisingly, the speed is not related to the calories burned. The actual number of calories utilized varies depending on body size; the heavier the person, the more calories used. The energy expended by walking or jogging 1 mile can be calculated by multiplying the body weight by 0.73. Of course it takes much less time to jog a mile than to stroll it. But if one does nothing more than park the car or get off the bus 6 blocks away from work or school and walk the rest of the way, or somehow make a real concerted effort to get that mile

in every day, a pound of fat will be lost every 35 days. In 20 months, all the excess weight will be gone without reducing any food from the diet at all.

Now the mathematics of weight loss becomes even more interesting. If every mile of walking uses a hundred calories, 35 miles of walking produces a 1-lb weight reduction. That sounds like a tremendous amount of walking, but at a very moderate pace, an hour's walk will cover 3 miles. Three miles per day means 35 miles in a week and a half. At the end of a year, assuming there has been no change in food intake, an incredible 36 pounds will have been lost! Walking does not require special shoes or any other kind of special equipment. It is one of the best exercises known.

If our hypothetical overweight woman decides to walk 3 miles a day and also cut down 500 calories in food intake, she will lose those 20 lb in 10 weeks.

The more vigorous the activity, the more calories that can be burned in less time. Twenty minutes of jogging is equivalent to an hour of walking. Walking will use energy as well as jogging, running, swimming, bicycling, cross-country skiing, fast tennis, or racquetball; it just takes a lot more of the walking. *Brisk* walking, in addition to using calories, will provide the same physiological benefits on the cardiovascular and respiratory systems as can be obtained by those other more active and intense exercises.

A very prevalent myth about increasing the energy expenditure is that it only increases the appetite so that one will end up gaining rather than losing weight. Any appetite stimulation as a result of exercise is likely to be a psychological rather than a physiological effect. Unfortunately, people who want to use exercise for weight reduction sometimes fall into the trap of wanting to reward themselves with extra goodies because of the virtuous exercise they are doing. Research studies have suggested that regular and moderate physical activity has no effect on increasing hunger and may actually decrease it. This is well known to many exercisers who program their daily activity into their lunch hours. They have observed that after exercising, they naturally want to eat less rather than more (Figure

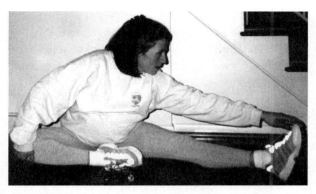

Figure 17–5 Lunchtime jogger. There is no medical reason to stop exercising during pregnancy if a woman wants to continue; physical fitness benefits the mother and the fetus.

17–5). There is also some evidence that the calorie-burning benefits of exercise may even extend for several hours beyond the actual exercise period.

EXERCISE AND HEALTH

Weight reduction and weight maintenance are welcome side effects of daily walking, jogging, running, swimming, cycling, tennis, rope jumping, calisthenics, or whatever form of physical activity fits into a lifestyle. Perhaps not every man or woman will end up with the figure of a movie star, but regular exercisers, even if they eat more than nonexercisers, are almost always leaner.

There are physiological and psychological benefits of working with the body that go beyond just making it more beautiful. Moderate regular exercise produces *physical fitness.* Being physically fit means having the superenergy promised but not delivered by swallowing vitamin pills. It means having strength and endurance, less fatigue, fewer aches and pains, and, possibly, even fewer colds and other infections. It means having flexible joints with the stretch and elasticity in muscles, tendons, and ligaments to produce an erect posture, a good carriage, and a smooth and easy gait. For long-term health and life expectancy, perhaps the greatest benefit of physical fitness is its significant effects on the cardiovascular and respiratory systems.

Not all exercises have an equal effect on all components of physical fitness. Yoga does a lot for flexibility but little for the heart and lungs. Running and walking do very little for flexibility but much for strength and endurance.

The kinds of exercises that produce the greatest number of physiological benefits are those that elevate the heart and breathing rate, raise the body temperature, and increase sweat production. Such exercises are called aerobics. The term was introduced by Kenneth Cooper, a physician and major in the U.S. Air Force. His book, *Aerobics,* first published in 1968, presents the concepts underlying the benefits of physical exertion. Aerobics, performed consistently and progressively, result in a conditioning or training effect. The heart muscle becomes stronger and able to pump out more blood with each beat, and the number of beats per minute of the heart at rest decreases. There is an increase in blood volume and in the arterial blood supply, not only to the heart itself through the coronary vessels but also to all the skeletal muscles of the body. The muscles become stronger. Their mass increases, their tone improves, and there is a more efficient exchange of oxygen and carbon dioxide. If the resting arterial blood pressure was originally elevated before the exercise program, the systolic and diastolic pressures will become decreased. Pulmonary function improves, and the oxygen uptake capacity increases. Another positive benefit of exercise of an endurance nature is that all blood lipids, such as cholesterol and triglycerides, are reduced.

Physical fitness can occur only with physical activity that is sufficiently demanding. This does not mean that the exercise must be overly strenuous, self-punishing, or boring. The whole key to choosing an exercise plan that can be maintained is to select one that can also be enjoyed. Anything is going to be hard at the beginning, but if there is not going to be any fun in the activity after one gets into condition, the exercise plan is likely to be dropped. The body, however, cannot store the benefits of exercise any more than it can store water-soluble vitamins. Unless the exertion takes place regularly and consistently, the physiological advantages will be lost.

Exercise classes, aerobic dancing, or working out at special exercise gyms have become very popular, especially if one can afford them, and provide a good incentive for keeping up an exercise program. The health and fitness shelves at the bookstores are crowded with celebrity-authored exercise books that tell us how to do a daily workout at home. Any of these activities are beneficial if done sensibly. Some of them, however, may not be completely without hazard. For example, belly dancing is great fun and good exercise, but the twisting movements are very hard on the knees. Some forms of aerobic dancing are overly vigorous, and not all the instructors are that knowledgeable about the limitations of tendons, muscles, and ligaments. Exercise is supposed to make one feel good, not crippled. Some of the exercise books, records, or tapes give nutritional misinformation or suggest that pain when exercising is a good thing. It is important to remember that pain is the body's way of saying that something is wrong. A good rule is, if it *hurts,* stop doing it.

Unless an individual is over 35 years of age, has a medical problem, or has never exercised at all, a medical checkup before initiating an exercise program is not necessary as long as the activity is begun slowly. For anyone who is over 35 and not accustomed to strenuous exercise, it is sensible to have a physical examination that includes a resting electrocardiogram. Over the age of 40, according to Cooper, the exam should include a stress test, or exercising electrocardiogram. If everything checks out all right, the only barrier left is the one in the mind that says, "I'll start tomorrow," or "next week," or "it's too hot," or "too cold," or the really negative "I don't have time to fit exercise into my schedule."

One can choose to be physically active, or one can choose not to, but those who make exercise a part of their lives make the better choice for wellness. People should exercise not only because it is so good physiologically but also because it *feels* so good. Further positive rewards of exercise are the relief of tension and strain; working out works out emotional stress as well.

Those who exercise describe their feelings as being on a natural high, of having a wonderful awareness of being fully alive and in complete control of their bodies. Bodies are designed to be active; they look and they work better when they are active. It is a pity that most people miss the joy of discovering the full physical potentials of their bodies and the realization of how truly healthy they can feel.

WOMEN, EXERCISE, AND SPORTS

How many of these statements sound familiar?

- Certain physical activities are simply too strenuous for women. Women can be damaged internally by exercise, although the damage may not show up for years. Besides, vigorous exercise is unfeminine. It causes unsightly bulging muscles, and women end up looking like one of those body-building addicts.
- Exercise during menstruation is unsafe. The performance of women athletes is bound to be adversely affected by competing while menstruating.
- Exercise causes a tilted uterus and makes it harder for a woman to conceive or deliver a child. Women should not jog, run, or compete in any athletic events while pregnant; it is too dangerous to the fetus.
- Physical activity or participation in contact sports may cause injury to the breasts. A blow to the breast can cause cancer. Even jogging or running makes the breasts jiggle and bounce, and they will become stretched out and saggy.
- Women are more vulnerable to sports injuries. They are smaller, their bones are softer, and they are more knock-kneed and loose jointed, making them especially injury prone.
- Female athletes are physically inferior to male athletes and can never complete on an equal basis. There are fundamental biological reasons why they cannot play games or excel in events as well as men.

The preceding are examples of the kinds of myths that have kept women sedentary. They have justified an inequality in physical education and instructional programs in school and a lack of community recreational facilities for women when they are adults. These fallacies have discouraged women from participating in sports and from getting the kind of training and coaching needed for competitive athletics. Fortunately, most of these myths have been recognized as untrue and are slowly fading out of the picture. Unfortunately, some of them still carry enough weight in some places to influence members of the International Olympics Committee.

There is no exercise that is too strenuous or too vigorous for women to perform, and there is no such sport for which they are physically unsuited. The only barriers to participation are cultural and social.

The thought of getting muscle bulges and turning into a "jock" has deterred many young women from pursuing vigorous physical activities, but since muscle hypertrophy is dependent on the amount of androgen present, the muscles in women who strenuously exercise become firmer, smoother, and stronger and do not balloon out in size. Studies have shown that even weight lifting, which causes increases in strength and muscle mass in men, results only in significant increases in strength in women. Pam Meister, 4 ft, 11½ in. tall and weighing 105 lb, won the Women's National Weightlifting Championship by lifting a deadweight 310 lb after just a year of weight training, a feat that would be an impossibility for most men. Meister's muscles possess great strength but no bulk. Unit for unit, the physiology of women's muscle—the contractile mechanism and the ability to exert force—is no different than that of men's.

All of the menstrual myths have now been disproved. Moderate exercise has no adverse effects on the menstrual cycle and may even regulate it. Exercise has a very beneficial effect on dysmenorrhea. Concerning the impairment of peak performance for women athletes during menstruation, it has been shown that women have competed, won events, and broken records during all stages of their cycles. Some have also won gold medals and championships when they were 6 months pregnant, although most stop competing after the fourth month. Heavy athletic training should not be *initiated* during pregnancy, but if an athlete wants to golf or play tennis until the day she delivers, there is no medical reason why she should not. One ranking tennis player competed in tournaments through her eighth month of pregnancy, claiming it was "great exercise" and that it "rocked the baby to sleep." Many nonpregnant women might be deterred by such strenuous activity, but Laurie Glenn Jacobson had no difficulty undergoing the rigors of a 21-week officer training course in the Marine Corps while pregnant. Shortly before completing the course, Laurie marched 21 miles over a rugged terrain while carrying a 7-lb rifle, a 25-lb pack, and a 5-month fetus.

Erdelyi's classic study of Hungarian women athletes showed that 87% of them had shorter labors in childbirth than women in a control group. There were also fewer complications in pregnancy and delivery in athletes. There has never been any evidence that women athletes have more difficulty conceiving children, and in many instances, their performance improves after pregnancy and delivery.

As described in Chapter 4, there is one menstrual difficulty that appears in some women who undergo intense physical training. Menstrual irregularity and, in certain individuals, amenorrhea or cessation of the menstrual periods, occur in marathon runners, ballet dancers, gymnasts, skaters, and other athletes who follow very strenuous training programs. Apparently, there are no lasting consequences of the menstrual irregularities; when the training stops, the disorder disappears. Even the accepted dogma that exercise-induced amenorrhea, by reducing the amount of circulating estrogen, may cause bone loss and set the stage for osteoporosis later in life has been disproved by a recent study. Researchers at the University of British Columbia studied 66 premenopausal women with bone loss and found that subtle and asymptomatic menstrual and ovulatory irregularities occurred in both exercisers and nonexercisers. Moreover, the bone loss was correlated not to the women's activity, but to the ovulation disturbances, even without amenorrhea. One-third of the women studied were training for a marathon, another third were runners, and the rest exercised less than 1 hour a week, but there were no statistical differences in ovulation disturbances between the three groups (Prior, Vigna, Schechter, & Burgess, 1990).

Participation in exercise or noncompetitive and competitive sports has no effect on breast sagging, stretching, or enlargement, which is primarily genetically determined. Large-breasted women may find that their breasts get in the way in contact sports but that they do not affect their athletic skills. All that women need are the same kinds of protection for their vulnerable areas that have been devised to protect exposed and vulnerable areas of the male anatomy. Christine Laycock, associate professor of surgery at New Jersey Medical School, has designed a protective "gym-bra" to reduce the possibility of breast problems during and after sport participation. Women who run or jog may find it difficult to get enough support from today's little-nothing nylon brassieres. Bras with a hook and eye closing may rub and cause irritation.

Proper training and preparation for sports activities are necessary to reduce injuries in women, men, or children who are active participants. Female bones may be smaller than those of the male, but unless a woman is postmenopausal and has osteoporosis, her bones are neither softer nor more fragile than a man's bones. The ligaments that give the joints stability may be more lax in some women, however, making them more loose jointed. This may result in a greater susceptibility to sprains and strains. Dr. James Nicholas, a sports physician, has written that knee sprains in female skiers, for example, can occur when the impact is less than violent. Ski injuries are likely to be more related to lack of experience, poor physical condition, and failure of the binding to release properly than to the sex of the skier. Anyone, male or female, who starts any activity and goes too far too rapidly without a slow, progressive buildup is likely to develop injuries. *Well-trained* women athletes are no more prone to injury than men athletes, and the kinds of injuries sustained by women are no different than those sustained by men.

Whether women athletes are inherently physically inferior to men athletes is still a moot point. Certainly, most of the world records for events are held by men. Men, however, have been at it longer, have had more training, better coaching and better facilities and have been expected to be better and continue to improve. As women athletes also receive these advantages and continue to gain in strength and endurance, female records may equal and even surpass male records in certain competitions. Right now, the best women swimmers are swimming faster in their events than the best male swimmers were in their events 25 years ago. Women marathon runners have improved their times by about 61% since 1955, while men's times in marathons have advanced by only 18%. The late U.S. track star Florence Griffith-Joyner's record time of 10.49 seconds in the 100-meter sprint at the Olympic trials was faster than that of the legendary Jesse Owens.

Women probably will never be able to compete with men across the board. They may always be at a disadvantage in certain competitions or contact sports where sheer force and size are factors. There is no physical reason, however, why the two sexes should not compete against each other in certain sports or play together on the same team in games such as baseball where agility and timing are more important than strength. Prejudice against women as professional major league players, not their lack of ability, is likely to keep them out of pro baseball for some time. The day of the female major league player may not be that far off, however. Even the legendary Hank Aaron gave approval for women on the same team as men, indicating that he saw no reason why they should not play pro baseball.

There are some events for which women may be physiologically better suited than men. Some researchers have suggested reasons why women may ultimately be better at long distance running. In the usual marathon race, where strength and speed are most important, men are likely to be more successful. Beyond the 26-mile marathon, when stamina may be more important than strength, it has been theorized that women may excel. Not only are they lighter, but there is evidence that they may be able to burn their body reserve of fat more efficiently than men.

Marathon running may truly be a woman's sport, but the barriers against women runners have only gradually been dropped. Before 1972, women had to enter under an assumed name and sneak into the Boston Marathon when no one was looking. Today, the Boston Marathon is open to women, and the Amateur Athletic Union has sanctioned marathon running for men and women in the same race. The AAU also sponsors a women's marathon national championship. For years there had been many women in the United States and several countries who could run a 26-mile marathon in less than 3 hours, a standard aimed for by the top male runners. But it took until the 1984 Olympics before there was any marathon event for women runners, or even a 3,000-meter (1.85-mile) competition.

Women athletes are obviously not going to be equal in all ways to men athletes in every sport, although there are bound to be similarities between some men and women athletes in strength, endurance, and even in body composition. Of course, all men athletes are not equal either, and it is evident that not everyone makes it to superstar status. Athletes of both sexes are, however, superbly fit people. They have become athletes because they have natural abilities for their particular sport, and they are endowed genetically with physical and physiological attributes that lead them to excel. That the gap between their abilities appears to be narrowing is significant, and perhaps closing it may be of benefit to women's sports. In our highly sports-conscious society, winning is what counts. When women athletes continue to win, break records, and become champions, when they, too, are perceived as superstars, then women's sports may be closer to generating the same audiences, money, and media coverage as men's sports.

While the difference in fitness between the male athlete and the female athlete is not very great, the difference between the trained woman athlete and the average woman is much greater, and it vastly exceeds the difference between the trained male and the average man. Females, after all, have never been encouraged from the time they were children to get out there after school and play competitive games, do push-ups and sit-ups, and in general, become active and stay active. Girls are socialized into becoming the cheerleaders, not the players. But with a push from Title IX of the Education Amendments of 1972, which prohibited discrimination on the basis of sex in any educational institution receiving federal funds, social and cultural attitudes have changed. A girl who wants to go out for sports is finding it easier. Formerly, she might have been derided by her contemporaries as a jock. Today, she is encouraged and admired. Schools are no longer permitted to allot a tiny fraction of the athletic budget to women's sports when half the student population is female (Figure 17–6). Today, girls and boys, women and men—separately—participate in basketball, baseball, volleyball, track, tennis, cross-

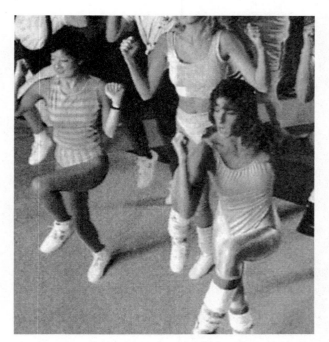

Figure 17–6 Active women are healthier, stronger, leaner women. Exercise is not only physiologically beneficial—it feels good.

country, and all the rest of the athletic programs offered in grade school, high school, and college. Twenty years ago, the National Collegiate Athletic Association (NCAA), which opposed the enactment of Title IX, was all male; now more than one-third of the participants in NCAA sports are women.

Physical fitness, however, is not only for athletes; it is for everyone, of any age and of either sex. Activity provides health benefits, whatever the activity and whenever it is initiated. But good exercise, like good nutrition, should be a lifetime habit to be of greatest benefit. The most logical time to establish good health habits is during childhood, in the home and in the school. Parents must demand a good exercise program in the schools for youngsters of both sexes, and they must make certain that athletic equality in training, equipment, and facilities exists. The emphasis should be on making physical activity attractive to all children, whatever their abilities. Often, programs that attempt to develop star athletes tend to discourage the less athletically gifted children. Unfortunately, too many of us have become lifetime bench sitters. We not only have to get off the sidelines ourselves, we have to see to it that everyone in the next generation becomes players.

REFERENCES

Adams, P. W., Rose, D. P., Folkard, J., et al. (1973). Effect of pyridoxine hydrochloride (vitamin B_6) upon depression associated with oral contraception. *Lancet, 1,* 897–904.

Barrett, S., & Knight, G. (1976). Rodale presses on. *Nutrition Notes, 9,* 6.

Bouchard, C., Tremblay, A., Despres, J., et al. (1990). The response to long-term overfeeding in identical twins. *New England Journal of Medicine, 322*(21), 1477–1482.

Broun, E. R., Greist, A., Tricot, G., & Hoffman, R. (1990). Excessive zinc ingestion. A reversible cause of sideroblastic anemia and bone marrow depression. *Journal of the American Medical Association, 264*(11), 1441–1443.

Browner, W. S., Westenhouse, J., & Tice, J. (1991). What if Americans ate less fat? A quantitative estimate of the effect on mortality. *Journal of the American Medical Association, 265*(24), 3285–3291.

Centers for Disease Control. (1990). Leads from the *Morbidity and Mortality Weekly Report. Journal of the American Medical Association, 264*(16), 2057.

Cochrane, W. A. (1965). Overnutrition in prenatal and neonatal life: A problem. *Canadian Medical Association Journal, 93,* 893–896.

Erdelyi, F. J. (1962). Gynecological survey of female athletes. *Journal of Sports Medicine and Physical Fitness, 2*(3), 174–179.

Henson, D. E., Block, G., & Levine, M. (1991). Ascorbic acid: Biologic functions and relation to cancer. *Journal of the National Cancer Institute, 83*(8), 547–550.

Herbert, V., & Jacob, E. (1974). Destruction of vitamin B_{12} by ascorbic acid. *Journal of the American Medical Association, 230*(2), 241–242.

Just what is a balanced diet anyway? (1992). *Tufts University Diet and Nutrition Newsletter, 9*(11), 3–6.

Kamil, A. (1972). How natural are those natural vitamins? *Journal of Nutrition Education, 4*(3), 92.

Kuczmarski, R. J., Carrol, M. D., Flegal, K. M., & Troiano, R. P. (1997). Varying body mass index cut-off points to describe overweight prevalence among U.S. adults: NHANES III (1988 to 1994). *Obesity Research, 5,* 542–548.

Lissner, L., Odell, P. M., D'Agostino, R. B., et al. (1990). Variability of body weight and health outcomes in the Framingham population. *New England Journal of Medicine, 324*(26), 1839–1844.

National Academy of Sciences. (1997). *Dietary Reference Intakes.* Washington, D.C.: National Academy Press.

National Center for Health Statistics. (1990). Health, United States, 1989. (DHHS Publication No. PHS90-1232). Washington, D.C.: U.S. Government Printing Office.

Ornish, D. (1990). Can lifestyle changes reverse coronary heart disease? *Lancet, 336*(8708), 129–133.

Prior, J. L., Vigna, Y. M., Schechter, M. T., & Burgess, A. E. (1990). Spinal bone loss and ovulatory disturbances. *New England Journal of Medicine, 323,*(18), 1221–1227.

Public Health Service. (1990). Healthy people 2000: National health promotion and disease prevention objectives.

(DHHS Publication No. PHS90-50212). Washington, D.C.: U.S. Government Printing Office.

Rexrode, K. M., Hennekens, C. H., Willett, W. C., et al. (1997). A prospective study of body mass index, weight change, and risk of stroke in women. *Journal of the American Medical Association, 277,* 1539–1545.

Rigotti, N. A., Neer, R. M., Skates, S. J., et al. (1991). The clinical course of osteoporosis in anorexia nervosa. *Journal of the American Medical Association, 265*(9), 1133–1138.

Shannon, I. L. (1974). Sucrose and glucose in dry breakfast cereals. *Journal of Dentistry for Children, 41*(5), 347–350.

Siegel, C., Barker, B., & Kunstadter, M. (1982). Conditioned oral scurvy due to megavitamin C withdrawal. *Journal of Periodontology, 53*(7), 453.

Snow, J. T., & Harris, M. B. (1989). Disordered eating in Southwestern Pueblo Indians and Hispanics. *Journal of Adolescence, 12*(30), 329–334.

Stunkard, A. J., Harris, J. R., Pedersen, N. L., et al. (1990). The body-mass index of twins who have been reared apart. *New England Journal of Medicine, 322*(21), 1483–1487.

Wolfe, S. (1989). Patients' diets which make doctors fat. *Health Letter, 5*(6), 12.

APPENDIX A

American Social Health Association www.ashastd.org
American Medical Association www.ama-assn.org
Center for Food Safety and Applied Nutrition http://vm.cfsan.fda.gov/list.html
Center for Science in the Public Interest www.cspinet.org
Food and Drug Administration www.fda.gov
Gay and Lesbian Medical Association www.glma.org
Herpes Resource Center www.ashastd.org/herpes/hrc/index.html
National Cancer Institute www.nci.nih.gov
National Center for Health Statistics www.cdc.gov/nchs
National Institute of Health www.nih.gov
National Women's Health Information Center www.4woman.gov/x/index.htm
National Women's Health Network www.womenshealthnetwork.org
Office on Women's Health of Health and Human Services
    www.4women.gov/owh/index.htm
Resolve: the National Infertility Association www.resolve.org
Women's Health Initiative www.nhlbi.nih.gov/whi

GLOSSARY

Abnormal uterine bleeding A change in the frequency, duration, or the amount of menstrual flow which may or may not indicate a medical problem.

Abortion The termination of pregnancy before the fetus is able to live independently.

Acne Localized skin inflammation as a result of overactivity of the oil glands at the base of hair follicles.

Acquired immunodeficiency syndrome (AIDS) The last stage of the progressive human immunodeficiency virus (HIV) infection.

Activin A peptide hormone that enhances FSH secretion.

Adrenal glands Located at the top of each kidney. Each gland has a cortex which surrounds the medulla. Each region of the gland is responsible for hormone production such as cortisol and aldosterone in the cortex and norepinephrine and epinephrine (adrenaline) in the medulla. The adrenal gland also produces sex steroids.

Amenorrhea The lack of menstruation during a woman's reproductive years; it is normal only during pregnancy.

American Medical Association (AMA) National organization that seeks to promote professionalism in medicine and sets standards for medical education, practice, and ethics.

Amniocentesis Withdrawal of amniotic fluid to obtain a sample for specimen examination.

Androgens The male sex hormones.

Anovulation Lack of ovulation.

Apgar score Method to assess newborn's status; a score of 0–10 rates the newborn's color, reflex irritability, muscle tone, respiratory effort, and heart rate.

Aphrodisiacs Substances that arouse an individual to increased desire and ability to engage in sexual activity.

Areola Characteristic wrinkled and pigmented skin of the nipple that extends out onto the breast for approximately 1–2 cm.

Axillary nodes A cluster of small, bean-shaped nodes in the breasts which play an important role in immunity by filtering out harmful substances. Also called pectoral nodes.

AZT A reverse transcriptase inhibitor; the first antiretroviral drug approved by the FDA.

Barr body Sex chromatin mass seen within the nuclei of normal female somatic cells.

Bartholin's glands Located in the cleft between the labia minora and the hymenal ring; these glands secrete a clear, viscid, odorless, alkaline mucus that improves the viability and motility of sperm along the female reproductive tract.

Basal body temperature (BBT) A daily chart of temperature taken upon awakening for the purpose of indicating the time of ovulation.

Braxton Hicks contractions Uterine contractions that are irregular and painless; also known as false labor.

Calorie Also called kilocalorie; with a capital *C*, it is the amount of heat required to raise the temperature of a kilogram of water from 14.5 degrees Celsius to 15.5 degrees Celsius; the calorie (with a small *c*) is really 0.001 Calories, but it is used so often in association with food that it is usually understood to mean the kilocalorie.

Candidiasis A name for vaginitis caused by genus *Candida,* primarily by the species *Candida albicans.*

Carcinogens Substances or agents that are known to cause cancer.

Carcinoma A new growth or malignant tumor that occurs in epithelial tissue.

CD4 receptor A cell surface receptor molecule; the target cells in the body attacked by HIV are those that have a CD4 receptor.

Cervical cap A thimble-shaped rubber cap used for birth control that covers only the cervix; it is used with spermicide in the same way diaphragms are.

Cervix The narrow outer end of the uterus.

Cesarean section An abdominal and uterine incision to remove a fetus.

Chlamydia Chlamydia infection is an inclusive term that describes three major groups of diseases caused by 15 recognized serotypes or strains of *Chlamydia trachomatis.*

Cholesterol Lipid that is produced by the body and used in the synthesis of steroid hormones.

Chromosomes Composed of protein and an exceedingly long and thin filamentous molecule called DNA; found in the nucleus of a cell.

Clitoris One of the structures of the female genitalia, consisting of two crura, a shaft, and a glans; the homologue of the penis.

Coitus Sexual intercourse between a man and a woman by insertion of the penis into the vagina.

Coitus interruptus A method of contraception in which the male withdraws his penis completely from the vagina before orgasm and ejaculates well away from the vaginal orifice.

Colostrum A thin, milky secretion expressed by the breast during pregnancy and for a few days after parturition; it is rich in antibodies and colostrum corpuscles.

Condom A thin, usually transparent, and flexible sheath made of latex or animal membrane that is closed on one end and open on the other; it is rolled over an erect penis to fit tightly during intercourse in order to trap the ejaculate and prevent semen from entering the vagina.

Conjugated equine estrogens A type of estrogen, administered clinically, that is derived from the urine of mares.

Contraction stress test (CST) A diagnostic procedure performed to determine the fetal heart response under stress, that is, when contractions are induced by oxytocin.

Cooper's ligaments Supportive fibrous structures throughout the breast that partially sheathe the lobes shaping the breast.

Corpus luteum Small yellow endocrine structure that develops within a ruptured ovarian follicle and secretes progesterone and estrogen.

Corticosteroids Hormonal steroids excreted by the cortex of the adrenal gland.

Cystitis Inflammation of the bladder.

Deoxyribonucleic acid (DNA) The substance of heredity; a large molecule that carries the genetic information necessary for all cellular function, including the building of proteins.

Depo-Provera The injectable contraceptive manufactured by the Upjohn Company.

Dermis Corium, or the second layer of the skin.

Diethylstilbestrol (DES) A nonsteroid synthetic estrogen that has estrogenic properties, is effective when taken orally, and is less expensive than the real thing.

Ductal carcinoma in situ (DCIS) A preinvasive malignancy likely to progress to cancer if no treatment takes place; with treatment, the outlook for a cure is about 98%.

Dysfunctional uterine bleeding (DUB) Term used to describe bleeding after ruling out, through diagnostic tests and physical examination, all the other possible reasons for unpredictable, excessive, frequent, and/or prolonged bleeding.

Dysmenorrhea Pelvic pain or cramps that occur during menstruation.

Eclampsia Seizure associated with pregnancy-induced hypertension.

Endocrine glands Consist of the pituitary gland, the thyroid gland, the parathyroid glands, the adrenal glands, the islets of Langerhans of the pancreas, and the ovaries and the testes.

Endometrial cycle Occurs as tissue is shed monthly in response to the hormonal changes of the menstrual period.

Endometriosis A condition in which bits of functioning endometrial tissue are aberrantly located outside of their normal site, which is the uterine cavity.

Endometrium The mucous membrane that lines the uterus.

Enzyme-linked immunosorbent assay (ELISA) The most commonly used test that detects the presence of circulating antibodies to HIV virus proteins in blood serum.

Epidermis Multilayered outer covering of the skin, consisting of four layers throughout the body, except for the palms of the hands and soles of the feet, where there are five layers.

Epidural anesthesia Epidural anesthesia has become the most popular anesthetic during labor and delivery; it is achieved by an injection into the epidural space, which lies between the dura mater of the spinal cord and the ligaments that connect the dura and the vertebrae, and gives complete relief from pain with fewer effects on the mother and infant than most other types of medication.

Episiotomy A small incision in the perineum that is performed on a woman during childbirth to prevent the perineum from tearing.

Estradiol An estrogen that occurs naturally in the body; it is the major hormone produced by the ovaries during the reproductive years.

Estriol An estrogen that occurs naturally in the body.

Estrogen-receptor-alpha (ER-alpha) One of the two estrogen receptors.

Estrogen-receptor-beta (ER-beta) One of the two estrogen receptors.

Estrogen replacement therapy (ERT) Administration of estrogen to menopausal and postmenopausal women.

Estrogens Estrogens and progesterone are the female sex hormones.

Estrone An estrogen that occurs naturally in the body and is found in postmenopausal women.

Fallopian tubes Site of fertilization; they extend from the cornu of the uterus to the ovaries and are supported by the broad ligaments.

Fetal alcohol syndrome (FAS) Condition in which fetal development is impaired by maternal consumption of alcohol.

Fibrocystic disease A term for several benign (non-cancerous) conditions of the breast characterized by lumpiness and cyclic pain.

Fibroids Benign masses of muscle and connective tissue in the uterus; the most common gynecological tumor.

Follicles Ovarian follicles are spherical structures in the cortex of the ovary consisting of an oogonium or an oocyte and its surrounding epithelial cells.

Follicle-stimulating hormone (FSH) Stimulates the growth and development of the primary follicles and results in hormone production in ovaries and sperm production in testes.

Follicular phase The first of the three phases of the ovarian cycle.

Gamete intrafallopian transfer (GIFT) A technique in which female germ cells required to begin formation of a human embryo are injected into a woman's fallopian tubes for fertilization.

Genital warts/condylomata Caused by the human papillomavirus (HPV); condylomata is Greek for warts.

Genome The term for all the DNA in an organism.

Genotype Genetic constitution.

"Gonadostat" hypothesis Theory that postulates that the immature hypothalamic-pituitary unit functions during childhood as a "gonadostat," is set at a particular level, and is extremely sensitive to the feedback action of the small amounts of circulating estrogen produced by the ovaries and to inhibin, a glycoprotein.

Gonadotropin-releasing hormone (GnRH) Causes the release of both follicle-stimulating hormone (FSH) and luteinizing hormone (LH).

Granulosa cells A layer of cells in the thera (outer layer) of an ovarian follicle. It produces sex steroids.

Growth hormone (GH) Controls the growth of all the cells of the body capable of growth, resulting in an increase in the numbers of cells and in enlargement of existing cells.

Health maintenance organizations (HMOs) A type of health plan in which enrollees pay a fixed monthly premium and are required to receive all health care from HMO providers; generally operates its own clinics and hospitals.

Herpesvirus A viral infection of the genital or perirectal skin by herpes simplex.

Highly active antiretroviral therapy (HAART) Therapy for those with HIV that includes three major classes of antiretroviral treatment.

Hormone replacement therapy (HRT) The combination therapy of estrogen and progestin.

Hormones Endocrine secretions.

Human chorionic gonadotropin (HCG) Hormone whose function is to preserve the corpus luteum and its progesterone production so that the endometrial lining of the uterus, and hence pregnancy, is maintained.

Human immunodeficiency virus (HIV) The agent that causes acquired immunodeficiency syndrome (AIDS).

Human papillomavirus (HPV) A papovavirus that causes genital warts.

Hymen A small, insignificant membrane around the vaginal opening that has no known function.

Hyperplasia An excessive proliferation of epithelial cells.

Hypothalamus Located in the basal region of the brain underneath the cerebral hemispheres; a key portion of a group of brain structures collectively called the limbic system, which is believed to be the part of the brain concerned with emotional behavior.

Iatrogenic disease Disease that is doctor induced.

Impotence Inability to achieve or maintain an erection.

Infertility The inability to conceive a child during the course of 1 year of regular sexual intercourse unprotected by contraception.

Inhibin A peptide hormone that suppresses FSH secretion from the pituitary gland.

Intercytoplasmic sperm injection A technique in which a single sperm is injected into a single egg to fertilize it.

Intrauterine device(IUD) A device inserted into the uterus (womb) to prevent conception (pregnancy). The IUD can be a coil, loop, triangle, or T-shape made of plastic or metal.

Introitus An opening or entrance into a canal or cavity, such as the vagina.

In vitro fertilization Fertilization outside of the body.

Kaposi's sarcoma A vascular malignancy whose incidence has risen dramatically along with the incidence of AIDS; characterized by obvious, colorful lesions.

Karyotype Manner of viewing chromosomes in which the chromosomes are cut out of an enlarged photograph of chromosomes in metaphase, arranged in pairs, and systematically grouped.

Kilocalorie   See *Calorie.*

Labia majora   Major lips; the two longitudinal folds of skin that extend down from the mons pubis, narrowing to enclose the vulvar cleft and meeting posteriorly in the perineum.

Labia minora   The delicate inner folds of skin that enclose the urethral opening and the vagina.

Lactiferous duct   Opening at the nipple through which milk and colostrum are excreted.

Lamaze method   Method of childbirth education that stresses education to remove the fear of pain, exercises to prepare muscles and joints for delivery, and muscle relaxation and breathing techniques to relieve tension.

Laparoscopy   The examination of the pelvic cavity by an instrument inserted through a small incision in the abdominal wall.

Lithotomy position   Position in which a woman lies for a gynecological exam, with feet in stirrups, buttocks hanging over the end of the table, and sheet draped like a tent over the knees and the upper part of her body.

Lobular carcinoma in situ (LCIS)   While it carries a risk of progression to cancer, it is generally not viewed as a true malignancy.

Luteal phase   The third phase of the ovarian cycle, during which the corpus luteum secretes estrogens, progesterone, and androgens.

Luteinizing hormone (LH)   Responsible for ovulation, corpus luteum formation, and hormone production in the ovaries; the stimulus for hormone production from the interstitial cells of the testes.

Mastectomy   Complete removal of the breast.

Melanocytes   Cells that produce pigmented substances that provide color to the hair, skin, and choroid of the eye.

Menarche   The term for the onset of the menstrual periods; ovulation generally does not take place for a year or more afterward.

Menopause   The cessation of the menstrual periods; considered complete after 1 year of amenorrhea.

Menstrual phase   Day 1 to day 4 of the endometrial cycle.

Menstrual synchronization   Phenomenon of women living in close proximity tending to menstruate at approximately the same time.

Menstruation   The periodic discharge of a bloody fluid from the uterus, occurring at more or less regular intervals during the life of a woman from the age of puberty to menopause.

Minipill   Small-dose progestin pill.

Mons pubis   The cushion of fatty tissue and skin that lies over the pubic symphysis and that is covered with pubic hair after puberty.

Mutagens   Anything capable of causing a gene change. Among the known mutagens are radiation, certain chemicals, and some viruses.

Nail   A cornified curved plate of hard keratin that rests on a thickened surface of epidermis called the nail bed.

National Institutes of Health (NIH)   Primary federal granting agency for research.

Nonsteroidal anti-inflammatory drugs (NSAIDs)   Drugs used to control, stop, or regulate abnormal uterine bleeding.

OB/GYN   A doctor who specializes in obstetrics and gynecology.

Oligoovulation   Irregular ovulation.

Oncogenes   Genes that have the ability to induce a cell to become malignant.

Oocyte maturation inhibitor   A peptide hormone in follicular fluid that suppresses final maturation of the dominant follicle until the time of ovulation.

Oral contraceptive   Common called "the Pill," the most commonly used form of reversible birth control in the United States. The form of birth control suppresses ovulation (the monthly release of an egg from the ovaries) by the combined actions of the hormones estrogen and progesterone.

Orgasm Contractions of the muscles that line the wall of the outer third of the vagina as a response to sexual arousal and stimulation. In women, an orgasm is a purely pleasurable experience that provides sexual satisfaction.

Orgasmic platform The muscles that make up the outer third of the vaginal wall and those surrounding the turgid tissues of the vulva.

Osteoporosis Disease characterized by reduced bone mass.

Ovarian cyst A sac that develops in the ovary proper; consists of one or more chambers containing fluid.

Oviducts See *Fallopian tubes.*

Ovulation The periodic ripening and rupture of the mature graafian follicle and the discharge of the ovum from the cortex of the ovary.

Oxytocin A very powerful stimulant of uterine contraction, especially of a pregnant uterus; also affects the flow of milk from the breasts in a nursing mother in response to the sucking stimulus from the baby.

Parturate Give birth.

Parturition Childbirth.

Pathology A condition produced by disease.

Pectoral nodes A cluster of small, bean-shaped nodes in the breasts which play an important role in immunity by filtering out harmful substances. Also called axillary nodes.

Pelvic exam A gynecological procedure in which a health professional palpates a woman's abdomen; and then inspects her internal genitalia. Cell smears of the cervix are usually taken for diagnostic analysis.

Pelvic inflammatory disease (PID) Infection of the uterus, fallopian tubes, and adjacent pelvic structures that is not associated with surgery or pregnancy.

Pituitary gland Oval and about the size of a pea, it is attached to the hypothalamus of the brain by a stalk called the infundibulum; it secretes a number of hormones that regulate many bodily processes, including growth, reproduction, and various metabolic activities.

Placenta The special structure for fetal-maternal exchange; it is delivered from the uterus after the baby.

Placenta previa The result of implantation of the fertilized ovum in the lower part of the uterus instead of its more usual site higher up in the fundus; late in pregnancy or at the time of delivery, a part of the lower edge of the placenta may separate from its attachment to cause characteristically painless bleeding that is bright red in color.

***Pneumocystis carinii* pneumonia** A type of pneumonia sometimes seen in AIDS patients that was previously seen only in cancer patients with profoundly suppressed immune systems.

Preeclampsia A disorder in pregnant women that is a combination of symptoms, including hypertension, edema, and proteinuria (protein in the urine) and is categorized as mild or severe.

Preferred provider organizations (PPOs) A type of health plan that contracts with selected doctors, clinics, and hospitals, which then constitute the PPO's network.

Premature ejaculation Inability to exert enough voluntary control to delay ejaculation, resulting in the attainment of orgasm too rapidly.

Premenstrual syndrome Premenstrual difficulties, either physical, psychological, or behavioral, that some women experience, causing a disruption in their personal and professional lives and resulting in limitation of their usual activities.

Progestational phase See *Secretory phase;* the changes that occur in the superficial layer of the endometrium in this phase are the result of the action of progesterone.

Progesterone Progesterone and estrogens are the female sex hormones.

Progestins A general term referring to chemical agents, both natural and synthetic, that produce changes in the uterine endometrium after it has previously been primed by estrogen.

Proliferative phase The part of the endometrial cycle that occurs after day 4 and lasts until a day or two after ovulation.

Prostaglandins (PGs) A closely related group of fatty acid derivatives with a variety of effects; belong to a group of compounds called eicosanoids.

Prostate A single gland that surrounds the urethra as it leaves the bladder; it secretes a milky, alkaline fluid to neutralize the acidity of the vagina during intercourse and enhance sperm motility.

Puberty Transition period between childhood and adulthood when physical and psychological changes that are associated with the ability to reproduce take place.

Receptors Sites located on the cell membranes or in the cytoplasm of the target cells; their job is to transmit the message of the hormone's arrival to the area of the cell that is involved in the response.

Reproductive neuroendocrinology The study of the integration of the nervous system and the endocrine organs of reproduction.

Retroviruses A viral class composed of a core of RNA surrounded by a protein coat, which is further surrounded by a protein envelope; they produce a unique enzyme called reverse transcriptase.

Sebaceous glands Sebum-producing glands that are found almost everywhere in the dermis except for the palmar and plantar surfaces.

Secretory phase The second half of the endometrial cycle, also called the progestational phase; the glands of the endometrium become dilated as they fill up with secretions of substances such as glycogen and fats, and the endometrium becomes twice as thick as it was in the previous phase, forming a hospitable site for implantation of a fertilized ovum.

Selective estrogen receptor modulators (SERMs) "Designer estrogens" which possess some, but not all, of the actions of estrogen and are used therapeutically in the treatment of complications of menopause and against some breast cancers.

Semen Consists of sperm suspended in a semigelatinous fluid that contains substances to nourish and protect the sperm and facilitate their movement.

Seminal vesicles Located at the base of the bladder in males, these saclike structures produce a viscous, alkaline fluid rich in fructose to provide a direct source of energy for sperm.

Sepsis The spread of an infection from its initial site to the bloodstream, initiating a systemic response that adversely affects blood flow to vital organs.

Seroconversion The production of antibodies to HIV.

Skin cancer The most common forms are basal cell and squamous cell; a third type, melanoma, is highly dangerous but much less common.

Speculum An instrument used to examine body canals.

Steroid General term applied to a group of substances that all have a common structural nucleus; found in both plants and animals and include a large number of body constituents, vitamins, and drugs, as well as sex hormones.

Steroid hormones Sex hormones and hormones of the adrenal cortex.

Sunscreen preparations Products designed either to reflect the rays of the sun or to absorb them, mimicking the body's own defenses against radiation.

Superovulation Giving fertility drugs to a woman to increase follicle production and ovulation.

Sweat glands Epidermal derivatives located in the dermis and widely distributed over the entire body surface except on the nail beds of the fingers and toes, the margins of the lips, and on certain parts of the external genitalia.

Teratogens Substances that can cross the placental barrier and impair normal growth and development of the embryo.

Testes Oval, smooth organs about 4–5 cm long and 2.5 cm in diameter that are suspended in the scrotum.

Testosterone The androgen produced by the interstitial cells of the male testes.

Theca externa The outer fibrous layer of an ovarian follicle. It produces sex steroids.

T-helper lymphocytes A lymphocyte population; T-helper cells help other lymphocytes combat foreign antigens.

Thrombus An abnormal blood clot that forms in an unbroken blood vessel.

Toxic shock syndrome (TSS) A rare and sometimes fatal disease caused by the toxin produced by the bacterium Staphylococcus aureus, a bacterium that is commonly present on the skin and mucous membranes. Although TSS was linked with "superabsorbent" tampons (which are no longer on the market), about half of the total cases reported occur in men, menstruating women who are not using tampons, and women who do not menstruate.

Trichomoniasis Infestation with a parasite of the genus *Trichomonas.*

Tubal ligation Female sterilization.

Uterus Inverted pear-shaped, hollow, muscular organ in which the impregnated ovum develops into a fetus.

VACTERL syndrome A combination of abnormalities that includes vertebral, anal, cardiac, tracheal, esophageal, renal, and limb defects.

Vagina A tube that passes upward to the uterus at an approximate 45° angle from the vulva.

Vaginal diaphragm A soft, rubber dome surrounded by a metal spring; it is used in conjunction with a spermicidal jelly or cream and is inserted into the vagina to fit between the nooks of the anterior and posterior fornices to cover the cervix.

Vaginitis Generic term that means inflammation and infection of the vagina.

Vasectomy Male sterilization; removal of all or a segment of the vas deferens.

Vasocongestion The engorgement of the vaginal blood vessels which result in vaginal lubrication, a consequence of sexual arousal.

VDRL The test for syphilis.

Vulva Term used for a female's visible external genitalia; sometimes called the pudendum.

Women's Health Initiative A $625 million study involving between 100,000 and 200,000 women to gather data on the prevention and treatment of the major causes of death in middle-aged and older women.

Zygote Fertilized egg.

Zygote intrafallopian transfer (ZIFT) A technique in which a woman's egg is fertilized outside the body, then implanted in one of her fallopian tubes.

INDEX

follicular phase, 82–84
luteal phase, 82, 84–85
ovulation, 82, 84
Ovarian cysts, 295–96
Ovarian ligaments, 57
Ovaries, 50–52, 66
    atresia, 50
    changes during pregnancy, 326
    cortex, 50
    factors in infertility, 406–7
    follicles, 82
    germinal epithelium, 50
    malignant neoplasms of, 296–97
    medulla, 50
    oogonia, 50
    primordial germ cells, 50
    stroma, 50
    tumors of, 295–97
Overnutrition, 592, 593
Overweight and obesity, 600–607
    body mass index, 600–601, 603
    causes of, 601–4
    media-promoted ideal appearance, 600
    parental obesity, 602
    problems associated with, 601
    weight reduction, 604–7
Oviducts. See Fallopian tubes
Ovulation, 84, 412
Owens, Jesse, 612
Oxidation dyes, for hair, 559, 560–61
Oxytocin, 74, 202, 358, 368, 370, 388
Oxytocin-challenge test (OCT), 370–71

PABA. See Para-amino benzoic acid (PABA)
Pads, for menstruation, 34, 86
Paedomorphism, 120
Pantothenic acid, 582, 587
Papanicolaou, George, 21, 283
Papillary serous cystadenomas, 296
Pap smear, 21, 283–84, 457
    classification of, 283
    as preventive medicine, 284
Papulopustule, 548
Para-aminobenzoic acid (PABA), 530, 588
Paraaminophenol, 560
Paracervical block, 362

Paraphenylenediamine (PPD), 560
Paraplegia, 184–85
Parathyroid glands, 66
Parental obesity, 602
Parietal peritoneum, 49, 57
Parlee, Mary Jane, 110
Partial birth abortion, 475
Parturition, 121, 353
Pauling, Linus, 587
Pavlov, Ivan, 365
PBSCT. See Peripheral blood stem cell transplantation
        (PBSCT)
Pearson, Cynthia, 236
Pectoral nodes, 197
Pediculosis, 276–77
Pelvic brim, 25
Pelvic diaphragm, 53–54
Pelvic examination. See Gynecological examination
Pelvic girdle, 21–26
    ilium, 22–24
    ischium, 24
    position of reproductive organs within, 22
Pelvic inflammatory disease (PID), 271, 438, 448–49
Pelvic inlet, 25
Pelvic outlet, 25
Pelvic tilt, 27–29
Pelvic viscera
    coccygeus, 56
    iliococcygeus, 56
    ligaments, 57–58
    peritoneum, 57
    pubococcygeus, 54–56
    structure of pelvic floor, 53–54
    support of, 53–58
Pelvimetry, 26–27
Pelvis
    backache and its relation to, 29–30
    classification of, 26–27
    false or greater, 25
    sex differences in, 26–30
    true or lesser, 25–26
Penis, 61
Penis captivus, 56
Percutaneous umbilical blood sampling, 144–45
Perimenopause, 490
Perineal muscles, 53